"Radically open dialectical behavior therapy (RO DBT) is a truly innovati[ve] translation of neuroscience into clinical practice, integrating various inflt[...] therapy (DBT), mindfulness-based approaches, emotion, personality and developmental theory, evolutionary theory, and Malamati Sufism. RO DBT is applicable to a spectrum of disorders characterized by excessive inhibitory control or *overcontrol* (OC). This is the first treatment that directly targets social signaling and nonverbal aspects of communication not only in clients but also in therapists."

—**Mima Simic, MD, MRCPsych,** joint head of the child and adolescent eating disorder service, and consultant child and adolescent psychiatrist at the Maudsley Hospital in London, UK

"A new and comprehensive statement from one of the more creative minds in evidence-based clinical intervention today, RO DBT brings together a contemporary focus on a limited set of key transdiagnostic processes, with new assessment and intervention techniques for moving them in a positive direction. Emphasizing flexibility, openness, connection, and attention to social signaling, RO DBT specifies the details that can matter, from how you arrange your consulting room furniture to how nonverbal cues signal social information. RO DBT seems destined to make an impact on evidence-based care in many corners of clinical work. Highly recommended."

—**Steven C. Hayes, PhD,** codeveloper of acceptance and commitment therapy (ACT); Foundation Professor of psychology at the University of Nevada, Reno; and author of *Get Out of Your Mind and Into Your Life*

"RO DBT offers an intriguing reconceptualization of traditional views of internalizing and externalizing disorders, and provides the clinician with valuable new tools to address a number of problems that have been particularly resistant to standard CBT approaches. I will definitely include RO DBT theory and techniques in my graduate-level intervention class. I know beginning clinicians in particular will be grateful to have a systematic way to approach these slow-to-warm-up clients who are difficult to establish rapport with. Their early termination from therapy and failure to respond to traditional approaches often leaves clinicians befuddled and critical of their own skills. RO DBT provides a compassionate way for clinicians to view this type of resistant client, as well as to work on some areas that are likely to benefit them. A very welcome addition to any clinician's toolbox."

—**Linda W. Craighead, PhD,** professor of psychology and director of clinical training at Emory University, and author of *The Appetite Awareness Workbook*

The
SKILLS TRAINING MANUAL *for*
RADICALLY OPEN
DIALECTICAL
BEHAVIOR THERAPY

A CLINICIAN'S GUIDE *for*
TREATING DISORDERS *of* OVERCONTROL

THOMAS R. LYNCH, PhD

CONTEXT PRESS
An Imprint of New Harbinger Publications, Inc.

Publisher's Note

This publication is designed to provide accurate and authoritative information in regard to the subject matter covered. It is sold with the understanding that the publisher is not engaged in rendering psychological, financial, legal, or other professional services. If expert assistance or counseling is needed, the services of a competent professional should be sought.

Library of Congress Cataloging-in-Publication Data

Names: Lynch, Thomas R. (Professor of clinical psychology), author. | Complemented by (work): Lynch, Thomas R. (Professor of clinical psychology). Radically open dialectical behavior therapy
Title: The skills training manual for Radically open dialectical behavior therapy : a clinician's guide for treating disorders of overcontrol / Thomas R. Lynch.
Description: Oakland, CA : New Harbinger Publications, Inc., 2018. | Companion volume to Radically open dialectical behavior therapy / Thomas R. Lynch. 2018. | Includes bibliographical references and index.
Identifiers: LCCN 2017040505 (print) | LCCN 2017043166 (ebook) | ISBN 9781626259324 (pdf e-book) | ISBN 9781626259331 (ePub) | ISBN 9781626259317 (paperback)
Subjects: | MESH: Behavior Therapy--methods | Compulsive Personality Disorder--therapy | Behavior Therapy--education | Self-Control--psychology
Classification: LCC RC489.B4 (ebook) | LCC RC489.B4 (print) | NLM WM 425 | DDC 616.89/142--dc23
LC record available at https://lccn.loc.gov/2017040505

Printed in the United States of America

25   24   23

15   14   13   12   11   10   9   8

This book is dedicated to the the most important people in my life—
my wife Erica and our daughter Kayleigh

If I know anything, it is that I don't know everything and neither does anyone else.

—Michael P. Lynch, *True to Life: Why Truth Matters*

Contents

Lesson 11   Mindfulness Training, Part 1   **233**
Overcontrolled States of Mind

Lesson 12   Mindfulness Training, Part 2   **254**
The "What" Skills

List of Radical Openness Handouts and Worksheets

Basic Principles, Treatment Overview, and Global Structure of Skills Training Classes

Radically open dialectical behavior therapy (RO DBT) is an evidence-based treatment targeting a spectrum of disorders characterized by excessive inhibitory control, or overcontrol (OC). It is intended for clinicians treating clients with chronic problems such as refractory depression, anorexia nervosa, and obsessive-compulsive personality disorder. Radical openness (RO) is the core philosophical principle and core skill in RO DBT. The feasibility, acceptability, and efficacy of RO DBT are evidence-based, supported by more than twenty years of clinical translational research experience as well as by five published trials and one large multicenter randomized controlled trial; for an overview, see *Radically Open Dialectical Behavior Therapy: Theory and Practice for Treating Disorders of Overcontrol* (T. R. Lynch, 2018; this core source, to which the manual you are reading is the companion, will be cited frequently throughout the manual, and so I will refer to it simply as "the RO DBT textbook"). RO DBT research, training, and clinical work have been extended to differing age groups (adolescents, older adults, young adults), differing disorders (anorexia nervosa, chronic depression, autism, OC personality disorders, treatment-resistant anxiety), differing cultures and countries (Europe, North America), differing settings (forensic, inpatient, outpatient), and a wide range of differing providers (psychologists, nurses, social workers, psychiatrists, family therapists, occupational therapists); a range of differing modalities has also been developed and applied (skills alone, multifamily training, RO couples therapy). The primary aims of this manual, in contrast to those of the RO DBT textbook, are to provide a detailed overview of underlying treatment principles and clinical guidelines for assessing, targeting, and intervening with problems of overcontrol and to provide a hands-on practical guide and the supporting materials needed to teach RO skills (referred to throughout this manual simply as "RO skills"). The manual includes step-by-step teaching instructions, class exercises, and clinical tips on how to manage maladaptive behavior in class, with a brief overview of the underlying theory and interventions that are detailed more fully in the RO DBT textbook. The client handouts and worksheets for each RO skills lesson plan, available at http://www.newharbinger.com/39317, can be printed for distribution to clients and/or modified as needed for a particular setting.

This chapter begins with a definition of overcontrolled coping, followed by a description of the RO DBT therapeutic stance used when teaching RO skills. Next, principles for gaining commitment to attend RO skills training classes are described, followed by a description of the overall structure for each RO lesson plan and an overview of RO skills.

What Is Overcontrol?

Self-control—the ability to inhibit competing urges, impulses, behaviors, or desires and delay gratification in order to pursue distal goals—is often equated with success and happiness. Indeed, inhibitory control is highly valued by most societies, and failures in self-control characterize many of the personal and social problems afflicting modern civilization. However, too much self-control can be equally problematic. Overcontrol has been linked to social isolation, poor interpersonal functioning, hyperperfectionism, rigidity, risk aversion, lack of emotional expression, and the development of severe and difficult-to-treat mental health problems, such as chronic depression, anorexia nervosa, and obsessive-compulsive personality disorder.

Maladaptive overcontrol is posited to represent a personality style that results from transactions between temperamental predispositions (nature) and family/environmental/cultural influences (nurture) that create a style of coping characterized by excessive inhibitory control and aloof relationships (OC coping) that functions to limit new learning, flexible responding, and the development of close social bonds. There are four dimensions of infant temperament relevant to the "nature" component of this model:

1. Negative affectivity (threat sensitivity)

2. Positive affectivity (reward sensitivity)

3. Effortful control (self-control capacity)

4. Detail-focused (versus global) processing of stimuli

Children at risk for overcontrolled coping and social isolation are likely to have high threat sensitivity, low reward sensitivity, high detail-focused processing, and high effortful control and are characterized by being behaviorally inhibited, shy, timid, risk-avoidant, emotionally constrained; by having hyper-detail-focused processing; and by and showing aloof/socially withdrawn behavior. By contrast, children at risk for pervasive emotion dysregulation and behavioral dyscontrol (that is, undercontrolled coping) are likely to have high threat sensitivity, low effortful control (Linehan, 2015a), and high reward sensitivity (T. R. Lynch, Hempel, & Clark, 2015).

Yet, despite these inherent difficulties, overcontrolled coping is not always problematic. For example, innate capacities to inhibit impulses, plan ahead, and delay gratification make OC clients the doers, savers, planners, and fixers of the world. They are the guests who help clean up after the party and the people who save for their retirement so as not to burden others. They strive for moderation in all aspects of their lives and value honesty, fairness, and doing the right thing. They are the people you see working late at night and then rising early to ensure that things work properly; they are the reason why trains run on time (see table 1.1). The problem is that overcontrolled coping works well when it comes to sitting quietly in a monastery or building a rocket, but it creates problems when it comes to social connectedness.

Table 1.1. Overcontrol Is Fundamentally Prosocial

OC Characteristic	Prosocial Attribute
Ability to delay gratification	Enables resources to be saved for times of less abundance
Desire to be correct, exceed expectations, and perform well	Essential to communities' ability to thrive and grow
Valuing of duty, obligation, and self-sacrifice	Helps societies flourish and ensures that people in need are cared for
Valuing of rules and fairness	Helps societies remain balanced and enables resistance to powerful but unethical individuals and harmful societal pressures
Detail-focused processing and quick pattern recognition	Increases precision and thus the likelihood that problems will be detected and solved so that everything functions properly

For OC clients, their greatest strength is their greatest weakness. Too much self-control depletes the very resources needed to override habitual self-control when doing so would be adaptive. A type of catch-22 emerges: excessive self-control exhausts the resources needed to *control* excessive self-control, making it harder for alternative ways of coping (such as taking a nap or asking for help) to emerge. Internally, OC clients may feel like prisoners of self-control, and their natural tendency to inhibit (control) their expressions of emotion makes it harder for others to know they are distressed and to offer assistance. Plus, maladaptive OC coping is expressed discreetly. For example, an overcontrolled client is likely to downplay personal distress when queried, making identification of the problem more difficult for clinicians (see the material about the "I am fine" phenomenon in chapter 6 of the RO DBT textbook). The OC client feels like a stranger in a strange land, always watching yet rarely participating.

Four Core Deficits

Maladaptive overcontrol is characterized by four core deficits:

1. *Low receptivity and openness*, manifested by low openness to novel, unexpected, or disconfirming feedback, avoidance of uncertainty or unplanned risks, suspiciousness, hypervigilance for potential threat, and marked tendencies to discount or dismiss critical feedback

2. *Low flexible control*, manifested by compulsive needs for structure and order, hyperperfectionism, high social obligation and dutifulness, compulsive rehearsal, high premeditation and planning, compulsive fixing and approach coping, rigid rule-governed behavior, and high moral certitude (that is, the belief that there is only one right way of doing something)

3. *Pervasive inhibited emotional expression and low emotional awareness*, manifested by context-inappropriate inhibition of emotional expression (for example, exhibiting a flat face when complimented) and/or insincere or incongruent expressions of emotion (for example, smiling when distressed, showing concern when not feeling it), consistent underreporting of distress, and low awareness of body sensations

4. *Low social connectedness and intimacy with others*, manifested by aloof and distant relationships, feeling different from other people, frequent social comparisons, high envy and bitterness, and reduced empathy

RO DBT Therapeutic Stance

Rather than focusing on what's wrong with hyper-detail-focused perfectionists who tend to see mistakes everywhere (that is, OC clients), radically open dialectical behavior therapy begins by observing what's healthy (about all of us) and uses this to guide treatment interventions. Psychological health or well-being in RO DBT is hypothesized to involve three core transacting features:

1. Receptivity and openness to new experience and disconfirming feedback, in order to learn

2. Flexible control, in order to adapt to changing environmental conditions

3. Intimacy and social connectedness (with at least one other person), based on premises that species survival required capacities to form long-lasting bonds and to work in groups or tribes

The core idea is that OC clients are more likely to benefit from treatment approaches that prioritize the value of seeking pleasure, relaxing control, and joining with others over approaches prioritizing emotion regulation, nonavoidance, correcting deficits, and tolerating distress in order to achieve long-term goals.

Plus, the primary downsides of maladaptive overcontrol are social in nature. For example, both low openness and pervasive constraint of emotional expression have been repeatedly shown to exert a negative impact on the formation of close social bonds, leading to an increasing sense of isolation from others. OC clients suffer from emotional loneliness—not lack of *contact* but lack of *connection* with others. Rather than focusing on how to do better or try harder, the primary aim in RO DBT is to help OC clients learn how to rejoin their tribe and establish strong social bonds with others. Consequently, the role of the therapist in RO DBT can be likened to that of a tribal ambassador who metaphorically encourages socially isolated OC clients to rejoin their tribe by communicating, "Welcome home. We appreciate your desire to meet or exceed expectations and the self-sacrifices you have made. You have worked hard and deserve a rest" (see "The Therapist as Tribal Ambassador," in chapter 6 of the RO DBT textbook).

As ambassador, the RO skills instructor adopts a stance that models kindness, cooperation, and playfulness rather than fixing, correcting, restricting, or improving. Plus, ambassadors don't expect people they interact with in other countries to think, feel, or act the way they do, or to speak the same language. Ambassadors reach out toward those who are different and learn their customs and language, without expecting anything in return. Thus, RO skills training instructors are humble, working hard to find a common language with their clients, without assuming that their perspective as instructors is necessarily the correct one. Ambassadors are also face savers: they allow other people (or countries) to admit to some fault, without rubbing their noses in it. They take the heat off when things get extremely tense during negotiations by allowing others (and themselves) the grace of not having to understand, resolve, or fix a problem or issue immediately. Yet ambassadors also recognize that sometimes kindness means telling good friends painful truths in order to help them achieve their valued goals in a manner that acknowledges the ambassador's own potential for fallibility. "Therapist as tribal ambassador" principles are represented throughout the RO DBT treatment assumptions, described next.

Basic Assumptions

Broadly speaking, treatments differ by what is targeted for change (for example, neurochemical deficiencies, maladaptive schemas, lack of metacognitive awareness, dysregulated emotion, avoidant coping, childhood trauma, or, in the case of RO DBT, social signaling deficits). Yet treatments also differ philosophically (in terms of assumptions about the nature of reality, truth, free will, personal responsibility, optimal health, illness, morality, social responsibility, and the role of health care providers). Importantly, from an RO DBT perspective, assumptions about treatment are not truths but guiding principles of behavior. The following assumptions are most relevant to RO skills training.

- RO DBT defines psychological well-being as involving the confluence of three factors: *receptivity, flexibility,* and *social connectedness.*

- RO DBT highlights our tribal nature; it prioritizes the importance of social connectedness as essential for individual well-being and species survival.

- Social signaling matters! Deficits (not excesses) in genuine prosocial signaling represent the core problem for disorders of overcontrol and are posited to be the source of OC clients' emotional loneliness.

- Radical openness assumes that we don't see things as they are but that we see things as we are.

- Radical openness involves a willingness to question ourselves when challenged, in order to learn, by asking *What is it that I might need to learn?*

- RO skills instructors recognize that radical openness is not something that can be grasped solely via intellectual means, and they practice RO skills and self-enquiry themselves in order to model and teach key principles more effectively to their clients.

- RO skills instructors take responsibility for their emotional reactions, personal perceptions, and overt behavioral responses, without falling apart or automatically blaming themselves or others, in order to encourage their OC clients to practice similarly.

- RO DBT encourages clients to celebrate problems as opportunities for growth rather than obstacles that block personal well-being.

- RO skills instructors recognize that it is arrogant to assume that they can ever fully understand their clients, and yet they continue to strive to do so anyway.

- RO skills instructors recognize that OC clients are often suffering, even though they may not always show it.

- RO skills instructors recognize that OC clients take life too seriously and that, rather than needing to learn how to be better or work harder, they need to learn how to relax, play, and laugh at their mistakes, with kindness.

- RO skills instructors recognize that OC clients will not believe it is socially acceptable for someone to openly play, relax, or disinhibit unless they see their therapists model this behavior first.

- RO skills instructors recognize that alliance rupture repairs are best done outside of class—for example, during break or after class.

- RO skills instructors encourage class members to practice celebrating obstacles as opportunities for self-discovery and self-enquiry.

- RO skills instructors encourage engagement in conflict rather than automatic abandonment, and candid disclosure and uninhibited expression of emotion rather than constrained or carefully regulated expressions.

The Primary Mechanism of Change: Social Signaling

RO DBT introduces a unique thesis regarding the mechanism by which overcontrolled behavior leads to psychological distress by linking neuroregulatory theory and the communicative functions of emotional expression to the formation of close social bonds. A central component of this mechanism is that heightened biotemperamental threat sensitivity makes it more difficult for individuals with overcontrol to enter into their neurobiologically based social safety system (T. R. Lynch et al., 2013; T. R. Lynch, Hempel, & Dunkley, 2015). Feeling safe activates an area of the brain (the ventral vagal complex of the parasympathetic nervous system) associated with contentment, friendliness, and social engagement via innervation of muscles involved with modulating voice tone, making appropriate facial expressions, listening to human speech, and maintaining eye contact (Porges, 1995, 2001). When an organism feels safe, it naturally experiences a desire to affiliate with others and finds it easy to socially signal inner experience and empathically engage with others. However, when the environment is perceived to be threatening, defensive arousal and fight-or-flight responses become dominant, and social safety responses and capacities for signaling genuine cooperation become impaired (for example, when stressed out, we can only fake a genuine smile). Thus, overcontrolled biotemperamental threat sensitivity and sympathetic nervous system–mediated withdrawal of social safety responses, combined with overlearned tendencies to mask inner feelings, are hypothesized to engender social ostracism and loneliness, thereby exacerbating psychological distress. These observations help articulate the unique suffering associated with OC coping: natural tendencies to mask inner feelings lead to the very problem they were developed to prevent (that is, people prefer to not interact with OC individuals and see them as inauthentic). Thus, for OC clients, superior capacities for self-control represent both a blessing and a curse. OC clients' capacity for inhibitory control allows them to delay gratification and work harder than most others, yet compulsive self-control and hyper-detail-focused processing often negatively impact their relationships and their sense of well-being.

Importantly, RO skills instructors are no less susceptible to these reciprocal inhibitory influences than other people. Consequently, instructors must learn to go opposite to automatic urges to shut down, freeze, or mimic the inhibited expressions that can sometimes be exhibited by an OC client class. In my experience, the emotion most likely experienced by therapists in these situations is humiliation (that is, low-level shame), which triggers automatic action urges to hide and thoughts that one is behaving inappropriately (for example, when requesting group participation). Therapists should block automatic response tendencies to inhibit or constrict expressions when this occurs by freely revealing their emotions/thoughts to the group in a manner that signals to themselves and others that there is nothing to be ashamed of (for example, eyebrow wags, large gestures, half smiles, relaxed posture, use of humor). This approach, when used repeatedly by a skills instructor, is posited to reduce unjustified shame, signal to the group that emotional expression is not dangerous, and promote social safety via micromimicry.

Moreover, instructors are encouraged to practice outing themselves by demonstrating their willingness to not take themselves too seriously, via humorous or self-effacing revelations of personal quirks or fallibilities. Skills instructors should be mindful that biotemperamental predispositions make it harder for an OC client to benefit from the potentially rewarding experience of social interactions (see chapter 2). Thus, it is essential for instructors to encourage OC clients to use RO skills designed to activate the social safety system prior to practicing interpersonal skills (see Radical Openness Handout 3.1: Changing Social Interactions by Changing Physiology). Finally, instructors should be prepared to reference and encourage the use of other RO skills that are interpersonally focused when teaching interpersonal skills—for example, being open to critical feedback (Flexible Mind ADOPTS), revealing rather than masking inner feelings (Flexible Mind ALLOWs), forgiveness of self and others (Flexible Mind Has HEART), and learning how to validate others (Flexible Mind Validates). The vast majority of RO skills outlined in this manual have been derived from these core theoretical perspectives.

Treatment Structure and Targets

Although RO DBT has been researched and applied clinically in a wide range of settings (inpatient, day hospital, and skills alone), the approaches outlined in this manual are derived primarily from an outpatient model of treatment delivery. The RO DBT outpatient treatment protocol consists of weekly one-hour individual therapy sessions and weekly two-and-a-half-hour skills training classes occurring over a period of approximately thirty weeks. Telephone coaching of skills and/or availability of therapists outside of individual therapy and weekly therapist consultation/supervision meetings are recommended but not required. RO DBT recognizes that clinicians and treatment settings may need to adjust this recommended structure as a function of an individual client's needs and/or environmental constraints—for example, by adding individual therapy sessions, allowing clients to repeat skills training classes, or pragmatically adjusting to environmental/financial constraints.

The key for effective treatment targeting when treating problems of overcontrol is not to focus solely on inner experience (such as dysregulated emotion, maladaptive cognition, lack of metacognitive awareness, or past traumatic memories) as the source of OC suffering. Instead, RO DBT targets indirect, masked, and constrained social signaling as the primary source of OC clients' emotional loneliness, isolation, and misery. Robust research shows that context-inappropriate suppression of emotional expression or incongruent expression of emotion (that is, what is expressed outwardly does not match inner experience) is more likely to be perceived as untrustworthy or inauthentic (Boone & Buck, 2003; English & John, 2013; Kernis & Goldman, 2006) and to be associated with reduced social connectedness (Mauss et al., 2011). Indirect social signals interfere with social connectedness because they make it harder to know the sender's true intentions (for example, a furrowed brow can reflect intense interest or disagreement). Crucially, in comparison to nonsuppressors, chronic inhibitors of emotional expression report experiencing themselves as inauthentic and as misleading others about their true selves (Gross & John, 2003). Yet indirect or disguised social signals are powerful because they allow the sender to influence others without having to admit it—that is, they contain plausible deniability: "What? Me, angry? No, I'm just being quiet" or "Don't worry—I like you. The reason I never laugh at your jokes is simply because I don't find them funny."

RO DBT uses a three-step process to address indirect communication and disguised demands. First, the individual therapist introduces the problem of masking inner feelings during the orientation and commitment phase of treatment (ideally, in the third session; see the RO DBT textbook), thereby setting the stage for future targeting. Second, to facilitate the identification of indirect social signaling targets, therapists are encouraged to repeatedly ask themselves, throughout the course of treatment, *How might my OC client's social signaling impact social connectedness?* In addition, OC clients are encouraged to collaboratively join with their therapists (or skills trainers) in developing a sense of curiosity about their style of social signaling, using self-enquiry. Examples of self-enquiry questions relevant for OC clients include those that follow:

- To what extent am I proud of the way I communicate my emotions, intentions, and beliefs? Would I encourage another person or a young child to behave similarly? What might this tell me about my valued goals?

- What is it that I need to learn from how I communicate my needs, wants, and desires to others? To what extent am I willing to truly examine my social signaling behaviors? What might this tell me?

- What prevents me from directly asking the other person for what I need or want? What might this tell me about my relationship with this person or how I perceive myself? What is it that I might need to do differently, change, or learn?

Third, RO skills training classes explicitly address maladaptive indirect social signaling by teaching skills designed to specifically modify them (for example, Flexible Mind REVEALs skills; see lesson 16). Candid labeling and skills training publicly expose what is often a well-kept secret, making it harder for socially con-scientious OC clients to continue pretending (to others and themselves) that their indirect style of social sig-naling is nonexistent or not a problem (or perhaps an appropriate way to behave). Essentially, by naming the problem aloud, OC clients lose their shield of plausible deniability, prompting prosocial behaviors linked to values for truthfulness, fairness, and doing the right thing and motivating the practice of new RO skills linked to direct and candid expression of emotion.

Individual Therapy Treatment Target Hierarchy

Individual therapy treatment targets are organized hierarchically into three broad categories:

1. Severe and imminent life-threatening behaviors

2. Therapeutic alliance ruptures

3. Maladaptive OC social signaling linked to five OC behavioral themes (see figure 1.1)

The RO DBT textbook describes in detail treatment interventions for each level of this hierarchy.

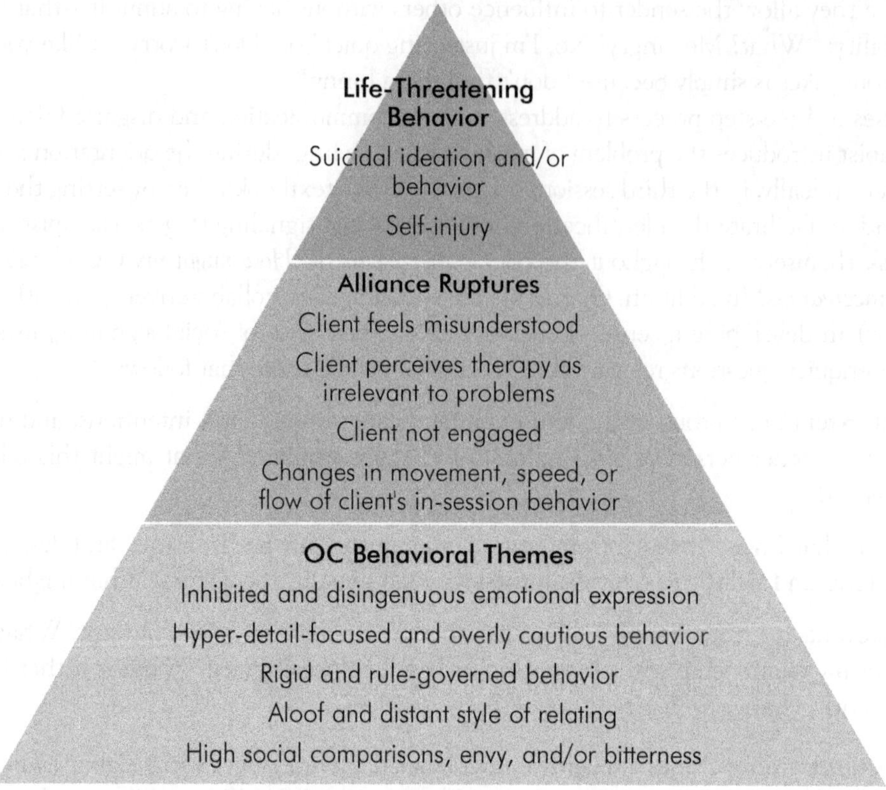

Life-Threatening Behavior

Suicidal ideation and/or behavior

Self-injury

Alliance Ruptures

Client feels misunderstood

Client perceives therapy as irrelevant to problems

Client not engaged

Changes in movement, speed, or flow of client's in-session behavior

OC Behavioral Themes

Inhibited and disingenuous emotional expression

Hyper-detail-focused and overly cautious behavior

Rigid and rule-governed behavior

Aloof and distant style of relating

High social comparisons, envy, and/or bitterness

Figure 1.1. Individual Treatment Target Hierarchy for Disorders of Overcontrol

RO Skills Training: Global Aims and Targets

The primary aim of RO skills training is to impart new knowledge and encourage self-discovery (that is, to educate rather than heal). RO skills training instructors are encouraged to adopt a teaching style that parallels the enthusiasm, passion, and curiosity exhibited by the best teachers around the world. The best teachers love to learn! They are both highly knowledgeable and humble about the subjects they teach. They encourage the student to challenge what they expound, and they are delighted when the student surpasses their personal understanding. From an RO DBT perspective, this requires RO skills trainers to practice what they preach (that is, to have direct experience with applying the RO skills in their own lives).

Since the primary aim of RO skills training is to teach skills, it occurs in a classroom, and the skills training component of the treatment is referred to as an RO skills training class, in order to differentiate it from group therapy or process groups. This use of language is purposeful. It helps remind reluctant OC clients of their prior success in educational settings (see "Orientation and Commitment," in chapter 4 of the RO DBT textbook, and "Enhancing Client Engagement via Orientation and Commitment," in chapter 5 of the RO DBT textbook).

Similar to individual RO DBT, treatment targets and aims in RO skills training classes can be arranged according to a hierarchy (see figure 1.2). The hierarchy helps guide instructors' behavior and attention, both during actual classroom teaching and outside of class. The hierarchy also discriminates among (maladaptive) behaviors that can be ignored, those that should be ignored in class but addressed in private, and those that must be addressed in class. For example, rather than publicly admonishing a late-arriving client or automatically assuming nonparticipation to mean nonengagement, an RO skills instructor is likely to give the client the benefit of the doubt in class while addressing the client's nonparticipation directly in private. In addition, RO DBT skills classes are not intended to provide a forum for class members to practice giving each other critical or interpersonal feedback, share unrelated stories, reminisce about the past, or tell others how they should cope with a problem (see chapter 3 for detailed strategies). Finally, in RO DBT there is not a formal list of class rules; indeed, it is considered unnecessary or even iatrogenic to formally review a list of rules regarding classroom behavior (see chapter 3 for a clinical example of how class rules can become a problem).

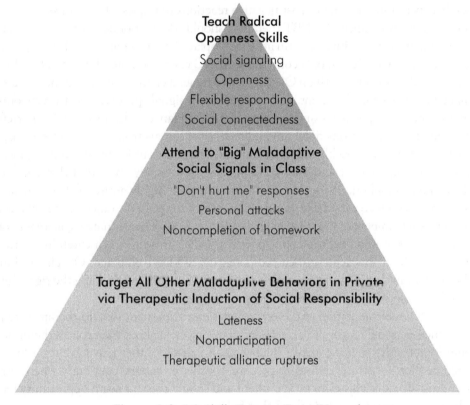

Figure 1.2. RO Skills Training Target Hierarchy

Orienting OC Clients to RO Skills Training

Clients should, ideally, begin attending RO skills training class in the third week of individual RO DBT therapy. Thus, during the second session, individual therapists should briefly outline the rationale and structure of RO skills training classes and obtain commitment to attend the very next scheduled class (see "Orientation and Commitment," in chapter 4 of the RO DBT textbook). Therapists should emphasize that the primary purpose of RO skills training is to learn new skills, not to process inner feelings, practice giving others feedback, or disclose highly personal information. It is important for therapists to refer to RO skills training as a class, not a group. Referring to RO skills training as a class not only more accurately reflects its primary function (that is, learning new skills) but also helps reduce automatic avoidance by an OC client who has negative memories of group activities and/or failed group therapy experiences.

Class attendance should be discussed in a manner that suggests that doing anything else would be irrational, since learning new skills and new ways of coping is the essence of the treatment. Therapists should adopt a stance that assumes class attendance rather than one that assumes they will need to convince or persuade the OC client to attend. The attitude needed is similar to one adopted by a nurse in a hospital who asks a client to undress and put on a hospital gown before surgery; despite the fact that most people experience anxiety or mild embarrassment when asked to do this, the nurse, via a relaxed and matter-of-fact tone, communicates that the request is a routine part of treatment, not a problem.

Well-intentioned attempts by a therapist to prepare an OC client who reports social anxiety at the thought of attending an RO skills training class (for example, by teaching emotion regulation or relaxation skills beforehand) can inadvertently signal that the client's fear is justified and can unnecessarily lengthen the commitment process, sometimes by months. It's like telling someone who has arrived for horseback riding lessons that horses aren't dangerous while placing full-body armor and a helmet on this person just prior to the first ride. Therapists' fears and concerns can be exacerbated by the opinions of other professionals, or by stories from family members pertaining to clients' past negative reactions to requests for change.

Rather than assuming resistance, RO DBT therapists should adopt a nondefensive, noncoercive, and non-apologetic stance, similar to the positive yet firm attitude displayed by the character Mary Poppins in the 1964 Disney film of the same name, that signals confidence in OC clients' innate ability to attend skills training classes. The core idea when working with an OC client is to remember that presuming the client's competence engenders competent behavior in the client. It works because it signals positive belief ("a spoonful of sugar") in the OC client's innate competencies and assumes class attendance ("the medicine") as irrefutable while ignoring (placing on an extinction schedule) any indirect social signals from the OC client suggesting otherwise (see the material about "pushback" and "don't hurt me" responses in lesson 16). Indeed, most OC clients are highly aware of their superior capacities for self-control—they already know that they can endure distress or physical pain without complaint, if they decide to, and they are highly aware of their innate capacities to resist impulses (such as desires to eat), delay gratification, or not to speak to someone they live with for hours, days, weeks, or even years, simply because they have decided to do so. Their innate capacity for control is what makes them difficult to treat and interpersonally powerful (albeit this may be a carefully guarded secret). In order to help reluctant OC clients achieve their full potential, RO DBT embraces OC clients' innate capacity for superior self-control while simultaneously noting their core values linked to doing the right thing, behaving with integrity, and honoring their prior commitments.

However, successful implementation of these principles can sometimes require therapists to practice self-enquiry regarding their personal reactions or the beliefs they may hold about their role as therapist, their beliefs about what comprises effective therapy, and/or the beliefs and attitudes they may have regarding their clients. Therapists should be alert for strong desires to prepare, soothe, or behave cautiously when introducing the necessity of attending RO skills classes to an OC client and should use this as an opportunity for self-growth. Examples of self-enquiry questions include those that follow:

- What do I fear may happen if I do not behave cautiously with this client?

- Is it possible that I am assuming the client is fragile or incompetent?

- Why do I believe it to be so important to prepare this client for class participation?

- Is it possible that I have been subtly shaped by my prior experiences or by this client to assume that skills classes will prove extremely difficult for the client?

In summary, rather than assuming incapability, therapists should remind OC clients that they already have a great deal of experience in similar situations (that is, they have attended school and participated in structured classroom activities). Attending an RO skills training class is like going back to school—the focus will be on the material being taught, not on the individual being taught. OC clients' superior capacities for self-control and their prior experiences in classroom settings function as proof of their ability to attend an RO class as well.

Finally, the structure of this manual assumes an outpatient setup, with either open or closed groups. In an open group setup, a client can join the skills group at any time (with the exception of RO Integration Week, lesson 30; see also chapter 4 for instructions on using this manual). In a closed group, all clients start with lesson 1 at the same time, and new clients wait until a new group starts. However, it should be noted that RO skills training lessons can be used flexibly to suit treatment providers' needs and/or limitations. For example, RO skills have been successfully applied in inpatient, day hospital, and forensic settings (T. R. Lynch et al., 2013; Keogh, Booth, Baird, & Davenport, 2016) as well as with adolescents and families (Simic, Stewart, Hunt, Konstantellou, & Underdown, 2016) and as an augmentation strategy (Chen et al., 2015).

Structuring RO Skills Training Classes

This manual contains twenty new skills compressed into thirty lessons (or weeks), with RO mindfulness skills repeated once (see table 1.2). Whenever possible, instructors should look for opportunities to link each new skill with clients' valued goals linked to social connectedness. For example, when reviewing homework, an instructor might ask a client the extent to which a new skill impacted the client's relationships.

Table 1.2. RO Skills Training, Weeks 1–30

Week/ Lesson	Title of Lesson
1	Radical Openness
2	Understanding Emotions
3	Activating Social Safety
4	Enhancing Openness and Social Connection via Loving Kindness
5	Engaging in Novel Behavior
6	How Do Emotions Help Us?
7	Understanding Overcontrolled Coping
8	Tribe Matters: Understanding Rejection and Self-Conscious Emotions
9	Social Signaling Matters!
10	Using Social Signaling to Live by Your Values: Flexible Mind Is DEEP
11	Mindfulness Training, Part 1: Overcontrolled States of Mind
12	Mindfulness Training, Part 2: The "What" Skills
13	Mindfulness Training, Part 3: The Core Mindfulness "How" Skill: With Self-Enquiry
14	Mindfulness Training, Part 4: The "How" Skills
15	Interpersonal Integrity, Part 1: Saying What We Really Mean
16	Interpersonal Integrity, Part 2: Flexible Mind REVEALs
17	Interpersonal Effectiveness: Kindness First and Foremost
18	Being Assertive with an Open Mind
19	Using Validation to Signal Social Inclusion
20	Enhancing Social Connectedness, Part 1
21	Enhancing Social Connectedness, Part 2
22	Learning from Corrective Feedback
23	Mindfulness Training, Part 1: Overcontrolled States of Mind (Repeated from Lesson 11)
24	Mindfulness Training, Part 2: The "What" Skills (Repeated from Lesson 12)
25	Mindfulness Training, Part 3: The Core Mindfulness "How" Skill: With Self-Enquiry (Repeated from Lesson 13)
26	Mindfulness Training, Part 4: The "How" Skills (Repeated from Lesson 14)

27	Envy and Resentment
28	Cynicism, Bitterness, and Resignation
29	Learning to Forgive
30	RO Integration Week

Each skills training session is designed to occur within a two-and-a-half-hour time frame, including homework review, a brief break, and new teaching. Paper copies of handouts and worksheets are considered essential to the learning process and should be made available during skills training classes. No later than the day of the first class, each participant should be provided with an RO skills training folder containing copies of all worksheets and handouts for the class. Pens and pencils should be supplied for notetaking. Instructors should remind class members to bring their personal RO skills folders with them to each class, and instructors should always have extra copies of the handouts and worksheets available for those who may have forgotten or misplaced their RO folders.

Skills instructors should also adopt a standard protocol for contacting missing class members. Typically this involves having the coinstructor briefly step out of the room at the beginning of class (for example, during the mindfulness practice) and make brief phone contact with all missing members, encouraging them to attend the day's class, if only a short period, while also assessing and blocking maladaptive behaviors. For example, if a client says he is too depressed to come to class, the coinstructor might say, "This is exactly the time you need to be practicing skills, by going opposite to your desire to isolate and by coming to class instead. So I would like you to get in your car now and come to class." The overall therapeutic stance is to strongly signal that attendance at skills training class is essential for genuine recovery and not an optional component of treatment. A general overview of the class structure is outlined here:

- *Beginning of class.* Instructors should establish a class norm of beginning class on time; delaying the start of class can make it more difficult to cover the lesson plan for the day and/or can imply that lateness is okay (because "we never start on time"). Indeed, delaying the start of class to wait for missing members can be interpreted as invalidating by those OC individuals who have arrived on time, and it may trigger feelings of unfairness, envy, or resentment, which can subtly undermine the class's functioning, influence attendance, and/or trigger alliance ruptures. Thus, as already noted, rather than delaying the start of class, the coinstructor should step out and telephone any members who have not arrived and encourage them to attend.

- *Brief mindfulness exercise (approximately one to ten minutes).* Each class begins with a short mindfulness exercise that, ideally, is linked to the new skill being taught during the day's class. The exercise can be followed by a brief discussion and sharing of observations, but discussion afterward is not required. Plus, rather than emphasizing silent practices involving dispassionate awareness (such as mindful breathing), RO mindfulness exercises prioritize repeated exposure to practices involving self-enquiry, outing oneself to a fellow practitioner, and participating without planning. When it comes to participating without planning, instructors are encouraged to use the "participate without planning" practices found in this manual rather than creating their own (see "Teach Directly from the Manual," later in this chapter).

- *Homework review (approximately forty minutes in total).* Next, the instructor or coinstructor reviews the homework that was assigned the previous week, making sure that participants have time to share how they did. Importantly, RO diary cards should *not* be reviewed in RO skills training classes. Although the RO DBT diary card includes a list of skills used during the previous week, it is intended solely for use during individual therapy.

- *Break (approximately ten to fifteen minutes).* After homework review, a short break is provided. One instructor should remain with class members during the break. This facilitates social interaction, provides opportunities for skills coaching, and cheerleads participation. A break also gives OC clients an opportunity to practice social engagement skills in a nonstructured setting. Plus, a class break is a core way for instructors to address maladaptive behaviors and/or potential alliance ruptures privately. In addition, the break provides important opportunities for instructors to shape prosocial classroom behavior (see "Protocol for Therapeutic Induction of Social Responsibility," in chapter 3) or manage potential alliance ruptures.

- *Teaching of new skills for the week or lesson (approximately fifty minutes).* After the break, the second half of the class begins, with one instructor taking the lead in teaching the new material for the week.

- *Assignment of homework (approximately five minutes).* Just prior to the end of the class, homework is assigned for the upcoming week (that is, the period before the next lesson). Participants are also encouraged to continue practicing their previously learned RO skills. Instructors should look for opportunities to augment required homework assignments with optional assignments for the entire class and/or individualized assignments targeting specific issues relevant for a particular client. Individualized homework assigned to a particular client should always be mutually agreed upon as useful and, ideally, should not be overly complicated or too time-consuming to complete. Instructors should keep a record of extra homework assignments and use it to remind themselves to ask clients about how things went with their completion of individualized assignments.

Composition of RO Skills Training Classes

Skills classes conducted with OC clients should consist, ideally, of seven to nine participants, with two instructors. Although it seems somewhat counterintuitive, given the socially anxious nature of overcontrol, OC clients actually experience a small class size (four or fewer members) as more difficult and/or anxiety-arousing than a larger class size. The reason for this apparent conundrum is that OC clients dislike the limelight. Most OC clients are uncomfortable being the center of attention during an interpersonal interaction, and a small class size naturally allows for more individualized attention, whereas a larger class size naturally takes the heat off anxious OC clients by making it easier for them to fade into the background for brief moments (for example, when they need time to reflect or downregulate), without disrupting the class or attracting unwanted attention.

Thus, on a day when there are four or fewer class members (regardless of the reason), it is recommended that only one instructor teach (as opposed to the normal two skills instructors present in a larger class). The presence of two instructors in a class with few members can be experienced as emotionally intense or exposing, causing learning to suffer and commitment to wane. Instructors should avoid the temptation to base their decisions on the opinions of class members; almost invariably, most participants will report that they are fine or even happy for both instructors to stay (recall the prosocial nature of OC) while privately believing otherwise and/or later regretting their consent, without letting it be known. Just as their natural tendencies to mask inner feelings make it less likely for them to reveal that a room is too hot, they are unlikely to reveal their discomfort about a small class size when queried (see "Maximize Learning by Maximizing the Physical Environment," later in this chapter).

Think Nondiagnostically to Enhance Class Size

The good news is that since overcontrol is a transdiagnostic problem cutting across a spectrum of disorders sharing similar biotemperamental features and behaviors, it is clinically appropriate to create multidiagnostic RO skills training classes rather than focusing solely on diagnostic status for class inclusion. Simply stated, as long as all the members of the class share overcontrol as their style of coping (and have agreed to work on it), their diagnostic status does not matter.* Thus, an RO skills training class might include a range of individuals presenting with differing problems and/or diagnoses, such as anorexia nervosa, chronic depression, autism spectrum disorder, chronic back pain, treatment-resistant anxiety, obsessive-compulsive personality disorder, and paranoid personality disorder. Indeed, our clinical experience suggests that multidiagnostic RO skills training classes may represent the ideal class composition because they provide a unique opportunity for OC clients to learn from diversity (recall that OC clients compulsively seek sameness) and lead to unexpected clinical benefits. For example, a young adult diagnosed with anorexia nervosa may suddenly find herself sitting next to an older adult diagnosed with chronic depression and obsessive-compulsive personality disorder. Both are likely to quickly recognize their OC bond, linked to shared qualities/values and struggles, and, ideally, the prospect of learning from someone who, on the surface, appears very different. Plus, it helps to not always swim in the same pool if one desires to genuinely see the world differently and/or make important life changes. Thus, the anorexic OC client is suddenly no longer surrounded solely by fellow "eating-disordered" classmates, who may communally trigger frequent body weight/body image social comparisons that function to reinforce restrictive eating or compulsive preoccupation with external appearance. Similarly, the chronically depressed older adult may find himself challenged by a young person anxiously engaged in learning how to cope and may feel excited about new possibilities rather than automatically assuming that nothing will change or that life is hopeless.

In addition, since a core goal of therapy is to help an OC client learn how to form genuine, honest, and mutually caring relationships with other people, RO DBT does not consider it a problem for class members to socialize together outside of class. Anecdotally, we have observed in our clinical trials that, without prompting, OC clients often independently form social networks composed of other class members upon completion of treatment, a practice that appears to facilitate continued use of core radical openness and social connectedness skills. These independently formed class tribes or aftercare groups typically meet weekly, do not involve clinical oversight, and are client-organized and client-run, with meetings most often taking place in such nonclinical settings as a client's home, a community meeting hall, or a local pub. Clients have been highly enthusiastic about these aftercare tribes, using them to stay connected, practice RO skills with like-minded people, and sometimes even find a lifelong partner. Thus, whenever an RO skills training class independently moves toward the creation of an OC tribe, the clinical program should celebrate clients' ingenuity and avoid the temptation to interfere with, direct, or manage client-generated aftercare unless specifically asked for help. Regardless of clients' initiatives, clinical programs are encouraged to integrate similar aftercare components, when possible, into existing treatment pathways. Although not required formally, the benefits derived from continued practice of RO skills can be enormous.

Maximize Learning by Maximizing the Physical Environment

The physical therapeutic milieu can be a critical factor in enhancing clients' engagement and achieving a successful outcome. The reason this is given such high priority in RO DBT pertains to the innate biotemperamental predisposition for heightened threat sensitivity that characterizes OC clients. OC clients are more likely to respond with low-level defensive arousal to environmental stimuli that might go unnoticed by other

---

* In some clinical settings, particularly those already using standard dialectical behavior therapy, there can be a temptation to collapse overcontrolled and undercontrolled (UC) clients into one class. In general, this is not recommended, for two reasons: first, RO skills address problems of overcontrol and fundamentally differ from the skills taught in standard DBT for problems of undercontrol; and, second, the talkative and effusive nature of most UC clients can inadvertently lead to domination of class discussions by UC clients' observations, with fewer contributions from their more restrained OC classmates. OC clients, if asked, may report being perfectly fine with this while secretly harboring judgmental thoughts or hoping that expectations for their own personal participation may be lessened.

people. They are also less likely to admit to anxious defensive arousal when queried. The primary goal of treatment is to help OC clients learn that social interactions can be intrinsically rewarding, and that it is possible to experience feelings of safety around others; it is not for OC clients to overcome, defeat, or control their social anxiety by braving it out or going opposite action.

Thus, it is helpful for therapists to proactively control the physical milieu in order to make it less likely for OC biology to interfere with clients' learning how to have fun, play, express themselves more freely, chill out, and be less serious. This means accounting for a range of often subtle physical and nonverbal factors that can enhance (or diminish) social safety experiences in OC clients. Therapists, even those who identify as leaning toward OC, should not dismiss these factors because they themselves are not bothered, or because a client denies discomfort.

OC clients generally have a greater need for personal body space relative to others. Close body proximity is a nonverbal signal of intimacy or confrontation (Morris, 2002). RO skills instructors should arrange seating in the classroom in a manner that maximizes physical distance. Ideally, this arrangement will include a long table, with chairs positioned around it in the style of a dining room, and with some type of whiteboard or flipchart in the front for instructors to write on (see figure 1.3). This classroom-type setting signals that the purpose of the group is to learn skills, in the same way that one learns algebra, for example; it is not a personal encounter or process group. The table and the room arrangement also provide a physical buffer between group members. This functions to reduce feelings in OC clients of being exposed while also providing space for note-taking, which can give OC clients time to regulate themselves in a less obvious manner. The skills class should, ideally, be conducted in a large and airy room, to accommodate up to nine people. A large room also allows clients greater freedom to adjust their seating or move their chairs farther away from others without calling attention to themselves.

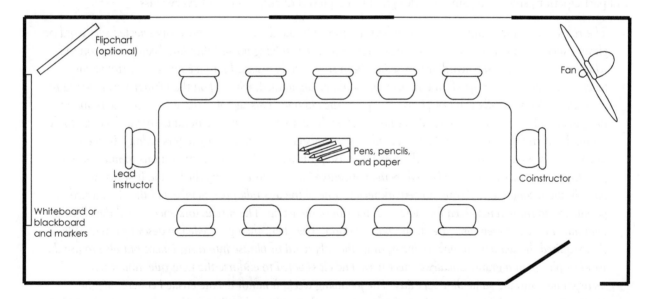

Figure 1.3. RO Skills Classroom Layout

It is also very important that room temperature be considered for skills training classes. A hot or very warm environment naturally triggers perspiration in most people. For many OC clients, sweating is a conditioned stimulus linked to anxiety and maladaptive avoidance. Instructors should set the temperature of the classroom lower than what might be normal, and there should be a fan or some other means of cooling the classroom, if necessary. In general, the rule is to keep the classroom cool. Class members who find the room too cool should be encouraged to wear extra layers.

Teach Directly from the Manual

Although a wide range of potentially valid reasons can be generated in support of therapists' personal and/or theoretical preferences to not explicitly follow this manual when teaching RO skills, my experience training and supervising thousands of therapists has repeatedly confirmed that deviating from the manual almost invariably creates more problems than it solves. The manual is designed to be used like a cookbook. When learning a new recipe, good cooks know that the tastiest outcome is most likely if they follow the recipe. Similarly, RO skills instructors are encouraged to follow the recipe, particularly when first learning RO skills. Plus, using the manual smuggles a core RO principle related to humility and fallibility, a core principle that OC clients need to learn.

The scientific, clinical, and ethical reasons for adhering to a manual, especially when first learning a new evidence-based procedure or treatment, become apparent when one considers how one might feel about being operated on by a heart surgeon who, one discovers, has decided to change or ignore certain parts of a new and recently learned surgical technique without ever having gained experience with the original protocol. The point is, people prefer heart surgeons who become experts in the delivery of a new procedure before deciding to change it. Similarly, RO skills instructors are encouraged to allow themselves time to learn the new skills and principles fully, and to gain expertise in teaching them, as described in the manual, before deciding to modify, omit, or create new skills or exercises.

The type of problem that can emerge when therapists and skills trainers go off model is illustrated by the following case. The instructors, both highly experienced therapists (albeit new to RO DBT), decided to introduce a new game into their RO skills training class. It was not included in the manual but was designed to creatively extend RO "participate without planning" exercises and, more broadly, to enhance classroom fun and participation, since the game was designed to be played during each and every class.

The rules of the game required class members to insert into the discussion a previously selected silly word or phrase, such as "broccoli," "boo-boo," "blessed art thou," or "talking horse," that had been written on the whiteboard. After the silly word or phrase had been successfully inserted into a comment or statement, teaching would be interrupted and the winner would be applauded, whereupon the winner was required to come up with a new silly word or phrase to replace the old one. This signaled the start of a new round of the game, and there could be several rounds per class. The instructors were careful to orient the class to the rationale behind the game, and they obtained class members' commitment before proceeding. To their delight, the class not only embraced the game but also provided several helpful suggestions to make it more fun. Enthusiasm was further bolstered by the noticeable increase in verbosity during the first two weeks of play. In the second week, during homework review, one of the less talkative members of the class asked permission to share a new idea for increasing the fun of the game. The instructors encouraged the client to continue, in order to reinforce the client's participation. The client then proceeded to describe a new rule that required the winner not only to incorporate the silly word or phrase into a statement but also to use the word or phrase in a grammatically correct way. The class voted to endorse the new rule, and it was incorporated into the game that very day. The following week, a minor debate ensued concerning the meaning of the word "grammatical," and two class members reported feeling anxiety about not being able to compete adequately. The skills instructors attempted to rectify the situation by using bigger gestures, expressing enthusiasm, and reminding the class that the game was not about being perfect. During class break, a different client revealed to an instructor that, although they remained enthusiastic about the game, they were finding it more difficult to concentrate in class because they kept thinking about the silly word. Moreover, the frequent minidebates about the game's rules, and interruptions to applaud the week's winners, limited the time available for the instructors to teach the RO skill that was supposed to be the main focus of the day. The instructors concluded that perhaps the new game was not such a good idea.

Upon reflection, it is easy to see that the game just described was bound to lead to difficulties. It encouraged competition among a highly competitive client population, without being explicit about it (that is, there were winners but no losers); it went counter to core RO "participate without planning" principles by making it impossible to win without some form of rehearsal or planning; and it reinforced OC maladaptive rigid and rule-governed behavior via the rules of the game. Core RO skills training principles and structural recommendations were ignored. For example, the game dominated a significant amount of class time. Not only did the instructors design the game so that it could be played each and every class, the rules also required RO skills teaching to stop in order for the winner to be applauded and have sufficient time to write the next silly word or phrase on the whiteboard. Plus, rather than encouraging "participate without planning" skills, the game encouraged multitasking and planning ahead.

Fortunately, the instructors in this real-life example quickly adjusted their teaching style and, with encouragement from their RO consultation team, outed their errors to their skills class the following week. The game was transformed into a class metaphor that symbolized the importance of self-enquiry and eventually became a class song titled "Isn't Arrogance Fun?" During supervision, the skills instructors used this experience as an opportunity for self-enquiry that led to important personal and professional growth. For example, self-enquiry practice led one instructor to realize that their desire not to follow the manual stemmed partly from exhaustion ("Oh no—not another treatment to learn!"), whereas others have reported resisting using the manual because they believed it would reflect incompetence or suggest that they were not intelligent enough to translate the core principles into their own words. Some have revealed choosing not to use the manual based on prior training contending that experienced therapists do better when not following manuals. Others have reported feeling embarrassed or uncomfortable with certain aspects of the treatment itself (such as a required teaching point necessitating role play or the dramatic reading of a story). Regardless, the main point of this section is to encourage instructors to practice self-enquiry whenever they find themselves desiring not to use the manual. Here are some examples of self-enquiry questions:

- To what extent do I actually follow the RO treatment manual? How much energy or resistance do I experience when asking this question? What might this tell me about my willingness to learn a new treatment? What is it that I need to learn?

- What am I afraid would happen if I were to comply with the manual?

- To what extent has my prior training influenced my behavior and/or openness to learn RO DBT? What might this mean for me as a health care provider?

- How open was I when first learning RO DBT? Has my openness changed? What does this tell me about myself? What is it that I might need to learn?

- What core RO principles or interventions do I disagree with or believe are wrong? To what extent am I holding on to an alternative treatment model? How might this impact my learning or delivery of the treatment? What does this tell me about myself?

- To what extent do I believe that it is unfair to require me to practice RO DBT as it was intended because of my exceptional status, training, or talent? What is it that I might need to learn?

Summary

Radically open dialectical behavior therapy (RO DBT) is an evidence-based treatment designed specifically for problems of overcontrol. In RO DBT, interventions emphasize the tribal nature of our species and the importance of prosocial signaling, self-enquiry, and social connectedness for emotional well-being. The aim of this chapter has been to provide a brief overview of core RO DBT principles and of the structural elements that need to be considered when an RO skills training class is introduced into a clinical program.

CHAPTER 2

Dialectics, Radical Openness, and Self-Enquiry

There are three core philosophical principles or ideas in RO DBT that strongly impact the manner in which a therapist delivers the treatment:

1. Dialectics

2. Radical openness

3. Self-enquiry

Dialectics in RO DBT provides a theoretically coherent means for a therapist to balance and switch between seemingly different therapeutic styles in one session—for example, playful irreverence versus compassionate gravity. *Radical openness* is the core underlying principle and skill in RO DBT. It represents the confluence of three capacities posited to be essential for emotional well-being: openness, flexibility, and social connectedness. *Self-enquiry* represents a core RO mindfulness skill that encourages the development of healthy self-doubt in order to learn. The primary aim of this chapter will be to provide an overview of the theoretical rationale underlying each principle and demonstrate how each influences the in-session behavior of an RO DBT therapist (or RO skills trainer).

Why Dialectics?

Dialectical strategies in RO DBT share roots with the existential and dialectical philosophies found in Gestalt therapy (Perls, 1969) and most prominently with the dialectical principles guiding interventions in standard DBT (Linehan, 1993a). Dialectical thinking involves three developmental stages: a thesis (such as "self-control is always necessary"), giving rise to its reaction, an antithesis (such as "too much self-control is always unhealthy"), which contradicts and seems to negate the thesis, while the tension between these two opposite perspectives is resolved via a synthesis of the two opposite perspectives that, ideally, results in higher-order functioning, not simply in a compromise (for example, a synthesis using the preceding example polarities might involve a willingness to flexibly relinquish control when the situation calls for it). Hegelian dialectics includes five key concepts or assumptions:

1. Everything is transient and finite.

2. Everything important in life is composed of contradictions (opposing forces).

3. Gradual changes lead to crises or turning points, when one force overcomes its opponent force.

4. The world is holistic, and everything is connected and in relationship.

5. Change is continual and transactional (that is, opposing perspectives influence each other and evolve over time).

In RO DBT, the therapist uses dialectical principles to encourage cognitively rigid OC clients to think in ways that are both more complex and more flexible.

An example of dialectical thinking can be seen within the RO mindfulness skill of self-enquiry. As described in detail later in this chapter, self-enquiry requires a willingness to question one's beliefs, perceptions, action urges, and behaviors without falling apart or simply giving in. The dialectical tension involves balancing trusting versus distrusting personal perceptions or ways of coping while remaining open to the possibility of learning from disconfirming feedback. For OC clients, who tend to automatically consider their interpretations of events as absolute truths or facts, the use of dialectical thinking is often an essential factor in embracing RO self-enquiry practices and viscerally learning the value of healthy self-doubt (discussed later in this chapter).

Dialectical thinking is also highly useful in helping to loosen OC clients' tendencies toward inflexible rule-governed behavior, rigid beliefs, and high moral certitude (that is, the belief that there is only one right way to do or think about something), which can interfere with the ability to flexibly adapt to change and with the formation of close social bonds. For example, many OC clients consider "dependence" a dirty word ("dependence makes you weak and vulnerable to abuse"). Yet, regardless of our personal preferences, all humans are dependent on something or someone, at least some of the time (for example, we depend on our grocer to provide us with fresh milk, our friends to tell us the truth, our rock-climbing instructor to show us how to tie a knot properly, and, as infants, on our parents' affection). Moreover, our dependence on others does not negate the value of independent living (as in standing up against moral wrongs, striving to go where no one else has gone, saving for retirement to avoid burdening others, or voicing an unpopular opinion). Thus, dialectical thinking is an important therapeutic tool in RO DBT. It allows a therapist to genuinely validate the client's perspective ("being independent keeps you from being hurt") while maintaining its opposite ("being dependent is essential for survival"), thereby creating the possibility for new ways of thinking and behaving (a new synthesis) to emerge. Finally, dialectical thinking also informs therapists' behavior during interactions with their clients. There are two dialectical polarities that I have found to most commonly arise when working with OC clients (see figure 2.1):

1. Nonmoving centeredness versus acquiescent letting go

2. Playful irreverence versus compassionate gravity

The next two subsections describe how they are used in RO DBT to enhance treatment.

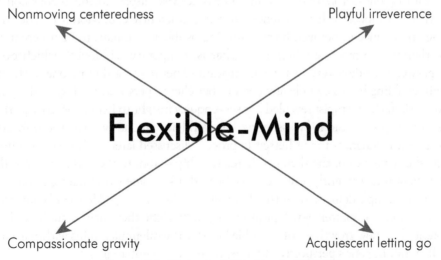

Nonmoving centeredness   Playful irreverence

Flexible-Mind

Compassionate gravity   Acquiescent letting go

Figure 2.1. Dialectical Thinking in RO DBT

Therapist's Use of Nonmoving Centeredness Versus Acquiescent Letting Go

Nonmoving centeredness versus acquiescent letting go is the dialectical dilemma of knowing when to hold on to rather than let go of a case formulation, a theoretical insight, or a personal conviction when working with an OC client, in order to model core RO principles, maintain the client's engagement, repair an alliance rupture, and/or spur new growth. It is informed by an overarching RO DBT principle positing that therapists as well as clients bring perceptual and regulatory biases into the treatment environment, and that these biases influence both the therapeutic relationship and treatment outcomes. Thus, being able to recognize and know when to let go of a bias represents an essential dialectical dilemma for therapists if they are (1) going to maximize the likelihood of forming a strong therapeutic alliance (RO DBT posits that a working alliance with an OC client does not appear until about the fourteenth session), (2) effectively model radical openness to their OC clients, and (3) provide alternatives for their clients' habitual ways of behaving and thinking. No small task! Unfortunately, mindful awareness of the dilemma will not necessarily lead to synthesis, nor will it necessarily mitigate the emotional distress that can accompany the therapist's attempts to grapple with it (for example, letting go of firmly held convictions and standing up for one's convictions can both be painful therapeutic choices). Plus, to make matters more complicated, therapists need to be biased; that is, the role of a health care provider necessitates professional opinions about a client's presenting problems and the best course of treatment, also known as a *case conceptualization*. Indeed, case conceptualization has been described as the "heart of evidence-based practice" (Bieling & Kuyken, 2003, p. 53). Therapists are usually trained to consider their case formulations as reliable and generally accurate descriptions of clients' behavior, despite research showing that therapists often formulate widely divergent case conceptualizations for the same client (Kuyken, Fothergill, Musa, & Chadwick, 2005). Yet, despite these difficulties, RO DBT posits that there is a way forward. It involves the creation of a temporary state of self-doubt whenever feedback from the environment or from the client suggests that one's case conceptualization may be in error.

Healthy self-doubt is a core construct in RO DBT (see lesson 13); it provides the therapist with a coherent means of relinquishing control without abdicating professional responsibility or needing to abandon a prior perspective (see also the material on Flexible Mind DEFinitely skills in lesson 1). As one example of the advantages of acquiescent letting go, a therapist in one of our research trials reported in consultation team that she was struggling with knowing how to resolve a potential alliance rupture with her OC client. Her client had been repeatedly dismissing any suggestion by the therapist that he was a decent human being or had prosocial intentions by saying, "You just don't know me. I am an evil person. I have a lot of resistance to joining the human race. I'm essentially not a very nice person, and my past is my proof." The therapist had attempted to address this by pointing out factors that discounted or otherwise disproved the client's conviction, yet each attempt appeared only to increase his insistence on being inherently evil. Moreover, the therapist reported feeling increasing angst, since in her worldview it was impossible for humans to be inherently evil. The team encouraged the therapist to practice self-enquiry (that is, temporary self-doubt), which eventually led the therapist to the personal self-discovery that it was arrogant of her to insist that no one in the world could ever be inherently evil, enabling her to be radically open to her client's perspective (despite the pain it generated). During the next session, the therapist revealed her self-enquiry insight to her client (that is, that she had been behaving arrogantly in prior sessions by assuming her worldview about evil was the only correct one). Her personal self-work and willingness to out herself (a process discussed later in this chapter) immediately functioned to change the dynamics of the therapeutic relationship—and, to the surprise of the therapist, several sessions later the client independently revealed, "I've been thinking lately that maybe I'm not so evil after all." This real-life clinical example demonstrates the therapeutic value of being able to radically give in, or let go of strongly held convictions no matter how logical or viscerally right they may seem. The dialectical tension enabling the potential for new growth is only possible because the dilemma retains within itself the therapeutic utility of doggedly retaining one's perspective (that is, nonmoving centeredness).

Consequently, nonmoving centeredness is the dialectical twin of acquiescent letting go. It refers to the importance of an RO DBT therapist holding on to a personal conviction or belief about a client, despite strong opposition from the client or the environment. The rationale for this stance may best be represented by the RO principle of *kindness first and foremost* (see lesson 17). Sometimes kindness means telling good friends a painful truth in order to help them achieve their valued goals in a manner that acknowledges the helper's own potential for fallibility. Thus, RO DBT therapists recognize that they may need to disagree with their OC clients to facilitate growth (albeit the vast majority of RO DBT confrontations involve asking, not telling, the client about his or her apparent problem; see "RO DBT Therapeutic Stance," in chapter 8 of the RO DBT textbook). This disagreement is usually combined with nonverbal nondominant social signals (such as a slight bowing of the head and a shoulder shrug along with openhanded gestures, a warm smile, an eyebrow wag, and direct eye contact; see Flexible Mind SAGE skills, lesson 8) to communicate equity and openness to critical feedback. Nondominance signals are especially important when a person is in a power-up position yet desires a close relationship (as in the therapist-client relationship). Importantly, this dialectical dilemma also allows for the possibility of less open-minded signaling (or urgency) and for the use of dominant assertions of confidence in order to block imminent life-threatening behavior (see "The RO DBT Crisis-Management Protocol," in chapter 5 of the RO DBT textbook).

Therapist's Use of Playful Irreverence Versus Compassionate Gravity

Playful irreverence versus compassionate gravity is the second most common dialectical dilemma encountered by therapists treating OC clients. It represents a dialectical means of challenging maladaptive behavior while signaling affection and openness. The stance of playful irreverence most often begins with the therapist's use of a nonverbal or verbal expression of incredulity and/or amused bewilderment, accompanied by a nondominant signal of openness and affection and triggered by a discrepant, odd, or illogical comment or behavior on the part of an OC client (for example, a client verbally indicates that she is unable to speak, or she reports a complete lack of animosity toward a coworker she has admitted to having lied about in order to get him fired).

Playful irreverence represents the therapeutic cousin of a good tease between friends. Friends playfully and affectionately tease each other all the time. Research shows that teasing and joking are how friends informally point out flaws in each other, without being too heavy-handed about it. Learning how to tease and be teased is an important part of healthy social relationships, and kindhearted teasing is how tribes, families, and friends give feedback to each other. Plus, a good tease is always kind. Most often it starts out with an unexpected, provocative comment that is delivered with an unsympathetic (expressionless or arrogant) voice tone and/or an intimidating facial expression (such as a blank stare), gesture (such as finger wagging), or body posture (such as hands on hips) that is immediately followed by laughter, gaze aversion, and/or postural shrinkage. Thus, a kindhearted tease momentarily introduces conflict and social distance but quickly reestablishes social connectedness by signaling nondominant friendliness. The nondominance signal is critical for a tease to be taken lightly (that is, as a friendly poke; see Keltner, Young, & Buswell, 1997). When teasing is playful and reciprocal, it is socially bonding, and people who can tease in a friendly manner and enjoy being teased are more likely to be mentally and physically healthy because they don't take life too seriously and can laugh at their foibles and learn from them.

Thus, when a therapist adopts a playful irreverent style with an OC client, the therapist sends a powerful social signal that says, "I like you, and I consider you part of my tribe." When interacting with friends, we are likely to use more colorful and less formal forms of language (such as slang or curse words), feel free to express our inner feelings, use more expansive gestures, adopt more relaxed postures (such as slouching), and tease or play with each other. However, the fun thing about a tease is that it also provides corrective feedback. This represents the essence of an RO DBT playful irreverent stance—that is, it incorporates some form of critical feedback (such as "Really? You don't ever desire to have a friend?") that is accompanied by nondominant body postures and facial expressions that communicate that the therapist likes the client and intends the client no harm. These nonverbal signals combine appeasement signals (such as a slight bowing of the head, a shoulder shrug, or openhanded gestures) with cooperative-friendly signals (such as a warm smile, eyebrow wags, and direct eye contact). Thus, playful irreverence in RO DBT encourages the therapist to drop his or her professional demeanor and adopt the behavior of a friend in order to provide socially relevant feedback to the emotionally lonely and isolated OC client and encourage the client to rejoin the tribe.

Compassionate gravity represents the dialectical opposite of a playful irreverent stance. Rather than aiming to tease and challenge, it seeks to understand and to signal sobriety (that is, that the therapist takes the client seriously). It also functions as a way of taking the heat off a client, whereas playful irreverence puts the heat on a client (see also "Heat-Off Strategies" and "Heat-On Strategies," in chapter 6 of the RO DBT textbook, and "Use Heat-On and Heat-Off Strategies to Shape Desired Behaviors," in chapter 3 of this manual). A stance of compassionate gravity is designed to slow down the pace of the interaction and signal social safety to the client. The most common nonverbal changes include slowing down the pace of speaking, speaking with a softer voice tone, slightly pausing after each utterance by the client in order to allow the client time to say more (if the client so desires), gentle eye contact (not staring), and a warm closed-mouth smile. It may also be accompanied by an involuntary therapeutic sigh of affiliation. Other common nonverbal signals that accompany a stance of compassionate gravity include leaning back in one's chair, raising one's eyebrows when listening to the client (or speaking), and signaling nondominant friendliness (especially during an alliance rupture repair) via a slight bowing of the head, a slight shoulder shrug, and openhanded gestures combined with a closed-mouth smile (see chapter 6 of the RO DBT textbook for details on each nonverbal signal). A stance of compassionate gravity can be used in a number of differing ways, including when therapists out themselves (as when a therapist's personal worldview may have interfered with the therapist's understanding of the client's perspective), repair an alliance rupture, signal intent listening, communicate warm friendliness, or balance a playful irreverent comment in order to ensure that the tease is not taken the wrong way. The overall aim is to communicate to the client, "I desire to know who you are from your perspective (not mine), and I am taking your situation seriously."

Why Radical Openness?

Openness and Well-Being

From my perspective, one of the most difficult challenges of being open is letting go of my personal perspective in order to experience the world from someone else's point of view (especially when I think I'm right). It is difficult because being correct matters (for example, for survival, success, job promotions, and for rockets to land on the moon) and it is a challenge because not every perspective is correct, making the choice of which perspective to believe a conundrum. The worry is "What if the source of new information is wrong?" (for example, one's grip on a spear is less important; what matters most when throwing a spear is that the shaft remains close to the body at all times during the throw) or "What if the source is trying to deceive us?" (for example, my so-called friend is giving me wrong advice on purpose so he can win the tribal spear-throwing contest). Indeed, when you take a moment to think about it, openness has a lot of downsides. It requires effortful control and valuable expenditures of energy, whereas habits not only demand fewer cognitive resources but can often be equally effective as or even more effective than deliberate control efforts (for example, driving my car doesn't require a great deal of cognitive effort, because I am an experienced driver; plus, I probably drive better when I don't think about it too much). So why bother being open at all?

One reason we may bother is because we instinctively recognize the value openness brings to relationships. We naturally admire open-minded individuals and desire to be close to them. For example, people yearn to meet the Dalai Lama (that is, he attracts large crowds of people), but not so much because of his eloquence as a speaker, his distinctive appearance, or his prior deeds (although these may contribute); they desire to be near him because his presence viscerally reminds them of what they already know—that is, as a species we are better when together, and open-minded living represents the way back home. Essentially, I contend that open-ness matters because tribe matters. When we feel part of a tribe, we feel safe. Our species survived because we developed capacities to form long-lasting bonds and share valuable resources with people who were not in our immediate family (that is, total strangers). Thus, for our very early ancestors living in harsh environments, being in a tribe was essential for personal survival. Indeed, we are constantly scanning the facial expressions and vocalizations of other people for signs of disapproval and are biologically predisposed to construe the intentions of others as disapproving, especially when social signals are ambiguous (see chapter 6 of the RO DBT textbook).

Open-mindedness evolved as a core means of ensuring that cooperative intentions were accurately per-ceived, especially during interactions involving conflict. Openness is a powerful social safety signal because it acknowledges our shared potential for fallibility and a willingness to learn from the world. It allows us the luxury of dropping our guard because we recognize that the open-minded person is willing to hear our point of view. Thus, despite its energy-depleting downsides, openness is posited to be a core part of a uniquely human evolutionary advantage that allowed for unprecedented cooperation among genetically unrelated individuals (see chapter 6 of the RO DBT textbook). In other words, open-mindedness is tribal glue—it binds together differences and creates new, unimagined accords.

Another reason we bother being open is because we innately recognize the value of learning new things. Tribes not only provided instrumental support (for example, helping a neighbor repair a fence after a storm, or collectively building a wall to keep out enemies) but also allowed individuals to benefit from the collective wisdom of their community through explicit instruction (for example, about the time of year to plant corn, or the type of stone best for making an axe), observational learning and modeling of successful others (for example, about how to ride a horse or throw a spear), and direct feedback ("You missed the target because you were gripping the spear too tight"). All three require the recipient to be open-minded to the new information or feedback for the lesson to be learned. Being open to new ideas or critical feedback from another member of the tribe ("That's not a cow—it's a tiger! Let's run!") provided a huge evolutionary advantage for both the open-minded individual and our species because our individual survival no longer depended solely on our personal perceptions; see "Fun Facts: The Story of Oog-Ahh (Sometimes a Cow Is Not a Cow)," lesson 19. The preceding observation may explain why we are so concerned about the opinions of others.

However, it can be extremely difficult to know when you are being open (versus actually closed). We tend to pay attention to things that fit our beliefs and to ignore or dismiss things that do not. We adamantly contend that we are open, only to discover later that we were actually closed (particularly common during arguments), and we don't know what we don't know, thereby making it doubly hard to notice closed-minded thinking, because our way of thinking feels so right! Moreover, being open to another person's perspective also necessitates a willingness to trust the good intentions of the person we are interacting with and/or to believe in the correctness of the source of collective wisdom (such as a tribal elder's memory or a written document). These issues highlight some of the difficulties in treating problems of overcontrol; that is, OC clients are char-acterized by low interpersonal trust and low openness to new experience and are expert at discounting or ignoring corrective feedback, often in very subtle ways.

Yet, despite these difficulties, RO DBT posits that there is a way forward. It involves the creation of a temporary state of self-doubt. This temporary state of mind is referred to in RO DBT as "healthy self-doubt." It begins with the assumption that we don't see things as they are but see things as we are, and it is based on notions that it is impossible for us to ever fully rid ourselves of our personal backgrounds or biogenetic predis-positions. Thus, it considers our perceptions of the world to be uniquely biased by who we are, and not to be accurate perceptions of reality. This core principle is manifested most clearly in the RO mindfulness skill known as self-enquiry, which is an essential component of the practice of radical openness more broadly (described next).

What Is Radical Openness?

Radical openness involves developing a passion for going opposite to where you are. It represents an intention to more deeply explore areas in your life that are difficult, painful, or disturbing. It means advancing courageously to the source of the unknown with proper humility and a willingness to sacrifice in order to learn more from what the world has to offer. However, being open to learning new things does not mean that we must reject our prior learning. Instead, RO recognizes that most often there are many ways to get to the same place or do the same thing (there are endless way to get to Paris and countless ways to cook potatoes), and that because the world is in constant change there is always something new to learn. The best scientists, for example, are humble because they realize that everything they know will eventually evolve or change into greater knowledge.

Radical openness is more than awareness or simply engaging in new behavior; at its most extreme, it involves actively seeking the things one wants to avoid or may find uncomfortable in order to learn. Thus, while it oftentimes involves trying out novel ways of behaving that may prove rewarding, it also involves purposeful self-enquiry, self-exploration, and discovery. It requires cultivating a willingness to be wrong and an ability to be open to new possibilities, with an intention to change, if change is needed. As Carl Jung might have described it, radical openness means seeking our shadow—the parts of our personality we are not proud of or might not wish to acknowledge. As such, it can sometimes be a difficult and scary endeavor. As a change strategy, it requires being open to corrective feedback, identifying what change(s) may be needed, and trying out new ways of behaving or relating to others. An important outcome for the practitioner of radical openness is an improved capacity for flexible responding to changing circumstances.

Thus, rather than automatically assuming that the world needs to change, RO considers an unwanted emotion, thought, or sensation in the body an opportunity for new learning. A practice of radical openness involves three sequential steps:

1. Acknowledging the presence of a disconfirming or unexpected event that triggers a feeling of tension, resistance, dislike, numbness, and/or desires to attack, control, or flee

2. Practicing self-enquiry by temporarily turning toward the discomfort and asking *What is it that I might need to learn?* rather than automatically regulating, distracting, explaining, reappraising, or accepting

3. Flexibly responding with humility by doing what's needed in the moment to effectively manage the situation and/or adapt to changing circumstances in a manner that accounts for the needs of others

Importantly, radical openness does not mean approval, naively believing, or mindlessly acquiescing. Sometimes being closed is what is needed in the moment, and/or change is unnecessary. Finally, radical openness is not something that can be grasped solely via intellectual means; it is experiential. It requires direct and repeated practice, and one's understanding evolves over time as a function of continued practice. Thus, RO DBT therapists and skills instructors are encouraged to develop and incorporate a personal practice of radical openness and self-enquiry into their lives. Strategies for integrating RO and self-enquiry into supervision and consultation team meetings are described in detail in chapter 7 of the RO DBT textbook.

Differentiating Radical Openness from Radical Acceptance

It is important to note that radical openness differs from the radical acceptance skills taught as part of standard DBT (Linehan, 1993a). Radical acceptance is letting go of fighting reality and is the way to turn suffering that cannot be tolerated into pain that can be tolerated, whereas radical openness challenges our perceptions of reality. Radical openness posits that we are unable to see things as they are, but instead that we see things as we are. This also contrasts with the concept of Wise Mind in standard DBT, which emphasizes the value of intuitive knowledge—the possibility of fundamentally knowing something as true or valid—and which posits inner knowing as "almost always quiet" and as involving a sense of "peace" (Linehan, 1993a).

From an RO DBT perspective, facts or truth can often be misleading, partly because we don't know what we don't know, because things are constantly changing, and because there is a great deal of experience occurring outside of our conscious awareness. Thus, RO encourages the cultivation of self-enquiry and healthy self-doubt in order to signal humility and learn from what the world may have to offer.

Why Self-Enquiry?

A core RO DBT precept is that it is impossible for us to ever be free of personal bias or be fully aware of every aspect of ourselves. For example, our brain is capable of being consciously aware of a thought, emotion, sensation, or image about every fifty milliseconds, making it theoretically possible for us to be consciously aware of about eighty discrete experiences in the span of one breath. (Phew!) Indeed, studies suggest that facial affect, especially among humans, most likely represents an evolutionarily hardwired unconditioned stimulus (from senders) that triggers an automatic unconditioned response in recipients—we need at least seventeen to twenty milliseconds to be consciously aware of an emotional face, yet our brain-body is already physiologically reacting at durations as low as four milliseconds (Williams et al., 2004, 2006). This process occurs at the preconscious sensory receptor level of emotional processing and is nonamenable to conscious emotion regulation. Plus, individual differences in learning and experience and in biotemperament make misappraisal of an evocative stimulus (such as interpreting a genuine offer of help as a manipulative ploy) a relatively common event. Essentially, truth in RO DBT is considered real yet elusive: "If I know anything, it is that I don't know everything and neither does anyone else" (M. P. Lynch, 2004, p. 10). It is the pursuit of truth that matters, not its attainment. Rather than assuming we can ever know reality just as it is, radical openness assumes that we all bring perceptual and regulatory biases into every moment, and that they interfere with our ability to be open and to learn from new or disconfirming information. This core principle of radical openness influences treatment interventions. For example, instead of automatically moving to regulate, rationalize, distract from, or accept aversive emotional arousal, RO prioritizes actively seeking the things one wants to avoid or may find uncomfortable, facilitated by a regular practice of self-enquiry (see lesson 13), in order to learn.

Self-enquiry involves a willingness to challenge our core beliefs—things we might normally consider facts or truths. It acknowledges that, on some level, we are responsible for our perceptions and actions, in a manner that avoids harsh blame of ourselves, others, or the world and encourages the cultivation of healthy self-doubt in order to learn and live by our valued goals. It involves a willingness to question ourselves when we feel threatened or challenged rather than automatically defending ourselves. Self-enquiry is not looking to solve a problem or avoid discomfort. It recognizes that each new insight or understanding we achieve is always fallible, limited, and/or potentially biased. Practicing self-enquiry is particularly useful whenever we find ourselves strongly rejecting, defending against, or feigning agreement with feedback that we find challenging or unexpected by first asking *What is it that I might need to learn?* rather than automatically assuming our perspective as correct or moving to emotionally regulate. It recognizes that in order to learn anything new, we must first acknowledge our lack of knowledge. Thus, although self-enquiry seeks self-discovery, it remains suspicious of quick answers, and this is why self-enquiry practices should be expected to last over days or weeks (see lesson 13).

Self-enquiry practices in RO DBT are based on assumptions that our brains are continually detecting discrepancies and evaluating environmental stimuli in order to adapt to changing contingencies. Our natural set point is one of calm readiness; however, when sensory inputs are evocative, or discrepant from expectations, a quick and typically unconscious evaluative process ensues, the primary function of which is to assign valence (positive or negative) and significance to such stimuli (that is, relevance to personal survival and/or well-being), a process that is moderated by biotemperament and past experience. When we evaluate a stimulus as threatening, our brain-body begins a process designed to defend itself, which naturally makes us more cautious about approaching the discrepant (that is, unknown or dangerous) stimulus. Self-enquiry considers defensive arousal helpful because it can alert us to areas in our lives where we may need to change or grow.

Thus, in RO DBT, defensive arousal (such as a feeling of resistance or dislike) is considered an opportunity for growth. Rather than automatically assuming that the world needs to change ("You need to validate me because I felt misunderstood by what you said") or automatically prioritizing regulation or acceptance strategies that functionally solve the problem, RO DBT posits that the truth hurts. This suggests that our most powerful moments of self-growth may stem from the very things we don't want to change or admit to as problems (that is, the point where our known makes contact with our unknown, which is referred to as *finding one's edge* in RO DBT). The emphasis on celebrating self-doubt in RO DBT stems from two observations:

1. We don't know everything; therefore, we will make mistakes.

2. In order to learn from our mistakes, we must attend to what we don't know.

Self-enquiry is not ruminating about a problem, because it is not looking to solve the problem or avoid discomfort. Indeed, the goal of self-enquiry is to find a good question, not a good answer. Quick answers are considered to most often reflect old learning and desires to avoid genuine contact with the pain associated with not having a solution. Thus, self-enquiry can be differentiated from other mindfulness approaches because it actively seeks discomfort to learn and blocks immediate answers rather than simply observing discomfort, metacognitively distancing from thoughts, and waiting for the experience to fade away. This is why most self-enquiry practices are encouraged to last for days or weeks and include opportunities to practice revealing to others what our self-examination has uncovered, a process referred to as *outing oneself* in RO DBT (see lesson 13).

Outing Oneself

RO DBT posits that we can enhance our self-knowledge through the eyes of our tribe by revealing our self-discoveries and inner experiences to another person. The importance of this when treating OC cannot be overemphasized, since revealing fallibility or weakness to another person goes opposite to OC tendencies to mask inner feelings. Importantly, since expressing vulnerability to another enhances rather than detracts from others' desires to affiliate with the self-disclosing person (see chapter 2 of the RO DBT textbook), the practice of outing oneself can become a powerful means for OC clients to rejoin the tribe. Plus, RO DBT posits that we need other people to reflect back our potential blind spots, since we carry perceptual and regulatory biases with us everywhere we go. Revealing to others our observations about ourselves and the world can enhance relationships because it models humility and willingness to learn from what the world has to offer. Moreover, it provides an enormous opportunity for self-growth because our individual well-being no longer depends solely on our personal perceptions. Skills instructors should be prepared to share observations from their own practices of self-enquiry in order to encourage clients to use self-enquiry more deeply (that is, OC clients are unlikely to believe it is healthy to redirect attention toward discomfort or reveal fallibility unless they see their therapists model this behavior first).

> Self-enquiry means finding a good question, not a good answer. may not be apparent.

The RO Self-Enquiry Journal

RO DBT strongly encourages therapists to practice and apply radical openness skills in both their personal and professional lives in order to be better able to model to their OC clients core RO concepts that can only be grasped experientially (that is, they are not accessible solely via rational thought or logic). This expectation includes an ongoing practice of self-enquiry and at least some experience with what is known in RO as *self-enquiry journaling*—that is, recording in writing, in a daily diary or journal, the thoughts, images, sensations, and emotions that arise during self-enquiry practices. This allows the therapist an opportunity to come into contact with what it feels like from the inside out to record self-enquiry experiences in a journal and potentially enhances the therapist's personal understanding of self-enquiry.

Thus, skills instructors (and RO DBT individual therapists), when first introducing self-enquiry principles, should encourage their OC clients to find a means of recording what has emerged during a practice of self-enquiry (usually by writing in a journal, such as a blank leather-bound book). What is actually written is up to the self-enquiry practitioner to decide. A core aim of an RO self-enquiry journal is to provide a means of privately recording struggles, insights, and personal questions about oneself that are expected to evolve over time as a function of continued self-enquiry practice. Thus, instructors should remind RO class members, as needed, that each person's RO self-enquiry journal is a private matter, meaning that its contents need not be shared with anyone, including therapists or other RO classmates (see also chapter 7 of the RO DBT textbook). Yet, at the same time, RO skills instructors should also look for opportunities to encourage class members to use their RO self-enquiry journals creatively.

Applying Self-Enquiry in RO Skills Class

Broadly speaking, a self-enquiry question posed by an RO skills instructor to an individual class member represents a heat-on technique. Yet heat-on is also how we all learn. Thus, when teaching RO DBT skills to OC clients, instructors should be alert for opportunities to incorporate brief moments of individualized self-enquiry into their teaching. Instructors should remind clients that the goal of self-enquiry is to find a good question, not a good answer. The best self-enquiry question brings a client face to face with his or her edge (the unknown, an inner secret that the client would prefer to avoid acknowledging, or the place where the client doesn't want to go). Similarly, whenever RO skills instructors experience frustration, confusion, or anxiety regarding how an OC client reacts to an RO skill being taught, rather than assuming that the problem lies solely with the client, they should use self-enquiry: *To what extent do I really know this skill myself? Who am I to assume that there is only one way to learn this skill? Is it possible that this skill makes no sense for a person with an OC style of coping? What is it that I might learn from this experience?*

Summary

The three guiding principles in RO DBT that strongly impact the manner in which a therapist delivers the treatment are *dialectics*, *radical openness*, and *self-enquiry*. The therapist uses dialectical principles to encourage cognitively rigid OC clients to think in ways that are both more complex and more flexible. The two most commonly used dialectical polarities in RO DBT are *nonmoving centeredness versus acquiescent letting go* and *playful irreverence versus compassionate gravity*. These dialectical stances can be used in combination with radical openness and self-enquiry principles.

Radical openness involves developing a passion for going opposite to where you are. It represents an intention to more deeply explore areas in your life that are difficult, painful, or disturbing. Radical openness posits that we are unable to see things as they are, but instead that we see things as we are—we all bring perceptual and regulatory biases into every moment, and these biases interfere with our ability to be open and learn from new or disconfirming information. This core principle of radical openness influences treatment interventions.

Being open to feedback may mean feeling threatened or challenged when the feedback doesn't match our perceptions of ourselves or the world. When this happens, RO DBT encourages self-enquiry practice. Self-enquiry involves a willingness to challenge our core beliefs—things we might normally consider facts or truths. It acknowledges that, on some level, we are responsible for our perceptions and actions, in a manner that avoids harsh blame of ourselves, others, or the world and encourages the cultivation of healthy self-doubt in order to learn and live by our valued goals. It involves a willingness to question ourselves when we feel threatened or challenged rather than automatically defending ourselves. The goal of self-enquiry is to find a good question, not a good answer.

Finally, RO DBT posits that we can enhance our self-knowledge through the eyes of our tribe by revealing our self-discoveries and inner experiences to another person, a process known as outing oneself. We need other people to reflect back our potential blind spots, since we carry perceptual and regulatory biases with us everywhere we go. Revealing our observations about ourselves and the world to others can enhance relationships because it models humility and willingness to learn from what the world has to offer.

CHAPTER 3

Managing Problematic Behaviors in RO Skills Training Classes

In general, skills training classes with OC individuals are not problematic or difficult, at least when it comes to the presence of chaotic and out-of-control displays of behavior. Indeed, if anything, OC skills classes are almost always well behaved, most likely because OC clients value structure, control, and restraint and tend to be disciplined, diligent, and dutiful during interactions with others in public. Unfortunately, being diligent or good all the time is not only exhausting but can also get you into trouble. OC clients are prisoners of their self-control, and their natural tendency to inhibit (control) their expressions of emotion makes it harder for others to know their true intentions and desire to socially connect. Rather than prioritizing regulated and controlled expression of emotion and non-mood-dependent behavior, RO skills prioritize candid expression of emotion, playfulness, and self-enquiry in order to enhance social connectedness with others.

Thus, RO skills training classes are designed to go opposite to the natural tendencies for constraint and control that characterize OC. Despite fears sometimes expressed by therapists first learning RO DBT, the vast majority of RO skills training classes are anything but quiet; they are characterized instead by frequent laughter, active sharing, a genuine sense of community support, and self-discovery. (My confidence in making this claim is based on more than twenty years of clinical and research experience in teaching, supervising, and refining the application of RO skills training classes in programs and independent research teams around the world, and with a wide range of ages and differing disorders; see chapter 1 of the RO DBT textbook.) Yet creating this type of excitatory learning environment requires not only awareness of core OC maladaptive behaviors, which can function to block communal activities (with plausible deniability), but also therapists' self-awareness regarding the behaviors and beliefs they may bring into the therapeutic environment that may inadvertently reinforce maladaptive overcontrol. The aim of this chapter is to provide an overview of the most common problems skills trainers are likely to encounter when working with OC clients and of how to manage them, using RO principles.

When a Classroom Goes Quiet

When an RO skills training class is quiet, nonresponsive, challenging, and/or seemingly nonengaged over repeated weeks or lessons, skills training instructors should use the experience as an opportunity to practice RO themselves. Sometimes a quiet or inhibited classroom reflects a similarly quiet or inhibited style of coping on the part of the skills instructor(s). Our research shows that the majority of therapists lean toward overcontrolled coping. Thus, skills training instructors leaning toward overcontrol can sometimes inadvertently reinforce cautious or perfectionistic tendencies in clients by striving too hard to get it right and/or by finding it difficult to participate without planning, express vulnerability, and play or be silly when the situation calls for it. Thus, rather than automatically assuming the difficulty lies with their OC clients, RO instructors are encouraged to practice self-enquiry and seek supervision (such as in RO consultation team meetings) in order to locate potential blind spots and maximize RO principle–based responding. Here are some examples of self-enquiry questions:

- What am I socially signaling or doing that might trigger nonparticipation, nonengagement, or distrust on my clients' part?

- How relaxed am I when I am teaching? To what extent do I truly know the material I am teaching? To what extent have I personally taken the time to practice the skills myself?

- Is there a part of me that does not believe this skill will work or that desires to dismiss it as irrelevant, silly, or inappropriate?

- To what extent am I willing to look at my own responses?

- To what extent am I expecting the world to change, or do I think that the treatment itself or the class or client is the problem? What is it that I might need to learn?

Yet simply telling oneself to practice self-enquiry, relax, or have fun in order to improve class participation is unlikely to work when one is surrounded by a classroom full of unresponsive, flat-faced, or disingenuous expressions. The reason for this is that we are evolutionarily hardwired to be hypersensitive to signs of social exclusion. For example, research shows that we can quickly spot the angry face in a crowd of people, and angry faces hold our attention (E. Fox et al., 2000; Schupp et al., 2004). For our ancestors living in harsh environments, the cost of not detecting a true disapproval signal was too high to ignore. Tribal banishment was essentially a death sentence for our primordial ancestors. Thus, we are biologically predisposed to be socially anxious, and we are hardwired to construe the intentions of others as disapproving, especially when social signals are ambiguous (as in a flat, neutral, or low-intensity facial expression). For example, simply reducing or limiting the amount of eye contact during interactions has been shown to trigger negative feelings associated with being ignored or ostracized (Wirth, Sacco, Hugenberg, & Williams, 2010).

Plus, in a situation where free expression of emotion is safe, customary, or expected (as in an RO skills training class, on a date, in an argument with one's spouse, or at a party), the discomfort triggered by flat (or disingenuous) facial expressions is not due solely to the absence of expression but also to the conspicuous lack of prosocial signaling and reciprocity (such as smiling and affirmative head nods). Thus, when OC clients pervasively mask or constrain their inner feelings during skills training classes, our brains are likely to automatically interpret this as a sign of distrust or disapproval. When nonengagement signals (for example, looking away when asked a question) or nonresponsiveness (for example, a few seconds of blank staring) are prolonged and displayed by several class members, we are likely to feel criticized and may start to feel self-conscious. Our body becomes tense, our breathing becomes fast and shallow, our heart rate increases, we may begin to sweat, and our facial expressions and body gestures feel constrained. We lose our easy manner and find it difficult to genuinely signal friendly or cooperative intentions without feeling phony. The problem for skills training instructors is that flat facial expressions are common when working with OC clients, thereby making discomfort and a low-level sense of embarrassment, shame, or self-consciousness a common experience.

To manage this, instructors must call upon their evolutionarily newer and nonemotional executive control systems to override automatic action urges to avoid shutdown or mimicking the flat expressions displayed by the class. Importantly, this does not mean attempting to talk oneself out of the dilemma via cognitive restructuring or admonishments to focus on the facts, yet it does take advantage of similar processes linked to language and executive control by using top-down processes and knowledge of social signaling to recognize that feeling excluded or ostracized by the class, or by some class members, represents bottom-up evolutionarily older signal-detection biases linked to survival of our species, and from there to use this knowledge to cheerlead the effortful control that will be needed to go opposite to automatic tendencies to hide or inhibit expansive expressions. Essentially, instructors must inhibit urges to inhibit emotional expressions when confronted with nonresponsive classes and should socially signal cooperative friendliness instead (via eyebrow wags, closed-mouth smiles, expansive gestures, and relaxed body postures). The good news is that expansive cooperative expressions are relatively easy to display physically, whereas the bad news is that they can be psychologically hard to display in the moment because they often go counter to a therapist's prior training and/or can feel out of place in the context of the instructor's internal feelings (such as annoyance, dislike, or shame). It is important for therapists to recognize that these reactions are unjustified, because the core goal of therapy with OC clients is to encourage open and vulnerable expression of emotion via the therapist's modeling, and because anxiety responses to nonprosocial signals by others are evolutionarily hardwired and impossible to fully control even for the most sophisticated of therapists. To change these dynamics, therapists must be willing to practice what they preach, as best they can, by going opposite to subtle internal urges to avoid, attack, inhibit, appease, or hide, and also by going opposite to prior professional training emphasizing the importance of restraint, by openly expressing vulnerability and the joy of self-discovery instead of adopting a reciprocally serious or somber tone. This signals to the entire class (and to the instructor, too) not only that there is nothing to be ashamed of when we express ourselves but also that expressions of vulnerability or playfulness can be intimacy-enhancing.

The following list provides additional approaches for managing quiet and nonresponsive classes and/or expands on the suggestions just made.

- **Practice radical openness by directly seeking critical feedback from the class.** For example, ask, "Has something just occurred to make it harder for everyone to participate or contribute to our work together?" This request for feedback is best delivered in a manner—balanced by compassionate gravity (via raised eyebrows, a warm smile, a slightly lowered voice volume, a slightly slower rate of speech, and eye contact, if possible, with each participant)—that celebrates criticism as a core means of learning rather than one that implies cause for alarm (via a furrowed brow and a somber expression).

- **Go opposite to urges to quiet down or behave in a solemn manner by purposefully employing big gestures to pull class participants into their social safety system.** As outlined earlier, a flat facial expression is a powerful social signal that indicates distrust or dislike and pulls for a reciprocal expression in the recipients. Instructors can reverse this process by engaging in nonverbal behavior that communicates affection and trust—for example, via a warm smile, a relaxed body posture, raised eyebrows when listening or speaking, and/or expansive gestures.

- **Randomly assign participants to read aloud the next point being covered in a handout or worksheet.** This breaks the barrier of silence and, because everyone is asked to take a turn, functions to smuggle the idea that classroom participation is expected. It is important for instructors not to allow a participant to skip a turn as reader, because this smuggles the idea that passing is okay and makes it more likely that others in the class will try to pass, too. Although nonparticipation may initially feel safe, the client who is not participating almost invariably experiences greater anxiety and feels like an outsider (albeit, admittedly, it is the client's decision not to join in that creates the problem in the first place). Instructors should be prepared to cajole, coax, sweet-talk, or entice a reluctant reader and must reward him or her for participation ("Great job" or "Well done"). Sometimes it can help to remind reluctant or shy participants that the heat (unwanted attention) will be taken off if they simply jump in and read aloud (recall that OC clients dislike the limelight). Thus, as soon as a client participates by taking a turn reading aloud (even if it is only one word), the instructor quickly responds with thanks and then matter-of-factly directs his or her attention away from the reader (that is, takes the heat off) and turns back to the class or to another participant while continuing with the lesson plan.

- **Use body movements and meaningless vocalizations to break the tension** (see the "participate without planning" mindfulness practices in lesson 12). For example, without warning, say, "Okay, everyone, clap your hands together." Raise your hands and begin to clap while smiling and engaging eye contact with class participants: "Okay, stand up." Stand and continue clapping: "Okay, now repeat after me!" Clap along while smiling encouragement: "Say *HA*" (*clap*), "say *HA*" (*clap*), "say *HO*" (*clap*), "say *HO*" (*clap*), "say *HA HA, HO HO, HA HA, HO HO!* Okay, now waggle your body all about…

and reach to the sky…say *HAAAA HAAAA HAAAA* and *HEE HEE HO!*" Reinforce participatory efforts, even when they are of low intensity (for example, wiggling a finger or whispering *HA*), by smiling and nodding approval yet simultaneously ignoring nonparticipatory signals (such as eye rolls and frowning). End the practice as abruptly as you began it by asking everyone to sit down: "Okay, well done. Now let's all sit down!" And then, with a big smile, sit down and say, "Yes?" Then, without pausing for discussion, return to the lesson plan. Importantly, as outlined later, all "participation without planning" practices should last no longer than thirty seconds to one minute (see lesson 12).

- **Bring the tribe to the client when the client refuses to participate with the tribe.** An RO skills training class is purposefully designed to function as a tribe. In the unlikely event that a class member refuses to stand up as instructed during a class "participate without planning" exercise like the one just described, instructors should simply reverse their instructions, saying to class members now standing, "Okay, good job! Now go ahead and sit back down again." The instructor should then, with eyebrows raised and a warm smile (and without further commentary), conduct the exercise from a seated position. Attempt to make eye contact with refusing class members as you continue to conduct the exercise (to communicate your genuine desire for them to join in with the class and to show that you do not disapprove of them). If they meet your gaze, quickly smile and perhaps give a little wave (this smuggles playfulness and affection; see also "Fun Facts: Teasing and Being Teased," in lesson 22). Importantly, instructors should conduct the next miniexercise as if nothing has happened—that is, starting with a request for everyone to stand up. Most often, nonconforming participants will reluctantly comply (they have learned that noncompliance doesn't work), whereupon the instructor can warmly smile (and even wink) in their direction to signal delight in their decision (during break or after class, the instructor can privately express appreciation for their participation). However, if they continue to refuse, instructors should simply follow exactly the same protocol already outlined. Our experience is that, over time, participants will eventually decide it is not worth continuing to refuse to participate (recall that they have voluntarily chosen to be part of the class), because the instructors make it nearly impossible to avoid. This functions to bring the tribe to the nonconforming member while simultaneously communicating several important messages, without making a big deal of it:

  - Class participation is expected.

  - If you don't join us, we will join you.

  - We are attached to you and respect you, which is why we are sitting back down.

  - We need you to participate so that we can all experience the joy of being part of a tribe.

- **Explain the dangerously attractive nature of nonparticipation.** Begin by noting that humans fear social embarrassment and humiliation to such an extent that we often decide not to participate in a community experience. OC clients are strongly motivated to avoid real or imagined social disapproval. Avoiding participation with others not only is common but also feels like a good idea because it appears to promise relief from imagined critical scrutiny—and yet, paradoxically, nonparticipation makes one's behavior more noteworthy because it is not a normal response among those desiring to remain part of a tribe. Thus, nonparticipation stands out in a crowd! For example, refusing to dance or sing at a party can often feel like independence, but in the long run it often leads to rumination when we realize that we are the only one not participating.

- **Encourage participation by reminding clients of valued goals related to helping others and contributing to society** (using the "Protocol for Therapeutic Induction of Social Responsibility," described later in this chapter). Recall that although OC clients' social signaling deficits make it difficult for them to experience social connectedness with others (and for others to experience social connectedness with them), OC behaviors, in general, are often prosocial in nature (for example, planning ahead contributes to society). This approach is best applied in private (for example, during the class break) rather than publicly with the entire class. The focus of the discussion is to encourage the client to use self-enquiry to examine how his or her lack of participation (that is, social signaling) may impact others in the class and to examine the extent to which this behavior fits with the client's valued goals (see "Lateness and Noncompletion of Homework," later in this chapter, for additional details on how to apply this approach).

- **Take the heat off by telling a story or using a metaphor** (for example, see the story that I sometimes refer to as "It Takes Only Thirty Seconds to Know," told in the next section). Overcontrolled clients are less likely to volunteer personal information or ask questions in a group setting, particularly when new to the class. Stories and metaphors help reestablish classroom participation by momentarily removing the expectation for it (that is, taking the heat off), but without entirely losing that expectation (that is, the story links back to the topic that was being discussed). Importantly, the actual storytelling itself should ideally be delivered in a dramatic yet lighthearted manner (that is, a slightly tongue-in-cheek fashion) that communicates to participants that the instructors don't take themselves too seriously and that joining in will be fun. OC clients tend to be overly serious about life and to compulsively strive, and yet research shows that the capacity to laugh at oneself (without putting oneself down) signals confident acceptance of one's problems or weaknesses and is associated with psychological well-being (Beermann & Ruch, 2011).

Finally, if problems with participation persist, they should be dealt with in private by one of the RO skills instructors, either during the break or at the end of class, and/or by the client's individual RO DBT therapist. For more details about how RO skills instructors can deal with participation problems, see "Protocol for Therapeutic Induction of Social Responsibility" and "Managing Alliance Ruptures and Repairs" later in this chapter).

Using Metaphor to Take the Heat Off: "It Takes Only Thirty Seconds to Know"

This story, a favorite of mine, is based on research conducted by Ambady and Rosenthal (1992, 1993) and is particularly helpful in breaking the ice whenever lack of participation appears to be due to class members' not knowing the instructor very well (for example, during the first class). To tell this story, begin by looking around and, if possible, making eye contact with each class member, with eyebrows raised and a warm smile.

You know, there was some really interesting research done at Harvard that I think you might find extremely helpful. The study involved asking a group of people to rate a five-minute film clip of a course taught by a professor the raters had never met. They were asked to evaluate the teacher's personality—for example, how dominant, empathic, honest, or warm the teacher was—and then the researchers compared their ratings to the same ratings completed by students who had just completed a three-month course with the same professor. To their surprise, the researchers discovered that the ratings between the two groups were nearly identical! So then, being clever researchers, they decided to try it again with another group of research subjects, but this time they only showed the subjects one minute of the lecture—and when they compared these subjects' ratings to the ratings of students taking a course from the same professor, what do you think happened? They matched again! Almost identical ratings!" [Pause dramatically.] *So what do you think happened next?* [Keep your eyebrows up; display a warm smile and, if possible, make eye contact with each class member.] *Yes!* [Nod happily, as if each member has replied.] *Those clever researchers said to themselves, "Let's make it harder—let's shorten the film clip to just thirty seconds." And what do you think happened? That's right. Another match—nearly identical ratings to those done by students spending an entire semester with the same professor! Wow! In just thirty seconds, people can know a great deal about a person they have only just met! Amazing!* [Pause, lean back in your chair, slow the pace of your speech, and adopt a tone of compassionate gravity.] *So I guess what I wanted to say is that although most of you have only just met me, you already know a great deal about me because we have been talking together for more than thirty seconds. For example, I am aware of imagining that you likely suspect that I am the type of person who enjoys hearing differing viewpoints or is okay with things not being perfect. Plus, perhaps…*[Use a nondominant social signal; see chapter 6 of the RO DBT textbook.]*…you might sense that I genuinely care about our work together.* [Pause.] *So, with that in mind, I'd like to go back to my earlier question.* [Pause.] *As I recall, we were talking about…*[Name the topic, and repeat the unanswered question or request for participation.]

Use Heat-On and Heat-Off Strategies to Shape Desired Behaviors

Contingency management (such as positive and negative reinforcement or extinction principles) is a core part of RO DBT used to reinforce target-relevant adaptive behavior and reduce target-relevant maladaptive behaviors (see the information about behavioral strategies in chapter 10 of the RO DBT textbook). Yet when it comes to treating OC, knowing what to reinforce or not can be difficult, since most OC dysfunctional behavior is expressed subtly. OC clients habitually mask or constrain inner feelings and work hard to maintain a public persona of normality, despite feeling miserable inside. Their indirect social signals and natural stoicism make them difficult to get to know. For example, when OC clients say "Maybe," they may mean "No," or "Hmmm" may really mean "I don't agree." The problem for the therapist (and others) is that OC social signaling has plausible deniability ("No, I'm fine—I just don't feel like talking" or "No, I'm not angry—I'm just thinking"), making direct confrontation of potentially maladaptive behavior more difficult, whereas the problem for OC clients is that their hidden intentions and disguised demands negatively impact their relationships (see lesson 15). Thus, rather than emphasizing emotion regulation, therapists working with OC clients should look for opportunities to reinforce open and candid expressions of emotion.

Plus, almost all OC clients strongly dislike the limelight (that is, being the center of attention), making the removal of scrutiny or attention a powerful reinforcer. Heat-on and heat-off techniques capitalize on this by using attention-management strategies (including, for example, the time the instructor spends focusing on a particular client) to shape OC clients' behavior. Heat-on strategies involve some form of social attention, such as eye contact, a question, or a request for participation. The "heat" pertains to how OC clients evaluate the attention. Their biotemperamental predisposition for heightened threat sensitivity, combined with family and cultural reinforcers prioritizing performance, functions to make attention or requests feel like critical evaluation of performance, leading to increased self-consciousness. For example, during homework review an instructor might ask a client, "Do you think you might have assumed that you already knew what they were going to say and that this might have made you less likely to actually listen?" This is an excellent self-enquiry question for the client, and at the same time it also represents a heat-on strategy because it functions to direct attention toward the client and necessitates some sort of response.

OC clients are likely to respond in three ways to an experience of having the heat turned on:

1. They may join with the instructor by directly answering the question in a manner that signals a willingness to openly explore the issue.

2. They may delay or pause before responding, which may be due to a wide range of reasons. For example, a client may delay responding because a classically conditioned shutdown response was triggered by the query (respondent behavior), they may be using Flexible Mind to inhibit an automatic "pushback"

response (adaptive response), or they may be blaming themselves for not already having the problem sorted out (maladaptive response).

3. They may exhibit behavior that is in between the two responses just described. That is, they may appear to be genuinely trying to reply or engage with the discussion, and at the same time their manner may appear to change once the heat is on. Skills instructors should avoid making assumptions that particular behaviors (such as sudden silence, gaze aversion, or an increased rate of speech) provide strong evidence of an OC client's inner experience. Even if the instructors are correct, behaving as if they know what is going on with an OC client (especially early in treatment) may be experienced as disrespectful, overly provocative, or inappropriate by the client (see "The Enigma Predicament," in chapter 10 of the RO DBT textbook).

It is also essential for instructors to know when and how to take the heat off a client during an RO skills training class. Heat-off strategies in RO DBT are primarily used to maximize engagement and reinforce newly acquired adaptive behavior. They work because they briefly move the focus of attention away from the client, but without changing the topic. This allows time for the OC client to downregulate, without making it obvious that he or she is doing so or calling attention to it. For example, during a client's homework review, a skills instructor noticed that a normally highly engaged and vocal client was struggling with a certain aspect of her homework, despite several helpful prompts from the class. Rather than continuing to focus on the client directly, either by repeating the question or by waiting for an answer, the instructor briefly took the heat off the client by rephrasing the question and redirecting it toward the entire class: "So, class, when you think about the various ways people react to compliments, like in Mary's homework, what do you think makes them so hard for some people to give?" This gave the client a breather, without making a big deal of it, while simultaneously retaining the cue by not changing the topic being discussed. The instructor then redirected attention to a now more regulated client so she could complete her homework. Sometimes simply removing eye contact for a few seconds is all that is needed for an OC client to regulate and reengage. Other heat-off techniques include telling a relevant anecdote or using a metaphor, having an instructor practice self-disclosure about a similar self-discovery, and writing a particular teaching point on the blackboard or whiteboard when it is relevant to the topic being discussed.

Finally, heat-on and heat-off strategies can be applied structurally. A good example is the RO DBT principle of letting new class members know that, after introducing themselves, they are not required to speak on their first day of class, although they are asked to participate (nonverbally, at least) in class exercises. This exception regarding verbal participation is made only for new class members attending their first class (that is, an open class that has been already running). The exception functions to structurally take some of the heat off a new client and works for the class dynamics because all the older class members had the same exception made for them on their first day. What is interesting is that taking the heat off by simply removing the onus of speaking seems, almost paradoxically, to lead to more speaking.

Maladaptive Social Signals That Cannot Be Ignored in Class

Most often problematic behaviors in class can be ignored, if they remain at a low level, or they can be dealt with privately during class break or at the end of class. The vast majority are not intended to disrupt the class, nor do they necessarily mean that a client is nonengaged. Nevertheless, among the problematic behaviors that can emerge during skills training classes with OC clients, there are a few that, if not immediately addressed, can interfere with the primary aim of skills training—that is, learning new skills—and, if ignored, they may shortly come to be assumed as appropriate classroom behavior. Consider, for example, the client who innocently decides to answer an incoming text message. If this behavior is not addressed, the classroom may soon be full of texting participants, or a client who has been asked an uncomfortable question may pretend to have received a text message in order to avoid answering (see the required teaching point "Hiding Intentions and Disguising Demands," in lesson 15).

Regardless of the client's intention, when a behavior occurs that clearly has the potential to interfere with learning skills, the best way to manage it, at least initially, is for the instructor to politely ask for it to stop. For example, an instructor might say, "Um…Joan and Sue, can you do me a favor…and not carry on private conversations during class? I find it hard to concentrate." Then, with a warm smile and an eyebrow wag, the instructor can say, "Thanks." Most OC clients, even when they are nonengaged or purposefully trying to niggle the instructor or a fellow classmate, will comply with this type of direct request. The instructor can then simply turn back to teaching and, later on, during the class break, approach the client to discuss the problematic behavior further, if necessary.

I am aware of imagining that some readers may be thinking that the problem behaviors just described—texting in class and holding private conversations—could easily have been prevented or dealt with if the instructor had simply provided each class member with a set of written rules or guidelines and reviewed them at the start of each class. Yet this is explicitly advised against in RO DBT—we like our therapists to have to work hard (tee hee). Seriously, though, although providing everyone with a list of rules may seem like a good idea, it most often creates more problems than it solves. Our experience is that providing lists of rules to OC clients is a bit like giving heroin to a junkie to calm him down, or using gasoline to try to put out a fire. Rules, once present, take on a life of their own with OC clients, regardless of how they are introduced (individually with a client or with the entire class). OC clients, despite their initial enthusiasm and indications of agreement with the use of rules proposed, are likely to carefully examine the new rules when alone, to determine whether they actually agree with them and/or how they may need to adjust their behavior in order to comply, and then plan accordingly (whereas undercontrolled clients are more likely to lose the list of rules and forget it ever existed). Plus, asking OC clients to review and approve a list of rules is likely to generate new rules, improved rules, and detailed analyses that uncover discrepancies or mistakes (such as grammatical errors and misspellings) that OC clients may feel morally obligated to discuss with the class and point out to instructors. The following scenario, described by an RO skills instructor, highlights just how quickly a list of rules can come to dominate the attention of OC clients and interfere with learning.

When our clinic first started to learn RO DBT, we were skeptical when our trainers informed us that RO skills training classes do not explicitly review class rules or expectations at any point in the treatment process. We decided to test out this recommendation by developing our own list of class rules, which were then introduced to the entire class. Reception was positive, with only a few suggestions. We were ecstatic! Unfortunately, our ecstasy was short-lived—problems started to emerge two weeks later, during the brief overview of the class rules at the start of the class. During this overview, one of the class members asked if she could make a comment about the rules, and she made a suggestion to the entire class, stating, "Although I will not mention any names, ha-ha, for several weeks now I have noticed that some class rules seem to be at least occasionally ignored by certain members of our class. So I would like to propose that we appoint a rule monitor to help out our busy instructors and ensure that the rules are applied fairly to all." This suggestion resulted in a forty-five-minute discussion about its potential merits that had to be tabled for later because it also triggered some colorful debates about word usage, grammatical errors, and the ethics of even having rules. It also spurred another class member to reveal that he had been working for several weeks on a new list of rules that better represented RO principles and would like to present it to the class the following week. However, before his request could even be addressed, the entire class suddenly became aware that the group's most reticent and least talkative member was silently raising her hand high in the air and appeared to be signaling that she had something important to say. The entire class held a collective breath as the instructor, recognizing the potentially enormous therapeutic significance of the moment, leaned toward the client and encouraged her to speak, whereupon she said, "I too have come up with an improved list of rules. I will bring them in next week." The class burst into exclamations of support while the instructors began to doubt the wisdom of class rules and wondered how they would ever cover the material that was planned for that day.

The moral of the story is "Don't give out written rules to OC clients." However, this is not the end of our story about problem behaviors in OC classes. There remain three additional broad classes of social signals that are important to address directly in class because of their potential for impacting both learning and class morale:

1. "Don't hurt me" responses

2. Harsh criticism directed at another class member

3. Noncompletion of homework

"Don't Hurt Me" Responses

"Don't hurt me" responses are operant behaviors that function to block unwanted feedback or requests to join in with a community activity (see chapter 10 of the RO DBT textbook). They are typically expressed nonverbally via behaviors—lowered head, face covered with the hands or hidden from view, slackened posture, lowered eyelids, eyes cast downward, avoidance of eye contact, slumped shoulders, postural shrinkage—that collectively are associated with self-conscious emotions. The underlying message of a "don't hurt me" response is as follows:

> You don't understand me, and your expectations are hurting me, since normal expectations of behavior do not or should not apply to me, due to my special status or talents, my exceptional pain or suffering, my traumatic history, the extreme efforts I have made to contribute to society, my hard work, and my self-sacrifices for the benefit of others. As such, it is unfair of you to fail to recognize my special status and expect me to participate, contribute, or behave responsibly, as other members of my community are expected to behave. Consequently, if you were a caring person, you would stop pressuring me to change, behave appropriately, or conform with norms. For example, stop expecting me to complete my homework, stop asking questions I don't like, and stop expecting me to participate in class discussions or exercises.

The final hidden or indirect signal in a "don't hurt me" response is "And if you don't stop, I will fall apart, and it will be your fault."

Another way to understand the maladaptive nature of "don't hurt me" responses is to examine the behavior from the perspective of a tribe, family, or community group, since the "don't hurt me" response always occurs within a social context (although its cousin, self-pity, often occurs alone and frequently precedes "don't hurt me" social signaling). What can often be missed by recipients of "don't hurt me" responses is that the sender has almost always willingly chosen to be part of the community, group, or tribe in which the behavior is exhibited; that is, the sender has not been forced into the community, group, or tribe but still expects special treatment. "Don't hurt me" responses have usually been intermittently reinforced by others' well-intentioned behavior, such as soothing, attending to, and taking care of the sender, or not bringing up potentially distressing topics in order to avoid further upsetting him or her. Yet this kind of walking on eggshells can engender social ostracism of the sender when the maladaptive signal is of long standing, pervasive, and nonresponsive to initial attempts by others offering assistance. Similar to pouting, "don't hurt me" responses are maladaptive because they function to signal disagreement and nonengagement indirectly and, as a consequence, over the long term they not only negatively impact the sender's sense of self but also interfere with the sender's formation of close social bonds (see information about problems associated with indirect social signals in lesson 15).

A "don't hurt me" response can be difficult to identify because it is usually subtly expressed and disguised to look like a respondent pain reaction (such as the cry of pain after twisting an ankle, or the sadness and grief upon losing a friend) or like an unwarranted self-conscious emotion (as in the lowered head and averted gaze that suggest an unjustified shame response after an appropriate self-disclosure in class). Plus, it can be engaged with conscious intent or can occur without conscious awareness (habitually). A good way to tell the difference between a "don't hurt me" response, on the one hand, and a respondent pain reaction or unwarranted self-conscious emotion, on the other, is that the "don't hurt me" response has a relatively long duration (the entire length of a skills training class, for example), with the intensity of the signal increasing and possibly developing into an extinction burst if recipients fail to respond in the desired way (such as by soothing, withdrawing a question, changing the topic, or apologizing; see the information about disguised demands in lesson 15). By contrast, a respondent reaction, justified or not, is naturally likely to match the intensity of the eliciting stimulus (the pain expressed when your foot is run over by a car is likely more extreme than when someone steps on your toe); the behavioral expression slowly fades, usually in minutes, once the eliciting stimulus has been removed, and it does not depend on the reactions of nearby others. Regardless, the good news is that the treatment intervention is essentially the same whether the behavior is operant or respondent, varying only as a function of context (that is, as a function of whether the behavior occurs during an individual therapy session or during a skills training class; see the information about interventions for individual therapy in chapter 10 of the RO DBT textbook). Since the focus of this manual is on skills training, the emphasis here will be on managing this type of response in skills classes.

A "don't hurt me" response is a big signal for an OC client to display in public (that is, outside of the immediate family or the individual therapy room). When "don't hurt me" responses occur in skills training classes and are prolonged and obvious, they send a powerful message suggesting that the signaler requires some form of help or attending to. A "don't hurt me" response in a skills training class is often accompanied by others' sense of moral obligation to assist the signaler in some way, and very quickly such signals, rather than the lesson, can subtly come to dominate the attention of the signaler's classmates (the only exception is when "don't hurt me" responses have inadvertently become a class norm). Most often this felt sense of moral obligation translates into expectations for the skills training instructors to do something about the "don't hurt me" response, since this is seen as their job. Unfortunately, if instructors attend to the sender of the maladaptive social signal by assessing what happened, problem solving, or soothing, they not only spend valuable class time on behavior unrelated to the lesson for the day but are also likely to reinforce the "don't hurt me" response (see "Behavioral Principles and Strategies," in chapter 10 of the RO DBT textbook). Yet if instructors completely ignore a prolonged and obvious "don't hurt me" response, they are likely to quickly find themselves confronted by a room full of nonengaged OC clients who feel increasingly distressed by their instructors' lack of action (recall that most OC clients feel it is their moral duty to help those in distress) but who may not explicitly reveal their distress (recall that OC clients mask inner feelings). Plus, completely ignoring a "don't hurt me" response can create a new class norm that it's okay to shut down in class, or pout, or behave as if you don't care. This in turn can trigger mimicry and contagion effects (particularly in classes with adolescents). The situation can quickly escalate until instructors face a classroom full of hanging heads, averted gazes, slumped shoulders, and faces covered with hands, hair, or clothing, with a nearly complete shutdown of learning for the entire class and premature dropout.

Thus, prolonged "don't hurt me" responses should not be ignored in RO DBT skills training classes. Steps for management include those that follow:

- The instructor should matter-of-factly acknowledge the behavior and, rather than exploring the factors that may have elicited it, simply ask the client to look up and join in with the class: "Molly, I am aware of imagining that something has happened that makes you either sad or upset in some manner. But can you do me a favor? Can you pick up your pen, sit up straight, and look at the material on the page in front of you?" The underlying tenor of the message is "Of course you can do this," without a direct statement—a stance that celebrates the OC client's capabilities rather than assuming that the client is unable to tolerate change, confrontation, or direct feedback.

- The instructor should be prepared to repeat the request for prosocial behavior in skills class, several times if necessary, and to reinforce compliance: "Thanks, Molly. I really appreciate that."

- The instructor should signal to the rest of the class the intention of further attending to the "don't hurt me" signaler's distress in private: "And, Molly, I want you to know that no matter what is going on, I think it is important to address it. So I would like to meet with you at break [or after class] to discuss what we might need to do in order to deal with what happened and enhance your learning. In the meantime, I would appreciate it if you would do the best you can to attend to the lesson, with the understanding that you and I will be able to address what's going on with you personally very shortly. Thanks." This message is followed by a warm closed-mouth smile from the instructor.

- If these strategies are ineffective, the instructor should say, "Okay. Well, thanks for trying. Tell you what—in the meantime, do the best you can to join with us as we go back to reviewing homework [or the lesson], and you and I can talk about this at break [or at the end of class]." The instructor should then carry on with teaching, without further discussion and with the knowledge of having done his or her job (at least from the perspective of the OC participants) by making an attempt to address the problem in class, an attempt that also includes a plan for dealing with the problem later.

During the break, or at the end of class, the instructor should invite the client who exhibited the "don't hurt me" response to have a little chat about what was going on and how best to deal with it. This would include a brief check-in about what triggered the client's "don't hurt me" signal in order to determine the extent to which it was respondent behavior (which would imply problem solving), represented a possible alliance rupture (which would call for an alliance rupture repair), or was a maladaptive operant behavior (that is, an indirect social signal). As mentioned earlier, when a "don't hurt me" response is prolonged, it is usually a maladaptive social signal and is also what is most common (until the behavior gets shaped out of the client's repertoire). Regardless of whether the behavior is respondent, indicates an alliance rupture, or is operant, the aim of this short discussion is to obtain the client's agreement to behave appropriately in class by reminding the client of several things:

- That he or she has a natural tendency to value doing the right thing (this is linked to high moral certitude in OC) as well as a sense of social obligation (the instructor points out that the client's in-class misbehavior—that is, the engagement in "don't hurt me" responses—is impacting the learning of other class members)

- That the client has a superior capacity for restraint and can therefore, unlike many other people, at least choose to appear okay and engaged in class, even when not feeling that inside

- That the client can discuss the issue further with the instructor, if necessary, as well as with his or her individual therapist

Finally, the RO skills training manual has an entire lesson targeting indirect social signaling, including "don't hurt me" responses (see the information on Flexible Mind REVEALs skills in lesson 16). Thus, instructors can remind clients who have already been through that lesson to use their Flexible Mind REVEALs skills, and clients who have not yet come to lesson 16 can be provided with handouts from the lesson, or the instructor can explain to them that the type of behavior they are exhibiting will be covered in an upcoming lesson. The following script shows how one instructor discussed these points with an OC client after checking in and conducting a brief assessment of what had triggered the client's "don't hurt me" response.

Instructor: Molly, one last thing before we go back to class. I would like to ask if you would be willing to do me a favor. Here's the thing. The problem from my perspective is that when you behave like you did earlier in class—hanging your head and not responding immediately to questions—you send a powerful social signal to everyone in class that may negatively impact the learning of your fellow classmates, even if you did not intend to do so. Yet one of the things I admire about you is that you actually are one of those people in the world who actually gives a damn. You care about things working out and doing the right thing. Am I right about that?

(Client nods yes.)

Instructor: That's what I thought, too. Plus, at the same time, I am aware of imagining that we would both agree that one of your talents pertains to superior self-control, meaning you can delay gratification, inhibit impulses, and tolerate distress in ways that others might find impossible. Would you agree?

(*Client nods yes.*)

Instructor: So what I would like to ask is that you use your superior capacities for inhibitory control, and your values linked to caring for others, to inhibit future urges to give up, hide, not participate, or hang your head during class, in order to help your fellow classmates and not impede their learning. (*Smiles warmly.*) Would you be willing to do this?

In summary, "don't hurt me" responses are big social signals for OC clients. They have been intermittently reinforced over time. If allowed to occur unchecked during skills training, they can subtly undermine the aims of the class itself. When "don't hurt me" responses occur in class, instructors should kindly and matter-of-factly ask clients exhibiting this behavior to put their heads up and direct their attention, as best they can, toward the lesson of the day. Instructors should also indicate that, regardless of what is going on, they would like to talk with these clients about the behavior during break or at the end of class (see "Protocol for Therapeutic Induction of Social Responsibility," later in this chapter). This functions to reassure other class members that they do not need to intervene themselves while also redirecting the class's attention to skills acquisition. Interestingly, OC clients who exhibit "pushback" responses in class (see "'Pushback' Responses," in chapter 10 of the RO DBT textbook) generally fail to elicit similar protective behaviors among their fellow classmates. Instead, "pushback" responses directed at an instructor are more likely to elicit urges to protect the instructor, usually because a "pushback" often feels like a personal attack. The next section explains how to manage personal attacks in class.

Personal Attacks

The second most common OC behavior requiring immediate attention pertains to personal attacks and harsh critical comments directed at another class member. OC clients' personal attacks toward other classmates rarely involve shouting, cursing, arm waving, foot stomping, finger pointing, fist shaking, table pounding, thrown objects, or physical contact (most OC clients consider an RO skills class a public arena, whereas OC emotional leakage is more likely in private settings). However, this does not mean that personal attacks do not occur. If personal attacks appear in an OC skills training class, they are much more likely to be delivered in a controlled manner and may have been rehearsed. Their controlled nature is what can make them disconcerting. They are likely to be delivered in a tone of voice that may be cold, clipped, sarcastic, exasperated, or even neutral, and they may or may not involve direct eye contact. The reasons why they may occur vary widely. For example, sometimes OC clients are critical of fellow classmates simply as a function of past experiences in group therapy, or because they believe that learning new skills related to interpersonal relationships and openness means they should practice giving feedback to others in class.

In addition, harsh judgmental comments often reflect fundamental attribution errors. An attribution bias is a way of thinking that affects how we determine who or what is responsible for having caused some event, or an action exhibited by someone else (Ross, 1977). The error has to do with a cognitive bias toward judging others' problematic behavior as revealing something fundamental about character or personality (we blame them), whereas when we exhibit the same behavior, we judge it to be the result of circumstances or believe that it is due to a context beyond our control (we are not to blame). For example, if Jack and Jill run up a hill to fetch a pail of water and Jill falls down, Jack may consider Jill careless or clumsy, but if Jack himself falls down and breaks his crown, he will be more likely to label his fall an accident and blame the uneven terrain. Theorists have proposed that one of the reasons for this type of bias is our desire for a "just world" (Lerner,

1997). A just world is one where actions and events have predictable and appropriate consequences—people get what they deserve according to how they behave. Thus, punishing a transgressor restores faith in a just world. For example, an OC client may believe it is her moral duty to correct errors or assist instructors in teaching others how to behave better.

Yet not every behavior exhibited by an OC client is morally motivated. Since being correct, winning, and achieving matter greatly to most OC clients, they are more likely to engage in social comparisons than are less performance-focused people. RO skills training classes can become yet another venue for OC clients to test their competence, and this makes social comparisons among class members commonplace. Thus, a personal attack directed at another class member may reflect unhelpful envy and premeditated revenge, motivated by a desire for the envied person to fail or experience pain (see the discussion of schadenfreude in lesson 27). The problem for the envious OC client is that winning by putting someone else down feels like a hollow victory because it is achieved not through personal merit but by blocking the merit of a rival.

The good news is that the intervention for an OC client's personal attack in class is always the same, regardless of the underlying motive. The first step is to discriminate helpful critical feedback from an unhelpful and harsh personal attack. There is no right answer, but a general rule is to intervene when the feedback is unkind and when it is characterized by a conspicuous lack of prosocial signaling (for example, not smiling, lack of head nods, blank stare). For example, a classmate saying to a fellow class member, "John, I am aware of imagining that you are in Fatalistic Mind" would most likely not be considered a personal attack, primarily because it includes a qualifier suggesting that the sender may be incorrect (that is, "I am aware of imagining…"). However, "You are behaving like a child" or "I don't believe you" or "I know what you are thinking" or "You are one of those users—*poor me*" are examples of feedback that is personally attacking. A personal attack is problematic because (1) often it doesn't take into account a context or circumstances that may be impacting someone else's behavior, (2) the attacker assumes that the attack is justified and/or accurate, and (3) it implies that the attacker has special knowledge of or insight into the recipient of the attack. To put it simply, a personal attack is identifiable by its conspicuous lack of humility.

When a personal attack is directed at another class member, instructors should immediately intervene to block further critical feedback. This also functions to remove the necessity of a defensive comeback from the recipient. In one RO skills class, for example, a client decided to tell a fellow class member that she found his tendency to repeat certain words really annoying. The instructor immediately recognized this as a personal attack and stepped in to block further unhelpful feedback:

Instructor: (*Smiles*) You know, June, there are groups where you can practice giving and receiving critical feedback. However, our class is not one of them. Rather than practicing critical feedback, our RO skills class is a group where we practice supporting each other in learning new skills. As such, I would like to ask that you work to avoid giving critical feedback to others in class and instead focus on helping others and yourself learn the RO skills. (*Smiles.*) Thanks.

Most often, simple direct instructions to clients about how to behave are all that is needed, especially when these instructions are delivered in a manner that does not make a big deal of the fact that feedback is being given. Any unresolved issues are discussed privately with clients during break or at the end of class. Finally, it is important to note that this protocol is designed to deal with a personal attack by an OC client that is directed at another class member, not a personal attack directed at a skills training instructor. When a client harshly criticizes an instructor, the instructor should view the attack as an alliance rupture and institute the alliance rupture repair protocol in private (that is, during the break or at the end of class).

Lateness and Noncompletion of Homework

The third most common problem behaviors likely to occur in an RO skills training class that require in-class intervention are noncompletion of homework and its cousin, not wanting to talk about homework (that is, passing). I have also included in this section a discussion of managing clients' repeated lateness, even though it does not require in-class intervention, because the strategies used to manage lateness share features with some of those used to manage issues concerning homework. Plus, from an RO perspective, noncompletion of homework and repeated lateness are considered social signals.

Instructors, rather than immediately assuming that a problem of lateness or noncompletion of homework lies solely in the client, should begin by asking themselves *What is this client trying to communicate to me or the class? Is it possible that the client is experiencing an alliance rupture?* This should be followed by a quick self-enquiry practice: *As a skills trainer, how may I have contributed to this problem? What is it that I might need to learn?* The good news is that, in general, issues concerning lateness and homework completion are of relatively low frequency in most well-functioning RO classes; indeed, most OC clients compulsively complete homework and are doggedly punctual.

The protocol for managing lateness is to take the heat off. Instructors should briefly acknowledge a late arrival without making a fuss, by saying, for example, "It's good to see you," smiling warmly, adding, "Take a seat—we are working on…," and then returning to teaching, with a brief check-in with the client during break. By not making a fuss about lateness, instructors make it more likely for hyper-threat-sensitive OC clients not to associate arriving at skills class (the tribe) with being put on the spot, being interrogated, being humiliated, or having to justify their actions (recall that OC clients dislike the limelight). Instructors can also circumvent some issues surrounding lateness by occasionally reminding participants that if they do arrive late for class, they should not wait outside the door and enter only at an opportune moment (such as the end of the mindfulness practice or the break) but instead should enter as soon as they arrive. Instructors can explain that lateness and interruptions are part of life and can be opportunities for practicing RO skills, not only for latecomers but also for the entire class (if "energy" arises around classmates' lateness, for example). At the same time, even though heat-off techniques are used when a client arrives late, the behavior itself is targeted for change, albeit not in class.

Protocol for Therapeutic Induction of Social Responsibility

Similar to some of the in-private interventions used to address "don't hurt me" responses and noncompletion of homework, change strategies targeting clients' lateness, noncompletion of homework, lack of participation, or any other form of nonengagement are carried out in private, usually during the break. As in a chat about a "don't hurt me" response or noncompletion of homework, the aim of this chat is to help OC clients motivate themselves to do the right thing by exhibiting behavior appropriate in a classroom setting by reminding them of their core values for fairness. The following transcript shows how one therapist actualized this idea.

Instructor: The thing is, although I am aware of imagining that you don't intend to disrupt the learning of your fellow classmates, I feel obligated to let you know that [showing up late, not doing homework, not participating in class exercises] sends a powerful social signal that is most likely subtly impacting the learning of the entire class. RO skills training classes are little tribes. Regardless of the reasons why, someone who repeatedly shows up late, doesn't participate, or doesn't complete homework is placing an unfair burden on classmates by making the source of practical examples stem primarily from individual efforts rather than from the class as a whole. We need the efforts of every person involved in our little tribe to make things work, not only to learn from each other but also to build the type of camaraderie that is needed to fight the social isolation and loneliness that characterize OC problems. Learning RO skills is a bit like joining the Three Musketeers—all for one, and one for all! (*Smiles.*) We depend on you to arrive on time, ready to go, having practiced your skills, and with a spirit of openness that encourages your fellow classmates to behave similarly. (*Smiles.*) I know this may sound a bit silly, but it really does matter. RO skills are not something we can learn alone, or simply by reading the text. To be fully grasped, they depend on the passionate participation of each and every one of us—and that means you. (*Smiles warmly.*) So my question to you...now that you are aware of the impact your behavior has on other people...is whether you would be willing to use your capacities for superior inhibitory control, and your values for giving a damn, to help out your fellow musketeers... and do your part by...[showing up on time, completing homework, participating when asked].

Managing Noncompletion of Homework

The protocol for dealing with noncompletion of homework combines the preceding heat-off strategy (a private discussion about the problem during the break) with a heat-on strategy that addresses the issue immediately in class. When an OC client reports not having completed his or her homework, the instructor, instead of ignoring or accepting the report, admonishing the client, assessing the situation, or problem solving, should keep the heat on the client by adopting a stance of playful irreverence (see chapter 2) that presumes commitment and ignores signs of nonengagement—in this case, by the instructor behaving "as if" the client always intended to complete the homework and will therefore leap at the opportunity to complete it in class (wink, wink and tee hee). Recall that playful irreverence, also known as therapeutic teasing (see "Fun Facts: Teasing and Being Teased," in lesson 22), is how friends give each other feedback.

Most often this is actualized when the instructor simply asks the OC client to complete the homework in the moment (that is, in class): "So, Tim, can you remind me what the homework assignment was for this week?" The question should be delivered in a manner that signals genuine yet irreverent curiosity (because it will be obvious to everyone in the room that the instructor and the client both already know the answer to what appears to be a silly question; tee hee). This strategy works because it requires the client to say something other than "I didn't do my homework" while also making it clear that a discussion about homework is impossible to avoid. After the client answers the question (most will), the instructor should start to go through at least some part of the homework in class, cheerfully carrying on in a manner that communicates the instructor's assumption of the client's competence and commitment, and ignoring any signs of reluctance from the client. For example, if the homework was to practice the Match + 1 skills that are part of Flexible Mind ALLOWs (see lesson 21), then the instructor can ask the client to demonstrate the way he would have used the skill if he had been able to do so during the preceding week. This approach both gives the client the benefit of the doubt and provides a mild aversive contingency for noncompletion of homework (puts the heat on) by asking the client to complete the homework (at least partially) in class—making noncompletion of homework less likely in the future (recall OC clients dislike the limelight).

The same playful irreverent approach should be adopted when a client has completed the homework but doesn't want to talk about it—that is, the client wants to pass when the time comes for everyone to take turns reporting on the homework. In this situation, when the client says, "I really don't want to talk about it" or "I want to pass," the instructor should adopt a playful irreverent stance, ignore what the client said, and simply ask instead, "Okay—so can you remind me what our homework assignment was for this week?" The following transcript demonstrates the key principles.

Instructor: Okay, Jane. So how did your homework go?

Client: I don't want to talk about it

Instructor: Okay. So can you remind me—what was the homework?

Client: I said I don't want to talk about it.

Instructor:	*(Displays a closed-mouth smile and performs an eyebrow wag)* Yeah, I get it. But can you just remind me again what it was? Just take a look down at your skills notebook, and read off the title on the page in front of you.
Client:	*(Pauses, looks down at notebook)* It says "Flexible Mind ALLOWs, Match + 1 skills."
Instructor:	Thanks. So, Jane, did you do your homework?
Client:	Yes, but I don't want to talk about it.
Therapist:	Sure. *(Nods; displays a closed-mouth smile.)* So who did you practice Match + 1 with? *(Performs an eyebrow wag.)*
Client:	It was someone I know at work.
Therapist:	Is this the same someone you've talked about before? Or was it someone new?
Client:	It was the same person.
Therapist:	*(Smiles and performs an eyebrow wag)* How cool! So, if I remember correctly, this is a person you have already decided to try to get closer to. Is that correct?
Client:	Yes.
Therapist:	That's what I thought. So…well done on practicing. *(Smiles.)* Okay, now, everybody take out your handout labeled "Match + 1 Intimacy Rating Scale." *(Briefly takes the heat off the client by asking the entire class to look together at an RO handout.)* Okay, Jane, when you look at this scale, what level do you think you got to when you practiced your Match + 1 skills?

From that point, the client shared more about what had happened during her homework practice, and it was discovered that her desire not to talk about her homework stemmed from her belief that she had not done a very good job. The instructor was able to use this information as a means of teaching more about the process of forming new relationships. Finally, the instructor purposefully chose to keep Jane's homework review shorter than what might have been typical, in order to reinforce her for successful homework completion and for making a direct request to pass instead of simply going quiet, pouting, or displaying a "don't hurt me" response. By ignoring the client's initial request to pass on the homework review, and by asking questions that were pertinent yet easy to answer, the instructor (1) sent a message to the client and the rest of the class, without being too heavy-handed, that passing on homework review is not acceptable in RO DBT; (2) gave the reluctant client an opportunity to receive positive feedback for having completed her homework, and an opportunity to practice being flexible by reporting on her homework even though she didn't want to; and (3) reinforced the client's willingness by giving her leeway and allowing her not to report on every step of her homework.

Very occasionally, OC clients may remain adamant about their requests not to talk about their homework, regardless of how proficient the instructor is in cajoling them to give it a go. After the instructor has attempted three times to get an OC client to join in and talk about the homework, and if the client's nonverbal and verbal signaling appear to show that the client is becoming increasingly distressed, tense, resistant, or adamant, the instructor should smile warmly and take the heat off, saying, "Okay, then—well done for being direct with me. I can see that, for whatever reason, you really don't want to talk about your homework today. So, first, I am really happy you did your homework—and, at least for today, let's move on to someone else, and you and I can chat at break. However, if you change your mind, you just let me know." The instructor should then smile and wink at the client, look around the room, and say, "Okay, who wants to go next?" During class break, the instructor should check in with the client, assess for the possibility of an alliance rupture (repairing it, if necessary; see the following section), and then implement the protocol for therapeutic induction of social responsibility in order to prevent future attempts to pass when it comes to reviewing homework in class.

Managing Alliance Ruptures and Repairs

Instructors should also consider the possibility that lateness and noncompletion of homework signal the presence of an alliance rupture. Instructors should not attempt to repair an alliance rupture in class; instead, they should assess and repair alliance ruptures in private (that is, at class break or at the end of class) and, if an alliance rupture is present, attempt to repair the rupture before the client returns to class (see "Alliance Ruptures and Repairs," in chapter 8 of the RO DBT textbook). This might seem like a daunting task, considering that classroom breaks are normally scheduled for fifteen minutes. In practice, however, most alliance ruptures can be repaired in a few minutes; and, as outlined in the alliance rupture protocol, a repair attempt should always be time-limited anyway (ideally, no longer than ten minutes), to avoid inadvertently punishing the client's efforts at self-disclosure by prolonging the repair attempt (keeping the heat on). Instructors can reengage a repair attempt the following week, if necessary, and the client should also be encouraged to discuss the issue with his or her individual RO DBT therapist.

Managing Suicidal Behavior

OC individuals appear composed and self-controlled on the outside, but suicidal and self-injurious behaviors occur at disproportionately high rates among overcontrolled clients. Chapter 5 and appendix 4 of the RO DBT textbook provide detailed assessment and intervention guidelines for suicidal behavior and nonsuicidal self-injury, including specific assessment questions and a crisis-management protocol for managing OC clients' imminent life-threatening behavior. OC life-threatening behaviors are often qualitatively different from those displayed by other clinical groups. A summary of these features is outlined here:

- OC clients' suicidal behavior and self-harm are usually planned—often hours, days, or even weeks in advance (and sometimes longer).

- OC self-harming behavior is usually a well-kept secret. It may have been occurring for years without anyone knowing, or knowledge about it may be limited to immediate family members (or very close friends, plus therapists). Thus, OC self-harm is rarely attention-seeking. The severity of self-inflicted injuries is carefully controlled in order to avoid medical attention, and scars are carefully hidden. An OC client may acquire medical training or training in first aid in order to treat self-inflicted wounds and avoid having to go to a hospital. Exceptions to hiding behavior can occur, most often among OC clients with a long history of psychiatric hospitalization, with dramatic displays of self-injury often intermittently reinforced (as when self-injury gets an OC client placed in a private observation room, which is preferable to the uncertainty of being placed in the general inpatient community).

- OC clients may attempt suicide to punish family members or close others ("When I'm gone, you'll be sorry") or to get even, expose moral failings, or make a rival's life difficult (as when the OC client hopes that his or her death will make it impossible for the rival to achieve an important goal).

- OC self-harm and suicidal behavior are more likely to be rule-governed than mood-governed (for example, OC clients may try to restore their faith in a just world by punishing themselves for their perceived wrongs).

- Some OC clients may romanticize suicidal behavior and may consider brooding or melancholy to be noble and/or creative.

The good news is that, in general, it is very rare for an RO skills instructor to have to manage imminent life-threatening behavior in class (or outside of class, for that matter) when working with OC clients. The primary exception is the RO skills instructor who is also the individual therapist for a suicidal client (this situation makes it more likely that the client will reveal a life-threatening problem to the therapist during class or at the break). The general rule for when a client reveals life-threatening ideation, plans, or actions in class is to thank the client for letting this information be known and then request to meet with the client during the break (or at the end of class), as necessary, to address the issue. This reassures the class that the instructor is taking the problem seriously, and the instructor can feel free to move on with teaching. Importantly, assessment or problem solving around suicidal behavior should not be conducted in class. During the break or after class, one of the instructors can conduct, in private, a brief assessment for imminent suicide risk. In addition, the RO DBT crisis-management protocol should be activated if the client is unwilling to provide a commitment to the instructor not to commit suicide before the next meeting with the individual therapist, or if it is determined that the risk is sufficient to warrant immediate intervention (see "Assessing OC Life-Threatening Behaviors" and "The RO DBT Crisis-Management Protocol," in chapter 5 of the RO DBT textbook). When risk is high and imminent, the following core elements of the RO DBT crisis-management protocol should be recalled.

- Focus on removing available lethal means and increasing short-term availability of social support.

- Remind the client of his or her prior commitments. If the client has previously made a commitment not to self-harm or commit suicide, then remind the client of that prior commitment and of his or her core values linked to doing the right thing, honoring prior commitments, and integrity.

- Arrange for emergency backup. Make sure the client has emergency contact numbers.

- Contract with the client not to engage in suicidal acts. If the client remains at high risk, ask the client to call someone for a ride home. If the client appears unwilling to make the call, offer to make the call for the client.

- For all class members, as a general rule, obtain contact information (such as phone numbers and email addresses) of people who are in their support networks, and keep this information in a place where it will be easily accessible to skills instructors.

- Accompany the client to the emergency room, or call emergency services or the police if suicidality cannot be reduced, risk is high, no other support can be found, and the client refuses help.

As mentioned earlier, it is extremely rare for an RO skills instructor working with OC clients to have to manage imminent life-threatening behavior in class. Nevertheless, instructors should be prepared to have one instructor remain with a suicidal client, either to complete a risk assessment or to problem solve, while the other instructor continues teaching the class. Instructors are advised to become familiar with the guidelines for managing imminent life-threatening behaviors with OC clients, as detailed in chapter 5 of the RO DBT textbook.

Summary

In skills training environments with OC clients, overt problematic behaviors are far less common than with other clinical populations, partly because of the nature of the OC personality itself. If problems do emerge, instructors are advised to recall their role as tribal ambassadors, not enforcers, when it comes to working with hyperperfectionistic OC clients. Heat-on and heat-off principles are essential means of shaping up classes to be fun, participatory, and educational. Most OC classes quickly develop a class norm that is supportive and participatory. Thus, if problems persist or become contagious, it is important for instructors to step back and conduct self-assessment and self-enquiry about how they may be contributing to the problem, and to use a consultation team or supervisor as an outside source of feedback.

CHAPTER 4

Using the RO Skills Training Manual

This manual contains twenty new skills compressed into thirty lessons (or weeks), with RO mindfulness skills repeated once. Each skills training session is designed to occur within a two-and-a-half-hour time frame, including homework review, a brief break, and new teaching. Prior to the start of each lesson, instructors should familiarize themselves with the overall aims of the lesson and should use the manual to plan the class exercises and/or mindfulness practices and to prioritize the required teaching points (see "Structuring RO Skills Training Classes," in chapter 1). It is important for instructors to teach directly from the manual (as a teacher of algebra or history might do). This smuggles to OC clients that it is okay to not know everything while ensuring that required teaching points and exercises are not missed or forgotten (see "Teach Directly from the Manual," in chapter 1). Each lesson begins with the main points for that lesson, and instructors should prioritize covering the required teaching points and exercises. Recommended and optional exercises and teaching points can be incorporated into the lesson plan if time permits and/or can be saved for use in the final lesson of the RO module (lesson 30, RO Integration Week).

Deciphering an RO Lesson Plan

The manual is organized according to lessons, and the headings that follow are like the legend on a map. Instructors should be completely familiar with them in order to maximize use of the material in this manual.

A lesson may start with a quote, and a quote can also form the basis of a class discussion. It is up to the discretion of the instructor whether or not to read the quote aloud.

Main Points for Lessons

At the start of each RO lesson, the main teaching points considered essential to be covered during the lesson are numerically listed. Main points should be used by instructors to organize lesson plans and are particularly helpful when time constraints make coverage of all the suggested material difficult to fully review with the class. Instructors should check prior to ending the class that all the main points have been covered. Main points do not need to be read aloud to the class; they are listed for the benefit of the instructor only.

Materials Needed

The key materials and specific worksheets and handouts that will be needed for the lesson are listed after the main points. At the start of each RO module, instructors should provide, ideally in a binder, a paper copy of each handout and worksheet for the entire module.

Required, Recommended, and Optional Mindfulness Practices, Teaching Points, Discussion Points, and Class Exercises

Skills classes consist of a number of topics, exercises, and/or discussion points for a specific lesson. Each of these exercises and discussion points is accompanied by an indication of whether it is required, recommended, or optional. Some lessons also include "fun facts," indicated with a star icon (★). The required sections are essential to teaching the skills and have to be completed for the lesson. The recommended sections can be covered in class, if time allows, and the optional sections can also be covered if time allows and the instructor thinks they are relevant to the learning that the class needs. The fun facts are meant to be read aloud and are, in general, optional material unless marked otherwise.

Required, recommended, and optional *mindfulness practices* can be found throughout the RO skills module. When marked as optional, these practices can be incorporated into the lesson plan in any manner that the instructor finds useful, including at the start of the lesson. Text in italics should be read aloud to the class.

Required, recommended, and optional *teaching points* are bulleted. The text in large print and bold italics should be considered the essential material and are designed to be read aloud verbatim by instructors, in order to maximize clarity and precision. Each specific bold italic teaching point typically has a number of smaller, nonbold teaching points attached to it. Nonbold teaching points provide important supplemental information and/or key discussion questions that can be used at the instructor's discretion.

Required, recommended, and optional *discussion points* are also distributed throughout the RO skills module. They provide instructors with a range of topics, examples, stories, metaphors, and key questions designed to spur class discussion. Discussion points are meant to augment teaching points, not replace them. Therefore, instructors should feel free not to ask all of the suggested questions under a discussion point when time is limited, regardless of whether the discussion point is required, recommended, or optional.

Required, recommended, and optional *class exercises* are scattered throughout the RO module as well. Instructors should strive to cover all the required exercises.

Notes to Instructors

Also scattered throughout the RO skills module are *notes to instructors*. The material in these notes is supplemental but nevertheless important. Most often, notes to instructors provide additional background about a specific point and/or additional scientific research that can be used to strengthen teaching.

Homework Assignments

Homework is assigned at the end of each class and includes both required and optional assignments. The homework assigned at the end of class should be reviewed during the first hour of the following class. Most homework assignments include worksheets, and instructors should encourage class participants to use them when completing homework assignments.

Additional Instructions for Using the Skills Manual

- *Planning lessons.* When planning the material that will be covered during each of the thirty lessons, instructors should schedule a "participate without planning" mindfulness practice for the beginning or middle of approximately fifteen lessons (or more, if possible). The emphasis on practices involving disinhibited expression, tribal participation, and publicly revealing inner experience cannot be overstated when working with OC clients. "Participate without planning" practices are a core means of helping risk-averse OC clients discover the rewards of tribal participation and break down overlearned inhibitory barriers.

- *Open groups.* Instructors running an open group should avoid having clients start during RO Integration Week (lesson 30) and allow them to start the following week instead (lesson 1).

- *Self-enquiry journal.* It is recommended that each client start a self-enquiry journal. An empty notebook can be used for this purpose. Clients should be made aware of the need for a self-enquiry journal before attending the first skills class.

- *Teaching from the manual.* Instructors are encouraged to "follow the recipe" when teaching RO skills.

- *Reading aloud and verbatim.* Instructors should get into the habit of reading aloud, and verbatim, the scripts provided throughout the RO manual because (1) doing so smuggles to hyper-performance-focused OC clients that appearing like a novice (that is, having to read aloud from a script) is okay, (2) reading aloud from a script ensures that all the key constructs are covered, and (3) the words used in most of the scripts throughout the manual have been purposefully chosen to maximize OC clients' receptivity (recall that the primary goal of RO skills training is to learn new skills).

- *Typographical indications.* Generally speaking, text printed in **bold** indicates an instruction to the instructor. Text printed in *italics* indicates that it should be read aloud to the class. Text printed in ***bold italics*** indicates that it should be read aloud and is the most important teaching point.

- *Keeping it light.* Throughout the manual, "tee hee," often combined with a smiley face (☺), signals that the point being made represents a therapeutic tease and should ideally be delivered with a playfully irreverent manner.

CHAPTER 5

The RO DBT Lesson Plans

Radical Openness

Main Points for Lesson 1

1. We tend to pay attention to things that fit our beliefs and ignore or dismiss those things that do not.

2. We don't know what we don't know, and this keeps us from learning new things.

3. To learn anything new, we must acknowledge our lack of knowledge and then behave differently!

4. RO DBT considers psychological health to involve three core features: (1) receptivity and openness, (2) flexible control, and (3) intimacy and connectedness.

5. There are pros and cons to being open, as well as to being closed.

6. We only need to practice radical openness when we are closed.

7. Radical openness involves actively seeking the things we want to avoid in order to learn. It requires courage and humility—it is painful and liberating. It is key for participating in the community. Radical openness does not mean approval, naively believing, or mindlessly acquiescing.

8. To practice Use Flexible Mind DEFinitely and the three steps needed for radically open living: (1) acknowledge the presence of an unwanted private experience, (2) practice self-enquiry by turning toward the discomfort in order to learn, and (3) flexibly respond by doing what's needed in the moment.

Materials Needed

- Handout 1.1 (Inkblot)
- Handout 1.2 (What Is Radical Openness?)
- Handout 1.3 (Learning from Self-Enquiry)
- (Optional) Handout 1.4 (Main Points for Lesson 1: Radical Openness)
- Worksheet 1.A (Myths of a Closed Mind)
- Worksheet 1.B (Flexible Mind DEFinitely: Three Steps for Radically Open Living)
- Worksheet 1.C (The Pros and Cons of Being Open Versus Closed to New Experience)
- Self-enquiry journal (*Note:* Clients will need to bring their own journal or notebook for this.)
- Whiteboard or flipchart with marker

NOTE TO INSTRUCTORS: Each RO class normally begins with a brief mindfulness exercise or practice prior to reviewing homework. Assuming that the RO class is an open group (that is, individuals enter the skills class at differing times), the recommended mindfulness exercise that follows would occur at the beginning of the class, just before reviewing the homework assigned from the previous lesson's class. Instructors should aim to keep practices and discussions afterward brief; in general, a mindfulness practice and sharing of observations afterward should last approximately six to eight minutes.

(Recommended) Mindfulness Practice

Mindfulness of Ambiguity

Refer participants to handout 1.1 (Inkblot).

Use the script and questions that follow to guide the practice.

To begin our practice, place the inkblot I just gave you in front of you, in a way that will allow you to gaze at it without having to move. Now, with awareness, take a slow deep breath and center your attention on your inkblot. Notice any patterns or images that arise from it—and when your mind wanders, as minds are prone to do, gently guide your attention back to the visual features or patterns you observe within your inkblot. [Pause approximately ten seconds.] Okay, now bring your attention back to the room and let's discuss what you observed.

- ✓ **Ask for observations.** *What did you observe when you examined your inkblot? Did you notice any familiar shapes or images—for example, did anyone see a bunny rabbit?*

- *Highlight the range and diversity of different shapes observed by different people.* Instructors should point out that there is no perfect way to see an inkblot, and this observation applies to much of life—that is, there is no perfect way to behave and rarely is there a perfect answer. For example, it is likely that everyone in the class drives slightly differently, yet everyone made it today on time to class. Radical openness begins by acknowledging our differences as opportunities for learning new things rather than seeing them as automatically wrong or potentially threatening.

- *Encourage self-enquiry.* (*Note:* Instructors should feel compelled to ask only the required question that follows; optional questions should be asked only if time permits.)

  - ✓ **(Required) Ask:** *To what extent do you believe that there is only one way to observe an inkblot? What might this tell you about how you see yourself and the world? What is it you might need to learn from this?*

  - ✓ **(Optional) Ask:** *To what extent did you notice yourself socially comparing your observations of the inkblot to the observations made by others? Were your comparisons judgmental? Of others? Of yourself? Of something else? What might this tell you about how you see the world? What might you need to learn?*

  - ✓ **(Optional) Ask:** *Do you ever find it difficult to see both sides of an issue?*

Additional discussion points might include playful challenges for the class to come up with as many ways as possible to solve a simple problem or complete a simple task like how to eat an apple or how to do the laundry.

(Required) Class Exercise

Our Perceptual Biases: How We Become Closed to New Information

The primary aim of this exercise is to help participants identify the potentially maladaptive ways they deal with disconfirming feedback while also understanding that all humans struggle with being open to feedback, to some degree.

Instructors should aim to spend approximately five to seven minutes on this exercise. Optional questions listed here should be asked only if time permits.

Begin by asking the two required questions that follow.

- ✓ **(Required) Ask:** *How do you respond when confronted with a different point of view about something important?*

- ✓ **(Required) Ask:** *What is your favorite strategy to avoid hearing a different perspective?*

- ✓ **(Optional) Ask:** *Do you think other people know when you use it? What might this tell you about yourself?*

- ✓ **(Optional) Ask:** *If you already believe you know everything about something, will you be more or less open to feedback suggesting you are wrong?*

- ✓ **(Optional) Ask:** *If you believe the world is flat, are you more or less likely to seek out information suggesting that the world is round?*

Next: Write on a whiteboard or flipchart a list of differing strategies generated by the class.

Examples: Rehearse a rebuttal, search for disconfirming evidence, ruminate about it, shut down, pretend not to listen, go on the attack, change the topic, behave as if one is bored, make a joke out of it, earnestly listen, begin to automatically doubt oneself, pretend to agree when you don't, take some time to think about it, change the topic.

Lastly: Place an asterisk (*) next to the strategies that the class agrees are most likely to be unhelpful or may lead to negative consequences.

(Required) Teaching Points

Perceptual Biases

- *We all create our own belief systems, like it or not.* Often our belief systems are so much a part of us that we do not recognize them as beliefs; it's like asking a fish to recognize the water!

- *We tend to pay attention to things that fit our beliefs and ignore or dismiss things that don't.*

- *Social psychologists call this a "confirmation bias."* For example, if you are conservative politically, you are likely to read or watch only conservative political newspapers or TV, and you will read something entirely different if the opposite is true.

  - ✓ **Ask:** *What type of confirmation biases do you think are most common among overcontrolled individuals?* For example, "The only way to get ahead is to make self-sacrifices," "Planning ahead is imperative," "Being correct is more important than being liked by others."

- *We don't know what we don't know, and this keeps us from learning new things.* Sometimes we think we know something but find out later that what we actually knew was only part of what we needed to understand.

  - For example, someone living in the United States might assume that they would know how to buy a car in France, only to discover that the laws surrounding the purchase of a vehicle in France require a wide range of documentation never needed in the USA (such as proof of residence, passport, utility bill, and so on).

  - Plus, sometimes we don't even know that we lack a skill and we need someone else to point this out to us (for example, a two-year-old doesn't know that they don't know how to use a microwave oven when they want their oatmeal heated).

  - Not knowing what we don't know becomes a problem when it blocks achieving important goals.

- *Whenever we believe we already know the answer or feel threatened by a differing point of view, we have already made a decision about the incoming information*—that is, it is potentially dangerous (because I feel threatened) or it is irrelevant (because I believe I already know the answer). As a consequence, we are less receptive to potentially valuable information.

- *To learn anything new, we must first acknowledge our lack of knowledge.*

- *To learn anything new, we must also behave or think differently!* This can be painful, anxiety-producing, and humbling.

(Required) Teaching Points

What Is Psychological Health?

- *Living well is not just about self-improvement—it also requires seeking what is healthy.*

  - ✓ **Ask:** *To what extent do you believe genuine psychological health or well-being is possible? What might your answer tell you about how you perceive the world or yourself? What is it you might need to learn?*

- *To seek psychological health, it helps to first know what it means.*

  - ✓ **Ask:** *What type of behaviors do psychologically healthy people display?*

  - ✓ **Ask:** *What features do psychologically healthy people share?*

- *RO considers psychological health to involve three core features:*

  1. **Receptivity and openness** to new experience and disconfirming feedback, in order to learn.

  2. **Flexible control** in order to adapt to changing environmental conditions.

3. *Intimacy and connectedness with at least one other person.* Our species survival depended on our ability to form long-lasting bonds and work together in tribes or groups.

- *Thus, more or less...according to this definition, a well-adjusted person is able to not only be open to disconfirming feedback but also to modify their behavior to be more effective in a manner that accounts for the needs of others.*

  ✓ **Ask:** *Can you think of examples of how these three points might manifest in a person's life? What is it that you might need to learn to be able to manifest these traits in your life?*

(Required) Teaching Points
To Be Open or Closed? That Is the Question!

- *Sometimes being closed-minded is exactly what is needed in a given moment, and/or a recommended change may not be necessary.* For example, being closed-minded about eating cottage cheese when one dislikes its taste is fine—assuming there is something else to eat. Closed-mindedness is highly useful when being attacked by a mugger or tortured when captured in war. Being closed-minded might help protect certain family traditions—for example, doggedly celebrating Christmas despite no longer believing in it.

- *The advantages of closed-mindedness almost always pertain to avoidance or dominance.*

  - Being closed-minded may help a person avoid a feeling—for example, of being out of control, awkward, embarrassed, stressed, or uncertain.

  - Being closed-minded may also help a person win a fight or an argument, defeat a rival, prove one's superiority, or achieve a goal.

  - Being closed-minded often seems like a good idea at the time—that is, when we are in the midst of doing it.

- *Closed-mindedness has short-term gains but most often results in long-term negative consequences.* For example, refusing to listen to feedback that smoking can cause cancer may allow you to continue smoking but eventually result in cancer, a stroke, and many hospital bills. Refusing to listen to feedback that you are arrogant may maintain your self-esteem but lead to a lonely and isolated existence.

- *Yet open-mindedness is not all fun and games!* It can be painful because it often requires sacrificing firmly held convictions or self-constructs in order to learn or live by one's values.

- *However, openness is the only way to learn something new.* Whether it is learning to play the violin, to ride a horse, or to maintain a marriage, learning anything or improving how we behave always requires openness.

- *Openness also enhances relationships because it models humility and willingness to learn from what the world has to offer.* Openness signals to another person that you are willing to hear their opinion without automatically discounting it. Importantly, openness does not mean approval, naively believing, mindlessly giving in, or resignation.

(Recommended) Class Exercise

Myths of a Closed Mind

Refer participants to worksheet 1.A (Myths of a Closed Mind).

Instruct the class to place a checkmark in the box next to each myth in worksheet 1.A that they believe to be true or somewhat true.

Divide participants into pairs. Have each member of the pair choose a myth that they strongly believe in and then take turns practicing self-enquiry and outing themselves about their respective myths. The steps for conducting this exercise are outlined here:

1. The revealing partner—that is, the person who is outing themselves—begins by reading aloud their myth three times in a row to their partner.

2. The listening partner then reads aloud several of the self-enquiry questions found on the worksheet. For example, *What is it that you need to learn from this myth? What might this myth be telling you about yourself and your life? Does the thought of reexamining this myth elicit tension? If so, then what might this mean? How open are you to thinking differently about this myth? If you are not open or only partly open, then what might this mean?*

3. Pairs should then switch roles, with the listener now taking the role of outing themselves by speaking aloud the images, thoughts, and memories linked to the myth they have chosen for their practice.

4. After each pair has played both roles at least once, instructors should encourage participants to share their observations about the exercise with the entire class.

Participants should incorporate questions they found most provocative into their daily practice of self-enquiry and record their resulting observations in the self-enquiry journal.

(Required) Teaching Point

What Is Radical Openness?

Refer participants to handout 1.2 (What Is Radical Openness?).

- Radical openness means being open to new information or disconfirming feedback in order to learn.

- Radical openness helps us learn to celebrate self-discovery—it is freedom from being stuck.

- Radical openness can be rewarding—it often involves trying out novel ways of behaving that may help us cope more effectively.

- Radical openness is courageous—it alerts us to areas of our life that may need to change.

- Radical openness enhances relationships—it models humility and readiness to learn from what the world has to offer.

- Radical openness involves purposeful self-enquiry and a willingness to acknowledge one's fallibility—with an intention to change (if needed). It can be both painful and liberating.

- Radical openness challenges our perceptions of reality. *We don't see things as they are—we see things as we are.*

- Being *open* to learning new things involves a willingness to consider that there are many ways to get to the same place.

- Radical openness takes responsibility for our personal reactions and emotions—rather than automatically blaming others or the world.

- Radical openness helps us adapt to an ever-changing environment.

- Radical openness is not…

  - Approval, naively believing, or mindlessly giving in

  - Assuming one already knows the answer

  - Something that can solely be understood intellectually—it requires direct and repeated practice

  - Rejecting the past

  - Expecting good things to happen

  - Always changing

  - Being rigid about being open

NOTE TO INSTRUCTORS: Use examples from your own life or others you may have collected over time to enhance the preceding teaching. For example, the best scientists realize that current knowledge will eventually change and evolve into greater knowledge. Science is a process of discovery: a more sophisticated idea eventually replaces old theory. Ask participants for examples of times they have been open to new things and this has led to new knowledge or skills. For example, numerous roads lead to Chicago; there are countless ways to cook potatoes. Trying to appear perfect, to never make a mistake, is not only impossible but also exhausting! Openness frees energy that in the past was used to protect oneself; it is the opposite of pretending. Importantly, radical openness does not mean approval, naively believing, or mindlessly acquiescing. Sometimes being closed is what is needed in the moment, and/or change is not necessary.

NOTE TO INSTRUCTORS: The extent of existing knowledge about self-enquiry and radical openness, both as concepts and skills, will vary depending on whether skills class is open (that is, participants can join the class at any time) or closed (that is, each skills class starts and ends with the same individuals, with new members joining at a later time). For closed groups, this will be the first time any of the participants will have likely encountered concepts of self-enquiry and radical openness. However, for open groups, many of the clients may have already been exposed to these concepts in other skills classes or via individual therapy.

- **Radical openness is the core skill in RO DBT.** It functions as the cornerstone for all other RO skills.

- **Small moments of closed-mindedness frequently offer just as many opportunities for self-discovery as big moments** (for example, disliking someone cutting you off in traffic may be just as important to practice RO with as an argument with your spouse).

(Required) Teaching Point

Flexible Mind DEFinitely: Three Steps for Radically Open Living

Refer participants to worksheet 1.B (Flexible Mind DEFinitely: Three Steps for Radically Open Living).

> NOTE TO INSTRUCTORS: When teaching Flexible Mind DEFinitely, you are essentially teaching the core skill for the entire RO skills training course. Participants should be encouraged to carry Flexible Mind DEFinitely and self-enquiry questions with them (if possible) to refer to when they find themselves in Fixed or Fatalistic Mind. Individual therapists may need to teach Flexible Mind DEFinitely in individual therapy if their client enters the sequence of skills training after lesson 1 has been taught (this ensures that the client does not have to wait until the skills cycle repeats itself to learn the skill). Teach directly from handout 1.3 (Learning from Self-Enquiry) and worksheet 1.B (Flexible Mind DEFinitely: Three Steps for Radically Open Living). The teaching points that follow do not cover all of the material that is on the worksheets (use the following points to supplement teaching). Since both are assigned as required homework, it is important for instructors to take the time to ensure that participants are familiar with both handout 1.3 and worksheet 1.B before requesting participants to use them on their own.
>
> NOTE TO INSTRUCTORS: When teaching Flexible Mind DEFinitely, write out the acronym (DEF) on a flipchart or whiteboard with each letter arranged vertically in a column but without teaching or naming the specific skill that each letter signifies. Next, starting with the first letter in the acronym (*D* in DEF), teach the skills associated with each letter in the acronym using the key points outlined here, until you have covered all of the skills associated with each individual letter. Importantly, only write out on the whiteboard or flipchart the global description of what each letter actually stands for when you are teaching the skills associated with its corresponding letter. This teaching method avoids long explanations about the use of certain words in the acronym and/or premature teaching of concepts. The meaning of each letter is only revealed during the formal teaching of the skills associated with it.

Flexible Mind DEFinitely

D	Acknowledge **D**istress or unwanted emotion
E	Use self-**E**nquiry to learn
F	**F**lexibly respond with humility

> NOTE TO INSTRUCTORS: Instructors should familiarize participants with how to use worksheet 1.B (Flexible Mind DEFinitely: Three Steps for Radically Open Living) and handout 1.3 (Learning from Self-Enquiry) in their upcoming homework assignment.

D *Acknowledge* **Distress** *or unwanted emotion (for example, annoyance, anxiety, tension in the body, numbness).*

- **Radical openness is the core skill in RO DBT.** In many ways, it underlies all others. So, you DEFinitely will want to practice your DEF skills (☺).

- *We only really need radical openness when we are closed.* Most often this occurs when we encounter a novel or uncertain situation, when we feel invalidated or criticized, and/or when our expectations and beliefs about the world, ourselves, and other people are challenged.

- **Unwanted emotions are often secretly wanted.** The drama of trying to regulate, control, accept, or change an unwanted emotion allows us to pretend we are so busy regulating that we just haven't had time to truly self-examine what the unwanted emotion may actually be trying to say (that is, teach us: "Oops—I was so busy regulating that I forgot to look at what I was avoiding" ☺). This can sometimes lead to a crash (for example, emotional leakage).

E *Use self-Enquiry to learn from the distress rather than automatically attempting to regulate, distract, change, deny, or accept.*

- **Turn toward the emotional distress and practice self-enquiry** in order to learn.

- **Self-enquiry in the heat of the moment** may simply mean silently asking oneself *What is it that I might need to learn from this unwanted experience?*

- **Remember to keep self-enquiry practices brief** (five minutes or less). Prolonged practices often (but not always) reflect strong (often hidden) desires to find some sort of solution. Of course, if this happens, use self-enquiry to explore your intense need for solutions ☺.

- **Remember to be slightly suspicions of quick answers or urges to justify your actions when practicing self-enquiry.**

F **Flexibly respond** *with humility by doing what's needed in the moment, in a manner that accounts for the needs of others.*

- **Flexible responding means taking responsibility for our personal reactions to the world** (including our unwanted emotions).

- **Be suspicious when you check the facts.** Recall that our perceptions cannot help but be limited (by our biology and personal experience). So what I consider a fact may not, in fact, be a fact to you. Okay, let's see if I can say that faster! (tee hee ☺)

- **Be careful not to overdo problem solving.** Remember that for most OC individuals their motto is "When in doubt, apply more self-control." Thus, most OC clients tend to be compulsive fixers.

NOTE TO INSTRUCTORS: Although for some in the class this may be their first exposure to the concept of self-enquiry, it will not be their last. Instructors can let participants know that RO mindfulness training also emphasizes self-enquiry and will be covered in greater detail in other lessons. That said, most participants quickly grasp the core idea of self-enquiry after looking over the self-enquiry questions provided in handout 1.3 (Learning from Self-Enquiry).

Lesson 1 Homework

1. **(Required) Worksheet 1.B (Flexible Mind DEFinitely: Three Steps for Radically Open Living).** Instructors should encourage participants to use handout 1.3 (Learning from Self-Enquiry) to facilitate their practice of step 2 of Flexible Mind DEFinitely. Ask if there are any questions about how to use the worksheet.

2. **(Required) Encourage class participants to carry a copy of handout 1.3 (Learning from Self-Enquiry)** with them, ideally for the entire duration of their treatment and wherever they go. Encourage them to use these self-enquiry question examples to kick-start their own practice or when they are finding it difficult to find a question on their own. Ask if there are any questions about self-enquiry or how to use the handout before assigning it as homework.

3. **(Recommended) Worksheet 1.A (Myths of a Closed Mind).** Quickly review the instructions on how to use this worksheet. Encourage participants to use this worksheet to enhance their practice of radical openness in the coming week.

4. **(Optional) Worksheet 1.C (The Pros and Cons of Being Open Versus Closed to New Experience).** Use worksheet 1.C to deepen participants' understanding about the advantages and disadvantages of open-minded versus closed-minded behavior.

Radical Openness Handout 1.1

Inkblot

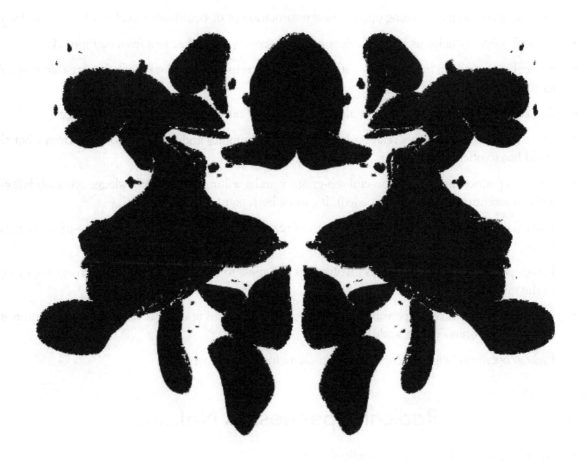

Radical Openness Handout 1.2

What Is Radical Openness?

- Radical openness means being open to new information or disconfirming feedback in order to learn.

- Radical openness helps us learn to celebrate self-discovery—it is freedom from being stuck.

- Radical openness can be rewarding—it often involves trying out novel ways of behaving that may help us cope more effectively.

- Radical openness is courageous—it alerts us to areas of our life that may need to change.

- Radical openness enhances relationships—it models humility and readiness to learn from what the world has to offer.

- Radical openness involves purposeful self-enquiry and a willingness to acknowledge one's fallibility—with an intention to change (if needed). It can be both painful and liberating.

- Radical openness challenges our perceptions of reality. *We don't see things as they are—we see things as we are.*

- Being *open* to learning new things involves a willingness to consider that there are many ways to get to the same place.

- Radical openness takes responsibility for our personal reactions and emotions—rather than automatically blaming others or the world.

- Radical openness helps us adapt to an ever-changing environment.

Radical Openness Is Not...

- Approval, naively believing, or mindlessly giving in

- Assuming one already knows the answer

- Something that can solely be understood intellectually—it requires direct and repeated practice

- Rejecting the past

- Expecting good things to happen

- Always changing

- Being rigid about being open

Radical Openness Handout 1.3

Learning from Self-Enquiry

Instructions: Use the sample questions that follow to enhance your practice of radical openness; see worksheet 1.B (Flexible Mind DEFinitely: Three Steps for Radically Open Living).

Carry a copy of this list with you and write down in your RO self-enquiry journal new questions you discover.

➢ *Is it possible that my bodily tension means that I am not fully open to the feedback? If yes or possibly, then what am I avoiding? Is there something here to learn?*

➢ *Is the resistance, dislike, and tension I am feeling helpful? What is it that I might need to learn from my closed-mindedness?*

➢ *Do I find myself wanting to automatically explain, defend, or discount the other person's feedback or what is happening? If yes or maybe, then is this a sign that I may not be truly open?*

➢ *Am I finding it hard to question my point of view or even engage in self-enquiry? If yes or maybe, then what might this mean?*

➢ *Am I talking more quickly or immediately responding to the other person's feedback or questions? Am I holding my breath or breathing more quickly? Has my heart rate changed? If yes or maybe, then what does this mean? What is driving me to respond so quickly? Is it possible I am feeling threatened?*

➢ *Am I able to truly pause and consider the possibility that I may be wrong or may need to change? Am I saying to myself "I know I am right" no matter what they say or how things seem? Or do I feel like shutting down, quitting, or giving up? If yes or maybe, then is it possible that I am operating out of Fixed or Fatalistic Mind? What is it that I fear?*

➢ *Am I resisting being open to this feedback because part of me believes that doing so will change an essential part of who I am? If yes or maybe, then what might this mean? What am I afraid of?*

➢ *Am I automatically blaming the other person or the environment for my emotional reactions? If yes or maybe, then is it possible this could represent a way for me to avoid being open to the feedback?*

➢ *Do I believe that I know what the intentions are of the person giving me the disconfirming feedback? For example, am I assuming that they are trying to promote themselves? Or do I believe that they are trying to manipulate, coerce, or intimidate me? If yes or maybe, then is it possible that I am not really giving them a chance? What am I afraid might happen if I were to momentarily drop my perspective?*

➢ *Do I think it is unfair to fully listen to someone who I believe is not listening to me? If yes or sometimes, then is it possible this is occurring now? If yes or maybe, then why do I need things to be fair?*

➢ *Do I feel invalidated, hurt, unappreciated, or misunderstood by the person giving me the disconfirming feedback? Is there a part of me that believes it is important for them to acknowledge (or apologize) that they do not understand me before I would be willing to fully consider their position? If yes or maybe, then why do I need to be understood? Why do I need to be validated? Is it possible this desire might subtly block openness on my part by requiring the other person to change first?*

> ➤ *Do I believe that further self-examination is unnecessary because I have already worked out the problem, know the answer, or have done the necessary self-work about the issue being discussed? If yes or maybe, then is it possible that I am not willing to truly examine my personal responses? Why do I feel so convinced that I already know the answer? What do I fear I may lose?*

> ➤ *Do I desire to capitulate, give up, or agree with the feedback? If yes or maybe, then is it possible that my agreement is disguised avoidance? Am I agreeing in order to avoid conflict, not because I truly believe they are right? What might this mean?*

> ➤ *Is the feedback I am being given something that I have heard from others before? If so, what might this mean? Is it possible that there is something to learn from this feedback?*

If you find yourself resisting self-enquiry or feeling nothing, use self-enquiry to explore this further by asking…

> ➤ *What might my resistance be trying to tell me? What is it I need to learn?*

> ➤ *What does my resistance tell me about myself or my willingness to engage in learning this new skill?*

> ➤ *What am I resisting? Is there something important for me to acknowledge or recognize about myself or the current moment?*

> ➤ *Is it possible that I am numbing out or shutting down in order to avoid taking responsibility or make important changes? What is it that I need to learn?*

Use the following space to record new self-enquiry questions that emerge for you over time.

_____

_____

_____

_____

_____

Radical Openness Handout 1.4

Main Points for Lesson 1: Radical Openness

1. We tend to pay attention to things that fit our beliefs and ignore or dismiss those things that do not.

2. We don't know what we don't know, and this keeps us from learning new things.

3. To learn anything new, we must acknowledge our lack of knowledge and then behave differently!

4. RO DBT considers psychological health to involve three core features: (1) receptivity and openness, (2) flexible control, and (3) intimacy and connectedness.

5. There are pros and cons to being open, as well as to being closed.

6. We only need to practice radical openness when we are closed.

7. Radical openness enhances relationships because it models humility and a willingness to learn from the world. Yet, it can be both painful and liberating because it often requires sacrificing firmly held convictions or beliefs in order to learn or connect with another.

8. To practice Use Flexible Mind DEFinitely and the three steps needed for open living: (1) acknowledge the presence of an unwanted private experience, (2) practice self-enquiry by turning toward the discomfort in order to learn, and (3) flexibly respond by doing what's needed in the moment.

Radical Openness Worksheet 1.A

Myths of a Closed Mind

Instructions: Place a checkmark in the box next to each myth you believe is true or somewhat true.

- ☐ Being open means others can use you. Only idiots are open.
- ☐ If you don't have an opinion on how things should be, you'll get hurt.
- ☐ Planning ahead is always imperative.
- ☐ There is a right and wrong way to do things and that's the way it is.
- ☐ Behaving correctly is the most important thing in life.
- ☐ I have tried everything there is to try. There is nothing new out there.
- ☐ Even if I tried something new, it won't help.
- ☐ You can't teach an old dog a new trick.
- ☐ If I try something new and it works, I was a fool for not trying it before.
- ☐ If I try something new, then it means I was wrong.
- ☐ New things are for gullible fools.
- ☐ Doing something different means giving up my values.
- ☐ It doesn't matter what you say or how things seem, when I am right about something I know I am correct.
- ☐ Doing what I always do just feels right.
- ☐ It is always important to do things properly.
- ☐ Rules are there to be followed—especially mine.

In the following space, write out any other myths you may have about emotions that were not mentioned.

_____

_____

_____

Next: Pick one of the preceding myths that you strongly believe in and practice self-enquiry about the myth over the next week.

- **Remember to keep your self-enquiry practices short in duration**—for example, not much longer than five minutes. The goal of self-enquiry is to *find a good question* that brings you closer to your edge or personal unknown (the place you don't want to go), in order to learn. After a week, move to another myth and repeat your self-enquiry practice.

- **Remember to record** in your RO self-enquiry journal the images, thoughts, emotions, and sensations that emerge when you practice self-enquiry about your myths.

- **Remember to practice being suspicious of quick answers** to self-enquiry questions. Allow any answers to your self-enquiry practice to emerge over time.

- **Remember, self-enquiry does not automatically assume that a myth is wrong, bad, or dysfunctional.** Use the following questions to enhance your practice.

  ➤ *What might I need to learn from this myth?*

  ➤ *What might this myth be telling me about myself and my life?*

  ➤ *Am I feeling tense doing this exercise?*

  ➤ *Am I feeling tense right now? If so, then what might this mean? What is it that I might need to learn?*

  ➤ *How open am I to thinking differently about this myth or changing the myth?*

  ➤ *If I am not open or only partly open, then what might this mean?*

  ➤ *How does holding on to this myth help me live more fully?*

  ➤ *How might changing this myth help me live more fully?*

  ➤ *What might my resistance to changing this myth be telling me?*

  ➤ *Is there something to learn from my resistance?*

  ➤ *What does holding on to this myth tell me about myself?*

  ➤ *What do I fear might happen if I momentarily let go of this myth?*

  ➤ *What is it that I need to learn?*

Use the following space to record additional self-enquiry questions or observations that emerged from your practice.

_____

_____

_____

Radical Openness Worksheet 1.B

Flexible Mind DEFinitely: Three Steps for Radically Open Living

Flexible Mind DEFinitely

D   Acknowledge **D**istress or unwanted emotion

E   Use self-**E**nquiry to learn

F   **F**lexibly respond with humility

Instructions: Look for a time in the coming week when you find yourself feeling tense, irritated, annoyed, uncertain, invalidated, criticized, fearful, judgmental, numb, shut down, closed, resisting, ruminating, or disliking something and then use the following skills to practice radical openness.

- **Remember, we only need to practice radical openness when we are closed**—plus, small moments are just as important as big ones (for example, disliking someone cutting you off in traffic may be just as important to practice RO with as an argument with your spouse).

D *Acknowledge* **Distress** *or unwanted emotion (for example, annoyance, anxiety, tension in the body, numbness).*

Place a checkmark in the boxes next to the questions that best address your unwanted experience.

☐   Were you in a novel or uncertain situation?

☐   Did you feel invalidated, misunderstood, or criticized?

☐   Were your expectations or beliefs about the world, other people, or yourself being challenged?

Other circumstances.

_____

_____

_____

Describe in the following space what happened. Where were you when it happened? Who were you with? What did you feel inside your body?

_____

_____

_____

E   *Use self-Enquiry to learn from the distress rather than automatically attempting to regulate, distract, change, deny, or accept.*

Place a checkmark in the boxes that best describe the skill you practiced.

☐ In the heat of the moment, I turned toward my discomfort and asked *What do I need to learn?* rather than automatically regulating, distracting, fixing, or trying to accept.

☐ Made a commitment to practice self-enquiry on multiple days after the event had passed.

☐ Remembered that self-enquiry means *finding a good question* that brings me closer to my edge (my personal unknown), not finding a good answer.

☐ Found my edge by turning my mind to the very thing I don't want to think about or admit having.

☐ Celebrated finding my edge as an opportunity for growth.

☐ Recorded my edge in my RO self-enquiry journal and used it to focus my self-enquiry practice.

☐ Pinpointed a question that elicited my edge.

☐ Used a self-enquiry question from handout 1.2 (What Is Radical Openness?) to enhance my practice.

☐ Remembered that the best self-enquiry question is the one I dislike the most.

☐ Set aside five minutes per day over a period of several days to ask my self-enquiry question and recorded what emerged each day in my RO self-enquiry journal.

☐ Purposefully kept my self-enquiry practices brief (five minutes or less) by recognizing that prolonged practices are often disguised attempts to prove I am working hard, punish myself, or solve the problem in order to feel better.

☐ Practiced being slightly suspicious of quick answers or urges to justify my actions when asking my self-enquiry question.

☐ Remembered that ruminating or brooding is not self-enquiry—it is me trying to *solve the problem or regulate/avoid my discomfort.*

☐ Blocked blaming myself, others, or the world during my practice of self-enquiry.

☐ Noticed secret attempts to avoid my edge or downregulate during a self-enquiry practice and used this to deepen my understanding rather than as another opportunity to get down on myself.

☐ Blocked attempts to be perfect at self-enquiry.

☐ When I found myself resisting self-enquiry, I used self-enquiry to explore my resistance, using the questions from handout 1.3 (Learning from Self-Enquiry).

Record in the following space the self-enquiry question(s) you found most useful.

_____

_____

_____

F Flexibly respond *with humility by doing what's needed in the moment, in a manner that accounts for the needs of others.*

Place a checkmark in the boxes next to the skills you practiced.

- ☐ Acknowledged that flexible responding is freely chosen by me; no one can force me to be flexible.

- ☐ Activated my social safety system to maximize my flexible responding (for example, by closed-mouth smiling with eyebrows raised while slowing and deepening my breathing).

- ☐ Used stall tactics to block automatic, habitual, and quick responding. **Check all that apply.**

  - ☐ Reminded myself it is okay to take time to reflect—not every problem needs immediate fixing.

  - ☐ Let two to three days pass before making a decision or responding to an emotionally evocative event (for example, an email, request, or telephone call).

  - ☐ Communicated to another person that I needed some time to reflect on what had just happened—including how I may have contributed to it—before making a decision about what to do or discussing it further, and then used this time to practice self-enquiry.

  - ☐ Reminded myself that stalling does not mean walking away or abandoning the problem, my responsibility, or the relationship. It means taking a short break to practice self-enquiry and then reengaging with the issue.

- ☐ Practiced living according to my values by taking responsibility for my personal reactions and responses to the world. **Check all that apply.**

  - ☐ Blocked my automatic tendency to blame others or expect the world to change when things did not go as expected.

  - ☐ Reminded myself that no one can force me to feel something.

  - ☐ Practiced outing myself about secret desires to pout, stonewall, walk away, or obstruct another person or an event instead of pretending that I was not upset, that the other person made me do it, or that they got what was coming to them.

  - ☐ Gave others the benefit of the doubt (for example, by assuming that they mean well and/or are doing the best they can to cope effectively).

  - ☐ Challenged my rigid belief that I was correct or right by reminding myself that we don't see things as they are, but that we see things as we are.

  - ☐ Reminded myself that it is arrogant to assume that the world or other people should conform to my expectations or beliefs.

  - ☐ Remembered that I don't know what I don't know, in order to be more receptive to what was happening in the moment.

  - ☐ Practiced a willingness to be wrong without falling apart or giving up.

  - ☐ Practiced surrendering arrogance (for example, by acknowledging the fallibility inherent in all humans or by recalling times when my convictions were proven wrong).

  - ☐ Practiced letting go of desires to control or dominate other people.

☐ Practiced celebrating diversity by recognizing that there are many ways to live, behave, or think.

☐ Practiced celebrating problems as opportunities for new learning rather than obstacles preventing me from enjoying my life.

☐ Practiced seeing the big picture and letting go of detail-focused processing by asking...

    ☐ *Does what I noticed really matter in the long run?*

    ☐ *What are the downsides of holding on to my detailed observation?*

    ☐ *What other valued goals may be negatively impacted by my insistence on this?*

☐ Used my desired level of intimacy to guide how I would respond by asking...

    ☐ *Should I persist or suspend the behavior I had been engaging in prior to the unwanted experience?*

    ☐ *Should I inhibit or disinhibit my action urges?*

    ☐ *Should I express or constrain what I am feeling inside?*

    ☐ *Should I reveal or edit what my beliefs, expectations, or inner thoughts are?*

☐ Practiced being flexible about flexibility; sometimes being closed may be what is needed in the moment, and/or change is not necessary.

Describe other ways you may have practiced flexible responding in the following space.

_____

_____

_____

Radical Openness Worksheet 1.C

The Pros and Cons of Being Open Versus Closed to New Experience

Make a list of pros and cons for being open to new experience, trying out new things, tolerating the distress of not having an answer, or being seen as inexperienced. Also make a list of pros and cons for being closed to new experience or solely basing a decision on the past.

	Being open to new experience	Being closed to new experience
PROS		
CONS		

Understanding Emotions

Main Points for Lesson 2

1. Our neurosensory system is constantly scanning the world and ourselves for the presence of cues or stimuli relevant to our well-being.

2. Our brains are hardwired to detect and react to five broad classes of emotionally relevant stimuli or cues.

3. Safety cues are stimuli associated with feeling protected, secure, loved, fulfilled, cared for, and part of a community or tribe.

4. Novel cues are discrepant or unexpected stimuli that trigger an automatic evaluative process designed to determine whether the cue is important for our well-being.

5. Rewarding cues are cues appraised as potentially gratifying or pleasurable.

6. Threatening cues are cues appraised as potentially dangerous or damaging.

7. Overwhelming cues trigger our emergency shutdown system.

8. We are never unemotional, because we are always in one of the five emotional-mood states.

9. Broadly speaking, when one emotional system is on, the other four are off, or inhibited.

10. Finally, when an emotional response tendency is ineffective, we move to another neuroregulatory response.

Materials Needed

- Handout 2.1 (The RO DBT Neuroregulatory Model of Emotions)
- (Optional) Handout 2.2 (Main Points for Lesson 2: Understanding Emotions)
- Worksheet 2.A (Identifying the Different Neural Substrates)
- Whiteboard or flipchart with marker

(Recommended) Mindfulness Practice
Participate Without Planning

Pick a "participate without planning" exercise from one of the examples provided in the RO mindfulness skills training module in lesson 12. For example, practice "I am NOT pouting!" (also known as "Let's Have a Temper Tantrum") or "Yippee, I'm a Puppet!" Remember that a "participate without planning" practice should not begin with an orientation to or forewarning about the practice, and it should be of short duration (thirty seconds to four minutes).

NOTE TO INSTRUCTORS: Instructors can refer back to this mindfulness practice when teaching handout 2.1 (The RO DBT Neuroregulatory Model of Emotions) to help participants start practicing using the model to label their emotional experience. For example, ask participants to see if they can identify the cues that may have triggered their novelty-evaluative system during the mindfulness practice at the start of the class and to identify the behaviors that suggest this system was active. This process can be repeated as each section of the model is taught—for example, when teaching about reward cues—asking whether anyone noticed their reward system being activated during the practice and use their experience to augment teaching points. Instructors should be ready to share which system they had activated during the mindfulness practice, too, and use their personal experience as possible teaching examples.

(Required) Teaching Point

Five Emotionally Relevant Cues

Refer participants to handout 2.1 (The RO DBT Neuroregulatory Model of Emotions).

- *Our neurosensory system is constantly scanning the world and ourselves for the presence of cues or stimuli relevant to our well-being.* Cues can occur inside the body (for example, a thought or image), outside the body (for example, a loud bang), or contextually (for example, a time of day evokes urges to smoke a cigarette).

- *This scanning process, known as neuroception in our model, is what defines our emotions and is constantly being updated or modified by experience.*

> ★ **Fun Facts:** *Neuroception Occurs in Milliseconds!*
>
> *Neuroception can occur in milliseconds and without conscious awareness: we don't even know we are doing it. Our brains are constantly scanning our environment for cues. For most people the natural set point is a state of safety, of calm readiness, of openness to new stimuli, with ongoing, low-level processing of environmental inputs. However, when our brains detect something different or new in the environment or within our body or mind, a quick and typically unconscious evaluative process ensues, the primary function of which is to assign valence and significance to such stimuli—more specifically, to classify them as safe, novel, rewarding, threatening, overwhelming, or some combination thereof, such as when a stimulus has both rewarding and threatening aspects (imagine a hive dripping with honey and swarming with bees).*

- *Our brains are hardwired to detect and react to five broad classes of emotionally relevant stimuli or cues.*

1. *Safety cues are stimuli associated with feeling protected, secure, loved, fulfilled, cared for, and part of a community or tribe.*

  - **Our natural set point is one of safety, a state of calm readiness and openness,** which includes an ongoing low-level processing of environmental inputs or stimuli.

    - *Safety cues are stimuli that trigger this set point: a calm-friendly state linked to a brain-neural substrate known as the* **ventral vagal complex** (VVC), which is part of the parasympathetic nervous system (PNS; Porges, 2011).

- *Our calm-friendly or PNS-VVC social safety system controls how we communicate nonverbally,* that is, via our facial muscles (allowing us to effortlessly make facial expressions), our voice box muscles (allowing us to have a musical tone of voice), our middle ear muscles (allowing us to tighten our ear drum so we can hear human speech better), and our neck muscles (allowing us to direct our gaze and ears).

- *Social safety activation is characterized by feelings of contentment, well-being, receptivity, curiosity, and desires to socialize.*

- *When the social safety system is on, our body feels relaxed, our heart rate slows, our breathing slows and deepens, and we feel that it is safe to openly express our emotions (for example, via facial expressions).* We feel approachable, sociable, and receptive. We are more likely to make eye contact, we more accurately hear what others are saying, and we are more likely to want to touch and be touched by another person. Plus, we can hit the high notes in a song! (Recall the muscles innervated by the PNS-VVC.) We are also more likely to explore our environment with curiosity, thereby maximizing our potential for discovery and learning.

  - **Examples of safety cues:** a warm cup of milk, a stroll in the park, a laughing child, a hug, a person's voice, a warm smile, stroking a beloved pet, sitting by a warm fire, a happy memory, an image of a loving parent, a thought of a good friend, a pleasant meal with a friend, and so forth

  - ✓ **Ask:** *What cues trigger feelings of safety in you? How often do you think you feel social safety?*

2. **Novel cues are discrepant or unexpected stimuli that trigger an automatic evaluative process designed to determine whether the cue is important for our well-being.**

   - *When something unexpected occurs, our calm-friendly state is briefly withdrawn.* We don't feel aroused, but neither are we relaxed.

   - *We freeze, hold our breath, our heart rate and blood pressure increase, and we turn our attention toward the novel cue.* Our body is immobile but prepared to move (Bracha, 2004; Schauer & Elbert, 2010).

"A Story of Two Friends." **Read the following text aloud:** *Imagine you are walking with a friend down your neighborhood street, having just finished a nice cup of tea. You both comment on the unusual quiet—traffic seems nonexistent. You notice ahead in the distance, on the other side of the street, what looks like a large crowd of people. Both of you stop and stare, holding your breath as you strain to discern what's happening. Something is peculiar; many of the people are standing in the middle of the street. You can see that some people are laughing as if something's hilarious; others are shaking their heads as if in disapproval. You continue to stare—your brain is trying to figure out what the significance of this unexpected event is. Is this a good thing or a bad thing? Will it be helpful or harmful to move closer?*

- *The story illustrates how, when unexpected, novel, or discrepant things occur, our brain quickly tries to determine whether what is happening is important to our well-being.*

- *This evaluative process is automatic: it can happen so fast (in milliseconds) that we often have no awareness of it.*

- **Examples of novelty cues:** a barking parrot, a loud bang in a church, a teacher slapping a student, a lottery ticket with a winning number, a spacecraft landing in our backyard, a book misaligned, a critical comment by a friend

- ✓ **Ask:** *What are recent examples of novel cues in your life? How did you evaluate them (that is, safe, rewarding, threatening)?*

3. **Rewarding cues are cues appraised as potentially gratifying or pleasurable.**

Continue "A Story of Two Friends" by reading the following text aloud: *Let's return to our story about the two friends. As you recall, our story concluded with you and your friend unexpectedly encountering a crowd of people in the middle your neighborhood street. Your novelty-evaluation system was triggered by this event, which momentarily deactivated your social safety system. You both stopped and stared intently at the crowd, trying to ascertain its significance. Now let's imagine that your friend is delighted by this new discovery! They want to approach it. They smile broadly, turn to you, and excitedly exclaim, "Wow, it's a parade! Let's go see!" They begin tugging on your sleeve and urge you to move closer.*

- *Your fictional friend in the story evaluated the novel cue (the unexpected crowd of people) as a potential reward.*

  ✓ **Ask:** *In real life, how do you think you would have responded? Would your evaluation of the event have been the same as your fictional friend's? What might your answer tell you about yourself?*

- **When we evaluate a novel cue as rewarding, our sympathetic nervous system (SNS) excitatory approach system is activated.** See handout 2.1 (The RO DBT Neuroregulatory Model of Emotions).

- *We experience a sense of anticipation that something pleasurable is about to occur.*

- *We feel excited and elated—our heart rate goes up and we breathe faster.*

- *We experience urges to approach or pursue the potential reward.*

- *Our conversations are more animated, making us more fun to be around.*

  ✓ **Ask:** *What cues trigger rewarding or pleasurable experiences for you? How often do you feel excited and animated?*

- *However, there are some downsides to reward states.*

  - *The more extreme or strongly activated a reward state is, the less active is the PNS-VVC social safety system.* We may find it hard to rest or relax. For example, under high reward states a person may feel so excited that they cannot sleep, which can lead to mental and physical exhaustion if it persists.

  - *We can become hyper-goal-focused and less open to non-reward-related stimuli.* For example, we may be unaware that our conversations solely focus on describing how we will achieve our desired goal or may feel bored/disinterested if someone tries to talk about something unrelated to our reward state.

  - *We may lose our ability to read subtle (and sometimes not so subtle) social cues.* For example, we may fail to notice that another person appears to be in pain, or that they may be feeling angry or sad about something, or that they look bored and may want to change the topic.

  - *We may become overly expressive.* For example, we may express emotions or feelings that are context-inappropriate (for example, begin to giggle during a funeral), may become self-focused or dominating during social interactions (for example, exclaim exceptional knowledge of Asian cooking to the owner of a Chinese restaurant and then order food for everyone at our table without their permission), and/or may be unaware that we are speaking louder and faster than others.

★ **Fun Facts:** *Not All Aggression Is Due to Anger*

Although most textbooks use the term "fight or flight" when describing the emotional action urges triggered by threat, to be more accurate, the order of the wording should probably be reversed (that is, "flight or fight"). When threatened, an animal's first response is to run away (flight); only after the animal is trapped does defensive attack behavior emerge (fighting). Although "fight" addresses many of the types of aggressive behavior we may occasionally witness or read about (or sometimes engage in), it doesn't explain aggressive behavior that feels pleasurable—that is, it does not account for nondefensive aggressive-approach behaviors. Nondefensive aggressive attacks also involve heightened SNS activation, but in this case, the active SNS system is the reward system (not the defensive system). Reward activation and pursuit behaviors are commonly seen in predatory species (for example, imagine the behavior of a fox in a henhouse). Thus, the aggressive energy of the champion boxer, the bloodlust of a soldier during battle, the satisfaction of revenge, and the pleasure associated with winning are not a consequence of defensive anger. Although anger may spur us to attack, we generally dislike experiencing it, because feeling threatened is not fun, whereas winning, control, and power are pleasurable.

✓ **Ask:** *What are other examples of aggressive pursuit behaviors? What might this tell us about desires to dominate? To what extent do you like to dominate, win, or control situations or other people? What might this tell you about yourself?*

NOTE TO INSTRUCTORS: For OC clients, differentiating between anger and aggression can be important. It is common for OC clients to deny feeling anger, yet most will admit to desires to win, achieve, or dominate.

4. *Threatening cues* **are cues appraised as potentially dangerous or damaging.**

Continue "A Story of Two Friends" by reading the following text aloud: *Let's return again to our story of the two friends. Our last episode ended with your friend's SNS reward and excitatory approach system being activated, leading them to excitedly encourage you to join them in their pursuit of what they believe is a parade. Now let's imagine that your appraisal of the situation is different than your friend's. Rather than seeing the mass of people as potentially rewarding, your brain perceives it as potentially dangerous. While your friend excitedly smiles and urges you to join them, your body tenses, your heart begins to race, and your facial expression becomes flat. Your easy manner is long gone. You grab your friend and earnestly shout, "NO, it's not a parade, it's a riot. We need to get out of here! RUN!" You pull your friend toward you and begin running away from the crowd. You are sweating and breathing fast as you run, and you don't dare look back.*

• **In the final episode of our story—in contrast to your friend—you interpreted the crowd of people as a potential threat.**

• **The lesson of "A Story of Two Friends" shows that people can be in exactly the same situation yet interpret it in exactly opposite ways!** Both feel true to the person interpreting, which is why they can sometimes trigger arguments.

✓ **Ask:** *How often do you interpret things differently from other people? How often do you think your disagreements with others pertain to differing interpretations about events? What might this tell you?*

- *When we feel threatened, we experience a sense of anticipation that something bad may happen and/or that desired goals may be blocked.*

- *Our sympathetic nervous system is activated, triggering feelings of anxiety, irritation, and an urge to flee or attack.*

- *Our body feels tense; our breath is fast and shallow, and our heart rate speeds up as we prepare for flight or fight.*

- *Both our social safety–driven (PNS-VVC) empathetic perception and prosocial signaling become impaired.* For example, we can only force a fake smile, our facial expressions are constricted, our voice tone becomes monotonic, our gestures are tight and nonexpansive, and we are more likely to avert our gaze or stare with hostility and misinterpret what another person says.

  ✓ **Ask:** *What cues trigger threat for you? How often do you think you are in a state of anxious irritation?*

5. **Overwhelming cues trigger our emergency shutdown system.**

- *Imagine being chased by a hungry bear: you try to run away, but it is too fast; you try to fight it off, but it is too strong.*

- *When our emotion-based actions are ineffective or overwhelmed (for example, it looks like we are going to be dinner for a bear), our brain-body copes by turning off our flight/fight/approach behaviors* in order to conserve energy and maximize survival.

- *Our heart rate, breathing, and body movements slow down—we become immobilized. Our social safety signaling is deactivated—we lose all facial expression.*

- *It's like becoming one of those zombies you see in horror films.*

NOTE TO INSTRUCTORS: This can be a good time to smuggle in a brief "participate without planning" practice. Say: *It's like becoming one of those zombies you see in horror films.* Raise your eyebrows, smile warmly, and then, without further preamble say: *Okay, everyone stand up! Place your arms straight out in front of you, parallel to the ground. Now let your hands dangle. Great! Okay, now let's all practice being zombies!* Begin to moan loudly, and shuffle about with your arms held straight out in front of you while encouraging the class to do the same. After about thirty seconds, tell the class to sit down, smile broadly, and say: *Wow, that was fun!* or *Wow, I sure needed that!* Encourage a quick round of applause. Then immediately move back to teaching the next point, without further comment or discussion (see "Instructor Guidelines for 'Participate Without Planning' Practices," in lesson 12).

- *Our parasympathetic nervous system's dorsal vagal complex (PNS-DVC) is triggered.* Interestingly, this neural substrate is evolutionarily older than the other emotion systems— for example, frogs have a PNS-DVC shutdown response, too.

- *Like a zombie, we look and feel emotionally numb. Fear, anger, and other powerful emotions fade.*

- *We experience pain less intensely. We may dissociate or faint.*

  ✓ **Ask:** *What cues do you experience as overwhelming? How often do you think you are in this state? How often do you feel shut down? What triggers it?*

(Required) Teaching Point

Pulling It All Together

- *We are never unemotional, because we are always in one of the five emotional-mood states.* We always feel something, even when the duration of the emotional sensation is so low in intensity or so quick as to be barely noticeable.

- *Broadly speaking, when one emotional system is on, the other four are off, or inhibited.* For example, a person cannot feel both extremely angry and extremely contented at the same moment in time. That said, sometimes two (or more) neural substrates are coactivated (for example, that first date with someone you just met over the internet).

- *Finally, when an emotional response tendency is ineffective, we move to another neuroregulatory response.*

(Required) Story and Discussion

"So Close and Yet So Far Away"

> NOTE TO INSTRUCTORS: The following story is broken into chapters. Instructors should read aloud each short chapter and ask the underlying embedded questions before moving on to read the next chapter. Encourage participants to use handout 2.1 (The RO DBT Neuroregulatory Model of Emotions) to facilitate answering the questions.

Chapter 1: The Setting

Imagine a teenager named Sally, whose idol is Johnny Depp, the famous movie star. She is at the airport, traveling with her loving grandparents, who have decided to treat her to a special trip to a movie set in the Caribbean Islands. (Can you guess which movie?) Their plane isn't scheduled to depart for another two hours, so they have plenty of time. Grandfather buys everyone a cup of their favorite tea, and they all decide to enjoy it while waiting in the boarding area. Sally finishes her tea and then quietly rests her head on the shoulder of her grandmother, who gently strokes her hair. Just as her eyes begin to close, she remembers how her grandmother used to love reading her bedtime stories. Gently smiling, she takes a slow deep breath.

> ✓ **Ask:** *What neural substrate (part of the brain) has most likely been triggered in Sally? What eliciting cues helped you make your decision? What action tendencies, actions, and/or expressions further confirm your choice?*
>
> **Answer: The neural substrate is the PNS-VVC social safety system. The eliciting cues include** the airplane is on time; she is traveling with members of her family who deeply care about her; she had just finished a cup of her favorite tea; her grandmother is gently stroking her hair; and a comforting memory from childhood occurred.
>
> **The confirming action tendencies, actions, and expressions include** resting her head on her grandmother's shoulder; eyes beginning to close; smiling gently; and a deep cleansing breath upon recalling the memory.

Chapter 2: The Discrepancy

While resting quietly, Sally begins to notice that the noise level around her family's seating area is different—it suddenly seems unusually quiet.

✓ **Ask:** *What neural substrate (part of the brain) is likely to have been at least partially withdrawn, and what was the cue that triggered this?*

Answer: The PNS-VVC social safety system has been partially withdrawn due to the unexpected change in the ambient level of noise—her sensory system has detected a novel stimulus.

Chapter 3: "What Is It?"

Sally is feeling less drowsy; she lifts her head from her grandmother's shoulder, scans the area, and listens intently. The people in the seats next to her family are now standing—they appear to be staring intently at something. She looks to see what it is and spots a large crowd gathered around what appears to be an arrivals gate.

✓ **Ask:** *What neural substrate (part of the brain) is now fully activated? What cues triggered it? And what action tendencies, actions, and/or expressions further confirm its presence?*

Answer: Her novelty-orienting system is now fully activated and the social safety system has withdrawn. **The eliciting cues include** staring behavior exhibited by nearby others; unexpected presence of a crowd of people all looking in the same direction.

The action tendencies, actions, and/or expressions confirming this include she feels alert but not aroused, and she adjusts her body posture from one of relaxation (head down) to one of alertness (head up). Without necessarily even being aware, Sally's brain is working to assign significance to the novel stimuli—that is, to what extent may it be relevant to her personal well-being? Is it unimportant (that is, safe, meaning she can return to resting) or is it important (that is, potentially rewarding/threatening, meaning she might need to get active)?

> NOTE TO INSTRUCTORS: Instructors can use the preceding section of the story to point out how the behavior of others influenced the behavior of Sally—that is, she directed her gaze in the same direction as those nearby. Research shows that we are hardwired to experience urges to direct our gaze in the same direction of a person staring intently in a different direction from our own. This provided us with a huge survival advantage because our individual survival no longer depended solely on our personal perceptions. In the story, without conscious awareness, Sally used the gaze direction of her neighbors to enhance her awareness of her environment. It also helps explain why we are so concerned about the perceptions of others—because deep down we know that what others see may impact our personal well-being.

Chapter 4: The Mad Dash

Without warning, the crowd suddenly breaks into applause. A few people seem to be excitedly shouting. With a smile, Sally turns to her grandparents and says, "Let's go see what's happening!" The applause continues; her heart begins to race, her breath quickens, and she feels flushed. As she gets closer she spots the source of the crowd's applause. It's Johnny! It's Johnny Depp! Here in person—right now! She squeals with delight and sprints toward him shouting, "Johnny, Johnny, Johnny—I love you! I love you!" She fails to notice the stern looks she is getting from others as she pushes them aside, leaps over them, or steps on their toes. She only has eyes for her Johnny! Her grandparents hurry to catch up.

✓ **Ask:** *What neural substrate (part of the brain) is now fully activated? What cues triggered it? And what action tendencies, actions, and/or expressions further confirm its presence?*

Answer: *Her SNS excitatory arousal system has been strongly activated* and her social safety system (PNS-VVC) is disengaged. **The eliciting cues include** the sound of applause and, of course, spotting her idol—Johnny Depp!

The action tendencies, actions, and/or expressions confirming this include her body is animated; heart and breath rate increase; she feels flushed; she excitedly approaches her reward and becomes hyper-goal-focused; her empathetic perception becomes impaired—for example, she ignores stern looks and appears to not realize that she is pushing and stepping on people in her single-minded pursuit of her desired goal.

Chapter 5: The Crash

Sally is determined to get to her Johnny! She hurdles three startled elders and vaults two picture-snapping reporters. She gets within five feet of her beloved, only to smack into three muscle-bound bodyguards blocking her way. She cannot move them—they are impassable. But her Johnny is right there—within arm's reach! He is turning toward her and looking right at her! And then he does the unimaginable—he looks directly at her and smiles! She feels light-headed, her knees go wobbly. It's like she's peering down a long tunnel—she can no longer hear the roar of the crowd. It looks like Johnny is trying to say something to her…is he perhaps trying to say…. "I love you"? She suddenly feels numb all over—and then faints!

✓ **Ask:** *What neural substrate was activated? What cues helped you determine this? Why did she faint?*

Answer: *The parasympathetic nervous system's dorsal vagal complex (PNS-DVC) shutdown system was activated. The eliciting cue was overwhelming reward.* Although experiences of overwhelming reward are rare, when they occur the brain responds in the same way it would to overwhelming threat. In Sally's case, a DVC shutdown response was triggered after her high-energy-consuming SNS excitatory approach behaviors were blocked by the three bodyguards. Plus, the reward value of the stimulus did not dissipate but instead increased in intensity (for example, when Mr. Depp smiled at her).

Why fainting? Acquisition and consumption of her reward (presumably a hug and a kiss) became not only impossible but a waste of valuable energy. As a consequence, her evolutionarily older emergency shutdown system (PNS-DVC) was triggered, manifested by fainting. Real-life examples of this can be found in 1960s film clips showing teenagers fainting during press conferences given by the Beatles.

NOTE TO INSTRUCTORS: Rather than triggering reward responses, the preceding event triggered threat and avoidance responses in Sally's grandparents. Instructors can use this to illustrate how the same or a similar stimulus can trigger a completely different response among different people as a function of differing experiences and biotemperaments. Despite this, the grandparents used self-control to overcome their automatic urges to run away, and by doing so they were able to ensure their granddaughter's well-being (for example, they were able to convince a nearby police officer not to arrest her and were able to catch her when she fainted).

NOTE TO INSTRUCTORS: The preceding story also illustrates how our neuroregulatory system normally operates: from safety to novelty to reward/threat activation or back to safety, and finally to shutdown if the threat/reward increases in intensity and/or does not dissipate *and* the evolutionarily prepared flight/fight/approach response tendencies are ineffective or blocked. Examples of times when shutdown responses can be observed include the zoned-out and numbed expression seen among victims of kidnapping or torture, the blank look of someone who is starving or severely dehydrated, the person who is afraid of flying who faints upon entering an aircraft.

Lesson 2 Homework

1. **(Required) Worksheet 2.A (Identifying the Different Neural Substrates).** Ask if there are any questions about how to use the worksheet.

2. **(Optional) Encourage participants to practice self-enquiry when they observe an unwanted emotion, using the sample questions in handout 1.3 (Learning from Self-Enquiry) to facilitate their practice.**

Radical Openness Handout 2.1

The RO DBT Neuroregulatory Model of Emotions

	Neuroception[a] of Evocative Cues[b]				
	Safety Cue	Novelty Cue	Rewarding Cue	Threatening Cue	Overwhelming Cue
Primary neural substrate response	PNS[c]-VVC[d] engaged	PNS-VVC withdrawn without SNS[e] activation	SNS-E[f] (excitatory) engaged	SNS-D[g] (defensive) engaged	PNS-DVC[h] engaged
ANS system triggered	Social safety engagement system (*adaptive function*: enhances intraspecies communication, facilitates social connectedness)	Orienting and primary appraisal system (*adaptive function*: provides a quick means to identify and appropriately respond to environmental threats or rewards)	Excitatory approach system (*adaptive function*: promotes goal-pursuit behaviors that maximize goal attainment)	Defensive avoidance system (*adaptive function*: promotes defensive fight and flight behaviors that maximize harm avoidance)	Emergency shutdown systems (*adaptive function*: conserve vital energy reserves needed for survival when SNS fight/flight/approach responses are ineffective)
Primary action urge	Socialize	Stand still	Approach or pursue	Flee or attack	Give up
Automonic responses	Body is relaxed / Breathing is slow and deep / Heart rate is reduced	Body is frozen / Breath is suspended / Orientation is toward cue	Body is animated and vivacious / Breathing is faster / Heart rate is fast	Body is tense and agitated / Breathing is fast, shallow / Heart rate is fast / Sweating	Body is immobile / Heart rate and breathing is slowed / Increased pain threshold
Emotion words associated with interoceptive experience[i]	Relaxed, sociable, contented, open, playful	Alert but not aroused; curious, focused, evaluative	Excited, elated, passionate, goal-driven	Anxious or irritated, defensively aroused	Numb, unresponsive, trancelike, nonreactive, apathetic, insensitive to pain

	Safety Cue	Novelty Cue	Rewarding Cue	Threatening Cue	Overwhelming Cue
Impact on social signaling	Social signaling enhanced	Social signaling capacities momentarily suspended	Empathic perception impaired; individual still expressive	Empathic perception capacities and prosocial signaling capacities both impaired	SNS fight/flight/approach responses withdrawn; social signaling irrelevant
Action or expression (overt behavior or social signal)	Effortless eye contact and facial expressions Listening to and touching others Appearing approachable, sociable, receptive, open to exploration	Orienting response ("What is it?") Stopping, looking, listening	Excitatory approach Goal-driven behavior Expansive gestures Insensitivity to others' facial expressions and subtle social cues	Constrained facial expressions, tight gestures Monotonic voice Averted gaze or hostile stare Fight-or-flight response	Flat, unexpressive face Monotonic voice Slow speech Dissociation, swooning, fainting

[a] The term *neuroception* denotes how a person appraises or assesses evocative stimuli. Primary appraisals are quick evaluations, elicited without conscious awareness and originating at the sensory receptor level. Secondary appraisals are slower, top-down reappraisals of primary evaluations; they involve evolutionarily newer central cognitive and conscious levels of emotional processing.

[b] A *cue* is an emotionally evocative stimulus that occurs inside the body (a happy memory, for example), outside the body (an unexpected loud noise), or as a function of context (the time of day).

[c] PNS = parasympathetic nervous system.

[d] PNS-VVC = ventral vagal complex ("new" vagus) of the parasympathetic nervous system; social safety system.

[e] SNS = sympathetic nervous system; activating system.

[f] SNS-E = SNS excitatory approach system.

[g] SNS-D = SNS defensive avoidance system.

[h] PNS-DVC = dorsal vagal complex ("old" vagus) of the parasympathetic nervous system; shutdown system.

[i] The term *interoceptive* refers to emotion-based phenomena and sensations occurring inside the body.

Radical Openness Handout 2.2

Main Points for Lesson 2: Understanding Emotions

1. Our neurosensory system is constantly scanning the world and ourselves for the presence of cues or stimuli relevant to our well-being.

2. Our brains are hardwired to detect and react to five broad classes of emotionally relevant stimuli or cues.

3. Safety cues are stimuli associated with feeling protected, secure, loved, fulfilled, cared for, and part of a community or tribe.

4. Novel cues are discrepant or unexpected stimuli that trigger an automatic evaluative process designed to determine whether the cue is important for our well-being.

5. Rewarding cues are cues appraised as potentially gratifying or pleasurable.

6. Threatening cues are cues appraised as potentially dangerous or damaging.

7. Overwhelming cues trigger our emergency shutdown system.

8. We are never unemotional, because we are always in one of the five emotional mood states.

9. Broadly speaking, when one emotional system is on, the other four are off or inhibited.

10. Finally, when an emotional response tendency is ineffective, we move to another neuroregulatory response.

Radical Openness Worksheet 2.A

Identifying the Different Neural Substrates

Instructions: During the coming week, be on the lookout for experiences and events linked to changes in body sensations and mood states (for example, felt suddenly very hot, unexpectedly felt keyed up, without warning was suddenly very tired, a headache rapidly came on, all of a sudden began to sweat). Use the following skills to identify which of the five emotional response systems may have been involved and to pinpoint the name of the emotion you may have been experiencing.

Step 1. Describe the cue that triggered your emotional response.

Use the following questions to facilitate your description.

- *Did the cue occur inside your body*—for example, a memory about an ex-partner?
- *Did the cue occur outside your body*—for example, a loud bang, a beautiful sunset?
- *To what extent did contextual factors matter*—for example, time of day, season of the year?

Describe other features of the emotion-eliciting cue.

_____

_____

_____

_____

Step 2. Use your body to identify the emotional system triggered by your cue.

Place a checkmark in the box next to the statement that best describes how your body felt.

- ☐ My body felt relaxed and calm (social safety cue).
- ☐ My body felt alert and focused (novelty cue).
- ☐ My body felt energized and powerful (rewarding cue).
- ☐ My body felt tense, agitated, and hot (threatening cue).
- ☐ My body felt numb and detached from reality (overwhelming cue).

Describe other body sensations.

_____

_____

_____

_____

Step 3. Observe how you socially signaled.

Place a checkmark in the box next to the questions that best address your experience.

- ☐ Was it easy to make eye contact or express your emotions? Was your voice tone easygoing? Did you touch or reach out to someone? (likely the parasympathetic social safety system)

- ☐ Did you suddenly find yourself standing still and gazing intently? Or listening carefully? (likely novelty-evaluative system)

- ☐ Were you highly expressive, talkative, or using expansive gestures? Did it require effort to listen to others? Did it seem like you had missed something important that another person had said or done during an interaction but you were unable to identify it? (likely SNS excitatory arousal system)

- ☐ Did you find it difficult to smile without feeling phony? Was your facial expression flat or stony? Did you avert your eyes or stare intensely? Did your voice tone sound flat or strident? Were your gestures tight and constrained? (likely SNS defensive arousal system)

- ☐ Were your face and body expressionless? Were your body movements slow? Was your speech rate slow and your voice tone flat? Did you stare vacantly? (likely parasympathetic shutdown system)

Describe other social signals you observed.

_____

_____

_____

_____

Step 4. Describe if there was someone with you who experienced the same external cue or trigger but signaled a different response to you.

_____

_____

_____

_____

Record other emotional response tendencies or reactions.

_____

_____

_____

_____

Activating Social Safety

Main Points for Lesson 3

1. Overcontrolled individuals are biotemperamentally (genetically) threat-sensitive, making it more likely for them to unintentionally carry defensive moods and behaviors (hunting dogs, shields, and swords) with them into social situations that can lead to social ostracism.

2. One can naturally improve social connectedness by changing one's physiology by activating the brain's social safety system.

3. Effective emotional expression is always *context*-dependent—that is, sometimes not expressing an emotion is the most effective way to manage a given situation.

Materials Needed

- Handout 3.1 (Changing Social Interactions by Changing Physiology)

- Handout 3.2 (Closed-Mouth Cooperative Smile)

- (Optional) Handout 3.3 (Main Points for Lesson 3: Activating Social Safety)

- Worksheet 3.A (Activating Social Safety)

- Whiteboard or flipchart with marker

(Required) Discussion Point

Hunting Dogs, Shields, and Swords

"The Story of the Disliked Friend"

Read the following text aloud.

There once was a man who believed no one liked him.

His friend said, "Just go to the village and spend time in the square. You will see that none avoid you."

The man said, "You don't understand—people really hate me. They look at me as if something is wrong with me. I don't see how this would work."

Finally his friend convinced him to try, and so he did.

The next week his friend asked, "How did it go at the village?"

The man replied, "I did just as you said. I went to the village with my three hunting dogs—restrained of course—my shield on my back, and my sword in my belt. You never can be too cautious! What might you think happened? The mothers in the village picked up their children and took them inside. The fathers glared at me with contempt, and not a soul came to speak to me on the bench I sat on in the center of the square. My dogs weren't even barking that much! And you think people like me?"

✓ **Ask:** *What do you think are the main points of this story?*

Answer: The point is that overcontrolled individuals are likely to bring moods and behaviors (hunting dogs, shields, and swords) into social situations that make those situations worse. This can range from relatively subtle behaviors, such as neutral facial expressions and fake smiles, to more obviously problematic behaviors, such as accusing others of nefarious motives. Though these strategies are designed to protect them from harm, they damage relationships and most importantly the reactions of others tend to reinforce their beliefs and habits.

✓ **Ask:** *What types of hunting dogs, shields, and swords do you take with you when you go to the village?* For example, it is not uncommon for participants to report that they exhibit blank facial expressions or habitually force smiles even when distressed. They may remain on the outskirts of conversation circles, unknowingly scowl when they go to a party, or be overly apologetic (or never apologize).

✓ **Ask:** *Is it possible that your tendency to control emotions may have social consequences that you do not intend? How has this impacted your interpersonal relationships?*

NOTE TO INSTRUCTORS: Broadly speaking, the brain system that arouses us (the sympathetic nervous system, or SNS) and the brain system that calms us (the parasympathetic nervous system, or PNS) operate as antagonists; when one is on, the other is off (Berntson, Cacioppo, & Quigley, 1991).

NOTE TO INSTRUCTORS: Instructors should be aware that the SNS and PNS can also be coactivated, with one being dominant. For example, when going to a job interview one hopes to be in one's social safety system yet it is likely that one will also feel somewhat anxious (see lesson 2).

(Required) Teaching Point
The Social Safety System

- *When we perceive the world as unsafe our defensive-threat system goes on the alert.*

- *We lose our ability to flexibly interact with others and our facial expressions become frozen because our body is preparing for action* (fight/flight).

- *For example, when we feel anxious or threatened, smiling is likely to feel false, inauthentic, or forced.* This is true for everyone.

  ✓ **Ask:** *Have you ever noticed that it is harder to sing, listen, or genuinely express positive feelings toward others when distressed or tense?*

- *The good news is that we can turn off or minimize defensive arousal by activating an area of our brain linked with social safety* (Porges, 1995). For example, activating our social safety system automatically alters frozen facial expressions because we feel naturally more easygoing and flexibly expressive.

- *When the social safety system is on, the defensive-threat system is off or minimized.* This is because our brain is hardwired such that when one emotional system is on (for example, excitatory reward system), the others (for example, defensive-threat system, social safety system, novelty-orienting system) are downregulated in order to allow full expression of the emotional system being activated (see lesson 2).

✓ **Ask:** *Have you ever noticed that you cannot feel both calm and fearful at the same time? Similarly, we cannot simultaneously experience genuine joy and real anger at the same moment in time.*

- **The social safety system promotes social connectedness.** When activated, we experience a sense of calm readiness and a desire to affiliate with others—we are naturally more open, playful, and curious about the world.

- **Our social safety system contains nerves that govern the muscles in our body needed to communicate and form close social bonds.**

- **These social safety muscles help us to...**

  - **Hear better what others are saying** by tuning in to the higher-frequency sound vibrations associated with human speech (middle ear muscles)

  - **Communicate warmth and friendliness to others** via a musical tone of voice (laryngeal and pharyngeal or voice box muscles)

  - **Signal authenticity and trustworthiness to others** by openly revealing (rather than hiding) our facial expressions of emotion (facial muscles)

(Required) Class Exercise
Playing with Eyebrows

Teach: An eyebrow wag involves raising both eyebrows and universally signals affection and liking. It is our friendly signal. It most often occurs without awareness and is usually accompanied by a slight smile and warm eye contact. Without words it says to another person "I like you" and "You are in my tribe." It can often be seen when friends initially greet each other. For example, when a person greets someone they have affection for they are likely to quickly and unconsciously raise their eyebrows during the greeting. And their friend is likely to do the same.

Instruct class members to pair up with a partner. Instructors may need to partner up with someone (it is very important to have everyone participate).

Begin the exercise by reading the following text.

> *Imagine that your partner is a long-lost best friend and you happen to run into them unexpectedly at an airport. You are delighted and ecstatic at seeing them again—it has been maybe ten years since you last saw them! Wow, what a lucky break! So, with this in mind, turn toward you partner and greet them as your long-lost friend, just like you would in real life. Go! Go! Greet your long-lost friend now!* [Encourage everyone to turn to their partner and practice greeting them.]

After approximately one minute, stop the exercise, and exclaim, *Well done!* Without discussion, **immediately begin the next practice** by reading aloud the following text.

> *Now we are going to do the same thing—we are going to greet our long-lost friend in the airport! Only this time, when you greet them, make sure that you **do not** use any eyebrow wags! Meaning, this time greet them, just like before, but with eyebrows down. Okay, Go! Go! Greet that friend— remember to keep those eyebrows down!*

After approximately one minute, stop the exercise and solicit observations from the class about the differences between the two greetings. Then use the following required teaching points to explain the significance of the exercise.

✓ **Ask:** *What were the differences between the two interactions? Which way felt more natural? What did you notice in your body? When your eyebrows were down, did it change your experience? Did you notice any changes in your voice tone? (Usually most people notice that they lost their musical tone of voice, that they became monotonic.) Did you notice any differences in desires to spend time with them or feel close or trusting toward them? How easy was it to smile with eyebrows down? Did it influence the words you used? Did you feel more or less like touching them? What else did you notice?*

(Required) Teaching Points

Talking Eyebrows

- *It's important to know where your eyebrows are when you are talking because their placement (up or down) matters when it comes not only to how we feel inside but how we impact others.*

- *What's amazing is that our social safety system can be turned on or turned off simply by how we move our facial muscles and/or position our body* (see lesson 2). This is because our neuroregulatory system is bidirectional, meaning our facial expressions, the gestures we use, and our body movements can alter how we feel about ourselves, other people, and the world.

- *The bidirectional nature of our neuroregulatory system also highlights how social signaling impacts our desires to socially connect with each other.*

- *Our next set of skills will build on these observations.*

(Required) Teaching Point

Activating Our Social Safety System

Refer participants to handout 3.1 (Changing Social Interactions by Changing Physiology).

NOTE TO INSTRUCTORS: The social safety system can just as easily be switched off. We can easily reactivate our threat system simply by thinking about something unpleasant or simply talking to someone using a flat facial expression or by inhibiting an eyebrow wag when greeting someone (see "Playing with Eyebrows" class exercise). Thus, instructors should remind participants that they will need to reactivate their social safety system repeatedly, particularly when in a threatening environment.

> NOTE TO INSTRUCTORS: When teaching each of the following strategies, instructors should create opportunities for minipractices in class using the examples provided or by creating new ones. For example, instructors should lead participants in a progressive muscle relaxation exercise, or bring in soft furry objects and ask participants to stroke their face with the object, and ask participants to practice hugging themselves. Importantly, instructors should encourage everyone to participate. See "Instructor Guidelines for 'Participate Without Planning' Practices," in lesson 12, for tips on how to introduce (or not introduce— tee hee ☺) each miniexercise.

- *The Big Three + 1 skills.* There are three + 1 (conditional) ways to activate our social safety system that work almost anywhere and anytime, regardless of how stressful the situation may feel. I call these four behaviors the Big Three + 1. When we engage them, our brain reacts as if all is well.

  - *If you are sitting down, start with the (+ 1)—this step involves leaning back in your chair (rather than sitting forward).* It is a bit like slouching or relaxing on a big couch—it says to your brain, "I'm chilled out." The + 1 can only be used when sitting, which is why it is separated from the other three.

  - *Next, engage the Big Three by taking a slow deep breath, displaying a closed-mouth cooperative smile, and using an eyebrow wag.* The Big Three can be done at the same time, whether one is sitting, standing, or lying down.

    - *A slow deep breath tells your brain "all is well."* It works by moving a band of muscle beneath your lungs, known as the diaphragm muscle, that helps facilitate deep breathing during states of rest or relaxation. The diaphragm muscle is innervated by the nerves in your PNS-VVC social safety system. Taking a slow deep breath moves your diaphragm muscle in such a way that it signals to your brain that "all must be well" (because when we are threatened we either hold our breath or breathe faster and more shallowly). It can be likened to a "sigh of contentment."

    - *Closed-mouth cooperative smiles:* A closed-mouth cooperative smile involves turning both corners of the mouth upward, stretching the lips over the teeth but keeping the mouth closed so that your teeth are not exposed **(refer participants to handout 3.2)**. It almost always is accompanied by direct eye contact, a slight constriction or narrowing of the eyes, and crow's-feet wrinkles that characterize genuine smiles of pleasure (that is, *orbicularis oculi* muscle activation).

    - *An eyebrow wag involves raising both eyebrows and universally signals affection and liking.* Eyebrow wags are almost always accompanied by a slight smile, eye contact, and a musical tone of voice. They can be seen when friends initially greet each other and/or during interactions among people who find each other attractive, or interesting.

- *The social safety system comes on fast and can go off just as fast (in milliseconds).* Therefore, when stressed or in a threatening situation, it is very important to repeat the Big Three + 1 multiple times and to not be discouraged if the effects seem to go away. Repeating them will just as quickly bring them back. Plus, the Big Three + 1 have the added advantage of signaling friendliness, which may help reduce stress for all involved.

NOTE TO INSTRUCTORS: Contrary to other consciously produced smiles, the closed-mouth cooperative smile can be held static for relatively long periods of time without feeling contrived or phony. The closed-mouth smile is more likely to be experienced by both the sender and receiver as a genuine smile of pleasure and as a consequence trigger reciprocal smiling and/or social safety responses (for example, via PNS-VVC activation). Often an automatic sigh of contentment accompanies or occurs immediately after engaging a closed-mouth cooperative smile, suggesting PNS-VVC social safety activation. This can be used to confirm successful engagement of closed-mouth cooperative smiles and can be especially helpful when first learning how to use them. The closed-mouth cooperative smile differs from the averted gaze and bowed head that characterizes the closed-mouth appeasement smile or smile of embarrassment (Sarra & Otta, 2001). It also differs from what is known as the *half smile* (see Linehan, 1993b). The half smile is less expressive—that is, it does not involve stretching the lips, it is less wide, and it is less likely to be associated with crow's-feet wrinkles around the eyes. Instead, the half smile is more physically similar to a burglar smile and as a consequence can be easily misread. Half smiles and burglar smiles are associated with a wide range of differing emotions and intentions, ranging from contentment to strong dislike and feeling pleasure in another's misfortune. The world's best-known half smile—that is, Leonardo da Vinci's painting known as the *Mona Lisa*—is intriguing precisely because the elusive smile on the woman's face is so subtly shadowed that the exact nature of the smile cannot be determined, with interpretations ranging from pleasure to disdain (see Livingstone, 2000).

(Required) Class Exercise
The Big Three + 1

Let's practice. To start, we need to get our body into a position that normally signals to our brain that we are anxious, tense, or uptight. To do this, everyone should adopt a very erect sitting posture that leans forward slightly (almost as if ready to run), adopt a frozen or flat facial expression, and then slightly tense as many muscles as you can throughout your body without making it obvious (this mimics bodily tension).

Use the *Big Three + 1* to activate your social safety system: (1) sit back in your chairs, lean away, and adopt a relaxed sitting posture; (2) take a slow deep breath (3) while closed-mouth smiling, and (4) add an eyebrow wag (raise your eyebrows). Instructors should demonstrate how this looks—and then have the class mimic it.

Play While You Teach

Instruct the class to mimic your sitting posture, gestures, and facial expressions. For example, instructors can exaggerate chilled-out, relaxed, and loafing sitting positions, pretend to be asleep then suddenly sit upright, then fall back again into a different relaxed pose, or pretend to be drunk or stoned, or encourage everyone to practice while speaking with an exaggerated hippie voice: *Hey man, let's just chill out and lay back—put those eyebrows up, sit back, and just let the world roll by. Get that closed-mouth smile on and breathe in the love. Let it all hang out. Feeling groovy and letting it be. Yeah, this is the life.*

Ask participants to adopt their best laid-back posture and then go around and adjust the posture for those having difficulty.

Make being laid back a contest—that is, who has the most chilled-out posture? Or who has the best eyebrow wag? Or let's play the "Who Can Be Less Competitive?" game! The only problem is, if you win, you lose—but when you lose, you win…hmmm. This should be fun.

- **Then discuss:** What did it feel like to do the Big Three + 1? What did you notice? Did you notice anything different in your body? Which of the four actions did you find easy to do? Which was more difficult? Remember to practice the difficult one until it becomes easy.

NOTE TO INSTRUCTORS: Some OC clients will report feeling awkward when engaging in the preceding practice. Most typically this occurs when they try to lean back in their chair. Most often this is because they don't normally sit like this (particularly in public) and they may have been told by parents or teachers "Sit up straight!" or "Don't slouch!" Instructors can play with different postures to help loosen up overlearned inhibitions about body posture.

(Required) Teaching Point

Expansive Gestures Communicate Safety

- Expansive gestures communicate safety via the facilitative component of emotions. Recall that humans reciprocally mimic the facial expressions of others, which triggers similar emotional experiences in them. When we use expansive gestures and facial expressions, we not only trigger our own social safety system but we send an important social signal to others—that is, that we trust them, thereby facilitating activation of social safety in the person we are interacting with (via micromimicry and mirror neurons). When we are defensively aroused, we tend to tighten up; our gestures and body movements are more likely to be smaller and closer to the body (for protection). So, when feeling tense, move your facial muscles, and use big expansive gestures with open hands rather than keeping your arms and hands close to your body. Open your hands (rather than clenching), place your palms upwards (rather than palms down), and practice talking with your hands. When alone and tense, scrunch your face muscles, stick your tongue out as far as it can go while opening your eyes wide, flap your arms and legs about, and make frequent eyebrow wags. All of these body movements will send the message to your brain that all must be well because otherwise you wouldn't be moving like this (that is, we are not expansive in our gestures and facial expressions when uptight).

(Required) Class Exercise

Practice Big Gestures

Instructors should ask the class to mimic their body gestures as they teach the preceding points, and purposely exaggerate them. For example, make your eyebrows go up and down, then scrunch your eyes together, pucker your mouth and then stretch your lips as wide as they can go, open your mouth and eyes as wide as they can go, stick out your tongue as far as it can go, raise your eyebrows and stretch all of these muscles as much as you can at the same time. Now close your eyes as hard as you can and scrunch up all of the muscles in your face—tense them all as hard as you can—then release the tension.

Tense and release as many different facial muscles as you can and see if you can find all of them. Rotate your head from side to side, up and down, stretching and tensing each muscle. Use your hands to massage the muscles in your face. Stretch your arms up to the ceiling, open your hands palms-upward, and try to make up gestures that incorporate palms up. Be creative—pretend you are talking with someone, and try to come up with as many new gestures as you can think of; purposefully exaggerate your body movements. The idea is to make this fun and a communal exercise—it need only last a few minutes, albeit ideally it is repeated multiple times, either throughout the current lesson or as an ice-breaker at the start of teaching or prior to other RO "participate without planning" practices. Participants should be encouraged to practice big gestures in front of a mirror at home and to incorporate these facial and body exercises into their daily routine with as much repetition as possible throughout their day (for example, tensing and relaxing facial muscles while driving).

(Required) Teaching Point

The "Slow Your Breath" Skill

- **The "slow your breath" skill: Deliberately breathe more deeply and slowly; use long, slow exhalations.** Hyperventilation is highly associated with extreme fears when under threat. Slowing breathing to approximately six breaths per minute (one complete breath cycle lasting ten to twelve seconds) is effective at reducing emotional arousal. Normally most people breathe at a much higher rate. Instructors should emphasize abdominal breathing (breathing that moves the diaphragmatic muscles in the abdomen) rather than shallow chest breathing.

(Required) Class Exercise

Slowing Our Breath

Instructors should conduct a brief mindfulness practice that emphasizes the importance of slow and deep breathing. Time the practice to last one minute. Instruct participants to count one inhalation-exhalation cycle as one breath. Encourage participants to slow down their rate of breathing to approximately six breaths per minute. Remind them the goal is not to be perfect (that is, that they must have only six breaths) but to slow the rate down substantially. The belly should rise on the inbreath and not the chest. Ask each participant to report the number they had during the one-minute practice, then conduct the practice again.

(Required) Teaching Point

The Tense-and-Relax Skill

- **The tense-and-relax skill: Deliberately tense and relax large muscle groups.** This is one of the most commonly used methods of relaxation. It consists of first tensing an entire limb and holding the tension for a brief moment, then relaxing the tension. There are progressive muscle relaxation scripts available on the internet. Participants should be strongly encouraged to look for commercially produced relaxation tapes. Body-scan mindfulness practices may share some features with progressive muscle relaxation techniques, because of their focus on the body, and may also be used.

(Optional) Class Exercise
Muscle Relaxation Exercise

Conduct a progressive muscle relaxation exercise during class. Record it and give the audiorecording to participants as a means for practice, or ask participants to record it themselves (most mobile phones have an audiorecorder nowadays). Start with the toes and feet, asking participants to tense the muscle, hold the tension, and slowly release. Move then to legs and torso, then to arms and neck, and finally the facial muscles.

(Required) Teaching Point
Using Touch, Chewing, Hearing, and Vision Skills

- *Using touch, deep pressure, massage, and hugs.* For humans, body sensations linked to physical closeness and touch are universally experienced as comforting because they signal to our brain that we are back in the tribe and therefore safe. You can use touch to trigger social safety, even when others are not around. For example, practice touching or hugging soft objects (furry pets, stuffed toys, pillows); lightly stroke your face and neck; massage the muscles of your face, scalp, and neck. Participants should also be encouraged to stroke pets, ask for hugs from a close friend or partner, get a neck or back massage, buy a massaging machine, wrap themselves tightly in blankets or towels (swaddling), hug themselves by wrapping their arms across their chests, stroke their own faces or necks, and hold warm water bottles against their stomachs.

- *Using the chewing skill.* Our brains associate eating and chewing with rest and digestion. Chewing moves the muscles of the face linked to social safety and has been shown to facilitate memory and reduce stress (Weijenberg & Lobbezoo, 2015). Swallowing food naturally calms the body; it is difficult to swallow when really upset. Look for your favorite calming foods and incorporate them into everyday living. Chewing gum is another means to accomplish the same thing but without needing to actually ingest food. (*Note:* Chewing gums without laxative properties should be suggested when working with anorexia nervosa.)

- *Using sounds to enhance social safety.* The muscles of our inner ear that allow us to hear human speech are linked to the brain regions of our social safety system. When we feel threatened, our ability to hear others literally diminishes. Music can modulate brain activity in emotion-processing areas. When stressed you can use calm, soothing music to activate your social safety system. Avoid music that is arousing, disturbing, or exciting. Because the human voice can calm, use vocal music you find soothing.

- *Using vision to enhance social safety* by gazing at pictures of loved ones, pets, or landscapes. You can trigger your social safety system by gazing at pictures linked to warmth, expansion, or a sense of peace. These might be pictures of a friend, your child or grandchild when young, a favorite pet, or your partner in a place that brings back warm memories. Use pictures you can carry with you and look at when you feel threatened or tense. As you gaze, breathe deeply and notice what happens.

(Optional) Teaching Points

Downregulating Defensive Arousal via Activation of Other Neural Substrates

Activation of other autonomic nervous systems (such as the SNS-appetitive or SNS-excitatory and the PNS-DVC) has been shown to operate in similar neuroinhibitory ways as activation of the social safety system (the PNS-VVC; see lesson 2)—that is, they function to inhibit or turn off defensive arousal. Two examples:

1. *The dive reflex or ice-cold water on face.* A forehead cold-pressor test (for example, placing forehead and eyes in a bowl of ice water and holding one's breath) replicates the dive reflex and increases vagal activity (Hughes & Stoney, 2000; Khurana, Watabiki, Hebel, Toro, & Nelson, 1980; Linehan, Bohus, & Lynch, 2007). The dive reflex slows heart rate and produces a feeling of slowing down, and we posit that the dive reflex likely activates the PNS-DVC (see lesson 2). The dive reflex should be used only by those for whom there is no cardiac risk or with doctor approval for those with any history of cardiac difficulties (Houk, Smith, & Wolf, 1999; Linehan et al., 2007). For example, the dive reflex should not be recommended to individuals with anorexia nervosa without medical approval, since a low body mass index (BMI) has been shown to be associated with bradycardia (slow heart rate) and electrolyte imbalances that can influence cardiac health.

2. *Intense exercise.* Intense physical exercise (for example, sit-ups or running) activates the appetitive emotional system (the excitement or pleasure part of the brain) and inhibits the defensive emotional system. In general, intense exercise should *not* be recommended to severely underweight individuals (for example, those with anorexia nervosa).

> NOTE TO INSTRUCTORS: Instructors should be aware that activation of the sympathetic nervous system, either threat or reward, is posited to inhibit activation of the PNS-VVC-mediated social safety system linked to contentment and desires for social engagement. Thus, when SNS activation occurs (either positive or negative), we lose our ability to empathetically read social signals from others and prosocially signal cooperation to others, manifested by loss of our ability to read facial affect in others, monotone voices, reduced abilities to hear human speech accurately, and loss of facial expressivity (see Porges, 2003; see also lesson 2).

Lesson 3 Homework

1. **(Required) Worksheet 3.A (Activating Social Safety).**

2. **(Optional) Build a personal contentment box.** Instructors should encourage participants to begin creating their own personal contentment box that is designed to activate the social safety system. The contentment box can be constructed over time; the idea is to start the process via a homework assignment. Encourage participants to share their box with their individual therapist.

3. **(Recommended) Bring an audiorecorder to the next lesson.** Encourage participants to bring an audiorecorder or mobile phone to the next lesson so they can record the loving kindness script that will be practiced next week.

Radical Openness Handout 3.1

Changing Social Interactions by Changing Physiology

- Our bodies are hardwired with a special regulatory system for social safety. This system calms and relaxes us.

- We have another regulatory system for defending against threats and for exciting us. This system alerts and arouses us.

- When the social safety system is activated, we feel open, flexible, and relaxed; we are more likely to want to explore, play, and socialize—it's our friendly state.

- When our social safety system is on, our defensive system is off or muted. We can't be relaxed and angry, afraid and content, or excited and calm at the same time.

- The good news is that when stressed or anxious, we can turn our social safety system on and our threat-emotion system off by doing certain behaviors that our brain naturally links to safety.

- Thus, we don't have to *think* our way out of anxiety; we can *do* our way out.

- So if you want to feel less tension, let your body do the work!

Practice These Skills

- *Use the Big Three + 1.* Lean back in your chair, take a slow deep breath, make a closed-mouth smile, and use an eyebrow wag.

- *Use big expansive gestures with open hands* rather than keeping your arms and hands close to your body.

- *Move your facial muscles.* When threatened or tense, our facial muscles naturally become frozen and we lose our ability to flexibly communicate via facial expressions. By deliberately moving our facial muscles, we send safety signals to our brain. Facial movement tells our brain, "I must be safe because I am not trying to mask my inner feelings." In front of a mirror at home or elsewhere, when alone, practice tensing, releasing, and stretching your facial muscles. Exaggerate your facial expressions. Make your eyebrows go up and down; then scrunch your eyes together; pucker your mouth; then stretch your lips as wide as they can go, open your mouth and eyes as wide as they can go, stick out your tongue as far as it can go; then raise your eyebrows and stretch all of these muscles as much as you can at the same time. Now close your eyes as hard as you can and scrunch up all of the muscles in your face, and tense them all as hard as you can—then release the tension. Tense and release as many different facial muscles as you can—see if you can find all of them! Repeat whenever possible throughout your day.

- *Deliberately breathe more deeply and slowly; use long, slow exhalations.* Purposely exhale longer than normal. Slow your rate of breathing to six breaths per minute; on inbreath, focus on raising the belly, not the chest.

- *Deliberately tense and relax large muscle groups.* Start with your toes and feet, then to legs and torso, then to your arms and neck, and then to your facial muscles. Tense each set of muscles, hold the tension, then slowly release the tension and notice the difference.

- *Use touch, deep pressure, massage, and hugs.* Practice touching or hugging soft objects (furry pets, stuffed toys, pillows); lightly stroke your face and neck; massage the muscles of your face, scalp, and neck. Locate the spot directly beneath the beginning of each eyebrow in the uppermost corner of each eye socket; use both thumbs to press this spot in an upward direction, and notice what happens. Wrap yourself tightly in blankets or towels (swaddling). Place a small heavy beanbag or sandbag over your forehead and thighs—notice what happens. Hug yourself by crossing both arms over your upper chest until your hands can reach your upper back, then rock your body slowly back and forth. Rub your tummy in a clockwise direction. Wrap a hot water bottle in a towel, lie on the floor, and place a cushion under each knee, then place the hot water bottle over your belly—notice what happens. Gently but firmly press the space in between the webbing of your thumb and pointer finger—notice what happens. Purchase a commercially available massaging machine or vibrating/massaging chair. Take a warm bath or shower; use the jet sprays in hot tubs to massage your back and neck. If you have a partner or friend to practice with, ask for a neck or foot massage; ask for a hug and squeeze firmly—practice hugging each day, if possible. Lie down on the floor and allow your friend to gently support your head in his or her hands; then, with your fingers, gently rub the point directly above the bridge of your nose adjacent to each eyebrow. Experiment with using the sensation of touch—be creative—and incorporate touch into each day.

- *Chewing and eating food.* When anxious, our bodies are tense and ready for action. Our brain associates eating and chewing with resting and digesting, not fleeing or fighting. Chewing moves the muscles of the face linked to social safety. It is difficult to swallow when really upset; chewing and swallowing food naturally calms the body. Look for your favorite calming foods (for example, milk and cookies) and incorporate these into everyday living. Carry sugar-free chewing gum, sweets, or snack bars with you. When stressed, rather than restricting intake, start chewing and moving those facial muscles.

- *Hearing—music and the human voice.* When stressed, use music that you find calming or soothing and/or recordings of the human voice that you find calming to activate your social safety system. Avoid listening to music that is arousing, disturbing, or exciting.

- *Vision—gazing at pictures of loved ones, pets, or landscapes.* You can trigger your social safety system by gazing at pictures linked to warmth, expansion, or a sense of peace. These might be pictures of a friend, your child or grandchild, a favorite pet, or your partner in a place that brings back warm memories. Use pictures you can carry with you and look at when you feel threatened or tense. As you gaze, breathe deeply and notice what happens.

Radical Openness Handout 3.2

Closed-Mouth Cooperative Smile

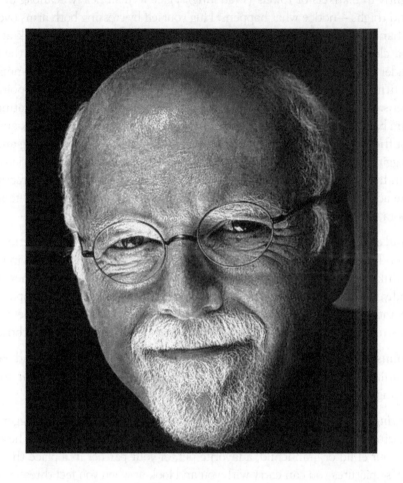

Radical Openness Handout 3.3

Main Points for Lesson 3: Activating Social Safety

1. Overcontrolled individuals are biotemperamentally (genetically) threat-sensitive, making it more likely for them to unintentionally carry defensive moods and behaviors (hunting dogs, shields, and swords) with them into social situations that can lead to social ostracism.

2. One can naturally improve social connectedness by changing one's physiology by activating the brain's social safety system.

3. Effective emotional expression is always *context*-dependent—that is, sometimes not expressing an emotion is the most effective way to manage a given situation.

Radical Openness Worksheet 3.A

Activating Social Safety

Look for opportunities to practice activating your social safety system. Describe the event you chose.

_____

_____

_____

_____

Observe and describe any hunting dogs, shields, or swords that you may have wanted to bring into a social situation—for example, frowning when entering a room, pretending to feel okay when not, and so forth.

_____

_____

_____

_____

Place a checkmark in the box next to each strategy you practiced, and in the spaces following each strategy, briefly describe your emotional experience, and rate the intensity of the emotion or body tension **before and after trying the strategy** (using a scale from 1 to 10, with 1 signifying low intensity, 5 moderate intensity, and 9 or 10 extremely intense).

☐ Adjusted my body posture by using the Big Three + 1—leaned back, took a deep breath, made a closed-mouth smile, and used an eyebrow wag.

_____

Intensity before _____   Intensity after _____

☐ Used big gestures with open hands rather than keeping my arms and hands close to my body.

_____

Intensity before _____   Intensity after _____

☐ Deliberately practiced exaggerating facial expressions and moving facial muscles.

_____

Intensity before _____   Intensity after _____

☐ Deliberately slowed my breath and used long slow exhalations.

_____

Intensity before _____   Intensity after _____

☐ Deliberately tensed and relaxed large muscle groups in my body.

_____

Intensity before _____   Intensity after _____

☐ Used touch, deep pressure, hugs, and massage.

_____

Intensity before _____   Intensity after _____

☐ Ate calming food(s) or chewed gum.

_____

Intensity before _____   Intensity after _____

☐ Used hearing by listening to soothing music and soothing voices.

_____

Intensity before _____   Intensity after _____

☐ Used vision by gazing at pictures of loved ones, pets, or landscapes.

_____

Intensity before _____   Intensity after _____

Describe other social safety activation skills you used.

_____

_____

_____

_____

_____

Enhancing Openness and Social Connection via Loving Kindness

NOTE TO INSTRUCTORS: Loving kindness meditation (LKM), when taught in skills class, will often be a review for the majority of participants, since it is also taught in RO DBT individual therapy (ideally, about the seventh individual therapy session). This allows for some flexibility in teaching; for example, if all class members are already using LKM, then instructors can quickly review the main principles, conduct an LKM practice, and then troubleshoot problems that participants may be experiencing applying LKM in their lives. If there is additional class time available, instructors should use the time to ask how overall use of RO DBT skills is going and address problems, ask for any questions about material covered in prior lessons, conduct one of the optional class exercises, or teach other optional material that had not been covered.

Main Points for Lesson 4

1. Loving kindness meditation (LKM) is a type of mood induction that activates our brain's social safety system.

2. LKM practices in RO DBT are designed to be used prior to social encounters (social safety effects have been reported to last from twenty minutes up to four hours).

3. Importantly, the overarching goal of LKM practices in RO DBT is not to improve a person's ability to experience love or kindness toward themselves or other people but instead to trigger a mood state associated with contentment, curiosity, and desires for social engagement by activating an area of the brain linked with social safety responses.

4. RO DBT LKM differs from other LKM practices. Since many OC clients can find it difficult or even distressing to consider extending feelings of warmth, kindness, or love toward themselves, LKM practices in RO DBT involve only three steps: (1) creating an experience of warmth/love/kindness, (2) extending warm feelings toward someone the client already cares about, and (3) extending warm feelings toward a neutral person.

Materials Needed

- Handout 4.1 (A Script for Loving Kindness Meditation)
- (Optional) Handout 4.2 (Main Points for Lesson 4: Enhancing Openness and Social Connection via Loving Kindness)

- Worksheet 4.A (Daily Practice of Loving Kindness Meditation)

- Digital audiorecorder: Ideally, each participant has brought with them some type of audiorecording device (for example, a mobile phone) to record the instructor's voice during the upcoming loving kindness practice.

NOTE TO INSTRUCTORS: Instructors should be alert for participant responses that may be judgmental, dismissive, or uncomfortable with concepts related to love, kindness, or compassion. For some OC participants, the idea of love is fake or phony or they may believe that those who desire love are naive or childish. Since LKM is derived from Buddhist traditions, many may find this off-putting because it may imply that we are pushing religion or trying to make them spiritual. Instructors should remind participants that the overall aim of LKM practices in RO DBT is to reduce SNS-mediated defensive arousal by inducing a positive mood state linked to the social safety system.

(Required) Teaching Points

Loving Kindness Meditation

- **Loving kindness meditation is a way of enhancing kindness and positive mood states as well as social connectedness.** LKM has been shown to increase feelings of warmth and care for self and others (Hofmann, Grossman, & Hinton, 2011; Salzberg, 1995). The practice of LKM has led to shifts in people's daily experiences of a wide range of positive emotions, including love, joy, gratitude, contentment, hope, pride, interest, amusement, and awe. Loving kindness has been beneficial in reducing pain, anger, and psychological distress in participants (Carson et al., 2005). Positive effects can occur even if the practitioner has little prior experience and with only a few minutes of training. Short practices of LKM (about seven minutes) have been shown in experimental studies to significantly increase positivity and social connectedness toward others (Hutcherson, Seppala, & Gross, 2008).

- **RO DBT practices of LKM are designed to activate the neurobiological social safety system** (PNS-VVC; see lesson 2). Changing physiology prior to social interactions is essential for threat-sensitive OC individuals in order to enhance social bonds. The goal is to develop a new habit that will allow one to induce a mood state associated with safety and contentment prior to social interactions. A minipractice can take four minutes or less and may simply involve repeating a few phrases that generate feelings of safety, kindness, or warmth while closed-mouth smiling and breathing slowly.

- **Even small amounts of generated love, warmth, kindness, or tenderness appear to be all that is needed to begin this work.** Research suggests that with continued practice one develops the ability to more easily generate these feelings (Carson et al., 2005).

NOTE TO INSTRUCTORS: Unlike many traditional LKM practices, RO DBT has purposely removed LKM steps that involve extending love or kindness toward oneself, a difficult person, or the world. Our reasoning is simple. The primary goal of LKM is to activate the social safety system in order to enhance social connectedness. Many OC clients find LKM practices that involve extending kindness or warmth toward themselves (or problematic individuals) to be difficult, thereby activating SNS-mediated defensive arousal rather than social safety. Therefore, we have purposefully removed three of the steps common among traditional LKM practices as a means of preventing this. In addition, some participants may ask why the words "love" and "kindness" are used if the primary goal of RO DBT LKM is to activate a mood state linked to the neurobiologically based social safety system. Instructors can explain that the words used in RO DBT LKM are those that have been researched and shown to most reliably activate social safety (that is, if saying "bloop" activated social safety, then it could be used, too). Thus, if someone strongly objects to certain words used in the LKM script (see handout 4.1), then participants should be encouraged to work with their individual therapist on finding wording that works for them (see phrases suggested later to help facilitate this). Lastly, instructors should encourage participants to establish a daily LKM practice. With repeated practice over time, many participants are able to trigger their social safety system whenever and wherever they are by simply repeating a few of the core LKM phrases (for example, "May they feel a sense of peace," "May they feel safe and secure").

(Required) Class Exercise

Loving Kindness Meditation Practice

Refer participants to handout 4.1 (A Script for Loving Kindness Meditation).

NOTE TO INSTRUCTORS: Prior to the start of reading the LKM script, instructors should ask those participants who have brought an audiorecorder (see lesson 3 homework assignments) to start their recording. Alternatively, instructors should digitally record the LKM practice (not the discussion afterward) and make this recording available to the participants. This recording can then be used by the client as a means to augment their LKM work.

Use the script provided in handout 4.1 to guide the practice. Since LKM in RO DBT is designed to generate warm feelings and activate the social safety system (PNS-VVC), instructors should feel free to adopt a calm and relaxed tone of voice while conducting the practice. Indeed, research shows that warm human voice tones can activate the PNS-VVC (Porges, 2007). The book comes with several versions of LKM audiorecordings. Participants can use these, too. However, the recordings that come with the book should not replace an in-class LKM practice (that is, do not play the book audiorecording as a replacement for a live practice).

(Required) Discussion Points
LKM Practice

After completing the loving kindness meditation, instructors should ask for observations and discuss experiences. Use the following questions as a guide. Instructors should be familiar with the obstacles outlined here and use these to facilitate teaching around any difficulties with the practice.

- ✓ **Ask:** *What did you experience during this practice?*

- ✓ **Ask:** *Were there any difficulties locating a memory or prior experience linked to loving kindness? (Instructors should validate this as normal and use the teaching points under common obstacles to help participants make sense of their experience.)*

- ✓ **Ask:** *Were you able to generate a feeling of warmth or kindness during the practice? Are you feeling more peaceful or content following this practice? If not, what was your experience?*

- ✓ **Ask:** *Did anyone experience a sense of sadness in addition to or instead of warmth?*

- ✓ **Ask:** *What are the steps you need to take to make this practice more alive for you and/or more beneficial?*

Lesson 4 Homework

1. **(Required) Handout 4.1 (A Script for Loving Kindness Meditation).**

2. **(Required) Worksheet 4.A (Daily Practice of Loving Kindness Meditation).** During the next lesson (and for the remainder of RO DBT treatment), participants should develop a daily practice of LKM (if they do not already have one). LKM can be most beneficial when practiced prior to social interactions. Participants should record their observations using worksheet 4.A. Participants can use handout 4.1 as a script or guide during their practices. However, ideally, they will use an audio-recording from either the practice done during lesson 4, an LKM practice conducted and recorded during individual therapy, or one of the several audio versions of LKM that came with the book. **Importantly,** LKM practices, scripts, or audiorecordings from other sources should not be used. The script provided in handout 4.1 is purposefully designed to promote social safety, and non–RO DBT LKM practices often have different goals and wording. Finally, participants should be encouraged to make personal audiorecordings and to involve their individual therapists in creating an LKM practice that suits them.

Radical Openness Handout 4.1

A Script for Loving Kindness Meditation

Remember, the goals of LKM practices are to induce a positive mood state associated with social safety.

- **Use the following script to make an audiorecording.** It is designed to be read aloud. We recommend that you do not change the wording. Practice using the script as it is currently written first. Research has demonstrated this script to be the most useful for people in RO DBT skills classes. If you decide you would like to make changes to the script, work with your individual therapist or skills instructor before doing so.

- **Commit to a daily practice.**

Getting seated

Find a comfortable seated position in a chair, on the floor, on the sofa. The most important thing is that you find a position in which you feel alert and the chances of you drifting off to sleep are minimal. For the practice of loving kindness you can keep your eyes open or closed—the choice is yours—with the understanding that our goal is to remain awake, as best we can.

Noticing the breath

Once you find that position, begin by simply taking a breath—with awareness. Not trying to change the breath or fix it in some way, just being fully present with the full duration of the inbreath and the full duration of the outbreath. You may notice it most strongly in the nose and the throat. Some people notice the breath in the chest or the belly. Wherever the breath is most alive for you, just allow yourself to rest your awareness there. If your mind wanders away from the breath, which it is prone to do, then, without judgment, just simply bring yourself back to the next natural inhalation or exhalation.

Finding our heart center

And now, very gently, allow your awareness to move from your breath to your heart center. Into that place, right there, in the middle of the chest. Not as much the physical heart but that place where we tend to feel warm emotions. If you would like to do so, sometimes people find it helpful to gently place their open hand over the location of their physical heart as this can help facilitate the practice.

As best you can, try and find a memory or feeling sense of a time when you experienced a strong sense of loving kindness, either from someone or toward someone. It might have been the first day you met your life partner; the day a child or grandchild was born; it might have even been a particular afternoon with your favorite pet, or a time when you felt warm appreciation after helping or being helped by someone. The idea is not to find the perfect experience or image, nor should you be concerned if you find yourself thinking of many different events or experiences. The idea is—as best you can—to re-create the warm, tender, or positive feelings associated with prior experiences of loving kindness, and to allow these feelings to grow in your heart center. For just a moment, allow these feelings to grow.

Sending loving kindness to a person we care about

And now, in your mind's eye, gently bring into focus an image of someone you care about, a person you already have existing warm feelings for, may feel love toward, or may feel a sense of positive connection with. It doesn't have to be a perfect relationship or one without conflict—the idea is to find an image or feeling sense of someone you know whom you already have warm feelings for. As best you can, hold this image or a feeling sense of this person in your heart center. And now, from the feelings of loving kindness in the center of your chest, extend warm wishes to this person you care about. Using these phrases, silently repeat to yourself…

> *May this person be at ease.*
>
> *May they be content with their life.*
>
> *May they be joyful.*
>
> *May they feel safe and secure.*

Again, extending warm wishes of loving kindness to this person you care about…

> *May they be at ease.*
>
> *May they be content with their life.*
>
> *May they be joyful.*
>
> *May they feel safe and secure.*

And again, from the source of loving kindness in your own heart, extending well wishes to this person you already care for…

> *May this person be at ease.*
>
> *May they be content with their life.*
>
> *May they experience joy.*
>
> *And may they feel safe and secure.*

And now, gradually allow the image or feeling sense of this person you care for to gently dissolve from your mind's eye, resting your attention back in your heart center, back into those feelings of warm loving kindness—as best you can.

Sending loving kindness to a person we feel neutral about

Bring to mind an image of someone who you don't really know, who you've at least seen once but don't feel any connection with one way or another. It could be your postman, or a supermarket clerk you've seen, or someone else of that sort. And again, as best you can, from your own heart, extending warm wishes of loving kindness toward this person you hardly know about, saying silently…

> *May this person be at ease.*
>
> *May they be content with their life.*
>
> *May they be joyful.*
>
> *May they feel safe and secure.*

Again, extending warm wishes of loving kindness to this person you hardly know at all…

> *May they be at ease.*
>
> *May they be content with their life.*
>
> *May they be joyful.*
>
> *May they feel safe and secure.*

And again, from the source of loving kindness in your own heart, extending well wishes to this person you barely know…

> *May this person be at ease.*
>
> *That they be content with their life.*
>
> *That they be joyful.*
>
> *That they feel safe and secure.*

And now, with warm loving care, gently turn your attention back to the sensations of your breath and your heart center, allowing the image or feeling sense of this person you hardly know to be released—allowing yourself to rest here, in this moment, with your feelings of warmth and kindness. Remembering that you can carry with you throughout your day these warm feelings of love and kindness that you were able to generate, knowing that you can always find your heart center when needed and making a kindhearted commitment to integrate this practice of loving kindness into your life, as best you can. And when you are ready, you can open your eyes and bring your attention back into the room.

End of practice

Radical Openness Handout 4.2

Main Points for Lesson 4: Enhancing Openness and Social Connection via Loving Kindness

1. Loving kindness meditation is a type of mood induction that activates our brain's social safety system.

2. LKM practices in RO DBT are designed to be used prior to social encounters (social safety effects have been reported to last from twenty minutes to up to four hours).

3. Importantly, the overarching goal of LKM practices in RO DBT is not to improve a person's ability to experience love or kindness toward themselves or other people but instead to trigger a mood state associated with contentment, curiosity, and desires for social engagement by activating an area of the brain linked with social safety responses.

4. RO DBT LKM differs from other LKM practices. Since many OC clients can find it difficult or even distressing to consider extending feelings of warmth, kindness, or love toward themselves, LKM practices in RO DBT involve only three steps: (1) creating an experience of warmth/love/kindness, (2) extending warm feelings toward someone the client already cares about, and (3) extending warm feelings toward a neutral person.

Radical Openness Worksheet 4.A

Daily Practice of Loving Kindness Meditation

- Loving kindness meditation is a type of positive mood induction that activates our brain's social safety system, our "friendly system" that is linked to feelings of calmness, contentment, and an easy social manner.

- Use LKM practices before social interactions to increase positivity and social connectedness toward others.

- A short six-minute exercise is all that is needed; research shows that the more you practice, the stronger the effects. Make it part of your daily ritual.

- Remember, LKM in RO DBT involves only three steps: (1) creating an experience of warmth/love/kindness, (2) extending warm feelings toward someone you already care about, and (3) extending warm feelings toward a neutral person.

- Remember, LKM in RO DBT is less about extending love or kindness and more about activating our social safety system.

- Use the script in handout 4.1 as a guide for practice or in making a digital recording of a loving kindness practice to use on a daily basis. Practice each day prior to leaving your house. Record your experiences using the following daily practice log.

Day	What did I notice during the practice? How long did the social safety experience last? How did it impact my day?
Sunday	
Monday	
Tuesday	
Wednesday	
Thursday	
Friday	
Saturday	

Were there any obstacles that arose while practicing loving kindness meditation? Describe these and how you used radical openness skills to deal with them.

_____

_____

_____

Engaging in Novel Behavior

✳   *If it's not fun, then it's not play.*   ✳

Main Points for Lesson 5

1. Discovery requires openness and willingness not to always have an answer. The most effective people in the world learn something new every day!

2. Learning new things usually involves making a mistake.

3. There are four stages we all go through when learning something new: unconscious incompetence, conscious incompetence, conscious competence, and unconscious competence.

4. Use Flexible Mind VARIEs skills to try new things.

5. OC clients need to let go of always trying to perform better or try harder. Relaxing, playing, and being nonproductive are skills that OC individuals need to practice.

6. Doing something new or different every day helps break down old habits and encourages spontaneity. New behavior often opens up new horizons. It teaches our brain that it's okay to not have everything planned.

Materials Needed

- Handout 5.1 (Engaging in Novel Behavior: Flexible Mind VARIEs)

- Handout 5.2 (Using Experience to Examine Willingness to Learn)

- Handout 5.3 (The Art of Nonproductivity and Being Just a Little Bit Silly)

- Handout 5.4 (Are We Having Fun Yet? Self-Enquiry About Humor and Play)

- (Optional) Handout 5.5 (Main Points for Lesson 5: Engaging in Novel Behavior)

- Worksheet 5.A (Engaging in Novel Behavior: Flexible Mind VARIEs)

- Worksheet 5.B (Nonproductive and Novel Behavior Monitoring Log)

- Whiteboard or flipchart with marker

(Recommended) Mindfulness Practice
The Oompa-Loompa

NOTE TO INSTRUCTORS: The Oompa-Loompa chant or dance is a "participate without planning" mindfulness practice. In RO DBT, "participate without planning" practices do *not* begin with an orientation or forewarning of the upcoming practice. This is because talking about what is going to happen usually triggers anticipatory anxiety and rumination, resulting in a greater chance for a client to refuse to participate (see "Instructor Guidelines for 'Participate Without Planning' Practices," in lesson 12). Participating without planning is an essential skill for OC clients to learn how to join in with the community and feel like part of a tribe. Importantly, the Oompa-Loompa chant should be time-limited—ideally it should last no longer than one minute. Use the following instructions as a guide.

- Begin the Oompa-Loompa by saying to the class (without any warning): *OKAY...EVERYONE STAND UP! NOW, DO WHAT I DO! NOW, BEND YOUR ARMS AND PUT ONE FORWARD AND ONE BACK. Like this! Now start to move them back and forth!*

- The instructor should then start to gently rock their arms from side to side and say: *Now repeat what I say next!* The instructor should chant *Just because you think it, doesn't mean it's true* while continuing to signal for everyone to join in.

- The coinstructor can demonstrate what is meant by immediately joining in with the movements and chant.

- The instructor should continue to repeat the chant—*Just because you think it, doesn't mean it's true*—while continually changing their body movements (for example, raising their hands above their head, shaking them about, waving arms side to side like seaweed swaying in the ocean current, slowing the speed and then speeding up). Pat the table lightly, then harder and louder while increasing the volume of the chant, then slow everything down and slowly lower the volume to a whisper.

- Keep the chant and movement going the entire practice, with eyebrow wags and a warm smile.

- End the practice by raising your arms above your head and shouting *Just because you think it, doesn't mean it's TRUE!*

- Celebrate with the class: *Well done! Applause to all! Let's give ourselves a hand!* That is, encourage class members to applaud their practice.

- Then say: *Okay, everyone can sit down.*

- Solicit observations and teach.

After the practice, ask participants to share what they observed, with a focus on thoughts they may have had or predictions they may have made. For example, instructors can say, "Raise your hand if you had a thought before or during the practice that said something like 'I just won't or I just can't do this!'" Invariably, several hands will be raised. The instructor should smile warmly and gently whisper, "Just because you think it, doesn't mean it's true." (*Note:* This highlights the importance of everyone in the class participating, at least to some degree; otherwise, for those who did not participate, their prediction was actually accurate.) Instructors can continue by saying, "What other thoughts did people have during the practice?" Examples might include "I thought you were going to have us sing" or "I thought that I was going to die of embarrassment" or "I thought someone would walk by outside and call the police." After each inaccurate prediction or unwarranted thought, instructors should simply repeat with a warm smile, "Just because you think it, doesn't mean it's true." Instructors should be prepared to share examples of their own inaccurate or unwarranted thoughts (for example, "I had a fleeting thought of my boss walking in and wondering what I was up to") and to then encourage the class to reply by repeating the chant. Instructors should highlight that despite everyone thinking a wide range of things (for example, bad things), most predictions did not actually occur (for example, despite thinking I would die, amazingly I am still alive). The phrase *Just because you think it, doesn't mean it's true* should be remembered and used as a cue to remind participants that internal experiences (that is, thoughts, sensations, images, or emotions) are not *facts* or *truths*.

(Required) Teaching Point
Why Engage in Novel Behavior?

⁂   *We learn the most when approach what we fear the most.*   ⁂

✓   **Ask:** *What are the advantages of trying out new things? What are the disadvantages?*

- *You can never learn anything new if you don't take a risk.*

- *Novelty is the spice of life.* For example, eating porridge every breakfast, doing laundry on Sunday, driving the same way to work, wearing the same clothes, walking the same speed on the treadmill can sometimes get a little monotonous!

  ✓   **Ask:** *What type of behaviors do you always do the same? How many of the behaviors are based on rules? What are the consequences of always doing the same thing repeatedly?*

- *Discovery requires openness and willingness not to always have an answer.* The most effective people in the world learn something new every day!

- *Learning new things usually involves making a mistake.*

(Required) Teaching Point
How Do We Learn Something New?

- *There are four stages we all go through when learning something new:*

  1. **Unconscious incompetence, or *not knowing that we don't know.*** For example, all of us, at one time in our life, did not know that we did not know how to tie our shoes. This is unconscious incompetence.

  2. **Conscious incompetence, or *knowing what it was that we didn't know but not knowing what to do about it.*** Eventually we became aware of the fact that shoes have bits known as laces and, when tied together in what your big sister keeps referring to as a "knot" (not to be confused with "snot," tee hee ☺), they keep our shoes firmly attached to our feet! An amazing discovery that has moved us to the second stage of learning a new skill: conscious incompetence, or becoming aware of one's lack of knowledge.

  3. **Conscious competence, or *knowing what to do but not being very proficient at it when we do it.*** We can now tie our shoes! All by ourselves! But we are really slow. We have to concentrate really hard on the steps involved, and sometimes we get it wrong. Plus, our big sister's smirk upon seeing one of our more creative knot-tying attempts is not particularly helpful.

  4. **Unconscious competence, or *"We are so proficient, we don't have to think about it,"* also known as "the expert."** Our hard work has paid off: we can tie our shoes like an expert without ever having to think about it! We can tie our shoes in our sleep, in the dark, when upside down, or even when talking to our big sister about how big her nose is (tee hee ☺)—without ever missing a step! We are on top of the world!

- *For many adults, the only stage they ever desire to experience or acknowledge being in is the fourth stage*—that is, the stage where it is often assumed that new learning is no longer necessary.

  - ✓ **Ask:** *What are the downsides of being an expert?* (Hint: Experts may be more closed-minded because they assume they already know what the correct answer is when their knowledge is challenged.)

  - ✓ **Ask:** *To what extent are you okay with the earlier stages of learning? What might this mean?*

  - ✓ **Ask:** *What behaviors do you always do the same? How often do you think you keep things the same in order to minimize the stress of not knowing? What is it that you might need to learn?*

  - ✓ **Ask:** *How often have you thought that trying something new would be an awful experience, only to discover that it wasn't as bad as you had expected and/or that you might have even liked it (Oh my! ☺)—for example, eating oysters, riding a horse, going for a walk at night with your partner, giving a toast, saying hi to someone?*

- *Remember, the goal of doing something you are not used to doing is to do something you are not used to doing (tee hee ☺).*

- *Plus, "There's nobody here but us chickens!" We are all scared when we try something new, but we are also scared when we don't.* Not doing impacts our well-being just as much as doing. We can't escape being affected by our own actions.

- *Doing something new requires a willingness to tolerate uncertainty.*

  - ✓ **Ask:** *How comfortable are you with uncertainty? With chaos? With disorder? What might your answer tell you about what you need to learn?*

- *The good news is that we naturally feel more solid when we take on those things we fear the most, and then learn from them.*

- *Practice Flexible Mind VARIEs to learn how to learn from novelty and reap the benefits from behaving courageously* (albeit without getting too uptight about it—tee hee ☺).

(Required) Teaching Point
Engaging in Novel Behavior: Flexible Mind VARIEs

Refer participants to handout 5.1 (Engaging in Novel Behavior: Flexible Mind VARIEs).

NOTE TO INSTRUCTORS: Write out the acronym (VARIE) on a flipchart or whiteboard, with each letter arranged vertically in a column, but *without* teaching or naming the specific skill that each letter signifies. Next, starting with the first letter in the acronym (V in VARIE), teach the skills associated with that letter, using the key points outlined in the following sections until you have covered all of the skills associated with each individual letter. Importantly, only write out on the whiteboard or flipchart the global description of what each letter actually stands for when you are teaching the skills associated with it. This teaching method avoids long explanations about the use of certain words in the acronym and/or premature teaching of concepts. The meaning of each letter is only revealed during the formal teaching of the skills associated with it.

Flexible Mind VARIEs

V   **Verify** one's willingness to experience something new

A   Check the **Accuracy** of hesitancy, aversion, or avoidance

R   **Relinquish** compulsive planning, rehearsal, or preparation

I   Activate one's social safety system and then **Initiate** the new behavior

E   Nonjudgmentally **Evaluate** the outcome

V   **Verify** *one's willingness to experience something new.*

- *The most effective people in the world learn something new every day!* They learn by being open to change and trying out new things. Successful people are adaptive; they learn to adjust to changing circumstances. (Instructors can use examples from competition TV, like *American Idol* or *Dancing with the Stars.* For example, sometimes the judges with the toughest feedback are those who the contestants can learn the most from, whereas the judges who say nice things to everyone don't really give contestants anything to go on.)

- *Trying out new things involves active learning and practice.* After falling off a horse, one must ride again multiple times before feeling comfortable again. Similarly, to learn that new things can be interesting, educational, or even fun, one must try them out first.

- *To learn from something new, a person must be willing to open-mindedly experience it.* A genuine commitment for change represents the core difference between engaging in a new behavior and simply thinking about it.

- *Practice self-enquiry of willingness by asking...*

  ➢ *Will trying out this new behavior get me closer or farther away from my valued goals? What are my expectations or predictions of what might happen if I tried out the new behavior? What do I fear might happen if I did something different?*

  ➢ *To what extent do I really want to change or try something new? If low, what might this mean?*

- *With a closed-mouth smile, eyebrows raised, and slow deep breath, open and soften while you imagine engaging in the new behavior,* rather than tensing and resisting.

A   Check the **Accuracy** *of hesitancy, aversion, or urges to avoid engaging in the new behavior in order to determine whether your emotions are warranted.*

- *Remember that self-discovery requires a willingness not to always have an answer.*

- *Remember that taking risks and making mistakes is how one learns.* Learning new things usually involves making a mistake; otherwise, you would already know how to do it! For example, when truly engaged in learning how to play the violin, dance, or do calculus, one constantly discovers new or better ways to perform the new behavior.

- *Practice self-enquiry by asking...*

  ➢ *Do I believe that I already know the outcome of what might happen if I tried the new behavior?*

> ➤ *Do I believe that I know all of the facts in the situation I am in? Do I find myself wanting to automatically explain or defend my perceptions of the facts or discount the other person's perceptions of the facts? If yes or maybe, then is this a sign that I am in Fixed Mind?*

> ➤ *Am I saying to myself that I have already tried out the new behavior in the past and believe it useless to try again? Do I believe it is unfair that I must do something different? If yes or maybe, then, what might this mean? Is it possible I am operating from Fatalistic Mind?*

> ➤ *Is there a possibility that I may not really want to change how I behave or think? Do I secretly hope I will fail when trying the new behavior? If so, how might this influence my ability to achieve my valued goals?*

> ➤ *Is it possible I am minimizing the positive consequences?*

R Relinquish *compulsive planning, rehearsal, or preparation prior to trying out the new behavior.*

> NOTE TO INSTRUCTORS: Most OC clients obsess about social events before they occur, especially those that may require spontaneity or intimate exchanges (for example, a date, a party). Excessive planning and rehearsal when unneeded is energy-consuming; it can lead to burnout and exhaustion.

Discuss the pros and cons of planning and rehearsing beforehand.

> ✓ **Ask:** *What types of behaviors or events is it best to plan or rehearse beforehand (for example, sky-diving, horseback riding, a major speech, a presentation at a meeting)? What types of behaviors or events is it best to not rehearse or plan beforehand (for example, a date, a party, lunch with a friend)?*

> ✓ **Ask:** *Is preparation really needed for me to engage in this new behavior?*

> ✓ **If so:** Mindfully research the steps needed to engage in the new behavior and prepare, with an aim of not getting it perfect.

> ✓ **If not:** Purposefully decide to let go of planning and rehearsal. Practice turning your mind to unrelated activities (for example, read an amusing book, take a soothing bath or nap, practice mindful breathing, conduct a loving kindness meditation) and use the following skills.

- **Remind yourself that compulsive planning or rehearsal may feel like wisdom but in reality may masquerade as avoidance** (for example, "I just need to read one more article, and then I will be ready").

- **Practice loving your perfectionist tendencies rather than trying fix them or get rid of them.** Trying to rid oneself of perfectionistic thinking is like *using mud to wash mud off your car*—it just makes matters worse. Be kind to yourself.

- **Extend feelings of loving kindness toward the part of you that wants to rehearse or plan ahead, rather than berating yourself.** Repeat silently to yourself: *May my perfectionistic mind be at ease, may my perfectionistic mind be content, may my perfectionistic mind be safe and secure.*

- **Practice mindfully urge-surfing desires to rehearse what to say or do** (see the material on urge-surfing in lesson 12). Outside of formal lectures or speeches, rehearsing what you will say beforehand often backfires—we stop listening to the people we are interacting with and become focused on remembering our lines.

I *Activate one's social safety system and then* **Initiate** *the new behavior.*

- *Activate your social safety system before you engage in the new behavior.* Use skills from lesson 3; see handout 3.1 (Changing Social Interactions by Changing Physiology). Use a loving kindness mediation to induce a long-lasting social safety mood state (see lesson 4).

- *"Don't think—just do!"* Passionately participate by throwing yourself fully into the experience, and keep turning your mind back to the experience. Remind yourself that you are learning how to participate in life without always having to have everything planned. Turn your mind away from judgmental or worry thoughts.

- *When engaging in the new behavior, repeatedly use the Big Three + 1 skills to keep yourself in your social safety system* (that is, lean back, deep breath, closed-mouth smile, eyebrow wag).

- *Feeling awkward when trying something new means you are learning, not that you are doing something wrong or failing.* New experience is the only way to grow—it is the opposite of complacency.

- *When experiencing discomfort, use this as an opportunity to practice self-enquiry by asking* **How might I learn from this?** rather than automatically falling apart or blaming the world.

- *If possible, repeat the new behavior, again and again,* before you evaluate your performance.

E *Look back over what happened, and nonjudgmentally* **Evaluate** *the outcome.*

- *After initiating the new behavior, allow time to nonjudgmentally examine how things went and what you learned from the experience.* Use the Awareness Continuum (see lesson 12) to describe what happened, including the emotions, thoughts, or sensations you experienced during the event.

- *Practice noticing what went well and how you benefited from the experience,* rather than what you could have done better or what went wrong.

- *Focus on the objective evidence supporting your observations when evaluating the reactions of others.* Remember that we can only imagine what another person is thinking or feeling inside (if they have not revealed them to us).

- *Practice self-enquiry by asking…*

  ➢ *What objective evidence do I have to support my conclusions about the event or the other person, other than gut feeling or opinion?*

  ➢ *Is there a chance that I might be mistaken?*

  ➢ *To what extent am I willing to question my personal perceptions?*

  ➢ *What do I need to learn?*

- *Loosen Fixed Mind thinking by recalling "We don't see the world as it is—we see the world as we are."*

- *Block automatic tendencies to blame others or the world.* This means taking responsibility for our personal reactions and responses instead of automatically expecting the world to conform to our wishes.

- *Block Fatalistic Mind thinking by reminding yourself, without falling apart or harsh self-blame, that you choose how you respond to the world.* RO recognizes that for the most part we choose how we feel (that is, no one can force me to feel a particular emotion).

- *Remember to practice frequently. Doing something new every day for overcontrolled individuals is like brushing one's teeth—it represents good mental health hygiene.* Whenever we do something new or different, we acquire new learning (for example, that it is okay not to have everything planned, that making mistakes or embracing uncertainty is how we learn).

- *Practice self-enquiry to examine how open you are to trying out new things, and discover any potential obstacles for growth.*

Refer participants to handout 5.2 (Using Experience to Examine Willingness to Learn).

Instructors should randomly pick class members to read aloud a self-enquiry question (of their choosing) from this handout and then briefly discuss the question. Then pick another class member to read aloud another question, and so forth. Importantly, it is not necessary to cover (that is, read aloud) all of the questions; a few are usually sufficient to help expose participants to the handout (which is the point of reviewing it). Encourage participants to get into the habit of using this handout after they practice Flexible Mind VARIEs to further enhance their growth.

- *Make time to reward yourself for trying something new, regardless of how you evaluated your performance.* Get into the habit of rewarding yourself every time you do something new or different, whether you feel like you deserve a reward or not. The goal of Flexible Mind VARIEs is not to be perfect but to learn.

- *Experiment with new rewards rather than doing the same thing over and over again.* Examples include curling up for half an hour with a nonserious book, having a glass of wine, eating one of your favorite chocolates, taking a long hot bath with aromatic candles, taking a nap, listening to your favorite music while enjoying your favorite beverage, watching your favorite TV show, sitting out in your garden and enjoying the sunshine. Of course, now that you have rewarded yourself for doing something different, you need to reward yourself for rewarding yourself! (☺)

(Required) Teaching Point

Remembering How to Play: The Art of Nonproductivity and Being Just a Little Bit Silly

> ★ **Fun Facts:** *Born to Be Wild!*
>
> *Humans are born with an innate capacity for play, and family/environmental/cultural experiences shape how it is expressed over time. Indeed, play is a natural behavior among mammals (think of a small kitten playing with a ball of yarn). Many OC clients consider play or having fun childish or selfish. Archaeological records have shown that play and games have been a core part of human experience since prehistoric times, supported by the existence of dice, gaming sticks, gaming boards and various forms of ball-play material made of stones, sticks, and bones [S. J. Fox, 1977; Schaefer & Reid, 2001]. Play allows us to focus on the means (that is, what we are doing) rather than the ends (where we want to go) [Pellegrini, 2009]. It allows us a chance to repeat, practice, rehearse, exaggerate, or experiment with a new behavior before it really matters (for example, war games). Thus, play subsumes a vital role in the development of problem-solving skills in primates, and for humans it also provides the practice grounds for a range of higher-order cognitive and social-emotional skills essential for our success. One important caveat: If it's not fun, then it's not play. Be careful to not take your play too seriously.*

NOTE TO INSTRUCTORS: OC clients are unlikely to genuinely believe it is socially acceptable for an adult to play, relax, or openly express emotions *unless* they *see* their therapist *model* it first. Thus, therapists (especially those leaning toward OC) may need to practice the skills outlined in the following section first if they are going to effectively teach them.

Refer participants to handout 5.3 (The Art of Nonproductivity and Being Just a Little Bit Silly).

- *"All work and no play makes Jack a dull boy!"* Overcontrolled individuals don't need to learn to be more serious, try harder, or strive to do better! They are experts at this.

- *If you are overcontrolled, you need to learn how to chill out and have a little fun!*

- *Being able to nonjudgmentally chuckle at our foibles is a sign of mental health and essential for healthy relationships.* It signals to the world that we don't take ourselves too seriously and that we will likely be open to feedback.

- *Yet relaxing and playing can feel like hard work for an overcontrolled person!*

  - ✓ *Ask: When was the last time you remember having fun, laughing freely, or being silly? What are the benefits of play, laughter, or relaxing? How might playfulness benefit relationships? What do you find amusing in life?*

  - ✓ *Ask: What are the signs that tell you that you may need to take a break? What changes occur in your body (for example, headaches)? Are there changes in how you relate to others (for example, more aloof, isolation)?*

  - ✓ *Ask: What does taking a break mean to you? Do you always do the same thing to reward yourself? How much time do you allocate in your life for nonproductive activity (for example, taking a nap, reading a novel, enjoying a walk)?*

- *The good news is that it is possible to relearn how to not always take life so seriously, and to laugh and play!*

- *In the meantime, our motto can be "Fake it until you make it!"* (tee hee ☺)

  ✓ **Ask:** *Why do you think I said that?*

  Answer: Because doing some new or different may feel phony or fake at first, but it is the only way to learn.

- *Practicing new ways of expressing ourselves and moving our bodies helps break down overlearned inhibitory barriers that impair social connectedness.* Recall that research shows that we become anxiously aroused when interacting with a nonexpressive person *and* we prefer not to affiliate with them, whereas open expression of emotion—even when the emotion is negative— signals genuineness and trustworthiness, and research shows that people prefer to spend time with people who reveal their inner feelings to others.

- *Plus, joining in communal activities sends a powerful message to our brain—namely, that we are part of a tribe and have done nothing to be ashamed about,* even when it feels scary inside.

NOTE TO INSTRUCTORS: After reviewing handout 5.3 (The Art of Nonproductivity and Being Just a Little Bit Silly), instructors should immediately begin the following exercise, without any forewarning or orientation.

(Required) Class Exercise
The Extremely Fun Extreme Expression Workshop

NOTE TO INSTRUCTORS: Unless absolutely necessary, it is essential *not* to orient OC clients to this exercise or forewarn them about it (see "Instructor Guidelines for 'Participate Without Planning' Practices," in lesson 12). If they are forewarned, they will be more likely to worry, focus on their anticipatory anxiety, or go numb than listen to instructions, and their genuine participation will be less likely.

NOTE TO INSTRUCTORS: Instructors should plan for five brief "participate without planning" practices, distributed randomly, during lesson 5. Each practice should last only thirty seconds to one minute, ending with applause to celebrate tribal participation; see "Instructor Guidelines for 'Participate Without Planning' Practices," in lesson 12. Importantly, the practices used in the Extremely Fun Extreme Expression Workshop should be *randomly distributed throughout the lesson*, not bunched together. The idea is to provide multiple brief exposures to participating with others and being part of a tribe without thinking much about it beforehand.

Extremely Fun Extreme Expression Practices

- With a warm smile say to the class: *Okay...EVERYONE STAND UP! NOW, LET'S CLAP OUR HANDS AND SAY HA HA...HO HO HO!* Rhythmically clap your hands in

123

time with each sound of laughter: *Ha ha…ho, ho, ha…ha ha…ho, ho, ho…ha, ha…ho, ho, ho…ha, ha…ho, ho, ho!* Repeat once. Encourage eye contact, use large gestures, and move with your clapping sounds while encouraging the class to join you. Smile and use an eyebrow wag while you look briefly into the eyes of every participant. Stop after thirty seconds to one minute and say: *Well done! Applause to all!* Encourage all class members to give each other a round of applause. Then quickly move to the next minipractice, before anyone has a chance to comment or evaluate.

- **Say to the class: *Ohhhh, I'm a balloon!*** (Mimic blowing air into a balloon.) *Phoof…phoof…phoof…* Say: *Come on, blow up your balloon! Phoof…phoof…no, make it bigger…phoof…phoof…phoof…OH NO…I'm deflating!* Make movements of a balloon deflating… run around the room in random ways…*Phmmmm…blmmmm…sssssssss….Ha ha ha ha ho ho ho ho…ha ha ha ho ho ho.* Be sure to make eye contact with every member of the class as you encourage them to blow themselves up and then deflate. Then stop, have class members give themselves a round of applause, and quickly move on to the next exercise, before anyone has a chance to comment or evaluate.

- **Practice "I'm NOT arrogant, I'm just better than you!"** Say to the class: *Okay…EVERYONE STAND UP! NOW, DO WHAT I DO! Put your chin up in the air, shoulders back, and hold your head high! Put a swagger in your gait!* Instructors should start swaggering about and say: *Now shout **Out of my way! Don't you know who I am? I am a very important person! Just who do you think you are? Hrrmmph!*** Keep marching about and *hrrmmph*ing for another ten to fifteen seconds. Instructors should end by clapping their hands in celebration, encouraging class members to give themselves a round of applause, and saying: *Well done! Okay, sit down, and let's share our observations about our mindfulness practice.*

- **Practice "Ouch, that hurts!"** Instructors should demonstrate with a class member first. Have them lightly touch the instructor's arm, without telling them how you will respond. Immediately upon being lightly touched, the instructor should exclaim: *Ouch! That really hurt! I'm in excruciating pain! Waaahhhh!* Then have the entire class partner up and take turns practicing the same—that is, each partner takes turns lightly touching the other's arm—with similar raucous responses by the one being touched. Encourage participants to ham it up, waving their arms in the air and wailing, snarling with pain and gnashing their teeth. Say things like these: *My arm is going to fall off! Quick, call an ambulance! I hope you have insurance!* To end, instructors should celebrate with the class, smiling and saying: *How nice! Well done! Applause to all!* Encourage class members to give each other a round of applause. Then say: *Now, on to the next practice!*

- **Do the volcano.** Say to the class: *Let's do the volcano!* Take in a huge breath and dramatically hold it. Motion for the class to do the same, then say: *Hold it, hold it…let those bubbles rise…they are rising up…then they BURST! Blub, bla, blubble, blob! Ha ha…ho ho ho…ha ha…ho ho ho…ha ha ha ha hee hee hee ho ho!* Now grab the hand of the person next to you…take a huge breath again…now HOLD IT, HOLD IT…come on, HOLD IT—OKAY, LET IT GO—bloo bloo—ha ha ha…ho ho…hee hee ho ho…Raise your arms up above your head…Blub blub bubbling blub…Ha ha…ho ho ho…hee hee ha ha.* Smile, and be sure to make eye contact with each participant while you laugh and encourage the class to mimic your movements. Then stop, have class members give themselves a round of applause, and quickly move on to the next exercise, before anyone has a chance to comment or evaluate.

- **"Let's be Italian!"** Say to the class: *Okay…EVERYONE STAND UP! Now let's all talk with an Italian accent!* Say: *Mamma mia! My name is Marco Marconi, and I'm an Italian painter! Which* *means I am Italian! But I am very sad to say that I work with the evil Vissario, who likes to make my life miserable. He thinks he is so great! But he is NOT Marco Marconi! Ahhh, mamma mia—what am I to do?* Instructors should really ham it up, using big gestures and encouraging smiles and making eye contact with all class members. End with applause all around.

- **"Let's do funny faces together!"** Say to the class: *Okay, everyone do what I do! Let's make funny faces! Make a funny face, like this!* Change expression. *And this!* Change expression again. *Now try this one!* And so forth. End the exercise with applause all around.

- **"Time to mow the lawn."** Say to the class: *Okay, we need to mow the lawn.* Then lean down and act as if you are pulling the starter cord on a lawn mower. Say: *Ha…ha…ha…ha* with each pull of the mower cord: *Ha…ha…ha…ha.* And again: *Ha ha ha ha…BRRROMMM! BRA BRA RHH RHH…Wow, it started up!* Grab your lawn mower's handle. Begin randomly mowing, and say: *VRRRRMMMMM…VRRRMMMM!* Run into someone else's lawn mower and bounce off, or stall out. Keep it up, and encourage creativity. Be sure to make eye contact, if possible, with every participant while smiling and using eyebrow wags. Then stop, raise your arms high, and say: *HA HA HA HO HO HO HA HA HA HO HO HO!* Encourage a round of applause, and move on to the next exercise, before anyone has a chance to comment or evaluate.

- Solicit observations after at least one of the practices.

NOTE TO INSTRUCTORS: It is important to point out that what matters is not how big a person signaled when they participated in the preceding exercise but whether they had brought themselves to their edge (that is, their personal unknown) by going past their comfort zone. Small changes and attempts should be celebrated as much as big ones.

(Optional) Class Exercise
If It's Not Fun, It's Not Play

Refer to handout 5.4 (Are We Having Fun Yet? Self-Enquiry About Humor and Play).

NOTE TO INSTRUCTORS: The best way to make use of the handout is to randomly pick a class member to read aloud one of the questions (of their choosing) and then briefly discuss it as a group. Then randomly select a different class member to do the same. It is not necessary to read aloud each question. The aim is to provide some exposure to the handout in order to encourage participants to use it again later as a source of self-growth. Remind participants that the questions they find most uncomfortable may be the ones they need to learn from the most (see the information in lesson 29 about finding one's edge).

Lesson 5 Homework

NOTE TO INSTRUCTORS: Instructors should encourage participants to remember to activate their social safety system before initiating new behaviors; see handout 3.1 (Changing Social Interactions by Changing Physiology).

1. **(Required) Worksheet 5.A (Engaging in Novel Behavior: Flexible Mind VARIEs)**
2. **(Required) Worksheet 5.B (Nonproductive and Novel Behavior Monitoring Log)**
3. (Optional) Handout 5.4 (Are We Having Fun Yet? Self-Enquiry About Humor and Play)
4. (Optional) Encourage participants to use handout 5.3 (The Art of Nonproductivity and Being Just a Little Bit Silly)

NOTE TO INSTRUCTORS: Additional optional homework can be individualized. For example, participants who find pleasure in putting others down (assuming they admit it) can be encouraged to watch funny movies or TV shows where the humor is not sardonic, mocking, blaming, or demeaning (for example, the movie *Patch Adams*, starring Robin Williams; *Groundhog Day*, starring Bill Murray; *Ghostbusters*, starring Bill Murray and Dan Aykroyd). Participants who engage in competitive recreational activities can be encouraged to experiment with activities that are goal-oriented. Simple behavioral experiments (that include practicing activating their social safety system during the activity) can be assigned—for example, wearing different clothes to work, taking a bath rather than a shower, wearing a watch on the other wrist, taking a new route driving to the store, or trying a new type of food. Participants should be encouraged to experiment and be creative, and to remember that the Flexible Mind VARIEs skills are not about being the best at doing new things but instead learning to genuinely challenge oneself to break out of one's inhibitory shell.

Radical Openness Handout 5.1

Engaging in Novel Behavior: Flexible Mind VARIEs

Flexible Mind VARIEs

V	**Verify** one's willingness to experience something new
A	Check the **Accuracy** of hesitancy, aversion, or avoidance
R	**Relinquish** compulsive planning, rehearsal, or preparation
I	Activate one's social safety system and then **Initiate** the new behavior
E	Nonjudgmentally **Evaluate** the outcome

V **Verify** *one's willingness to experience something new.*

Notice what emotion arises when you imagine engaging in the novel behavior; rate the intensity of the emotion on a 1 to 10 scale (with 1 being low intensity and 10 highest). Notice any tendencies to avoid.

A Check the **Accuracy** *of hesitancy, aversion, or urges to avoid engaging in the new behavior in order to determine whether your emotions are warranted.*

- ✓ **Ask:** *What are my expectations or predictions of what might happen if I tried out the new behavior? Do I believe that I already know the outcome of what might happen if I tried the new behavior?*

- ✓ **Ask:** *Do I believe that I know all of the facts in the situation I am in? Do I find myself wanting to automatically explain or defend my perceptions of the facts or discount the other person's perceptions of the facts. If yes or maybe, then is this a sign that I am in Fixed Mind?*

- ✓ **Ask:** *Am I saying to myself that I have already tried out the new behavior in the past and believe it useless to try again? Do I believe it is unfair that I must do something different? If yes or maybe, then what might this mean? Is it possible I am operating from Fatalistic Mind?*

- ✓ **Ask:** *Is there a possibility that I may not really want to change how I behave or think? Do I secretly hope I will fail when trying the new behavior? If so, how might this influence my ability to achieve my valued goals?*

- ✓ **Ask:** *Is it possible I am minimizing the positive consequences?*

R **Relinquish** *compulsive planning, rehearsal, or preparation prior to trying out the new behavior.*

- **Remind yourself that compulsive planning or rehearsal may feel like wisdom but in reality may masquerade as avoidance** (for example, "I just need to read one more article").

- **Use self-enquiry to determine whether planning is actually needed. Ask:** *Is preparation actually necessary for me to engage in this new behavior?*

- **If yes:** Mindfully research what is needed while blocking obsessive rehearsals. Picture yourself doing the new behavior, memorize the steps needed, but block excessive planning.

- **If no:** Purposefully decide to not plan ahead and then let go of urges to practice further by turning your mind to an unrelated activity (for example, read an amusing book, take a soothing bath or nap, practice mindful breathing, conduct a loving kindness meditation).

- **Use urge-surfing to not respond to compulsive desires to plan ahead or excessively rehearse.** *Urge-surfing* means mindfully observing urges like a wave that crests and then passes away. Remind yourself of times you have been successful at urge-surfing in the past (for example, if you ever quit ciga-rettes, you surfed the urge to smoke repeatedly; eventually urges to smoke fade away with repeated practice). In the same way, repeatedly practice observing urges to plan ahead or rehearse (and the thoughts, emotions, or images accompanying them) like a wave that rises and falls. *As best you can, observe these urges without giving in to them—not trying to make them go away, but simply allowing them to crest and fall—knowing that they are transitory experiences that don't require an immediate response. Rather than dwelling on them, keep turning your attention to the sensations of your breath when they arise. Repeat the practice again and again every day until your brain learns that urges to plan or rehearse are not mandates for action.*

- **Practice radically accepting that no one knows what will happen in the future; mindfully live in the here and now.**

- **Remember that learning new things usually involves making a mistake;** otherwise, you would already know the skill!

I *Activate one's social safety system and then* **Initiate** *the new behavior.*

- **Activate your social safety system** *before* **you engage in the new behavior.** Use skills from lesson 3 (changing social interactions by changing physiology). Use a loving kindness mediation to induce a long-lasting social safety mood state (lesson 4).

- **When actually doing the new behavior, repeatedly use the Big Three + 1 skills to keep yourself in your social safety system** (that is, lean back, deep breath, closed-mouth smile, eyebrow wag).

- **Mindfully participate fully in the experience while letting go of judgmental thoughts.** Carry out the behavior again and again until anxiety begins to pass.

- **Remember that behaving differently is the only way to learn something new.** Feeling awkward tells you that you are learning, *not* that you are failing.

E *Look back over what happened, and nonjudgmentally* **Evaluate** *the outcome.*

- ✓ **Ask:** *What have I learned from this experience? Am I finding it hard to feel a sense of accomplish-ment because I did not perform perfectly?* If so, practice accepting your perfectionist tendencies rather than trying to fix them. Trying to rid oneself of perfectionistic thinking is like using mud to wash mud off your car—it just makes matters worse.

- **Open and soften into your style and practice loving kindness toward the perfectionistic part of you.** For example, "May my perfectionist self be happy, may my perfectionist self be content, may my perfectionist self be safe and secure."

- **Remind yourself that striving to meet or exceed expectations is needed for societies to flourish** (without it, trains would never run on time; we would never have landed on the moon, and so forth).

  ✓ **Ask:** *Do I find myself wanting to automatically discount positive feedback or praise from others about how well I did?* If yes or maybe, remind yourself that accepting praise from others when you believe that you could have done better lays down new learning that opposes your habitual tendencies to value only a perfect performance.

- **Practice saying "Thank you" to people giving compliments, without further explanation or minimization of your efforts.**

- **Reward yourself for trying out new things and create a list of potential rewards to be used in the future**—for example, curl up for half an hour with a nonserious book, have a glass of wine, eat one of your favorite chocolates, take a long hot bath with scented candles, take a nap, listen to your favorite music while enjoying your favorite beverage, watch your favorite TV show, sit out in your garden and enjoy the sunshine. Get into the habit of rewarding yourself every time you do something new or different, whether you feel like you deserve a reward or not. Then reward yourself for rewarding yourself! Experiment and remember that celebrating one's successes is a core means for preventing burnout and exhaustion.

Radical Openness Handout 5.2

Using Experience to Examine Willingness to Learn

- After engaging in a new behavior, evaluate your experience with self-enquiry.

- Use the following questions to examine how open you are to trying out new things and discover any potential obstacles for growth.

  ➤ *To what extent did I find myself enjoying the new experience?*

  ➤ *Am I more OR less inclined to try out this behavior again? What might my answer tell me?*

  ➤ *Am I dismissing or minimizing the positive benefits that occurred? What does this mean?*

  ➤ *If I am self-critical of my behavior—is there something important for me to learn?*

  ➤ *Have I allowed myself sufficient time to practice or try out the new behavior before I evaluated what happened?*

  ➤ *Am I finding it hard to feel a sense of accomplishment because I did not perform perfectly? If so, then what might this mean?*

  ➤ *Do I find myself wanting to automatically blame someone else for what happened when I tried out the new behavior? What might this tell me about my coping style? What do I need to learn?*

  ➤ *Am I secretly expecting myself to be perfect or for the new behavior to feel good when I first attempt it? If so, then what might this tell me about how I am feeling now?*

  ➤ *To what extent am I telling myself that my experience just proves I was right all along about the new behavior? What might this response tell me about my openness to new experience?*

  ➤ *Do I have urges to pout or give up because things didn't go as planned? If so or maybe, then what is it that I need to learn?*

  ➤ *Am I using this experience as another opportunity to beat up on myself or to prove to myself or others that I am worthless or unworthy? Is there a part of me that was hoping I would fail when engaging in the new behavior? If so or maybe, then what might this mean?*

  ➤ *Do I ever secretly fail or attempt to destroy others' expectations (even my own) so that I won't be expected to do things differently in the future? Do I ever harshly blame myself so that others will expect less from me?*

  ➤ *To what extent am I willing to change my behavior? What might I be doing to contribute to my personal suffering? How might I learn from this, without using it as another opportunity to prove to myself and others that I am a failure? What is it I need to learn?*

- Write other self-enquiry questions you found useful here.

_____

_____

_____

_____

Radical Openness Handout 5.3

The Art of Nonproductivity and Being Just a Little Bit Silly

- **Overcontrolled individuals don't need to learn how to take life more seriously.** Instead, those of us with overcontrolled tendencies need to learn how to chill out and take it easy. We need to practice relaxing, find time to be nonproductive, and learn how to take life (and ourselves) a little less seriously.

- **Relearning to laugh and play will require practice.** It involves a willingness to step outside of one's comfort zone.

- **Each day try to do something new or different.** Remember, whenever we do something new or different without judgment, we acquire new learning (for example, that it is okay not to have everything planned, that making mistakes or embracing uncertainty is how we learn).

- **Here are a few ideas.** Work at creating your own list that you add to each day. The idea is to increase your flexibility by changing old habits!

  - *Put your rings on different fingers.*

  - *Wear a watch on the opposite arm.*

  - *Use different bedding.*

  - *Do your hair differently.*

  - *Wear something different.*

  - *Use a purple (or silver) pen.*

  - *Write with your other hand.*

  - *Sit in a different seat during mealtime.*

  - *Listen to different music or radio stations.*

  - *Ask people to call you by a different name for a day (for example, shortened or longer form of name, nickname).*

  - *For fun, do the exact opposite of what you would normally do in a situation.*

  - *Read a different newspaper or watch a different newscast.*

  - *Talk to everyone wearing pink at a party.*

  - *Watch TV and repeat everything said in an Italian accent.*

  - *Go into a fancy restaurant and order a burger and fries.*

  - *Order a pizza and end the call with, "Remember, we never had this conversation."*

  - *Repeat every third word you say during a conversation with someone.*

  - *Walk backward.*

  - *Communicate in mime.*

  - *Drive a different way to work.*

- *Wear a Hawaiian shirt.*
- *Wear your underwear backward.*
- *Eat your dessert first, before your main meal.*
- *Ask someone else the best way to do a household chore and do it that way for the next few days.*
- **Make up your own list of novel behaviors and write your ideas here.**

_____

_____

_____

Radical Openness Handout 5.4

Are We Having Fun Yet? Self-Enquiry About Humor and Play

- **Remember, keep your self-enquiry practices short in duration**—that is, not much longer than five minutes. The goal of self-enquiry is to *find a good question* that brings you closer to your edge or personal unknown (the place you don't want to go), in order to learn.

- **Remember to record** the images, thoughts, emotions, and sensations that emerge when you practice self-enquiry about the following questions (or other questions that emerge) in your self-enquiry journal.

- **Remember to practice being suspicious of quick answers** to self-enquiry questions. Allow any answers to your self-enquiry practice to emerge over time.

- **Remember, the questions we dislike the most are usually the best.** They often hold some gem of truth or learning we may know is there but may wish to avoid. Be alert for questions that trigger bodily tension, annoyance, fear, urges to avoid or justify one's behavior, and/or urges to fall apart, attack or blame others, and/or get down on oneself.

- **Use the following questions to uncover your edge and facilitate learning.**

  ➤ *How many of my recreational activities are competitive in nature?*

  ➤ *If I am not winning, do I still find the activity enjoyable?*

  ➤ *How serious am I about my recreational activities?*

  ➤ *To what extent do the games, playtime, or recreational activities I engage in require preplanning (for example, parachuting requires careful checking beforehand that one's parachute has been packed properly).*

  ➤ *How often do I engage in recreation, relaxing, or fun that does not require any preplanning or preparation?*

  ➤ *How often do I read a book or watch a program on TV that is not teaching me something, about learning something new, and/or about self-improvement?*

  ➤ *Have I ever been given feedback that I work too hard or that I need to relax?*

  ➤ *Do I find it hard to self-soothe, relax, or experience pleasure without guilt?*

  ➤ *To what extent do I believe it immoral or selfish to engage in behaviors that are for pleasure and/or have no obvious productive value?*

  ➤ *How many of my recreational activities involve in-person contact with other people (that is, not over the internet or via telephone)?*

  ➤ *To what extent do I believe that relaxing, playing, or recreation must be earned?*

  ➤ *What do I find amusing?*

  ➤ *What is so amusing about what I find amusing?*

➢ What type of TV programs or movies do I find enjoyable or humorous? Am I proud of what I watch? If not or not always, what is it that I might need to learn?

➢ Do I consider myself to possess a cutting sense of humor? What might this say about my social interactions?

➢ Do I secretly pride myself on being able to make clever or barbed comments disguised as innocent jests? What prevents me from being more direct?

➢ Do I consider myself expert at the humorous put-down or the niggle?

➢ Do I like it when other people niggle me? What might this tell me about my values?

➢ How often do I laugh out of social obligation?

➢ Am I expert at the phony laugh? What might this mean?

➢ How free do I feel to express pleasure or laughter in public?

➢ Do I ever hide expressions of laughter from others? How might this impact my relationships?

➢ Do I pride myself on being able to make other people laugh?

➢ How much time do I spend memorizing or rehearsing funny stories or anecdotes?

➢ To what extent do I use a joke to avoid something serious? Has this ever caused problems for me? What might be the downsides?

➢ Do I ever feel like an impostor when telling someone a joke or a funny story? What might this tell me?

➢ What am I afraid might happen if I did not tell a joke?

➢ How often do I find myself laughing at other people's jokes?

➢ How often do I find myself laughing, chuckling, or giggling, without trying to?

➢ To what extent do I believe genuine laughter is even possible?

➢ When I hear the word "silly," what type of thoughts, emotions, or images arise?

➢ How often am I silly?

➢ Can I be silly? If not, what is preventing me?

➢ What do I fear might happen if I were silly?

➢ Who am I silly around?

➢ To what extent do I believe being silly is a silly thing to do (☺)?

• **Write here other questions that emerged.**

_____

_____

_____

_____

Radical Openness Handout 5.5

Main Points for Lesson 5: Engaging in Novel Behavior

1. Discovery requires openness and willingness not to always have an answer. The most effective people in the world learn something new every day!

2. Learning new things usually involves making a mistake.

3. There are four stages we all go through when learning something new: unconscious incompetence, conscious incompetence, conscious competence, and unconscious competence.

4. Use Flexible Mind VARIEs skills to try new things.

5. OC clients need to let go of always trying to perform better or try harder. Relaxing, playing, and being nonproductive are skills that OC individuals need to practice.

6. Doing something new or different every day helps break down old habits and encourages spontaneity. New behavior often opens up new horizons. It teaches our brain that it's okay to not have everything planned.

Radical Openness Worksheet 5.A

Engaging in Novel Behavior: Flexible Mind VARIEs

Flexible Mind VARIEs

V   **V**erify one's willingness to experience something new

A   Check the **Accuracy** of hesitancy, aversion, or avoidance

R   **R**elinquish compulsive planning, rehearsal, or preparation

I   Activate one's social safety system and then **I**nitiate the new behavior

E   Nonjudgmentally **E**valuate the outcome

V   **Verify** *one's willingness to experience something new.*

Notice what emotion arises when you imagine engaging in the novel behavior; rate the intensity of the emotion on a scale of 1 to 10 (with 1 being low intensity and 10 highest). Notice any tendencies to avoid.

_____

_____

_____

_____

A   *Check the **Accuracy** of hesitancy, aversion, or urges to avoid engaging in the new behavior in order to determine whether your emotions are warranted.*

Use the self-enquiry questions in handout 5.2 (Using Experience to Examine Willingness to Learn) to help with this. **Record here what you discovered.**

_____

_____

_____

_____

R Relinquish *compulsive planning, rehearsal, or preparation prior to trying out the new behavior.*

Check the skills you used.

- ☐ Reminded myself that compulsive planning or rehearsal may feel right but in reality might not be needed.

- ☐ Asked myself *Is preparation actually necessary for me to engage in this new behavior?*

  - ☐ **If yes:** Then mindfully planned or rehearsed what was needed and let go of urges to do more.

  - ☐ **If no:** Purposefully practiced not planning by engaging in an unrelated activity.

- ☐ Practiced urge-surfing compulsive desires to plan ahead or excessively rehearse; see handout 5.1 (Engaging in Novel Behavior: Flexible Mind VARIEs).

- ☐ Practiced radically accepting that I cannot predict or control what will happen in the future and turned my mind to living fully in the present moment.

- ☐ Remembered that taking risks and making mistakes is the only way to learn a new skill.

Other skills practiced.

_____

_____

_____

I *Activate one's social safety system and then* **Initiate** *the new behavior.*

Check the skills you used.

- ☐ Activated my social safety system *before* I engaged in the new behavior (write in the following space what skill or skills you used to do this).

_____

_____

- ☐ Used the Big Three + 1 skills while engaged in the new behavior.

- ☐ Mindfully participated in the experience while letting go of judgmental thoughts.

- ☐ Remembered that behaving differently is the only way to learn something new and that any feelings of awkwardness or discomfort are growth pains, not a sign of failure.

Other skills practiced.

_____

_____

_____

E *Look back over what happened and nonjudgmentally* **Evaluate** *the outcome.*

What have I learned by trying out the new behavior? What do I still need to do or practice when it comes to this new behavior? Was I able to allow myself to experience a sense of accomplishment or pride for having tried something new? **Write answers here,** and place a checkmark in the boxes next to the skills you practiced.

_____

_____

_____

☐ Remembered that behaving differently means new learning—*attaching new positive meanings to previously feared or avoided behaviors.*

☐ Practiced accepting my perfectionist tendencies rather than compulsively trying to ignore them, make them go away, or control them.

☐ Practiced extending loving kindness toward the perfectionistic part of myself rather than chastising myself for being a perfectionist.

☐ Reminded myself that striving to meet or exceed expectations (perfectionism) is needed for societies to flourish.

☐ Practiced saying "Thank you" and blocked automatic tendencies to dismiss praise or positive feedback about my performance.

☐ Rewarded myself for trying out the new behavior. Write here what you actually did.

_____

_____

Radical Openness Worksheet 5.B

Nonproductive and Novel Behavior Monitoring Log

Daily practice log: Each day practice trying out something new or different. Focus on behaviors that are not about self-improvement, work, or obligation. Stretch yourself—make it fun—but keep it real; use handout 5.3 (The Art of Nonproductivity and Being Just a Little Bit Silly) for ideas. Record what you did and what emotions, thoughts, and sensations you experienced in the spaces provided.

Use self-enquiry to enhance self-discovery. For example, *What type of new behaviors did I find myself resisting the most? Did I tend to choose behaviors that involved self-improvement? Did I find it difficult to not be productive? What might this mean? What skills would be useful for me to practice?* Record other self-enquiry questions that arose from this practice and describe where they led you.

	What did you do that was different? What emotions, thoughts, and sensations arose?	What self-enquiry questions did you use to enhance self-discovery?
Sunday		
Monday		
Tuesday		
Wednesday		
Thursday		
Friday		
Saturday		

1. **Describe any Fixed Mind or Fatalistic Mind behaviors that arose during the week.** How did they impact what you did? If you were able to get to Flexible Mind, what skills did you use?

_____

_____

_____

2. **What were the aftereffects of trying out something new or novel, behaving less seriously, being silly,** and/or practicing being less rather than more productive? What did you learn? What do you need to do to deepen your learning?

_____

_____

_____

3. **Describe how you will make this practice part of your life.** What are the obstacles that might make this difficult? What skills will you need to use to overcome these obstacles?

_____

_____

_____

LESSON 6

How Do Emotions Help Us?

Main Points for Lesson 6

1. Pure logic often fails when it comes to human relationships or making quick decisions.

2. Most of us carry myths about emotions with us that can bias how we respond to the world. Rather than challenging a myth about emotion to get rid of it, use self-enquiry in order to learn from it. Self-enquiry is able to enquire about a myth, but it does not automatically assume that a myth is wrong, bad, or dysfunctional.

3. Emotions exist for a reason. They have four primary functions or purposes: (1) they help us make decisions, (2) they motivate our actions, (3) they communicate our inner experience and signal our intentions to others, and (4) they facilitate the formation of strong social bonds.

4. Not everything that's important is emotional. OC individuals are characterized by superior self-control and detail-focused capacities, features that by nature are nonemotional yet have emotional consequences when they are excessively or compulsively used.

Materials Needed

-   Handout 6.1 (Emotions Are There for a Reason)
-   Handout 6.2 (Not Everything That's Important Is Emotional)
-   (Optional) Handout 6.3 (Main Points for Lesson 6: How Do Emotions Help Us?)
-   Worksheet 6.A (Overcontrolled Myths About Emotions)
-   Worksheet 6.B (Using Neural Substrates to Label Emotions)
-   Whiteboard or flipchart with marker

(Recommended) Mindfulness Practice

Deal an Emotion

Ask class participants to silently pick a number between one and ten. Next, "deal an emotion" by **assigning a different emotion word to each number** (for example, "If you picked number one, you have humiliation; if you picked number two, you have fear; if you picked number three, you have envy; if you picked number four, you have joy; if you picked number five, you have guilt; if you picked number six, you have anger; if you picked number seven, you have love; if you picked number eight, you have contempt; if you picked number nine, you have jealousy; if you picked number ten, you have contentment"). Next, instruct participants to silently repeat the emotion word they were dealt and to lean into the emotion they were dealt by consciously trying to generate it. Instruct participants to mindfully observe bodily sensations, thoughts, memories, and emotions that arise during the practice, and encourage them to be alert for desires to have a different emotion, envy directed to someone who had the emotion you wanted, resistance to participating in the practice, judgmental thoughts, feelings of numbness, and/or an inability to generate the emotion. The practice should be kept short, that is, about three minutes.

End the practice and then ask for observations. Use the following questions to facilitate discussion and self-enquiry.

- *Were you able to feel the emotion you had been dealt? If not, what might this mean?*

- *Did you secretly desire another emotion? What might this tell you about yourself? What emotion would you hate to have?*

(Recommended) Class Exercise
OC Myths About Emotions

Refer participants to worksheet 6.A (Overcontrolled Myths About Emotions).

Instruct the class to place a checkmark in the box next to each myth about emotion that they believe to be true or somewhat true.

Divide participants into pairs. Have each member of the pair choose a myth that they believe in strongly and then take turns practicing self-enquiry and outing themselves about their respective myths. **Use the following steps to structure how to accomplish this.**

1. The revealing partner—that is, the person who is outing themselves—begins by reading aloud their myth three times in a row to their partner.

2. The listening partner then reads aloud several of the self-enquiry questions found in worksheet 6.A (changing "I" to "you"). For example, the listening partner might ask: *What might you need to learn from this myth? What might this myth be telling you about yourself and your life? Are you feeling tense right now? If so, then what might this mean? What is it that you might need to learn? How open are you to thinking differently about this myth or changing the myth? If you are not open or only partly open, then what might this mean?*

3. Pairs should then switch roles with the listener now taking the role of outing themselves by speaking aloud the images, thoughts, and memories linked to the myth they have chosen for their practice.

4. After each pair has played both roles at least once, instructors should encourage participants to share their observations about the exercise with the entire class.

Participants should incorporate the questions they found most provocative into their daily practice of self-enquiry and record their observations that result from this in the self-enquiry journal.

(Required) Teaching

Emotions Are There for a Reason

Refer participants to handout 6.1 (Emotions Are There for a Reason).

> ✓ **Ask:** *What good are emotions? Why do you think we have them?*

- *For many people, an ideal life is one that is relatively emotion-free, where decisions are informed solely by logical reasoning.*

> ✓ **Ask:** *To what extent might you believe this?*

- *Unfortunately, pure logic often fails when it comes to human relationships or making quick decisions.* For example, if we depended solely on our abilities to logically calculate the probabilities of being hit by an oncoming speeding bus before moving out of the way, we would likely have been run over long ago. When it comes to making decisions about speeding buses, falling objects, buying or selling stock, or braking one's car, by the time logical calculations are complete, our fate has most often already been decided.

(Required) Story and Discussion

"The Logical Romantic"

Read the following story aloud.

> There once was a very logical person who decided that it would be advantageous to get married. Since they did not have a lot of experience in this area, they decided to begin this process by generating a list of the attributes they considered most important in a spouse—for example, conscientious, a hard worker, doesn't smell, is orderly, likes long walks, has good teeth, and so on. Next, they set about looking for their ideal mate. After some time, they finally located someone who matched all of their search criteria (checked all the boxes on their list). They then proposed marriage. And after the other person agreed, they married! But within two years they were divorced. Why? Because the very logical person discovered that they had never really liked their spouse in the first place! The moral of this story is that emotions matter when it comes to human relationships.

NOTE TO INSTRUCTORS: To further facilitate the preceding discussion, it can sometimes help to encourage participants to recall the various problems encountered by the characters made famous in the *Star Trek* science fiction series known for their impeccable logic—that is, Mr. Spock, Commander Data, and Seven of Nine.

NOTE TO INSTRUCTORS: Teach the next section directly from handout 6.1 (Emotions Are There for a Reason).

- *Thus, emotions are our friends. They have four primary functions or purposes:*

  - **They help us** *make decisions*—for example, who to marry.

  - **They** *motivate* **our actions**—for example, fight-or-flight behaviors.

- **They *communicate* our inner experience and signal our intentions.** For example, an angry facial expression signals that someone has crossed your boundaries without necessitating an actual physical attack to make this clear to the other person.

- **They *facilitate* the formation of strong social bonds.** For example, research shows that if I were to suddenly grimace in pain, all of you would mimic my facial expression. You would spontaneously microgrimace, without even knowing it, because it happens so fast (in milliseconds). Your microexpression then feeds back information to your brain, triggering neurons in your brain that mirror the same neurons being fired in my brain when I grimaced in pain. Thus, your micromimicry and mirror neurons allow you to literally feel my pain and know what I am experiencing inside my body.

- ***By being able to viscerally join with another person we are more likely to treat them as we would like to be treated*** (and be willing to risk our lives to save someone we may hardly know). This process underlies the development of empathy and altruism in our species and provided our species with a huge evolutionary advantage (Schneider, Hempel, & Lynch, 2013).

(Required) Teaching Point
Why Bother Labeling Emotions?

> NOTE TO INSTRUCTORS: OC clients frequently report diminished emotional experience in situations that most others might report as highly emotionally charged (for example, a funeral, a birthday party, a retirement celebration, a disagreement with a spouse). They often find it difficult to label or differentiate between emotional experiences and other body sensations.

- ***Labeling emotions makes it easier for us to predict the future*** because we are more likely to be aware of the thoughts, sensations, or action tendencies associated with a particular emotion.

- ***Labeling our emotions helps us communicate our inner experience to others, thereby enhancing social connectedness.*** For example, labeling an emotion as "plastic" or "tidy" may be perfectly understandable to you, but most people will find it hard to understand what you mean.

> NOTE TO INSTRUCTORS: Encourage participants to use worksheet 6.B (Using Neural Substrates to Label Emotions) and handout 2.1 (The RO DBT Neuroregulatory Model of Emotions) to help identify which of the five broad emotion-based systems may have been activated in order to help narrow down your search for an emotion label.

(Required) Teaching Point
Four Steps to Emotion-Labeling Bliss

Refer participants to worksheet 6.B (Using Neural Substrates to Label Emotions) and use this worksheet to augment the teaching points outlined here.

Step 1. Describe the cue that triggered the emotion by asking...

- *Did the cue occur inside my body?* (for example, a thought about failing a test)
- *Did the cue occur outside my body?* (for example, a mean-looking cow is staring at you)
- *To what extent did contextual factors matter?* (for example, Monday-morning blues)

Step 2. Identify which brain-body emotion system was likely triggered by the cue by observing body sensations.

- If your body felt relaxed and calm, the cue was likely linked to social safety.
- If your body felt alert and focused, the cue was likely linked to novelty.
- If your body felt energized and powerful, the cue was likely linked to reward.
- If your body felt tense, agitated, and hot, the cue was likely linked to threat.
- If your body felt numb and detached from reality, the cue was likely linked to overwhelming threat or reward.

Step 3. Ask how you socially signaled, to deepen your understanding.

- Was it easy to make eye contact or express your emotions? Was your voice tone easygoing? Did you touch or reach out to someone? (likely the parasympathetic social safety system)
- Did you suddenly find yourself standing still and gazing intently? Or listening carefully? (likely novelty-evaluative system)
- Were you highly expressive, talkative, or using expansive gestures? Did it require effort to listen to others? Did it seem like you had missed something important that another person had said or done during an interaction but you were unable to identify it? (likely SNS excitatory arousal system)
- Did you find it difficult to smile without feeling phony? Was your expression flat or stony? Did you avert your eyes or stare intensely? Did your voice tone sound flat or strident? Were your gestures tight and constrained? (likely SNS defensive arousal system)
- Was your face expressionless? Were your body movements slow? Was your speech rate slow and your voice tone flat? Did you stare vacantly? (likely parasympathetic shutdown system)

Step 4. Observe action urges and desires.

- This step uses action urges and desires that have been shown to be linked with differing emotions as a tool for accurate emotional labeling. The core idea is that each emotion has a discrete action urge, and this can be used to work backward to the emotion name. For example...

  - **Fear** triggers an urge to flee or run away.
  - **Shame** triggers an urge to hide.
  - **Guilt** triggers an urge to repair or make amends.
  - **Sadness** triggers an urge to isolate or deactivate.
  - **Disgust** triggers an urge to expel.
  - **Joy** triggers an urge to approach and jump up and down.
  - **Love** triggers an urge to relax and socialize.
  - **Curiosity** triggers an urge to explore.

See worksheet 6.B for complete details.

NOTE TO INSTRUCTORS: Neither the PNS-DVC shutdown response nor the SNS novelty-evaluative response has been linked to a discrete emotion by other emotion theorists or researchers. Extreme shame may represent the closest primary emotion label for a PNS-DVC shutdown response. In part, this may reflect biases by the majority of emotion theorists to not include motivational urges or action tendencies that have not classically been linked to what many consider primary emotions (for example, an urge for a cigarette, an urge to dominate, and so forth).

NOTE TO INSTRUCTORS: Steps 5, 6, and 7 are further detailed in worksheet 6.B (Using Neural Substrates to Label Emotions).

(Recommended) Teaching Point

Not Everything That's Important Is Emotional

NOTE TO INSTRUCTORS: There is consistent evidence, including recent systematic and meta-analytic reviews in the case of anorexia nervosa and autism (Happé & Frith, 2006; Lang, Lopez, Stahl, Tchanturia, & Treasure, 2014), showing that OC clients exhibit weaknesses on tasks requiring global processing, whereas they demonstrate superior capacities for detail-focused or local processing (Aloi et al., 2015; Lopez, Tchanturia, Stahl, & Treasure, 2008, 2009; Losh et al., 2009). Unfortunately for the OC client, exceptional perceptual abilities to notice small changes in the environment often come to dominate their daily routines, leaving little time for rest, relaxation, recreation, or socializing.

Refer clients to handout 6.2 (Not Everything That's Important is Emotional).

1. *It's all in the details!*

   - *The brains of overcontrolled individuals are hardwired to notice details rather than global patterns of information.* For example, they may often exhibit heightened memory for details and notice minor discrepancies (such as grammatical mistakes, a misaligned book in a bookcase).

   - *Research suggests that this way of behaving may be nonemotional.* That is, OC individuals appear to be very good at recognizing small details regardless of how they're feeling at the time.

   - *Yet the consequences of detail-focused processing may be emotional.* For example, noticing that a book is out of alignment on a bookshelf may be purely a nonemotional sensory receptor response. However, the obsessive need to straighten the misaligned item can trigger strong emotions.

   - *Plus, this superior ability to notice small changes may trigger emotionally driven social comparisons* (for example, frustration when a detailed observation is unappreciated by others or secret pride in being able to notice an error that no one else picked up on).

     ✓ **Ask:** *To what extent do you notice small changes or minor errors?*

     ✓ **Ask:** *What are the downsides of a superior capacity for detailed over global processing?* (Hint: Makes it harder to see the big picture, and compulsive needs for order and symmetry can come to dominate daily routines; compulsive needs to quickly fix uncertainties may lead to exhaustion from overwork or frequent experiences of irritation when the anomaly cannot be fixed; can lead to frequent social comparisons resulting in unhelpful envy or resentment.)

2. *Help! My self-control is out of control!*

- *By definition, overcontrolled individuals possess superior self-control capacities* (for example, being able to plan ahead, delay gratification, tolerate distress, and inhibit emotional action urges).

- *Self-control involves areas of the brain that are nonemotional by nature* (for example, dorsal lateral prefrontal cortex).

- *Despite being nonemotional, self-control is hard work!* It requires effortful control over emotion-based action urges and the delaying of gratification. Excessive self-control depletes energy resources (in the form of glucose).

- *Therefore, excessive self-control has emotional consequences.*

- *Too much willpower depletes the energy resources needed to override too much willpower,* making a person more emotionally vulnerable or reactive.

- *Superior capacities in self-control can lead to frequent emotionally based social comparisons* (for example, feeling proud that one can sit for hours during a meditation practice without coughing or twitching, and secretly judging those who can't; see the discussion of secret pride in self-control and the enigma predicament in chapter 10 of the RO DBT textbook).

- *Excessive self-control (for example, excessive rule-governed behavior) can result in a person being less open to changing circumstances and can damage important relationships* (for example, insisting my partner stack the dishwasher according to my rules might result in an argument, or compulsive planning may make it hard to be spontaneous in a relationship).

  ✓ **Ask:** *What are the emotional consequences of self-control in your life? How has your capacity for self-control emotionally impacted others?*

Lesson 6 Homework

1. **(Required) Worksheet 6.A (Overcontrolled Myths About Emotions).**

2. **(Required) Worksheet 6.B (Using Neural Substrates to Label Emotions).**

3. (Optional) Encourage participants to look for emotional responses throughout the coming week and see if they can identify the function of the response, using worksheet 6.B to help facilitate this.

Radical Openness Handout 6.1

Emotions Are There for a Reason

Emotions have **four** primary functions or purposes:

1. **They help us *make decisions*.**

   - Emotions help us make quick decisions about the world without having to spend a great deal of time thinking about it.

   - For example, if we depended solely on our abilities to logically calculate the probabilities of being hit by an oncoming speeding bus before moving out of the way, we would likely have been run over long ago.

2. **They *motivate* our actions.**

   - Emotions prepare us for action—each emotion has a unique action urge or response tendency that evolved to enhance our survival.

   - For example, fear prepares us to escape a threat, anger helps protect us from harm, and contentment helps us join with others.

3. **They *communicate* our inner experience and *signal* our intentions.**

   - Our species survival depended upon signaling cooperation to other members of our species in order to form tribes to fight enemies/predators, share valuable resources, and work together to achieve long-term goals that would be impossible in isolation.

   - We have more facial muscles than any other species and we are capable of making ten thousand different expressions.

   - Facial expressions communicate our intentions.

   - For example, an angry facial expression signals to another person that they have crossed our boundaries without necessitating an actual physical attack to make this clear.

4. **They *facilitate* empathic responding and the formation of strong social bonds.**

   - We automatically micromimic (that is, copy) the facial expressions of a person we are interacting with, which triggers the same brain areas and results in a similar emotional experience in the person who is watching the other person express an emotion.

   - This facial feedback process involves the mirror neuron system in our brain, and it happens so fast (in milliseconds) that we are rarely aware of it.

   - Thus, if we observe a person grimace in pain, we tend to, without conscious awareness, micro-grimace, and as a result, via the influence of the mirror neuron system, we can literally know in our body how the other person feels.

   - Emotions (and micromimicry) help *facilitate* the formation of strong social bonds because *knowing* how someone else feels means we are more likely to respond with empathy and even be willing to risk our lives to save (or fight for) someone we hardly know and *treat them as we would like to be treated*. A stranger can suddenly become part of the family.

Radical Openness Handout 6.2

Not Everything That's Important Is Emotional

1. *It's all in the details!*

    - **The brains of overcontrolled individuals are hardwired to notice details rather than global patterns of information.** For example, they may often exhibit heightened memory for details and notice minor discrepancies (such as grammatical mistakes, a misaligned book in a bookcase).

    - **Research suggests that this way of behaving may be nonemotional;** that is, OC individuals appear to be very good at recognizing small details, regardless of how they're feeling at the time.

    - **Yet the consequences of detail-focused processing may be emotional.** For example, noticing that a book is out of alignment on a bookshelf may be purely a nonemotional sensory receptor response. However, the obsessive need to straighten the misaligned item can trigger strong emotions.

    - **Plus, this superior ability to notice small changes may trigger emotionally driven social comparisons** (for example, frustration when a detailed observation is unappreciated by others, or secret pride in being able to notice an error that no one else picked up on).

2. *Help! My self-control is out of control!*

    - **By definition, overcontrolled individuals possess superior self-control capacities** (for example, being able to plan ahead, delay gratification, tolerate distress, and inhibit emotional action urges).

    - **Self-control involves areas of the brain that are nonemotional by nature.**

    - **Despite being nonemotional, self-control is hard work!** It requires effortful control over emotion-based action urges and the delaying of gratification. Excessive self-control depletes energy.

    - **Too much willpower depletes the energy resources needed to override too much willpower,** making a person more emotionally vulnerable or reactive.

    - **Superior capacities in self-control can lead to secret pride and frequent downward social comparisons** (for example, secretly looking down on people who are unable to sit for hours during a meditation practice without coughing or twitching).

    - **Excessive rule-governed behavior can result in a person being less open to change, which can damage important relationships** (for example, insisting my partner stack the dishwasher according to my rules might result in an argument, or compulsive planning may make it hard to be spontaneous in a relationship).

Radical Openness Handout 6.3

Main Points for Lesson 6: How Do Emotions Help Us?

1. Pure logic often fails when it comes to human relationships or making quick decisions.

2. Most of us carry myths about emotions with us that can bias how we respond to the world. Rather than challenging a myth about emotion to get rid of it, use self-enquiry in order to learn from it. Self-enquiry is able to enquire about a myth, but it does not automatically assume that a myth is wrong, bad, or dysfunctional.

3. Emotions exist for a reason. They have four primary functions or purposes: (1) they help us make decisions, (2) they motivate our actions, (3) they communicate our inner experience and signal our intentions to others, and (4) they facilitate the formation of strong social bonds.

4. Not everything that's important is emotional. OC individuals are characterized by superior self-control and detail-focused capacities, features that by nature are nonemotional yet have emotional consequences when they are excessively or compulsively used.

Radical Openness Worksheet 6.A

Overcontrolled Myths About Emotions

Instructions: Place a checkmark in the box next to each myth you believe is true or somewhat true.

- ☐ We make our best decisions when emotions are kept out of it.
- ☐ There is a right way to feel in every situation.
- ☐ Emotions should be controlled.
- ☐ Letting others know what I am feeling inside is a sign of weakness.
- ☐ Most people dislike emotional people.
- ☐ Negative feelings are bad and destructive.
- ☐ Feeling happy or excited is naive or childish.
- ☐ Love is only a chemical reaction.
- ☐ It is important to never let another person know what you are really feeling inside.
- ☐ Being emotional means being out of control.
- ☐ Most emotions are really stupid.
- ☐ All painful emotions are a result of a bad attitude.
- ☐ Painful emotions are not really important and should be ignored.
- ☐ People who feel happy are liars.

In the following space, write out any other myths you may have about emotions that were not already mentioned.

_____

_____

_____

_____

_____

Next: Pick one of the preceding myths that you believe in strongly and practice self-enquiry about the myth over the next week. Keep your self-enquiry practices short in duration, not much longer than five minutes. The goal of self-enquiry is to *find a good question* that brings you closer to your edge or personal unknown (the place you don't want to go), in order to learn. After a week, move to another myth and repeat your self-enquiry practice.

Keep a record in your self-enquiry journal of the images, thoughts, emotions, and sensations that emerge when you practice self-enquiry about your myths about emotions. Practice being suspicious of quick answers to self-enquiry questions. Allow any answers to your self-enquiry practice to emerge over time.

Remember, self-enquiry does not automatically assume that a myth is wrong, bad, or dysfunctional. Use the following questions to facilitate a daily practice. Record what emerges in your self-enquiry journal.

> ➤ *What might I need to learn from this myth?*
>
> ➤ *What might this myth be telling me about myself and my life?*
>
> ➤ *Am I feeling tense doing this exercise?*
>
> ➤ *Am I feeling tense right now? If so, then what might this mean? What is it that I might need to learn?*
>
> ➤ *How open am I to thinking differently about this myth or changing the myth?*
>
> ➤ *If I am not open or only partly open, then what might this mean?*
>
> ➤ *How does holding on to this myth help me live more fully?*
>
> ➤ *How might changing this myth help me live more fully?*
>
> ➤ *What might my resistance to changing this myth be telling me?*
>
> ➤ *Is there something to learn from my resistance?*
>
> ➤ *What does holding on to this myth tell me about myself?*
>
> ➤ *What do I fear might happen if I momentarily let go of this myth?*
>
> ➤ *What is it that I need to learn?*

Use the following space to record additional self-enquiry questions or observations that emerged from your practice.

_____

_____

_____

_____

_____

Radical Openness Worksheet 6.B

Using Neural Substrates to Label Emotions

Instructions: During the coming week, as you did last week, be on the lookout for experiences and events linked to changes in body sensations and mood states, and use the following skills to identify which of the five emotional response systems may have been involved. However, this week we go one step further, where the emphasis is on pinpointing the name of the emotion you may have been experiencing.

Step 1. Describe the cue that triggered your emotional response.

Use the following questions to facilitate your description.

- *Did the cue occur inside your body (for example, a memory about an ex-partner)?*

- *Did the cue occur outside your body (for example, a loud bang, a beautiful sunset)?*

- *To what extent did contextual factors matter (for example, time of day, season of the year)?*

Describe other features of the emotion-eliciting cue.

_____

_____

_____

_____

Step 2. Use your body to identify the emotional system triggered by your cue.

Place a checkmark in the boxes next to the statements that best describe how your body felt.

- ☐ My body felt relaxed and calm (social safety cue).

- ☐ My body felt alert and focused (novelty cue).

- ☐ My body felt energized and powerful (rewarding cue).

- ☐ My body felt tense, agitated, and hot (threatening cue).

- ☐ My body felt numb and detached from reality (overwhelming cue).

Describe other body sensations.

_____

_____

_____

_____

153

Step 3. Observe how you socially signaled.

Place a checkmark in the boxes next to the questions that best address your experience.

- ☐ Was it easy to make eye contact or express your emotions? Was your voice tone easygoing? Did you touch or reach out to someone? (likely the parasympathetic social safety system)

- ☐ Did you suddenly find yourself standing still and gazing intently? Or listening carefully? (likely novelty-evaluative system)

- ☐ Were you highly expressive, talkative, or using expansive gestures? Did it require effort to listen to others? Did it seem like you had missed something important that another person had said or done during an interaction but you were unable to identify it? (likely SNS excitatory arousal system)

- ☐ Did you find it difficult to smile without feeling phony? Was your facial expression flat or stony? Did you avert your eyes or stare intensely? Did your voice tone sound flat or strident? Were your gestures tight and constrained? (likely SNS defensive arousal system)

- ☐ Were your face and body expressionless? Were your body movements slow? Was your speech rate slow and your voice tone flat? Did you stare vacantly? (likely parasympathetic shutdown system)

Other social signals.

_____

_____

_____

_____

Step 4. Observe your action urges and desires in order to label your emotions.

Place a checkmark in the boxes next to the statements that best describe your experience.

- ☐ I wanted to run away (likely fear).

- ☐ I wanted to hide my face or disappear (likely shame).

- ☐ I felt an urge to repair or make amends (likely guilt).

- ☐ I wanted to isolate and deactivate (likely depression/sadness).

- ☐ I wanted to push away or expel (likely disgust).

- ☐ I desired to exert my superiority (likely dominance).

- ☐ I desired to harshly gossip about someone (likely unhelpful envy).

- ☐ I desired to reject help from another (likely bitterness).

- ☐ I desired to pursue (likely pleasurable dominance).

- ☐ I wanted to give up but blame it on others (likely bitterness).

☐ I wanted revenge (likely envy).

☐ I desired to block a person from getting to know someone I feel very close to (likely jealousy).

☐ I felt an urge to stand still or freeze (likely novelty).

☐ I desired to socialize (likely contented love).

☐ I wanted to explore my environment (likely curiosity).

☐ I desired to flee (likely fear).

☐ I experienced an urge to attack (likely anger).

☐ I wanted to explore (likely curiosity).

Record other emotional response tendencies or reactions.

_____

_____

_____

_____

Step 5. Identify the function of the emotion, remembering it may have more than one.

Place a checkmark in the boxes next to the phrases that best describe your experience.

☐ Helped me make a decision

☐ Motivated my actions

☐ Communicated my inner experience and signaled my intention

☐ Helped me get closer to someone and/or experience empathy with someone

Other functions of the emotion.

_____

_____

_____

_____

Step 6. Notice if the cue prompts a nonemotional reaction linked to OC tendencies to notice details, discrepancies, engage in rule-governed behavior, and or/superior capacity for self-control.

Place a checkmark in the boxes next to the statement that best describe your experience.

☐ I made a detailed observation missed by others.

☐ I noticed a discrepancy that no one else picked up on.

☐ My behavior was rule-governed.

☐ I engaged in compulsive planning behavior.

Other reactions.

_____

_____

_____

_____

Understanding Overcontrolled Coping

Main Points for Lesson 7

1. Excessive self-control is maintained because it is rewarding. For example, losing two pounds by not succumbing to urges to eat may trigger feelings of pride and a sense of achievement.

2. To break a habit, one must know how it is reinforced.

Materials Needed

- (Optional) Handout 7.1. (Main Points for Lesson 7: Understanding Overcontrolled Coping)

- Worksheet 7.A (Overcontrol Can Become a Habit)

- Worksheet 7.B (Finding Our Habitual Ways of Coping)

- Whiteboard or flipchart with marker

(Required) Teaching Point

Overcontrol Is a Habit That Is Hard to Kick!

> NOTE TO INSTRUCTORS: Most people believe that the source of their suffering stems from emotion. RO DBT emphasizes that although emotions may at times be painful, the problem is not what one feels in any given moment; it is what one does about it that matters. Excessive self-control and low openness negatively impact social connectedness. Instructors should look for opportunities to reinforce these observations while they are teaching.

- *Self-control = the ability to inhibit emotional urges, impulses, and behaviors in order to pursue long-term goals.*

- *It is highly valued (perhaps universally) by most societies,* and many see it as the secret for success and happiness.

- *Unfortunately, people with overcontrol have too much of a good thing: their self-control is out of control, and they suffer as a consequence (albeit quietly).* For example, for the overcontrolled individual, their motto is "When in doubt, apply more self-control," irrespective of circumstances or potential consequences. They tend to be perfectionists who see mistakes everywhere (mostly in themselves) and work harder than most to prevent future problems from occurring.

- *But if overcontrol is such a problem, why doesn't it just go away by itself?* The answer to this question underlies the skills we will learn today.

- *Overcontrolled coping persists because it gets rewarded (or reinforced), at least occasionally.* For example, pretending to be okay can sometimes prevent conflict, working long hours may sometimes result in a job promotion, planning ahead can often prevent a future problem, following rules usually makes life easier.

★ **Fun Facts:** *Occasional Rewards Make Habits Harder to Break!*

Perhaps somewhat counterintuitively, intermittent reinforcement or occasional rewards make habits harder to break. For example, a slot machine doesn't always pay—wouldn't it be wonderful if it did? (☺) It only occasionally reinforces us. Despite this, we keep feeding money into it! Why? Because our brain knows a reward is available, just not when it will arrive or how much effort—that is, money—will need to be spent obtaining it, that golden jackpot! Thus, when playing the Las Vegas slots, when we are not rewarded immediately, we try again, whereas when we don't immediately receive our reward when using another type of machine, such as a soda pop machine, we don't keep putting money in again and again to get the cold beverage—we tend to kick the machine instead (tee hee ☺). Why? Because our brain has learned to expect a reward from a soda pop machine each and every time, whereas a slot machine has shaped us up to expect a reward only occasionally. Intermittent reinforcement is what makes gambling so addictive and habits like overcontrol so difficult to break.

(Required) Teaching Point

Overcontrol Can Become a Habit

Refer participants to worksheet 7.A (Overcontrol Can Become a Habit).

NOTE TO INSTRUCTORS: The best way to use this worksheet is to draw each component of the model diagrammed in worksheet 7.A on a whiteboard or flipchart and then teach and obtain examples for that component before moving on to the next one. For example, start by drawing a box on the left side of the whiteboard and label this *CUES*. Next, solicit examples of how cue factors manifest in the lives of class participants (for example, uncertainty, being the center of attention, a skewed place setting at the dinner table, being asked an opinion, being criticized, making a mistake), and teach core concepts, using the teaching points that follow. Next, draw the box labeled *UNWANTED OR DISLIKED PRIVATE EXPERIENCE*, soliciting examples and teaching core concepts as before. Proceed similarly with each component until the entire diagram has been drawn and examples obtained for each. Participants should be encouraged to record in the blank spaces provided in worksheet 7.A the examples in each component that are personally relevant.

Step 1. Look for the cues that trigger overcontrolled coping.

- *Overcontrolled and closed-minded behaviors are most often triggered when the environment is perceived as disconfirming, unexpected, novel, or discrepant.*

  ✓ **Ask:** *What types of cues trigger closed-minded and overcontrolled coping in you?* Common cues include being in a situation that is new, being asked to perform, discovering a misspelled word in a document, making a mistake, and feeling exposed or vulnerable (for example, the center of attention). Instructors should ask participants to share their cues with the class and to write down the examples that pertain to them in the space provided in the *CUES* box on the worksheet.

Step 2. Describe the inner experience (thoughts, emotions, sensations, memories/images) linked to overcontrolled coping.

✓ **Ask:** *What unwanted private experience most often precedes my overcontrolled coping?* Examples include a stiff neck or sudden headache, thinking *They don't appreciate my self-sacrifices*, feeling annoyed, strong desires or urges to fix a discrepancy, feelings of anxiety or uncertainty, feeling numb, thinking *Rules must be followed*, feeling embarrassed.

Step 3. Identify the action urge triggered by the unwanted experience.

✓ **Ask:** *Did I desire to escape or dominate the stressful event?*

- *Overcontrolled individuals compulsively engage in approach coping.* For example, be driven to fix the problem; order a new washing machine immediately after the old one malfunctions; work late into the night to complete a to-do list for the day; immediately restrict all extra calories after gaining three pounds; feel compelled to answer every email before one can relax; or rather than avoiding a social event to escape feelings of anxiety, they may compulsively force themselves to attend even when avoidance might actually be more adaptive.

- *Excessive approach coping is usually driven by extreme desires to win, control, or dominate other people or situations,* which can become a precursor for OC self-hate. For example, when questioned they may attempt to put the other person on the defensive by answering the question with a question; may agree to a plan while inwardly knowing they will never comply or that they will sabotage it; may lie or cheat to win; may purposefully pretend they are confident or correct to control a situation; or may withhold important information to dominate a situation.

- *Overcontrolled individuals also engage in avoidance coping.* For example, by trying not to think about the problem; distracting oneself; walking away from the problem; abandoning the relationship; distracting one's attention; pretending not to hear what was said; changing the topic; attempting to suppress emotions linked to it; blaming others for the problem; insisting it is not one's responsibility or that the situation is impossible to deal with.

- *Both avoidance and approach coping can be helpful ways of coping, depending on the situation.* Problems arise when they are rigidly applied regardless of the circumstance. For example, someone might immediately order a new washing machine when the old one malfunctions, only to discover the next day that the problem was a clogged drainpipe and not something to do with the machine itself. Sometimes waiting to solve problems can be useful because we find out new information.

Step 4. Observe how overcontrolled coping manifests.

- *Examples include* shutting down; denying the problem; ignoring or pretending to not hear unwanted feedback; pretending everything is okay when it's not; abandoning a relationship rather than dealing with a conflict; pouting; sulking; walking away; redoing other people's work; using the silent treatment; going flat-faced; turning the tables by finding fault; sabotaging or disparaging other people's efforts or work; smiling when angry; compulsively caretaking others; being obsessed with details; losing the big picture; changing the topic; agreeing with someone while inwardly disagreeing; obsessive rehearsal or planning; pretending to cooperate while secretly sabotaging; thinking about death or suicide; engaging in self-harm; depriving oneself; punishing oneself; insisting things are the same;

telling others what to do or how to behave; insisting that there is only one way to do something or that one's perspective is the correct one; criticizing others who are dissimilar; showing concern when not feeling it; lying to someone to avoid social disapproval or to win; avoiding the limelight; desiring appreciation but never asking for it; persevering in a behavior or tolerating distress despite clear evidence that harm may result; pervasively attending parties or social events out of obligation or duty, not because one wants to; never or rarely allowing oneself to rest; masking inner feelings; downplaying one's successes; blocking compliments; rarely or never giving praise to others; blocking offers of help; planning or engaging in revengeful acts; harshly gossiping; engaging in social comparisons; isolating from others; saying yes but thinking no; obsessively working to solve a problem; blaming others or the world for one's emotions or reactions; having a hyperfocus on order and symmetry; overapologizing or never apologizing.

Step 5. Notice the consequences of overcontrolled behavior.

- *Overcontrolled behavior creates long-term problems.* For example, avoidance may prevent learning something new or a better way to fix a problem. Compulsive controlling or fixing can also result in exhaustion and burnout, which can be exacerbated if one's hard work or self-sacrifices are not appreciated (sufficiently) by others, leading to resentment and bitterness.

- *Despite its generally understated nature, overcontrolled behavior strongly impacts other people* (for example, the silent treatment is a subtle yet powerful social signal of disapproval or anger). At its core, OC is considered a problem of emotional loneliness, linked with deficits in social signaling and difficulties forming intimate social bonds.

  ✓ **Ask:** *How do you think your way of manifesting overcontrol impacts your relationships with others?*

- *Plus, overcontrolled behavior is maintained because it is rewarded (at least occasionally).* Planning ahead, striving hard, exceeding expectations, and delaying gratification can help a person achieve a desired goal. Working obsessively to address problems or repair mistakes may be reinforced by a promotion at work. Rehearsing beforehand helps improve performance. Changing the topic to something less emotional may be reinforced by relief.

  ✓ **Ask:** *What reinforces your overcontrolled behavior?*

Lesson 7 Homework

NOTE TO INSTRUCTORS: Prior to assigning homework for lesson 7, instructors should direct participants to worksheet 7.B and ensure that they understand how they should complete this in the upcoming week.

1. **(Required) Worksheet 7.B (Finding Our Habitual Ways of Coping)**

Radical Openness Handout 7.1

Main Points for Lesson 7: Understanding Overcontrolled Coping

1. Excessive self-control is maintained because it is rewarding. For example, losing two pounds by not succumbing to urges to eat may trigger feelings of pride and a sense of achievement.

2. To break a habit, one must know how it is reinforced.

Radical Openness Worksheet 7.A

Overcontrol Can Become a Habit

How did I socially signal my overcontrol?

Did I desire to escape or dominate the stressful event?

Action Urge

Overcontrolled Coping

Examples: Go quiet, pretend I'm okay, change the topic, walk away, work harder

How was my overcontrol reinforced?

Unwanted or Disliked Private Experience

Examples: Irritation, numbness, embarrassment, uncertainty, fear, a headache

Consequences

Cues

Examples: Unexpected event, critical feedback, a misaligned book, a compliment, an error

What was the cue that triggered my overcontrolled coping or closed-minded behavior??

What unwanted private experience preceded my overcontrolled coping?

Radical Openness Worksheet 7.B

Finding Our Habitual Ways of Coping

During the week, look for triggers that lead to an experience of stress or emotions that you do not like or want (aversive tension). They might be feelings of tension, irritation, impatience, annoyance, sadness, anxiety, or numbness. Use the following steps to identify what happened.

Describe the situation you were in. What was the trigger or cue for the emotion? For example, maybe your boss asked for your opinion about a new project, or a neighbor invited you over for tea, or you saw an email announcing the promotion of a competitor at work.

_____

_____

_____

Observe and describe your thoughts and emotions. Observe, then write down your thoughts and label the emotion. Rate the intensity of the emotion (on a scale of 1 to 10, with 10 being most intense). **Examples of thoughts:** _I am uncertain what is proper in this situation; they will think that I am a fool; they are being phony or fake or I am being phony or fake; they don't appreciate me; I must not show weakness; rules must be followed; being correct is more important than being liked by others._ **Examples of emotions:** anger, frustration, desire for revenge, fear, anxiety, despair, sadness, envious, jealous, shame, embarrassed, humiliated, cold or indifferent, numb, overwhelmed, spiteful, guilty.

_____

_____

_____

Describe what you actually did in the situation. For example, did you pretend that everything was okay? Agree with the person despite silently disagreeing? Avoid going to the event? Work very hard to find a solution to fix the problem? Quickly come up with a reason why the suggestion wouldn't work? Change the topic to something else? Point out the other person's error? Isolate yourself or avoid talking about the issue? Think of ways to make the other person fail? Stay in bed and sleep? Work to make things perfect?

_____

_____

_____

Describe the consequences of your behavior. For example, did you avoid having to go to the party and feel relieved? Work all night on the presentation and feel relieved to have made it perfect but miss your son's music recital? Feel relieved to have escaped thinking about the problem momentarily but later feel groggy and bad about yourself for sleeping all day?

_____

_____

Ask yourself: _How might the consequences have reinforced my behavior?_ In other words, did your behavior help you feel better in the short run? What are the long-term consequences of your behavior?

_____

_____

_____

Tribe Matters

Understanding Rejection and Self-Conscious Emotions

Main Points for Lesson 8

1. We are better when together: being part of a tribe was essential for personal survival.

2. A tribe can consist of just two people.

3. Tribal bonds begin when two people commit to make self-sacrifices for the other person when they are in distress, without expecting anything in return.

4. Most people belong to many tribes.

5. For our early ancestors, social exclusion from the tribe meant almost certain death.

6. We are biologically predisposed to care about whether we are in-group or out-group because tribal banishment was essentially a death sentence.

7. Self-conscious emotions include shame, embarrassment, humiliation, and guilt. When we become self-conscious, we doubt our status in the tribe.

8. Shame is warranted when we have intentionally harmed or deceived other tribal members for personal gain or we have engaged in a behavior that could threaten the well-being of the entire tribe.

9. Use Flexible Mind SAGE skills when feeling shame, embarrassed, rejected, or excluded.

Materials Needed

- Handout 8.1 (Tribe Matters: Understanding Rejection and Self-Conscious Emotions)

- Handout 8.2 (Prototypical Emotional Expressions)

- Handout 8.3 (Shaming Ritual)

- Handout 8.4 (Flexible Mind SAGE: Dealing with Shame, Embarrassment, and Feeling Rejected or Excluded)

- Handout 8.5 (The RO DBT Self-Conscious Emotions Rating Scale)

- Handout 8.6. Signaling Nondominance

- (Optional) Handout 8.7 (Main Points for Lesson 8: Tribe Matters: Understanding Rejection and Self-Conscious Emotions)

- Worksheet 8.A (Flexible Mind SAGE Skills)

- (Optional) Copies of the story "Better When Together" for class members so they can take turns reading a sentence aloud

- Whiteboard or flipchart with marker

(Optional) Teaching Point
Better When Together

> NOTE TO INSTRUCTORS: Instructors can either read this story aloud themselves or make copies and have the class members take turns reading a sentence aloud.

"Better When Together": Read this story aloud, ideally with a silly TV announcer's voice.

Imagine two Stone Age tribes, Tribe Clog and Tribe Roc, living millions of years ago. They are vaguely aware of each other's existence because they wander the same geographical area, but they have never actually met. Now imagine that there is a very large and nasty pride of lions in their area, lions that hunt and feed nightly on members of both tribes. The screams each night can be heard for miles. Fortunately, a very clever member of Tribe Clog, called Kowock—which meant "striver" because he was exceptional in being able to plan ahead and delay gratification—had an idea that involved trapping the lions, a plan that would rid Tribe Clog of its nemesis forever. Unfortunately, the plan, though excellent, could not be actualized because there were not enough members in Tribe Clog to complete the necessary work. The only way for the plan to work was if Tribe Clog had more tribe members. Kowock, being good at persistence, told the chief, "I suggest we meet Tribe Roc and ask them to join forces with us against the lions." The chief replied, "Kowock, there is a problem. How will Tribe Roc know that our intentions are cooperative and friendly?" After some deliberation, Kowock replied, "We must signal vulnerability. We must wash our faces clean of war paint and freely expose our bellies to Tribe Roc. We must not hide behind our shields but instead walk freely toward them with an open heart and a willingness to reveal our fears and joys. Tribe Roc will then know that we are their brothers and that only together will we be able to survive the lions."

Ask participants: *What is the point behind this story? What does it tell us about how our species survived? What might this tell us about what is needed to form close social bonds with people we don't know?*

> NOTE TO INSTRUCTORS: The major point of the preceding story is that our species' survival depended on our ability to form long-lasting bonds and work together in groups, or tribes, by signaling cooperative intentions to total strangers.

(Required) Teaching Point
Got Tribe?

Refer participants to handout 8.1 (Tribe Matters: Understanding Rejection and Self-Conscious Emotions).

- ***For humans, tribe matters!*** For example, compared to other species, we are not particularly fast, strong, or robust—we lack sharp claws, horns, thick hides, or protective fur. Even my dog can outrun me! Yet few would disagree that our species has not only survived but thrived and come to dominate the animal and much of the natural world (albeit perhaps a bit too much sometimes).

✓ **Ask:** *What factors do you think contributed to this?*

- *Our physical frailty is proof* that our survival depended on something more than individual strength, speed, or toughness.

- *Safety in numbers: We survived because we developed capacities to form long-lasting bonds and share valuable resources with other people who were not in our immediate family* (that is, total strangers).

- *Tribal bonds and intimate relationships are founded upon reciprocal exchanges* of vulnerability, openness, and affection.

- *We are better when together.* When we work together, we can accomplish tasks and overcome obstacles or achieve goals that would be impossible if attempted alone (for example, building a rocket to go to the moon, constructing an Egyptian pyramid, overpowering a ferocious, voracious lion).

✓ **Ask:** *What are some examples of tasks that can only be accomplished by working together?*

(Required) Teaching Point
What Does Tribe Mean?

✳ *I awoke to the sound of drums—and knew I was finally home.* ✳

- *What defines a tribe? From an RO DBT perspective, a tribe can consist of just two people.*

- *Tribal bonds begin when two people commit to make self-sacrifices for the other person when they are in distress, without expecting anything in return.* For example, they would drop everything in order to help you if you became injured, or you can trust them to be available when you need support. Research shows that we only need one other person who genuinely cares about our personal well-being to feel safe.

- *Higher levels of intimacy and commitment between tribal members equate to greater feelings of social safety.* See handout 21.2 (Match + 1 Intimacy Rating Scale).

- *Most people belong to many tribes* (for example, recreational clubs, work teams, family and kin, the nation we live in, a shared culture). Tribes are often built around shared values and goals, albeit some tribes we are born into (for example, our family, our nation) and others may be forced upon us (for example, an inmate in a prison). However, most of the time we choose our tribes. Our RO DBT skills class is a type of tribe—we share a common goal of learning new skills, and we strive to support each other in achieving this.

- *Tribes come with a cost: tribal groups expect members to make self-sacrifices for the common good.* This can include risking one's life (for example, firefighters entering a burning building, or going to war when two tribes are competing for the same goal).

(Required) Teaching Point

Humans Fear Social Exclusion

✳ *Lonely apes die.* ✳

- *For our very early ancestors living in harsh environments, being in a tribe was essential for personal survival.* Nonhuman primates who are socially isolated from their community die of exposure, lack of nourishment, or predation in a matter of days to weeks (Steklis & Kling, 1985). Similarly, isolation from a tribe meant almost certain death for our ancestors (from starvation or predation).

- *Our brains still respond as if we are living in primordial times.*

- *We are evolutionarily hardwired to be hypersensitive to signs of social exclusion.* For example, research shows that we can quickly spot the angry face in a crowd of people, and angry faces hold our attention (E. Fox et al., 2000; Schupp et al., 2004).

- *We are constantly scanning the facial expressions and vocalizations of other people for signs of disapproval,* that is, information about our social status, the extent to which our behavior is socially desirable, and/or the degree to which another person appears to like us.

- *The cost of not detecting a true disapproval signal for our ancestors living in harsh environments was too high to ignore.* Tribal banishment was essentially a death sentence for our ancestors.

- *Thus, we are biologically predisposed to be socially anxious and hardwired to construe the intentions of others as disapproving, especially when social signals are ambiguous.* Strong negative evaluations ("She hates me!") are formed quickly and on the basis of very little information. Fearful and aggressive facial expressions automatically trigger unconditioned defensive responses (Adolphs, 2008). Neutral expressionless faces are often interpreted as hostile or disapproving (Butler et al., 2003).

NOTE TO INSTRUCTORS: This helps explain why almost all people fear public speaking: speakers are subjected to a wide range of approval and disapproval signals from an audience, and their brain is hardwired to respond to them. Blank expressions, furrowed brows, or slight frowns are interpreted as disapproval regardless of the actual intentions of the listener (for example, some people frown or furrow their brow when intensely concentrating).

(Required) Teaching Point

Rejection: No, Thanks!

- ***Being rejected by a tribe hurts.*** Research shows that social ostracism triggers the same areas of the brain that are triggered when we experience physical pain (Eisenberger & Lieberman, 2004), whereas tribal acceptance feels good—for example, our self-esteem goes up (Leary, Haupt, Strausser, & Chokel, 1998; Murray, Griffin, Rose, & Bellavia, 2003).

- ***Rejection triggers self-conscious emotions such as shame, guilt, and embarrassment,*** frequently described as feeling uncomfortable, nervous, hesitant, timid, tentative, tongue-tied, unsure, sheepish, uneasy, disconcerted, flustered, mortified, discouraged, humbled, censured, chastened, discredited, disgraced, or dishonored.

- ***Shame is the most powerful and painful of the self-conscious emotions.*** It can involve extreme self-denigration and feelings of being different, inferior, abnormal, repulsive, or fatally flawed in comparison to others.

- ***Shame triggers submissive displays and gestures of appeasement*** designed to de-escalate aggression, elicit sympathy, and regain entry into the tribe (Keltner & Harker, 1998; Tsoudis & Smith-Lovin, 1998). The same expressions of shame seen in humans also occur in nonhuman primates and are known to serve similar social functions (De Waal, 1996; Gruenewald, Dickerson, & Kemeny, 2007; Keltner & Harker, 1998). Universal signals of submission among humans include lowering of the head, covering the face with hands or hiding the face from view, slackened posture, lowering eyelids, casting eyes downward, avoiding eye contact, slumping shoulders, and postural shrinkage.

- ***Humans will do almost anything to avoid feelings of shame, humiliation, or embarrassment.*** Examples include quick anger, immediately searching for someone else to blame, turning the tables on a real or imagined accuser via counteraccusations, walking away, distracting or confusing the issue by changing the topic or pretending ignorance, lying about what happened, shutting down, dissociating, or numbing out.

  ✓ **Ask:** *What do you do to avoid feeling shame or embarrassment?*

★ **Fun Facts:** *Shame Differs from Guilt*

Shame involves real or imagined disapproval of one's core sense of self by others, following public exposure or anticipated exposure of real or imagined failings or serious violations of tribal norms. Guilt, on the other hand, stems from one's own negative evaluation of oneself, arising whenever one fails to live according to one's values or idealized self, as opposed to real or imagined evaluations by others that characterize shame. In contrast to shame, there is no directly attributable body, facial, vocal, or physiological pattern of expression that uniquely characterizes guilt [Ekman, 1992b; Scherer & Wallbott, 1994]. Instead, guilt is expressed symbolically (for example, offering a gift as a repair) or with words (for example, apologies), suggesting that it is an evolutionarily newer emotion relative to shame. Plus, research shows that people distrust expressions of guilt (for example, saying "I'm sorry") if they are not accompanied by bodily displays prototypical of shame—for example, postural shrinkage, lowered gaze, and blushing [Ferguson, Brugman, White, & Eyre, 2007]. Signaling expressions of shame when making an apology communicates that the violator values the relationship because they are feeling viscerally distressed by their actions, making it easier for the person who has been wronged to trust they will not do it again.

(Required) Teaching Point

Despite Being Painful, Shame Is Prosocial

- *Shame evolved to "punish" extremely harmful acts that could damage tribal survival,* not punish innocent mistakes, differences in opinion or expression, new ways of thinking, challenges to authority, or victims of abuse.

- *When we feel ashamed, we desire to appease or submit to the other person (or the tribe)* in order to retain our social status, de-escalate aggression, and/or solicit sympathy.

- *Shame is the evolutionary solution of our species for making survival of the tribe more important* than older evolutionarily "selfish" tendencies linked to survival of the individual.

- *Most shame is unwarranted,* arising when low-intensity social signals are appraised as high-intensity social disapproval and/or by cues associated with past trauma that are unrelated to the current situation or actual behavior of the person experiencing the shame.

- *Shame is warranted whenever an individual* intentionally harms or deceives other tribal members for personal gain (for example, stealing a neighbor's cow, lying or cheating to get ahead or win, exploiting weaker members of the tribe), or when their behavior threatens the well-being of the entire tribe (for example, a guard falling asleep on their watch, the designated keeper of the fire misplacing the tribe's only source of firemaking, encouraging in-fighting among tribal members for personal gain).

- *Minor social transgressions call for embarrassment, NOT shame or guilt*—for example, exhibiting poor table manners, loudly farting during the tribe's daily practice of silent meditation, forgetting to put the toothpaste cap back on, forgetting to bow to a leader.

- *Embarrassment displays differ from shame displays.* **Refer participants to handout 8.2 (Prototypical Emotional Expressions).** Both involve downward head movements and gaze aversion. However, embarrassment involves smiling or inhibited smiling and sometimes nervous face touching, whereas shame expressions involve frowning and sometimes covering of the face with the hands. Plus, embarrassment is also more difficult to fake than shame—it is hard to blush on command.

★ **Fun Facts:** *There Is Nobody Here But Us Chickens!*

Shame and its counterpart—social exclusion—help us understand why people around the world care so much about in-group and out-group dynamics. Humans use expressions of shame and embarrassment by others as social safety detectors. Our brains have evolved and developed ways to reliably detect the extent to which another person is prosocial and likely to engage in reciprocal cooperative behavior. Research shows that we can recognize another's prosocial intent through emotion-based touching, smiling, and overall level of emotional expressivity [Boone & Buck, 2003; Brown & Moore, 2002; Hertenstein, Verkamp, Kerestes, & Holmes, 2006; Schug, Matsumoto, Horita, Yamagishi, & Bonnet, 2010].

✓ **Ask:** *What social signals do you use to determine whether you are in someone's tribe? To what extent do you feel part of a tribe?*

Plus, for the full social benefits of expressing shame or embarrassment, context matters! Research shows that signaling shame following a minor transgression is met with antipathy and coolness from observing others, whereas expressions of embarrassment trigger sympathy and warmth. The opposite also applies: when embarrassment is expressed following more serious transgressions, this is met with antipathy and less warmth, whereas, shame following serious transgressions is perceived prosocially and with greater warmth [Feinberg, Willer, & Keltner, 2012].

NOTE TO INSTRUCTORS: Shame and guilt have been shown to occur predominantly (about 80 to 90 percent of the time) when others are in close proximity (Tangney, Miller, Flicker, & Barlow, 1996). Shame that is triggered when a person is alone most often relates to memories of past rejecting or exclusionary experience (for example, sexual abuse, bullied as a child), rumination about recent exclusionary experience (for example, caught telling a lie earlier that day), or rumination about imagined or anticipated exclusionary experience (for example, being caught cheating). The elicitation of self-conscious emotions is also moderated by past learning and experience with exclusion and individual differences in biotemperament (for example, threat sensitivity), as well as the current context (that is, type of social situation). Finally, it is important to remind participants that social rejection signals are needed in order to provide corrective feedback *when the behavior warrants disapproval* (for example, lying, cheating, stealing). That said, it can be difficult to know for certain when a behavior crosses the line from unwarranted to warranted disapproval, explaining why we need courts of law and independent judges. The major point is that social rejection signals are not bad per se; their utility depends on how they are used.

(Required) Teaching Point

Self-Conscious Emotions Are Triggered During Social Interactions

- **Shame and other self-conscious emotions can be warranted, partially warranted, or completely unwarranted.** They most often occur when around other people (Tangney et al., 1996).

- *During social interactions, self-conscious emotions are triggered by...*

  - *Low-intensity or ambiguous social signals that can be easily misinterpreted* (for example, a blank stare)

171

- *A conspicuous absence or low frequency of expected or customary prosocial signals* (for example, lack of reciprocal smiling or head nodding)

- *Overt rejection signals or high-intensity social signals linked to shaming rituals* (for example, disgust eye rolls, lip curling, jeering)

- *Ambiguous signals are powerful because they are easily misinterpreted and easily denied.* Examples of ambiguous or low-intensity signals include a blank stare, a flat facial expression, a slight upturn of the mouth on one side of the face with a narrowing of the eyes (possible contempt), an expressionless tone of voice, a burglar smile or smirk when a person is stating their opinion, changing the topic or interrupting someone whenever they attempt to speak, a slight turning of the body or shoulders away from someone, a furrowed brow, a frown or compressed lips, a failure to acknowledge a person when they enter a room, yawning or closing eyes when someone voices their opinion.

- *Low-intensity signals can reflect expression habits or emotional leakage never intended as disapproving* (for example, the sender has a habit of closing their eyes when someone is talking, the sender has a painful toothache).

- *However, low-intensity signals can also reflect genuine disapproval, dislike, or envy that is intentionally disguised or restrained* in order to punish, dominate, or achieve an advantage over someone (for example, yawning when a rival speaks, pretending not to notice distress, a cold stare).

  ✓ **Ask:** *How would you read a furrowed brow displayed by a person who had just asked for your opinion about the weather, the possibility of space travel, or the color of a room?*

NOTE TO INSTRUCTORS: Most people would interpret a furrowed brow in the preceding context as a sign of unwarranted disapproval, particularly since they had cooperatively complied to a request from the other person that involved candidly revealing their opinion about a topic that does not have a correct answer. However, many people frown or furrow their brows when they are concentrating or listening intently to someone. Rather than disapproving, they may be intensely interested in what the other is saying. If this point does not naturally arise during the preceding discussion, instructors should make a point of bringing it up.

(Required) Mini–Class Exercise
Exploring Low-Intensity Signals

Instructors should use the following steps to conduct this exercise.

Begin: *Let's try out the example we just discussed ourselves! Get with a partner.* (Instruct class members to break into pairs. Instructors may need to pair up with someone if there is an odd number of participants in the class.)

Instruct: *Take turns. Have one person ask the other for their opinion—say, about the weather—and then, when your partner answers, frown, stare intently, and furrow your brow. Then discuss with your partner what it felt like to give an opinion to someone frowning and furrowing their brow. Then switch roles, and try it again. Okay, you can begin…and have fun!*

Discuss: Encourage participants to share what they learned and observed.

> ✓ **Ask:** *How often do you read furrowed brows or frowns as disapproval or criticism when you interact with others?*

> ✓ **Ask:** *To what extent do you think you might show furrowed brows or frowns during interactions? How might this impact your relationships?*

> ✓ **Ask:** *What other types of low-intensity signals do you use, either intentionally or unintentionally?*

- *An absence of prosocial signaling may be the most powerful: a behavior that involves a deficit or lack is easily denied because there is nothing to confront.*

- *Unfortunately, the intentions of the person exhibiting them (oops…I meant not exhibiting ☺) are frequently misinterpreted as hostile or disapproving* despite genuine intentions to signal otherwise.

- *Examples of absent prosocial signals that can trigger shame or other self-conscious emotions include* not smiling during greetings or interactions, a conspicuous lack of prosocial touching (for example, refusing to shake hands), a lack of affirmative head nods, absence of eyebrow flashes or eyebrow wags during greetings or conversations, low frequency of openhanded or expansive gestures, lack of eye contact, lack of facial affect or emotional expression during interactions, or a failure to reciprocally respond or match the level of emotional expression exhibited by the other person (for example, laughing when they laugh).

> ✓ **Ask:** *How often do you read expressionless faces, lack of affirmative head nods, or lack of eye contact during interactions as disapproving or critical?*

> ✓ **Ask:** *How often do you purposefully avoid displaying prosocial signals (for example, smile)? How might this impact your relationships?*

- *Overt rejection signals are linked to shaming rituals—they are less common but more overt.* Examples of high-intensity or overt shaming signals include taunting laughter combined with pointing; lip curling, rolling of eyes; hissing; booing; spitting; jeering, heckling; sarcastic voice tones; and rude gestures. *Yet these too can often be misinterpreted by recipients*—for example, a disgust expression may reflect self-condemnation rather than other-condemnation.

(Optional) Teaching Point
Tribes Punish

- *"The Emperor's New Clothes":* When the little boy in the story by Hans Christian Andersen (see H. C. Andersen, 1837/2004) exclaimed for all to hear that the emperor "was wearing nothing at all" (Lee & Pinker, 2010), he did not tell the onlookers anything that they did not already know; however, the little boy did change their perceptual state "because now everyone knew that everyone *else* knew that the emperor was naked, and this prompted them to challenge his authority through laughter."

- *When intentions, actions, or behaviors become public knowledge*—that is, become common, mutual, and/or accessible to all—*principles of equity or fairness dominate,* necessitating that the wrongdoing or antitribal acts be publicly exposed and punished; for example, see "(Not So) Fun (but Interesting) Facts: The Use of Shaming Rituals," later in this lesson.

- *Tribes most often punish shameful acts via rituals of humiliation, ostracism, and stigmatization.* Examples of shaming social signals include loud taunting, mocking, scoffing, name-calling, parodying, laughing, ridiculing, and rude gestures such as sticking out the tongue; see "(Not So) Fun (but Interesting) Facts: The Use of Shaming Rituals," later in this lesson, for more examples.

- *The most dreadful of all punishments for shameful acts, other than immediate death, was complete banishment from the tribe.* We strongly dislike forced isolation—this is why prisons use solitary confinement as one of their most aversive (and feared) punishments. For our early ancestors, social exclusion from the tribe meant almost certain death.

★ **(Not So) Fun (but Interesting) Facts:** *The Use of Shaming Rituals*

Shame has been used as a means of socialization in all communities throughout history, expressed through shaming rituals. Although expressed in widely divergent ways, shaming rituals all share one core feature that appears to cut across culture and time—they all involve some form of public humiliation and exposure of the offender's transgression to other members of the tribe. For example, most often in preindustrial communities, a criminal was placed in the center of town, whereupon the local inhabitants engaged in a form of mob justice, with the offender forced to act out their tribal offense in exaggerated caricature. [Refer participants to handout 8.3 (Shaming Ritual).] *Offenders were often forced to wear shame-stigmatizing clothes or conspicuous symbols in public (for example, striped prison uniforms, not allowed shoes, shaved head, forced to ride backward on a donkey, or dressed up like a clown) that set the offender apart from the tribe, symbolizing their loss of status and personal autonomy.*

(Required) Teaching Point

When Feeling Shame, Embarrassed, Rejected or Excluded, Practice Flexible Mind SAGE

Refer participants to handout 8.4 (Flexible Mind SAGE: Dealing with Shame, Embarrassment, and Feeling Rejected or Excluded).

NOTE TO INSTRUCTORS: When teaching Flexible Mind SAGE (in the following section of this lesson), write out the acronym (SAGE) on a flipchart or whiteboard, with each letter arranged vertically in a column, but *without* teaching or naming the specific skill that each letter signifies. Next, starting with the first letter in the acronym (S in SAGE) teach the skills associated with that letter, using the key points outlined in the following section, until you have covered all of the skills associated with each individual letter. Importantly, only write out on the whiteboard or flipchart the global description of what each letter actually stands for when you are teaching the skills. This teaching method avoids long explanations about the use of certain words in the acronym and/or premature teaching of concepts, since the meaning of each letter is only revealed during the formal teaching of the skills associated with it.

Flexible Mind SAGE

S   Use **Self-enquiry** to determine if shame is warranted

A   If shame is warranted or partially warranted, then **Appease**

G   If shame is unwarranted, then **Go opposite** to urges to hide

E   Show **Embarrassment** to enhance trust and socially connect

S   *Use* **Self-enquiry** *to determine if shame is warranted.*

- *Practice self-enquiry both during and after shame-evoking events* in order to enhance openness, alert yourself to areas in your life that may need to change, take responsibility for your behavior, and develop a kind sense of humor about your own unique foibles and habits. Research shows that people who can laugh at their personal habits or foibles (with kindness) are more likely to be emotionally healthy.

- *In the heat of the moment, when immersed in a shame-eliciting social interaction, get into the habit of asking What is it that I might need to learn from my emotion? before you do anything else.* Remember that the goal of self-enquiry is a good question, not a good answer. Allow an answer, if there is one, to emerge over a period of days or weeks. Use handout 1.3 (Learning from Self-Enquiry) or handout 16.2 (Using Self-Enquiry to Explore "Pushback" and "Don't Hurt Me" Behaviors) to deepen your self-enquiry practices.

- *After the event, use handout 8.5 (The RO DBT Self-Conscious Emotions Rating Scale)* to determine the extent to which your emotional reaction was warranted.

(Required) Mini–Class Exercise
Using the RO DBT Self-Conscious Emotions Rating Scale Effectively

Refer participants to handout 8.5 (The RO DBT Self-Conscious Emotions Rating Scale).

Ask participants to identify a recent interaction that triggered shame or another self-conscious emotion.

Explain to participants that for today's practice, the aim is to use a recent event that triggered shame, guilt, or embarrassment and involved other people. Although the same skills can be applied to shame experiences triggered by nonsocial cues (for example, the sight of a rose might trigger shame for a person who had suffered abuse in a flower shop), the emphasis for this practice will be social signaling cues.

Next: Ask participants to identify the specific behavior they displayed or failed to display during the event that they believe may have been the source of their shame or self-conscious emotional response.

Encourage participants to use the behavior and event they have identified as the template for answering the questions that will be read aloud by the instructor and to record on a piece of paper the number of YES responses they had.

Instruct: Participants should then add up the number of YES responses and use the scoring guidelines at the end of the handout to determine whether shame was warranted, partially warranted, or unwarranted, using the RO DBT Self-Conscious Emotions Rating Scale.

A *If shame is warranted or partially warranted, then* **Appease**.

- *Take responsibility by admitting your wrongdoing, without justifying or defending yourself.* First, to yourself. Second, to close others. Third, to those who you have harmed.

- *Signal integrity by not falling apart.*

  - *Falling apart, sulking, pouting, and harsh self-blame are phony responsibility behaviors*—they are Fatalistic Mind thinking and behavior (see lesson 11).

  - *Expect to suffer, and then decide to learn from it.* Warranted and partially warranted shame alert us to the very areas in our life that we may need to grow the most. Willingness to learn from shame (rather than avoid it) is an act of courage. Behaving courageously means living by your values. Use self-enquiry to enhance this process.

- *Out yourself by revealing your wrongdoing to others.*

  - *Cheerlead yourself—people who openly admit warranted shame or guilt are universally perceived as prosocial.* Outing your shame represents an important first step toward regaining trust, repairing a damaged relationship, and admittance back into your tribe.

  - *When you out yourself, block attempts by listeners to validate your behavior.* Explain that you are learning how to take responsibility for your actions and that outing yourself about warranted or partially warranted shame, without immediate validation, is a core means for accomplishing this.

  - *Use the Awareness Continuum when outing yourself* to block automatic tendencies to justify or explain your actions (see lesson 12).

- *Determine if you desire to maintain the relationship with the person(s) you have harmed. If yes, then...*

  - *Repair the transgression without expecting anything in return, using these eight steps for relationship repair to guide your actions.*

    1. *Signal deference and relinquish control when you make a repair by being polite, not talking over them, keeping voice volume low, allowing them control over the pace and content of the conversation.*

    2. *Accurately identify the harm done and communicate this to the person(s) involved.*

    3. *Confirm your perception of the harm done as valid from the person(s) harmed. Let go of arrogantly assuming you already know what it was—practice listening to their perspective without interrupting.*

    4. *Block automatic rationalization or justification of your behavior.*

5. *Make a genuine effort to repair the actual damage done (for example, not just saying "I'm sorry" if one has damaged a wall, but finding a way to repair the wall itself).*

6. *Commit to genuinely working to not harm the person again in a similar manner and promise to be more candid with them in the future.*

7. *Actively take steps to prevent future harm (for example, bring in an independent auditor to check on your progress; take a class or get professional help).*

8. *Forgive yourself for having harmed the other person(s), using Flexible Mind Has HEART skills to facilitate this (see lesson 29).*

- *Vary your social signaling to match the severity of your transgression.*

  - ***Signal shame if your shame was warranted*** by lowering your head, averting your gaze, and frowning when apologizing.

  - **Minipractice:** Ask participants to turn to a partner and take turns practicing shame displays. **Discuss:** *What did it feel like to display this behavior? What did it feel like to be on the receiving end? What might this tell you about your own social signaling?*

  - ***Signal appeasement and regret if your shame was only partially warranted*** by slightly bowing your head, displaying prolonged shoulder shrugs, and using openhanded gestures while maintaining eye contact with the other person in order to signal your confidence and commitment to change.

  - **Minipractice:** Ask participants to practice appeasement gestures with a partner. **Discuss:** *What did it feel like to display this behavior? What did it feel like to be on the receiving end? What might this tell you about your own social signaling?*

- ***Regularly signal nondominance and openness after you have successfully repaired the relationship by combining appeasement signals*** (for example, slight bowing of head, slight shoulder shrug, openhanded gestures) ***with cooperative-friendly signals*** (for example, warm smile, eyebrow wags, eye contact). Nondominance signals communicate equity, openness to critical feedback, and that you are not trying to manipulate the other person.

- ***Nondominance signals are especially important if you are in a power-up position*** to the person(s) harmed. **Refer participants to handout 8.6 (Signaling Nondominance).**

- ***Signal embarrassment when your transgression involves violation of a culturally specific social norm or convention*** (for example, misspeaking, stepping on someone's toe, poor table manners, forgetting to put the toothpaste cap back on, forgetting to bow to a leader, farting in church—oops! ☺).

- *The preceding skills are what you would need to practice if your shame is warranted or partially warranted. The next set of skills is for those times when your shame or other self-conscious emotions are unwarranted.*

G *If shame is unwarranted,* Go opposite *to urges to hide or appease.*

- *Behave as if you haven't done anything wrong—because you haven't.*

  - *Don't apologize or appease.*

  - *Signal confidence.* Stand or sit with your shoulders back, keep your chin up, maintain eye contact, speak with a matter-of-fact tone of voice and normal volume of speech (that is, don't whisper).

- **Minipractice:** Ask participants to practice signaling confidence with a partner.
  Discuss: *What did it feel like to display this behavior? What did it feel like to be on the receiving end? What might this tell you about your own social signaling?*

- *Balance signals of dominance (confidence) with signals of nondominance* in order to make it clear to others that, despite your shame being unwarranted, you remain open to critical feedback. **Refer participants once again to handout 8.6 (Signaling Nondominance).**

- *Out yourself to a friend about your shame experience being unwarranted in order to identify blind spots.* Be open to critical feedback or disagreement about your shame being classified as unwarranted; see handout 22.1 (Being Open to Feedback from Others: Flexible Mind ADOPTS).

- *Identify potential disguised toxic social environments that may trigger unwarranted shame, using the following questions.* If there are more NO responses then YES responses, then your environment may be toxic.

  1. *Do I trust the other person's or persons' true intentions or motivations?* YES/NO

  2. *Do I trust them to tell me what they really think?* YES/NO

  3. *When in their presence do I generally feel calm and safe?* YES/NO

  4. *Do I have any evidence or past experience suggesting that they have my best interests at heart?* YES/NO

  5. *Do they allow me time to express my inner feelings or ideas?* YES/NO

  6. *Are they open to me giving critical feedback or differing opinions?* YES/NO

- *If you believe the environment may be toxic, then...*

  - *Expect to experience more unwarranted shame.*

  - *If possible, talk to the person(s) involved about your feelings* (especially if you have never done this before). Use handout 22.1 (Being Open to Feedback from Others: Flexible Mind ADOPTS) to practice openness when (or if) you provide them with feedback.

  - *Ask an independent person to be present with you* when you speak to them, if you fear an extreme reaction.

  - *If the toxicity involves a long-term relationship, seek independent counsel* (for example, a marriage counselor).

  - *Use self-enquiry to examine how you may have contributed to the problem, without harsh self-blame.*

  - *Consider abandoning the relationship.* Some relationships can never be repaired. Make sure you seek independent counsel before taking this option.

  - *Don't try to outdo them in niggling* if you believe they are purposefully attempting to make your life difficult.

So far we have primarily focused on the problematic sides of shame and other self-conscious emotions. Our next set of skills in SAGE will focus more on the positive sides of self-conscious emotions.

E *Show **Embarrassment** to enhance trust and socially connect.*

- *Is there anything good in shame or other self-conscious emotions?*

- *The answer is embarrassing (tee hee ☺) because the answer is embarrassment.* Signaling embarrassment is what's good about shame and other self-conscious emotions.

- *Feeling embarrassed is nothing to be embarrassed about.*

- *Feeling embarrassed means you care about other people (and your tribe).* If you didn't really care about anyone, you could not experience embarrassment—you could only fake it.

- *People trust and like people who show embarrassment.* We feel more connected with people who show embarrassment because it signals they care about social transgressions (for example, hurting someone, being insensitive).

- *Expressing embarrassment is appealing.* For example, people display embarrassment signals when flirting (coy smiles, blushing). People prefer to spend more time with people who reveal intense embarrassment rather than inhibit it.

- *So if you try not to blush, STOP IT!* And start BLUSHING! Go on, BLUSH, BLUSH, BLUSH—people will like you and want to hang out with you!

- *The key point is: You don't have to feel safe on the inside to signal social safety and trust on the outside!*

Lesson 8 Homework

1. **(Required) Worksheet 8.A (Flexible Mind SAGE Skills).** Instruct participants to be alert for times they experience shame, embarrassment, guilt, humiliation, or similar self-conscious emotions, and to use worksheet 8.A in the coming week to practice Flexible Mind SAGE skills.

2. **(Recommended) Handout 8.5 (The RO DBT Self-Conscious Emotions Rating Scale).** Encourage participants to use handout 8.5 to determine whether self-conscious emotions are warranted.

NOTE TO INSTRUCTORS: Although SAGE skills can be used with both recent or long-past events that triggered shame or similar self-conscious emotions, encourage participants to practice SAGE skills in the coming week with events in which shame or other self-conscious emotions are at least partially warranted (that is, to learn the full range of skills from this lesson plan, it is best not to work only with unwarranted shame experiences).

Radical Openness Handout 8.1

Tribe Matters: Understanding Rejection and Self-Conscious Emotions

Tribes were essential for species survival

- **Safety in numbers.**

- **We are better when together.**

- **A tribe can consist of just two people.** Tribal bonds begin when two people commit to make self-sacrifices for the other person when they are in distress, without expecting anything in return.

- **Most people belong to many tribes** (for example, recreational clubs, work teams, family and kin, the nation we live in, a shared culture).

Social rejection and self-conscious emotions

- **For our early ancestors, social exclusion from the tribe meant almost certain death** from exposure, lack of nourishment, or predators in a matter of days or weeks.

- **We are biologically predisposed to care about whether we are in-group or out-group** because tribal banishment was essentially a death sentence.

- **We become self-conscious when we doubt our status in the tribe.**

- **Self-conscious emotions include shame, embarrassment, humiliation, and guilt,** emotional states often described as feeling uncomfortable, nervous, hesitant, timid, tentative, tongue-tied, unsure, sheepish, uneasy, disconcerted, flustered, mortified, discouraged, humbled, censured, chastened, discredited, disgraced, or dishonored.

- **Humans will do almost anything to avoid feelings of shame, humiliation, guilt, or embarrassment.** Examples include quick anger, immediately searching for someone else to blame, turning the tables on a real or imagined accuser via counteraccusations, walking away, distracting or confusing the issue by changing the topic or pretending ignorance, lying about what happened, shutting down, dissociating, or numbing out.

Despite being painful, shame is prosocial

- **Shame and similar self-conscious emotions evolved to provide painful corrective feedback** about behaviors that could potentially harm the well-being of the tribe.

- **When we feel ashamed, we desire to appease or submit to the other person** (or the tribe) in order to retain our social status, de-escalate aggression, and/or solicit sympathy.

Shame is warranted when...

- **An individual intentionally harms or deceives other tribal members for personal gain** (for example, stealing a neighbor's cow, lying or cheating to get ahead or win, exploiting weaker members of the tribe).

- **An individual's behavior threatens the well-being of the entire tribe** (for example, a guard falling asleep on their watch, the designated keeper of the fire misplacing the tribe's only source of firemaking, encouraging in-fighting among tribal members for personal gain).

Most shame is unwarranted or only partially warranted

- **Shame and other self-conscious emotions** can be warranted, partially warranted, or completely unwarranted.

- **We are evolutionarily biased to misinterpret the intentions of others as disapproving,** especially when social signals are ambiguous.

- **Shame evolved to "punish" extremely harmful acts that could damage tribal survival,** not to punish innocent mistakes, differences in opinion or expression, new ways of thinking, challenges to authority, or victims of abuse.

Radical Openness Handout 8.2
Prototypical Emotional Expressions

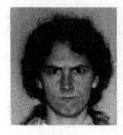 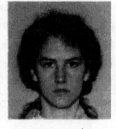 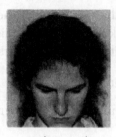 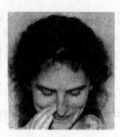 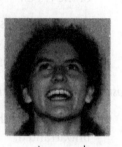

Angry   Neutral   Ashamed   Embarrassed   Amused

Adapted from Keltner, Young, & Bushwell, 1977, p 363.

Radical Openness Handout 8.3

Shaming Ritual

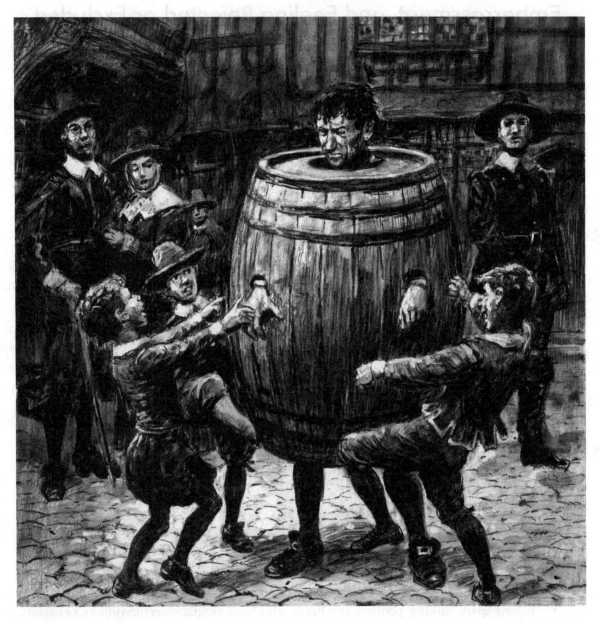

© Peter Jackson / courtesy Bridgeman Images.

Radical Openness Handout 8.4

Flexible Mind SAGE: Dealing with Shame, Embarrassment, and Feeling Rejected or Excluded

Flexible Mind SAGE

S   Use **Self-enquiry** to determine if shame is warranted

A   If shame is warranted or partially warranted, then **Appease**

G   If shame is unwarranted, then **Go opposite** to urges to hide

E   Show embarrassment to **Enhance** trust and socially connect

S   *Use **Self-enquiry** to determine if shame is warranted.*

- **Practice self-enquiry both during and after shame-evoking events** in order to enhance openness, alert yourself to areas in your life that may need to change, take responsibility for your behavior, and develop a kind sense of humor about your own unique foibles and habits.

- **In the heat of the moment, when immersed in a shame-eliciting social interaction,** get into the habit of asking *What is it that I might need to learn from my emotion?* before you do anything else. Remember that the goal of self-enquiry is a good question, not a good answer.

- **After the event, use the RO DBT Self-Conscious Emotions Rating Scale** (see handout 8.5) to determine the extent to which your emotional reaction was warranted.

A   *If shame is warranted or partially warranted, then **Appease**.*

- **Take responsibility by admitting your wrongdoing, without justifying or defending yourself.**
  - *First, to yourself*
  - *Second, to close others*
  - *Third, to those who you have harmed*

- **Signal integrity by not falling apart.**
  - **Falling apart, sulking, pouting, and harsh self-blame are phony responsibility behaviors.**
  - **Expect to suffer, and then decide to learn from it.** Warranted and partially warranted shame alert us to the very areas in our life that we may need to grow the most. Willingness to learn from shame (rather than avoid it) is an act of courage.

- Out yourself by revealing your wrongdoing to others.

  - Cheerlead yourself—people who openly admit warranted shame or guilt are universally perceived as prosocial.

  - **When you out yourself, block attempts by listeners to validate your behavior.** Explain that you are learning how to take responsibility for your actions and that outing yourself about warranted or partially warranted shame without immediate validation is a core means for accomplishing this.

  - **Use the Awareness Continuum when outing yourself** to block automatic tendencies to justify or explain your actions (see lesson 12).

- Determine if you desire to maintain the relationship with the person(s) you have harmed. If yes, then...

  - **Repair the transgression, without expecting anything in return, using these eight steps for relationship repair to guide your actions.**

    1. *Signal deference and relinquish control when you make a repair by being polite, not talking over them, keeping voice volume low, allowing them control over the pace and content of the conversation.*

    2. *Accurately identify the harm done and communicate this to the person(s) involved.*

    3. *Confirm your perception of the harm done as valid from the person(s) harmed. Let go of arrogantly assuming you already know what it was—practice listening to their perspective without interrupting.*

    4. *Block automatic rationalization or justification of your behavior.*

    5. *Make a genuine effort to repair the actual damage done (for example, not just saying "I'm sorry" if one has damaged a wall, but finding a way to repair the wall itself).*

    6. *Commit to genuinely working to not harm the person(s) again in a similar manner and promise to be more candid with them in the future.*

    7. *Actively take steps to prevent future harm (for example, bring in an independent auditor to check on your progress; take a class or get professional help).*

    8. *Forgive yourself for having harmed the other person(s), using Flexible Mind Has HEART skills to facilitate this (see lesson 29).*

- Vary your social signaling to match the severity of your transgression.

  - **Signal shame if your shame was warranted** by lowering your head, averting your gaze, and frowning when apologizing.

  - **Signal appeasement and regret if your shame was only partially warranted** by slightly bowing your head, displaying prolonged shoulder shrugs, and using openhanded gestures, while maintaining eye contact with the other person in order to signal your confidence and commitment to change.

- **Regularly signal nondominance and openness after you have successfully repaired the relationship** by combining **appeasement signals** (for example, slight bowing of head, slight shoulder shrug, openhanded gestures) with **cooperative-friendly signals** (for example, warm smile, eyebrow wags, eye contact). Nondominance signals communicate equity, openness to critical feedback, and that you are not trying to manipulate the other person(s).

- **Nondominance signals are especially important if you are in a power-up position** to the person(s) harmed. See handout 8.6 (Signaling Nondominance).

- **Signal embarrassment when your transgression involves violation of a culturally specific social norm or convention** (for example, misspeaking, stepping on someone's toe, poor table manners, forgetting to put the toothpaste cap back on, forgetting to bow to a leader, farting in church—oops! ☺).

G *If shame is unwarranted,* **Go opposite** *to urges to hide or appease.*

- **Behave as if you haven't done anything wrong—because you haven't.**

  - **Don't apologize or appease.**

  - **Signal confidence.** Stand or sit with your shoulders back, keep your chin up, maintain eye contact, speak with a matter-of-fact tone of voice and normal volume of speech (that is, don't whisper).

- **Balance signals of dominance (confidence) with signals of nondominance** in order to make it clear to others that, despite your shame being unwarranted, you remain open to critical feedback.

- **Out yourself to a friend about your shame experience being unwarranted in order to identify blind spots.** Be open to critical feedback or disagreement about your shame being classified as unwarranted; see handout 22.1 (Being Open to Feedback from Others: Flexible Mind ADOPTS).

- **Identify potential disguised toxic social environments that may trigger unwarranted shame, using the following questions.** If there are more NO responses then YES responses, then your environment may be toxic.

  1. *Do I trust the other person's or persons' true intentions or motivations?* YES/NO

  2. *Do I trust them to tell me what they really think?* YES/NO

  3. *When in their presence do I generally feel calm and safe?* YES/NO

  4. *Do I have any evidence or past experience suggesting that they have my best interests at heart?* YES/NO

  5. *Do they allow me time to express my inner feelings or ideas?* YES/NO

  6. *Are they open to me giving critical feedback or differing opinions?* YES/NO

- **If you believe the environment may be toxic, then...**

  - **Expect to experience more unwarranted shame.**

  - **If possible, talk to the person(s) involved about your feelings** (remember to stay open to any feedback).

- **Ask an independent person to be present with you** when you speak to them, if you fear an extreme reaction.

- **If the toxicity involves a long-term relationship, seek independent counsel** (for example, a marriage counselor).

- **Use self-enquiry to examine how you may have contributed to the problem, without harsh self-blame.**

- **Consider abandoning the relationship.** Some relationships can never be repaired. Make sure you seek independent counsel before taking this option.

- **Don't try to outdo them in niggling** if you believe they are purposefully attempting to make your life difficult.

E *Show* **Embarrassment** *to enhance trust and socially connect.*

- **Embarrassment displays** involve smiling or inhibited smiling and sometimes nervous face touching or blushing. Embarrassment is difficult to fake—it is hard to blush on command.

- **Feeling embarrassed is nothing to be embarrassed about.**

- **Feeling embarrassed means you care about other people (and your tribe).** If you didn't really care about anyone, you could not experience embarrassment—you could only fake it.

- **People trust and like people who show embarrassment.** We feel more connected with people who show embarrassment because it signals they care about social transgressions (for example, hurting someone, being insensitive).

- **Expressing embarrassment is appealing.** For example, people display embarrassment signals when flirting (coy smiles, blushing). People prefer to spend more time with people who reveal intense embarrassment rather than inhibit it.

- **The key point is: You don't have to feel safe on the inside to signal social safety and trust on the outside!**

Radical Openness Handout 8.5

The RO DBT Self-Conscious Emotions Rating Scale

Step 1. Identify the event, circumstance, or interaction triggering shame or other self-conscious emotions that you wish to evaluate.

Step 2. Identify the specific behavior you displayed or failed to display during the event that you believe may have caused or contributed to your shame or self-conscious emotional response.

Step 3. Use the event and specific behavior you have just identified to answer each of the questions that follow with YES or NO.

Step 4. Add up the number of YES responses, and use the scoring guidelines at the end of the handout to determine the extent to which your shame was warranted, partially warranted, or unwarranted.

1. *Did I purposefully lie, fabricate, or fail to disclose important information in order to achieve a goal or benefit myself?* YES/NO

2. *Did my behavior significantly damage an important relationship and/or result in serious injury to other tribal members or the community itself but benefit myself?* YES/NO

3. *Did my behavior result in severe physical or psychological injury to another person and/or my tribe as a result of my negligence, greed, envy, malice, or overconfidence?* YES/NO

Note: If you answered YES to any one of the three preceding questions, your shame or other self-conscious emotion IS WARRANTED. If you answered NO to all three questions, then answer the questions that follow to determine the extent to which your shame or other self-conscious emotion is likely warranted, partially warranted, or completely unwarranted.

4. *Have I been (or would I be) reluctant to make public and/or reveal, to the other persons involved, my hidden intentions during the event that triggered shame to get what I want or make things difficult?* YES/NO

5. *Have I avoided repairing the damage my behavior may have caused the other person(s) involved?* YES/NO

6. *Do I believe it would be important to correct a child if they had behaved similarly to how I did?* YES/NO

7. *Did my behavior betray or violate a prior agreement, commitment, or unspoken understanding between myself and the other person(s) involved?* YES/NO

8. *Was I in a position of power or authority over the person(s) involved when the event that triggered my shame or other self-conscious emotions occurred?* YES/NO

9. *Have I tried to justify or defend my actions or lack of action that resulted in harm or an unfair advantage with people who were not present at the event or who were at the event but are in a power-down relationship with me?* YES/NO

10. *Would my greater community or objective observers consider my behavior inappropriate, irresponsible, or unethical, given my position, my role, or my job at the time it occurred?*   YES/NO

11. *Does my shame, embarrassment, or guilt refer to the actual situation I was in rather than to similar past events?*   YES/NO

12. *Have I engaged in this type of behavior before and been told by others (or known myself) that it was inappropriate or morally/ethically wrong?*   YES/NO

13. *Have I in any way purposefully avoided answering YES to any of these questions?*   YES/NO

Scoring Guidelines

- **If a YES response was recorded for items 1, 2, or 3** (the first three questions), then shame or other self-conscious emotions are warranted.

- **Add up the YES responses for the remaining questions (items 4–13).**

  - **A score of 7 to 10 YES responses** = shame and other self-conscious emotions are *most likely warranted.*

  - **A score of 4 to 6 YES responses** = shame and other self-conscious emotions are *partially warranted.*

  - **A score of 0 to 3 YES responses** = shame and other self-conscious emotions are *most likely unwarranted.*

Radical Openness Handout 8.6

Signaling Nondominance

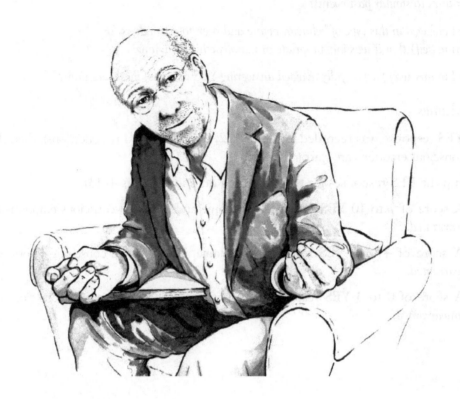

Radical Openness Handout 8.7

Main Points for Lesson 8: Tribe Matters

Understanding Rejection and Self-Conscious Emotions

1. We are better when together: being part of a tribe was essential for personal survival.

2. A tribe can consist of just two people.

3. Tribal bonds begin when two people commit to make self-sacrifices for the other person when they are in distress, without expecting anything in return.

4. Most people belong to many tribes.

5. For our early ancestors, social exclusion from the tribe meant almost certain death.

6. We are biologically predisposed to care about whether we are in-group or out-group because tribal banishment was essentially a death sentence.

7. Self-conscious emotions include shame, embarrassment, humiliation, and guilt. When we become self-conscious, we doubt our status in the tribe.

8. Shame is warranted when we have intentionally harmed or deceived other tribal members for personal gain or we have engaged in a behavior that could threaten the well-being of the entire tribe.

9. Use Flexible Mind SAGE skills when feeling shame, embarrassed, rejected, or excluded.

Radical Openness Worksheet 8.A

Flexible Mind SAGE Skills

Flexible Mind SAGE

S   Use **Self-enquiry** to determine if shame is warranted

A   If shame is warranted or partially warranted, then **Appease**

G   If shame is unwarranted, then **Go opposite** to urges to hide

E   Show embarrassment to **Enhance** trust and socially connect

Be alert for times you experience shame, embarrassment, guilt, humiliation, or similar self-conscious emotions. SAGE skills can be used with recent or past events that triggered shame and similar self-conscious emotions.

Pick an event to practice your SAGE skills.

Describe the event (for example, who was present, what their relationship was with you, and what the primary purpose of the interaction was).

_____

_____

_____

_____

_____

Describe the specific behavior you displayed or failed to display that you believe may have caused or contributed to your shame or self-conscious emotional response.

_____

_____

_____

_____

_____

S *Use* **Self-enquiry** *to determine if shame is warranted.*

Place a checkmark in the boxes next to the skill you practiced.

☐ **Used self-enquiry in the heat of the moment** before I attempted to regulate, accept, or deny my emotional experience by asking *What is it that I might need to learn from my emotion?* Record here what happened.

_____

_____

☐ Remembered that the goal of self-enquiry is a good question, not a good answer

☐ **Practiced self-enquiry** about my shame or self-conscious experience over several days to weeks.

Record here the question or questions that you found most helpful.

_____

_____

_____

_____

☐ Used the **RO DBT Self-Conscious Emotions Rating Scale** to determine whether my shame was warranted or unwarranted.

Record your score(s) here.

Total number of YES responses for questions 1–3 _____

Total number of YES responses for questions 4–13 _____

A *If shame is warranted or partially warranted, then* **Appease.**

Place a checkmark in the boxes next to the skills you practiced.

☐ Signaled integrity by not falling apart.

☐ Recognized that I did not wish to damage the relationship with the person I wronged and/or that I desired to regain entry into the tribe.

☐ Practiced outing myself about my transgression.

☐ Blocked attempts by others to explain away, justify, or validate my behavior or emotional reactions. I explained to the other person that my practice of outing myself is part of learning how to take responsibility for my actions and emotions without falling apart or immediately blaming others.

☐ **Repaired the transgression, without expecting anything in return, using the eight steps for relationship repair.** *Place a checkmark in the boxes next to the skills you practiced.*

   ☐ *Signaled deference and relinquished control.*

   ☐ *Accurately identified what I had done to harm the relationship or the other person and communicated this to them.*

   ☐ *Confirmed that my perception of the harm I caused was valid from the other person's perspective.*

   ☐ *Blocked automatic rationalization or justification of my behavior.*

   ☐ *Made a genuine effort to repair the actual damage done.*

   ☐ *Committed to genuinely work to not harm the person again in a similar manner.*

   ☐ *Actively took steps to prevent future harm.*

   ☐ *Forgave myself for having harmed someone or for having made a mistake.*

☐ **Varied my social signaling to match the severity of my transgression.**

   ☐ *Signaled shame if shame was warranted.*

   ☐ *Signaled appeasement and regret if shame was partially warranted.*

   ☐ *Balanced appeasement signals with cooperative-friendly signals after successfully repairing the transgression, to communicate openness and willingness to stand by my commitment to not harm again.*

Record here other observations or skills used.

_____

_____

_____

G *If shame is unwarranted,* Go opposite *to urges to hide or appease*

Place a checkmark in the boxes next to the skill you practiced.

☐ **Assessed whether I was in a toxic environment** and used Flexible Mind SAGE skills to work to improve the situation, protect myself, or end the relationship.

   Record here the specific skills you practiced.

_____

_____

☐ **Signaled confidence.** I purposefully stood with my shoulders back, posture straight, and chin up, and I maintained eye contact and spoke in a normal tone and volume of speech.

☐ Blocked apologizing or appeasing.

☐ **Balanced signals of dominance (confidence) with signals of nondominance** in order to signal openness.

☐ Outed myself to a friend about my unwarranted shame in order to identify potential blind spots.

Describe here any other skills you practiced, and the outcomes.

_____

_____

_____

E *Show* **Embarrassment** *to enhance trust and socially connect.*

☐ Signaled embarrassment when my transgression involved a violation of a social norm.

☐ Remembered that feeling embarrassed is nothing to be embarrassed about.

☐ Remembered that people trust and like people who show embarrassment.

☐ Revealed my embarrassment rather than hiding it.

☐ Practiced showing and loving blushing.

☐ Watched how my outing myself and expressing embarrassment impacted relationships.

Record here other observations or skills used.

_____

_____

_____

Social Signaling Matters!

Main Points for Lesson 9

1. People cannot know who you are unless you reveal who you are.

2. We trust what we see, not what is said.

3. People like people who openly express their emotions; they are perceived as more genuine and trustworthy, compared to those who suppress or mask.

4. Open expression does *not* mean simply expressing emotions without awareness or consideration; on the contrary, effective expression is always context-dependent.

5. To form long-lasting intimate bonds, you must reveal vulnerability.

6. Openly expressing vulnerability transmits two powerful social signals: (1) We trust the other person. When we don't trust someone, we hide our true intentions and mask our inner feelings. (2) We are the same because we share a common bond of human fallibility.

Materials Needed

*   Handout 9.1 (Open Expression = Trust = Social Connectedness)

*   Handout 9.2 (Emotions Communicate to Others)

*   (Optional) Handout 9.3 (Main Points for Lesson 9: Social Signaling Matters!)

*   Worksheet 9.A (Practicing Enhancing Facial Expressions)

*   Whiteboard or flipchart with marker

(Required) Class Exercise
What We Show on the Outside Matters!

Read each of the following stories aloud while acting out the voice tone and facial expression associated with each, and then discuss.

NOTE TO INSTRUCTORS: For story 1 it is essential for instructors to put on a phony smile that remains frozen during the entire time they are speaking the lines for the troubled coworker. *Seeing a phony face* enables participants to *viscerally experience* (in their body) what it would be like to interact with the person described in the story (via micromimicry and the mirror neuron system; see lesson 3). A phony smile involves moving only the lips, with eyes flat and without eyebrow wags. Instructors should exaggerate the phoniness of the smile, displaying teeth when they smile, but make sure the smile remains static or frozen throughout. This not only ensures the point of the story is made but it smuggles humor and the ability to not take oneself too seriously into the teaching.

Story 1: "'Twas a Lovely Affair"

Read aloud: *Imagine being in the following situation. You are out to lunch with a new coworker, and during the meal they reveal some very personal information. While smiling and nodding, they say...*

(Begin smiling) *"Last night I discovered that my husband was having an affair."*

(Keep smiling) *"Plus, I found out we are now bankrupt because he has spent all of our money on the other woman."*

(Keep smiling) *"So I decided to set fire to the house."*

(Keep smiling) *"So how was your evening?"*

Discuss story 1, using the following questions.

- *What would you think or feel if you interacted with someone who behaved like this? Did the coworker's description of her evening warrant smiling? In humans, what did smiles evolve to signal to other tribe members?* [Answer: Happiness, liking, contentment, desires to connect, cooperation, or appeasement.] *What did the smile in this instance communicate?*

- *Would you like to spend more or less time with this coworker after this interaction? What emotion was the coworker likely feeling but not showing?* [Answer: Most likely bitter anger.] *To what extent do you smile when you are actually angry or feeling an emotion other than happiness inside? Are you aware of times when this happens? When it does, what might you be trying to communicate to the other person (albeit indirectly)? How might this impact your relationships?*

NOTE TO INSTRUCTORS: For story 2 it is essential for instructors to put on a completely nonemotional and flat facial expression and voice tone for the story to be effective (behave like a zombie). *Seeing a flat face* enables participants to *viscerally experience* (in their body) what it would be like to interact with the person described in the story. As with story 1, reading the script for the story without adopting the facial expression described requires participants to intellectually imagine what it might be like to interact with the person in the story, making the learning less experiential. Playacting while reading the story aloud also nonverbally smuggles important RO principles to OC clients, such as it's okay to be silly and learning can still happen even (and perhaps especially) when you are having fun.

Story 2: "I Have Some Really Exciting News"

Read aloud: *Imagine being in the following situation. Similar to our last situation, you are out to lunch, but this time with a different coworker. During the meal, they reveal some very exciting news by saying…*

(Begin flat face and monotone voice) *"Last night I discovered that I won ten million dollars in the lottery. I was thrilled."*

(Continue with flat face and monotone voice) *"When my husband came home, before I could tell him the good news, the phone rang. It was Steven Spielberg, the movie director, calling from Hollywood. He had just read my script that I had sent him on a whim three months ago. He said he loved it so much that he was sending first-class tickets to fly me and my entire family to Los Angeles to discuss making my script into a movie. I was so happy."*

(Continue with flat face and monotone voice) *"Can you pass me the salt?"*

Discuss story 2, using the following questions.

- *What would you think or feel if you interacted with someone who behaved like this? Did the coworker's description of her evening warrant a flat face?*

- *When we are flat-faced, what are we signaling? To what extent do you display a flat face or monotone voice toward others? When does it happen? What are you usually trying to signal to the other person when you do so? How might this impact your relationships?*

NOTE TO INSTRUCTORS: For optional story 3, similar to story 2, it is essential for instructors to put on a completely nonemotional and flat facial expression and voice tone when speaking as subject 2 for the story to be effective (think zombie again). The following story is based on a research study by Emily Butler and her colleagues (2003), and a robust number of other studies have confirmed these results, using similar paradigms (see lesson 2).

(Optional) Story 3: "Let's Discuss the Movie We Just Watched Together"

Using a normal tone of voice, read aloud the following paragraph.

Imagine a psychology experiment involving two research subjects who have never met. They are asked to watch a movie together. The movie is full of funny, sad, scary, and disgusting pictures, sounds, and dialogue. After the movie, both are taken to another room and seated at a table directly opposite each other. A blood pressure cuff is then applied to each of them. They are handed written instructions and told to read them silently while being careful not to reveal the contents of their instructions to the other research participant. Subject 1's instructions say, "Talk about the movie with your partner, and express your thoughts, emotions, and feelings about the movie, just like you normally would." However, subject 2's instructions are slightly different; they say, "Talk about the movie with your partner, and express your thoughts, emotions, and feelings about the movie, just like you normally would, but do not show any emotion on your face while doing so." Both subjects' facial expressions are videotaped during the interaction, and neither knows what the other subject was instructed to do during the interaction. Now, imagine you are interacting with subject 2 (the one instructed to not show any emotion on their face), and they say…

Instructors should act out the suppressed-expression role for subject 2 by adopting a flat-faced expression and unemotional voice tone when they read aloud the next section.

(With flat face and monotone voice) *"I found this movie very exciting—some parts were really scary, but other parts were really funny. Like when the bad guy shot the lady in the pink dress, I was outraged, but when I realized that she had replaced the real bullets with ones made of Jell-O that started bouncing all over the room, I was giggling with delight. Plus, when the evil shooter fell into a vat of molasses, I was so giggly that I nearly peed my pants."*

Discuss, using the following questions.

✓ **Ask:** *What do you think the researchers discovered?*

Subject 2's blood pressure went up; this indicates they became more anxious when they inhibited expressions of emotion. Recall that subject 2 was the one instructed to suppress expression.

Plus, subject 1's blood pressure also went up, and when asked if they would like to spend more time interacting with subject 2, almost all of them declined.

✓ **Ask:** *What does this tell us about suppressing emotion?*

Keeping emotional expression out of your voice and face is seen as unfriendly and as a possible noncooperative danger signal by others. Plus, we become anxious when we're around others who are suppressing their emotions, especially when free expression would be okay. Robust research shows that people tend to avoid people who habitually mask their inner feelings. They are more likely to see them as untrustworthy, and this can lead to social exclusion, ostracism, loneliness, and severe mental health problems.

✓ **Ask:** *What might this research mean for those of you who tend to mask your inner feelings?*

Frozen or flat facial expressions negatively impact our relationships with others, whether we intend for this to happen or not!

NOTE TO INSTRUCTORS: Masking feelings is normal, but when pervasive it can damage relationships. Instructors should encourage participants to practice self-enquiry about their style of social signaling by asking *How might my style of social signaling impact others? How often does my facial expression match what I feel inside? What do I fear might happen if I were to reveal my true feelings to someone? What is it that I need to learn?*

(Required) Teaching Point

Open Expression = Trust = Social Connectedness

Refer participants to handout 9.1 (Open Expression = Trust = Social Connectedness).

- *People cannot know who you are unless you reveal who you are.*

- *We trust what we see, not what is said.* People prioritize nonverbal expressions as more truthful indicators of a person's inner state over verbal descriptions of the same. Research shows that people consider nonverbal expressions of emotion to be better indicators of a person's true feelings than verbal communications.

> ★ **Fun Facts:** *Botox—Pretty but Lonely*
>
> *Research suggests that Botox, a neurotoxin used widely to cosmetically reduce facial lines, results in users feeling inauthentic, less able to express their emotions, and less able to quickly and accurately respond to emotional situations [Havas, Glenberg, Gutowski, Lucarelli, & Davidson, 2010]. People interacting with a Botox recipient report them as less genuine or trustworthy (for example, facial expressions seem forced, smiles less genuine).*
>
> *Facial muscles are frozen or paralyzed by Botox, similar to the facial paralysis common among stroke victims (albeit less extreme), thereby impairing both the "transmit" and "receive" channels of communication. The feelings of inauthenticity reported by Botox users are analogous to what happens when we smile for the camera but the snapshot is delayed by a fiddling photographer. Our smile quickly freezes but feels false; we may frantically encourage the photographer to hurry up and take the picture because we inwardly recognize the inauthenticity of frozen or forced expressions.*
>
> ✓ **Ask:** *How might this research apply to overcontrol?*

- *Openness and cooperative intentions are evaluated by actions, not by words* (for example, facial affect, voice tone, rate of speech, eye contact, body posture, and gestures).

- *As we discussed in our last lesson, facial expressions are powerful nonverbal social signals.* During interactions, we closely examine the facial expressions of the other person. Modern humans possess more facial muscles than any other animal species. We can make over ten thousand different facial expressions. Yet most people have only ever used one hundred. **SO GET PRACTICING!** **You have ninety-nine hundred more expressions to try out!**

(Required) Class Exercise
Four Mini–Social Signaling Exercises

NOTE TO INSTRUCTORS: The next three miniexercises should be conducted in the same spirit as "participate without planning" mindfulness practices in RO DBT (see lesson 12), meaning there is no orientation, no prewarning, and no discussion beforehand of what will happen next. Instead, instructors should simply begin each new minipractice without commentary. A core goal of these minipractices is to smuggle that making big gestures with your tribe can be fun—plus, you can learn at the same time! Follow the scripts and teaching points exactly; they are purposefully designed to make these minipractices quick and entertaining (the easiest way to do this is simply to read the teaching points verbatim). Extending the amount of time or adding additional practices can imply that there is something that must be fixed, or that we must be serious about having fun. This can trigger intense self-conscious emotions that your OC clients are unlikely to report (OC clients are notoriously polite), thereby losing the primary aim of the practice. Thus, for a successful experience, **stick to the following scripts and teaching points, don't feel embarrassed to read directly from the text, and keep your discussions short.**

IMPORTANT ANCILLARY NOTE TO INSTRUCTORS: In the unlikely event of a class member refusing to stand up as instructed, instructors should simply reverse their instructions, saying to class members now standing, "Okay, good job! Now go ahead and sit back down again." The instructor should then, with eyebrows raised and a warm smile (and without further commentary), conduct the exercise from a seated position. This functions to *bring the tribe* to the *nonconforming member* while simultaneously communicating several important messages without making a big deal out of it: (1) class participation is expected, (2) if you don't join us, we will join you, (3) we are attached to you and respect you, which is why we are sitting back down, and (4) we need you to participate so that we can all experience the joy of being part of a tribe. Instructors should attempt to acquire eye contact with the refusing class member as they begin to conduct the exercise (to communicate your genuine desire for them to join in with the class and that you do not disapprove of them). If the client meets your gaze, quickly smile, and perhaps give a little wave (this smuggles playfulness and affection; see also "Fun Facts: Teasing and Being Teased," in lesson 22). Importantly, instructors should conduct the next miniexercise as if nothing has happened—that is, by starting with a request for everyone to stand up. Most often, the nonconforming participant will reluctantly comply (that is, they have learned that noncompliance doesn't work), whereupon the instructor can warmly smile (and even wink) in their direction, to signal delight in their decision (during break or after class, the instructor can privately express their appreciation for their participation). However, if they continue to refuse, instructors should simply follow exactly the same protocol just described. Over time, our experience is that participants will eventually decide it is not worth continuing to refuse to participate (recall they have voluntarily chosen to be part of the class), because the instructors make it nearly impossible to avoid. This can be an important moment of learning for many OC clients.

First Minipractice

Instruct class members to stand up. When everyone is standing, say, "Okay, everybody make a big gesture like this." The instructor should demonstrate by placing their hands high above their head and then make a large circular gesture by sweeping both arms downwards as far away from their body as possible, until both arms are parallel with their legs. Immediately encourage the class by saying, "Okay, your turn—make a big gesture" (that is, everyone should do their gesture at the same time, including instructors). "Okay, everyone can sit back down."

Discuss: *What did you notice? Did you make a big gesture, as wide as the one I demonstrated, or was your gesture more understated or smaller? What might this tell you about how you socially signal?*

NOTE TO INSTRUCTORS: Most OC clients will make a smaller circle with their arms than what has just been demonstrated by the instructor. Use this to enhance discussion.

Second Minipractice

✓ **Ask:** *How do people signal receptivity and openness? Let's try it out. Everyone stand up again. Okay, now follow my lead: raise your arms, extend them to your side, away from your body, and at waist level. Keep your hands open and palms facing forward.* Instructors should demonstrate.

Teach: *This openhanded gesture universally signals openness to another person. How does it feel when you do this?*

Practice: *Okay, let's try it again—place your arms back down at your sides and clench your fists tightly. Now let's signal openness—extend your arms away from your body, palms outward. Now, closed-mouth smile, and raise your eyebrows. Notice how you feel? Okay, everyone can sit down.*

Discuss: *What did you notice? Did signaling openness feel different than what you might normally feel? What does this tell us?*

Third Minipractice

Teach: *Expansive and open gestures with palms facing forward signal receptivity, safety, willingness, and are most often associated with positive mood states linked with contentment, joy, celebration, and triumph.*

Teach: *Recall how Olympic athletes socially signal after they have won a race or an event. Regardless of culture, we raise our arms high with our palms facing outward when we celebrate success. It's almost like we are embracing the world.*

Teach: *These types of social signals are not something we learn, nor do they vary across cultures. For example, blind athletes who have never seen another person's facial expressions or gestures in their life have been shown to express the same emotional facial expressions and gestures as athletes who are not blind when they win or lose.*

Practice: *Let's all try it together. Stand up. Okay, we have just won the 500-meter sprint. How do we socially signal? Like this! Raise your hands high, palms outward and embracing the sky, and chin up! Say "YES! We've WON!" Again, arms high, palms outward, and chin up! "We've WON!" Okay, well done. Everyone can sit back down.*

Fourth Minipractice

✓ **Ask:** *How do people signal defeat? What does their body do, what does their facial expression look like?*

Practice (with a monotone voice and flat/sad facial expression): *Okay, Let's all try looking defeated. Shall we stand up? Ohhh, I'm too defeated to bother. I can barely even stand up—why bother. I'm so miserable.* Instructors should then start to lower their head, slump their shoulders, and mope about. Then end the practice.

Discuss: *How did that feel? Did you notice a difference between what it felt like to signal triumph or celebration versus what it felt like signaling defeat? What did you notice? What might that tell you?*

(Required) Teaching Point

Humans Are Expert Social Safety Detectors

Refer participants to handout 9.2 (Emotions Communicate to Others).

- *Humans are expert social safety detectors.* We are able to sense whether another person is feeling genuinely safe and relaxed during interactions, based on voice tone, body posture, and facial expression.

> ★ **Fun Facts:** *Knowing Others Based on Thin Slices of Behavior*
>
> *Humans are expert social safety detectors; our brains are hardwired to detect the extent to which another person is feeling genuinely relaxed versus tense, uncomfortable, or self-conscious during interactions. For example, research shows that we are adept at knowing whether a smile is genuine or phony and that we can accurately detect tension in the voice of a person, even over the telephone [Pittam & Scherer, 1993]. Research shows that exposure to a few minutes of nonverbal behavior, or even just a picture of the face, leads observers to form reliable impressions of a stranger's personality traits, socioeconomic status, and moral attributes like trustworthiness and altruism [Ambady & Rosenthal, 1992; Kaul & Schmidt, 1971; Kraus & Keltner, 2009]. One of the most reliable first impressions we form about others is whether they are warm (for example, kind, friendly) or cool (aloof, prickly).*

- *We are suspicious of people who hide their inner feelings.* We feel tense when around them and are more likely to avoid them.

- *People like people who openly express their emotions.* They are perceived as more genuine and trustworthy, compared to those who suppress or mask them.

- *Open expression does not mean simply expressing emotions without awareness or consideration. Effective emotional expression is always context-dependent.* Sometimes constraint or controlled expression is what is needed to be effective, avoid unnecessary damage, and/ or live by one's values (for example, a police officer arresting a suspect; during a game of poker; a charged discussion with one's adolescent child).

NOTE TO INSTRUCTORS: Context matters when it comes to emotional expression. For example, sometimes inhibiting an expression of emotion can be an act of kindness (for example, a mother inhibiting a tear when telling their young son they have been diagnosed with cancer). At other times, inhibiting emotional expressions is necessary for survival (for example, inhibiting a desire to attack when captured in war) or to protect oneself or one's tribe (for example, not letting an opponent know you are afraid; pretending to enjoy a meal you normally dislike when it was cooked in your honor), and/or constrained emotions can be needed to achieve an important goal (for example, getting through passport control without delay).

- *Nor does it mean uncontrolled venting or blaming of others for one's emotions.* It involves openly revealing emotions in a manner that acknowledges our responsibility in creating them. It takes responsibility for what we have brought to the table rather than blaming our experience on others.

- *Plus, open expression does not mean pretending that everything is okay when it's not.*

★ Fun Facts: *"Stay Calm and Carry On" Wins Wars, Not Love*

When we distrust someone, we naturally hide our inner feelings because we don't feel safe. Appearing too controlled, too self-possessed, or too accepting in circumstances that call for open and uninhibited expression of emotions (for example, discovering your friend has just been diagnosed with cancer, dancing at a party, asking someone to marry you, praising a child for a job well done, going out for a beer with coworkers, or arguing with your spouse) can send the wrong message. A calm exterior can be (and often is) misread by others as arrogance, indifference, manipulation, or dislike. People like people who freely express their emotions, even when they are negative, more than people who habitually suppress them. As we learned earlier, expressing embarrassment (for example, blushing) is a particularly powerful prosocial signal—people like and trust those who display embarrassment. We feel more connected with people who show embarrassment because it signals they care about social transgressions—for example, hurting someone, or being insensitive. [See handout 8.4 (Flexible Mind SAGE: Dealing with Shame, Embarrassment, and Feeling Rejected or Excluded).]

- *Importantly, there is no right or optimal way to socially signal.* Each of us has our own unique style of expression.

- *What is important is for your style to actually function to communicate your intentions and inner experience* to the other person, especially when it comes to people you desire to have a close relationship with.

- *Effective expression accounts for the type of relationship* (for example, a competitor, a new boss, or the police versus one's best friend, one's spouse, or your next-door neighbor) *and the appropriateness of expression in a given context* (for example, getting through passport control, a business meeting, a high-stakes poker game versus going out on a first date, winning the lottery, or going to a party).

  ✓ **Ask:** *What are other examples of times when open expression may need to be regulated, masked, hidden, or qualified?*

- *Yet to form long-lasting intimate bonds, you must reveal vulnerability without demeaning yourself. This transmits two powerful social signals to the other person:*

  1. **We trust them.** When we don't trust someone, we hide our true intentions and mask our inner feelings.

  2. **We are the same because we share a common bond of human fallibility.** True friendship begins when two people are able to share not only their successes but their secret doubts, fears, and past mistakes with the other.

     ✓ **Ask:** *To what extent do you like know-it-alls?* (When surveyed, almost unanimously people say "Not at all" or "Not much" to this question.) *What is it about know-it-alls that people dislike?*

     ✓ **Ask:** *To what extent do you like sycophants and brownnosers?* (When surveyed, almost unanimously people say "Not at all" or "Not much" to this question.) *What is it about bootlickers, flatterers, and grovelers we dislike?*

     ✓ **Ask:** *How many people in your life do you see as your equal? How often do you pretend inferiority when inwardly you feel superior (or at least equal) to the other person? What might your answer tell you about what you might need to learn?*

NOTE TO INSTRUCTORS: It is important to emphasize genuine intimacy does not mean just expressing one's emotions without taking into account the experience of the other person. For example, research shows that people in power-up or dominant positions to an interacting partner are more likely to feel free to show anger. However, open expression does not mean simply expressing anger whenever one feels it. For open expression to be effective (and kind), it has to be appropriate for the relationship and the context.

> ★ **Fun Facts:** *Why Do We Like Our Friends?*
>
> *This may seem like a silly question, but it is important to know why we like our friends—at the very least for reasons of personal understanding. Ask yourself this: Do I like my friend because they have just returned from Hawaii with a great suntan after purchasing their second yacht and are about to complete their third PhD after being nominated for a Nobel Prize for humanitarian work with impoverished children? Maybe so, but it is more likely that your friendship is based not just on knowing the good things about them. It is more probable that you like your friend because they have revealed to you things they may struggle to share with others or are less proud of—for example, their doubts, their fears, their past mistakes, secret desires, as well as their successes. When we signal vulnerability without falling apart, we automatically make relationships more intimate and equitable because revealing weakness opens us up to being hurt by the other but also to the possibility of new learning when our friend provides us with helpful advice or a differing perspective. True friends (close bonds) know things about the other person that could hurt them, but they don't use it against them.*

NOTE TO INSTRUCTORS: Vulnerable expression of emotion increases attachment. Recall that when we feel attached to others, we feel part of a tribe; we feel safe. Our social safety system is activated (see handout 3.1; see Porges, 2003). Our body is relaxed and our breathing and heart rate are slower. We feel calm yet playful. We are less self-conscious and we desire to socialize. We can effortlessly make eye contact and flexibly communicate, using our facial muscles. We have a musical tone of voice. We enjoy touching and being touched. We are open, receptive, curious, and empathic toward the feelings of others.

Lesson 9 Homework

1. **(Required) Worksheet 9.A (Practicing Enhancing Facial Expressions).** Instruct participants to practice enhancing varying facial expressions when interacting with others. Encourage them to use eyebrow wags and head nods when listening, and to use larger hand/body gestures when speaking. Ask them to experiment with being more dramatic than might be normal for them, and to consider how this impacts their relationships.

2. **(Optional) Experiment with expressions.** Instruct participants to practice enhancing expressions one day and inhibiting expressions the next day. Encourage them to observe differences between their expressive and nonexpressive days, both internally (thoughts, emotions) and externally (degree of social engagement).

Radical Openness Handout 9.1

Open Expression = Trust = Social Connectedness

- **Humans are expert social safety detectors.** We are able to sense whether another person is feeling genuinely safe and relaxed during interactions, based on voice tone, body posture, and facial expression.

- **We are suspicious of people who hide their inner feelings.** We feel tense when around them and are more likely to avoid them.

- **People like people who openly express their emotions.** They are perceived as more genuine and trustworthy, compared to those who suppress or mask them.

- **Open expression *does not mean* simply expressing emotions without awareness or consideration.** Effective emotional expression is always *context*-dependent. Sometimes constraint or controlled expression is what is needed to be effective, avoid unnecessary damage, and/or live by one's values (for example, a police officer arresting a suspect; during a game of poker; a charged discussion with one's adolescent child).

- **Nor does it mean uncontrolled venting or blaming of others for one's emotions.** It involves openly revealing emotions in a manner that acknowledges our responsibility in creating them. It takes responsibility for what we have brought to the table rather than blaming our experience on others.

- **Plus, open expression does *not* mean pretending that everything is okay when it's not.**

- **Importantly, there is no right or optimal way to socially signal.** Each of us has our own unique style of expression.

- **What is important is for your style to actually function to communicate your intentions and inner experience** to the other person, especially when it comes to people you desire to be close to.

- **Yet to form long-lasting intimate bonds, you must reveal vulnerability. This transmits two powerful social signals to the other person:**

  1. **We trust them.** When we don't trust someone, we hide our true intentions and mask our inner feelings.

  2. **We are the same because we share a common bond of human fallibility.** True friendship begins when two people are able to share not only their successes but their secret doubts, fears, and past mistakes with the other.

Radical Openness Handout 9.2

Emotions Communicate to Others

Inhibited Expression | **Open Expression**

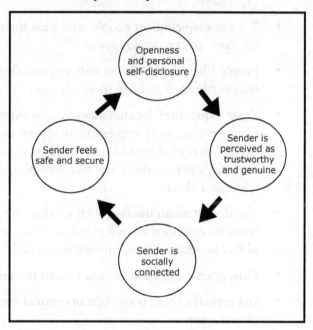

- Remember, open expression does *not* mean expressing emotions without awareness or consideration.
- On the contrary, effective emotional expression always depends on the situation.

Radical Openness Handout 9.3

Main Points for Lesson 9: Social Signaling Matters!

1. People cannot know who you are unless you reveal who you are.

2. We trust what we see, not what is said.

3. People like people who openly express their emotions; they are perceived as more genuine and trustworthy compared to those who suppress or mask.

4. Open expression does *not* mean simply expressing emotions without awareness or consideration; on the contrary, effective expression is always context-dependent.

5. To form long-lasting intimate bonds, you must reveal vulnerability.

6. Openly expressing vulnerability transmits two powerful social signals: (1) We trust the other person. When we don't trust someone, we hide our true intentions and mask our inner feelings. (2) We are the same because we share a common bond of human fallibility.

Radical Openness Worksheet 9.A

Practicing Enhancing Facial Expressions

In the next week, look for opportunities to try out various emotional expressions.

1. Notice the emotion you want to express to another person during an interaction.
2. Practice enhancing the expression of the emotion a little bit more than you normally would.
3. What did you do to enhance it?
4. Describe what happened after you enhanced your expression.

	Record the emotion you wanted to express.	What did you do to enhance it?	What happened after you enhanced your expression?
Monday			
Tuesday			
Wednesday			
Thursday			
Friday			
Saturday			
Sunday			

Using Social Signaling to Live by Your Values

Flexible Mind Is Deep

Main Points for Lesson 10

1. Emotional expressions in humans can be grouped into three broad functional domains: *status, survival,* and *intimacy.*

2. Use the primary expressive channel—*face, body,* or *touch*—linked with the emotion you wish to convey during the interaction, to maximize the likelihood that what is transmitted is what is actually received.

3. Use Flexible Mind Is DEEP to improve relationships and live by your values.

Materials Needed

- Handout 10.1 (The Three Channels of Emotion Expression)

- Handout: 10.2 (Face in the Crowd)

- Handout 10.3 (Using Social Signaling to Live by Your Values)

- (Optional) Handout 10.4 (Main Points for Lesson 10: Using Social Signaling to Live by Your Values: Flexible Mind Is DEEP)

- Worksheet 10.A (Flexible Mind Is DEEP: Identifying Valued Goals)

- Worksheet 10.B (Flexible Mind Is DEEP)

- Videoplaying equipment or screen with internet access to show YouTube videos

  - "Talking Eyebrows" clip from Michael McIntyre's *Comedy Roadshow*: https://www.youtube.com/watch?v=ZaO-llc_E64

  - "The Still Face Experiment," with Dr. Edward Tronick: https://www.youtube.com/watch?v=C8ZTx1AEup4

- Whiteboard or flipchart with marker

(Required) Teaching Point

The Three Functions of Emotions

Refer participants to Handout 10.1 (The Three Channels of Emotion Expression).

- *Emotional expressions in humans can be grouped into three broad functional domains: status, survival, and intimacy,* identifiable by a primary channel of expression specific to that domain (App, McIntosh, Reed, & Hertenstein, 2011). This area of research shows that…

  - *The body channel promotes social status emotions* (for example, embarrassment, humiliation, shame, and pride).

  - *The face channel supports survival emotions* (that is, anger, disgust, fear, enjoyment-happiness, and sadness).

  - *The touch channel supports intimate emotions* (for example, love, sympathy).

- *Thus, if you want someone to know your true intentions, use evolutionarily evolved social signaling channels linked to the emotional intention (status, survival, intimacy) you wish to communicate as your primary means of communicating.*

★ **Fun Facts:** *Survival Emotions Are Fast*

Refer participants to handout 10.2 (Face in the Crowd).

Survival emotions (that is, anger, disgust, fear, happiness, and sadness) are quickly expressed and quickly assessed (usually in milliseconds), and the unique facial expressions associated with each are universally recognizable [Ekman, 1993]. For example, we can quickly spot the prototypical downward slant of inner eyebrows and compressed frown characterizing the angry face in a crowd of people, even when the expression is a simple line drawing. Can you spot the angry expression in handout 10.2?

(Required) Teaching Point

Nonverbal Social Signals Matter!

- *Nonverbal signals matter! For example, raised eyebrows are universal signals of friendship and affection.* Eyebrow wags are nature's way of saying "I like you" or "You are in my tribe." Most often they are accompanied by a genuine smile, kind or happy eyes, and a musical tone of voice. They can be seen when friends initially greet each other and/or during interactions among people who find each other attractive or interesting (see also the required class exercise "Playing with Eyebrows," in lesson 3).

NOTE TO INSTRUCTORS: Eyebrow wags are conspicuously absent when we are greeted by someone who dislikes us or during interactions with rivals. However, lack of eyebrow wags during an interaction cannot be taken as definitive proof of dislike. For example, the other person may be in pain or feeling threatened by something that is unrelated to you (both pain and threat turn off social safety responses and prosocial signaling), or they may rarely exhibit eyebrow wags with anyone, regardless of context (that is, even when among friends).

> ★ **Fun Facts:** *Social Signaling Impacts Brains!*
>
> *Eyebrow wags not only communicate prosocial intentions, they also automatically trigger the social safety system in both the sender and the receiver* [via the bidirectional nature of our brain-body regulatory system in the sender and via micromimicry and mirror neurons in the recipient; see lesson 3]. *We automatically micromimic, in milliseconds, the facial expressions of others, which triggers the same brain structures, or mirror neurons, and physiological experience of the mirrored person* [Montgomery & Haxby, 2008; Van der Gaag, Minderaa, & Keysers, 2007]. *Thus, if we observe a person grimace in pain, we tend to, without conscious awareness, microgrimace and, as a result, via the influence of the mirror neuron system, can viscerally know how the other person feels inside* [T. R. Lynch, Hempel, & Dunkley, 2015; Schneider et al., 2013].

(Recommended) Class Exercise

Apollo Eyebrows!

Show "Talking Eyebrows," the 1.3-minute YouTube video clip from Michael McIntyre's *Comedy Roadshow.* Use this as a basis for discussing how the comedian's friendliness changes simply as a function of how he moves his eyebrows. We have found this video clip an invaluable teaching tool that viscerally demonstrates the importance of prosocial signaling.

Discuss the video clip, using the following questions.

- ✓ **Ask:** *What did you notice? What happened when the comedian lowered his eyebrows? Did his voice tone change? What might explain this?*

- **Teach:** Instructors should highlight how his voice tone changed from a musical tone (when he raised his eyebrows) to a flat/monotonic aggressive voice tone (when he lowered his eyebrows). Recall the bidirectional nature of our brain-body: the loss of his musical tone of voice when he lowers his eyebrows likely reflects withdrawal of the comedian's social safety system (parasympathetic ventral vagal system; see lesson 2).

Use the following question to introduce the next class exercise.

- ✓ **Ask:** *What might be the consequences for an infant or child if their parent habitually displayed a flat face or used an unexcited and monotonic voice tone when interacting with their child?*

(Required) Class Exercise
"The Still Face Experiment"

Show the 2.5-minute YouTube video clip "The Still Face Experiment," with Dr. Edward Tronick. Use this to discuss the powerful social signal flat or neutral facial expressions exert on others.

Discuss the video clip, using the following questions.

- ✓ **Ask:** *What does this video clip tell us about social signaling?*

- **Teach:** Instructors should highlight the research showing that among humans, facial expressions (for example, anger, fear, happiness) function as unconditioned stimuli, meaning that they automatically trigger emotional experience in the recipient. Facial expressions are evolutionarily prepared stimuli that we are hardwired to respond to, whether we like it or not (for example, similar to snakes, looming objects, spiders). Our reaction to them starts at the sensory receptor level, below conscious awareness.

- **Teach:** The baby in this video responds exactly as it is evolutionarily programmed. Despite being exposed for only two minutes to a flat-faced mom, the baby's reactions follow a prototypical pattern that can be observed across culture. First the baby tries to reengage the flat-faced mom via cooperative signals (that is, smiling, laughing, eyebrow wags, prior shared happy vocalizations, and pointing). When this fails, the baby becomes more desperate, engaging primal distress calls (screeching, crying, and writhing). When this fails, the baby then uses the only strategy it has left at its stage of development—that is, it literally attempts to turn away from the source of its pain (the mom).

- ✓ **Ask:** *What might be the consequences for an infant or child if their parent habitually displayed a flat face or used an unexcited and monotonic voice tone when interacting with their child?*

- **Reflect:** When interacting with babies, most people spontaneously adopt a musical and playful tone of voice ("baby speak"). What might this tell us about social signaling?

(Required) Teaching Point
Using Social Signaling to Live by Your Values: Flexible Mind Is DEEP

Refer participants to Handout 10.3 (Using Social Signaling to Live by Your Values: Flexible Mind Is DEEP).

NOTE TO INSTRUCTORS: As with other acronyms used in RO, write out each letter of the acronym (DEEP) on a flipchart or whiteboard, with each letter arranged vertically in a column, but *without* teaching or naming the specific skill that each letter signifies. Next, starting with the first letter in the acronym (*D* in DEEP), teach the skills associated with each letter in the acronym, using the key points outlined in the following sections, until you have covered all of the skills associated with each individual letter. Importantly, only write out on the whiteboard or flipchart the global description of what each letter actually stands for when you are teaching the skills associated with its corresponding letter. This teaching method avoids long explanations about the use of certain words in the acronym and/or premature teaching of concepts, since the meaning of each letter is only revealed during the formal teaching of the skills associated with it.

Flexible Mind Is DEEP

D   **Determine** your valued goal and the emotion you wish to express

E   **Effectively Express** by matching nonverbal signals with valued goals

E   Use self-**Enquiry** to **Examine the outcome** and learn

P   **Practice** open expression, again and again

Before the Interaction

Refer participants to worksheet 10.A (Flexible Mind Is DEEP: Identifying Valued Goals).

D **Determine** *your valued goal and the emotion you wish to express.*

- *Reflect on the level of intimacy you would like to have with the other person.* Use the Match + 1 Intimacy Rating Scale (see lesson 21) to rate both the current level of intimacy in the relationship and the desired level of intimacy.

- *Identify the valued goals you will need to live by in order to achieve your desired level of intimacy,* and use worksheet 10.A (Flexible Mind Is DEEP: Identifying Valued Goals) to help facilitate this process.

- *When there are multiple valued goals, determine the one most important for the type of relationship you desire in the current situation.*

- *Determine the emotion linked to your most important valued goal* (for example, guilt linked to a valued goal to behave ethically, sadness linked to a valued goal to admit when I am wrong, embarrassment linked to a valued goal to not violate social norms needlessly).

- *Identify the primary channel of expression needed to effectively communicate the emotion identified.*

  - *Social status emotions are expressed through the* **body** (for example, embarrassment, humiliation, shame, and pride).

  - *Survival emotions are expressed through the* **face** (that is, anger, disgust, fear, enjoyment-happiness, and sadness).

  - *Intimacy emotions are expressed through* **touch** (for example, love, sympathy).

During the Interaction

E Effectively Express *by matching nonverbal signals with valued goals.*

- *Practice expressing without expecting anything in return.* Give the other person time to react—don't assume that a lack of response means they didn't notice, they don't care, or they disliked what you did. They may be happily astounded by your change in behavior, may struggle with open expression themselves, and/or may simply have not known how to respond.

- *Give the other person the benefit of the doubt,* especially if you have had conflict in the past with the person you are being open with.

- *Use the primary expressive channel—body, face, or touch—linked with the emotion you wish to convey during the interaction* to maximize the likelihood that what is transmitted is what is actually received.

- *Match your nonverbal signals with your valued goals.* Instructors should model the nonverbal social signaling described in each of the following examples and encourage class members to mimic them.

  - *If your valued goal is to be taken seriously, signal gravity and confidence* (for example, by looking the other person in the eye, speaking calmly but firmly, keeping your shoulders back and chin up).

  - *If your valued goal is to establish a close social bond with someone, signal friendliness* (for example, via eyebrow wags, warm smiles, openhanded gestures, adopting a musical tone of voice, head nodding, taking turns when conversing, and/or gently touching them on the arm).

  - *If your valued goal is to be forthright and honest, then when the situation calls for it, express what you are feeling inside on the outside* (for example, when sad after a loss, cry; when uncertain about something, shrug; when you like what you hear, nod your head; when praised, smile warmly and express thanks).

  - *If your valued goal is to be fair-minded, signal openness* (for example, while listening to feedback, use an eyebrow wag; if sitting, lean back in your chair; slow the pace of the conversation by taking a deep breath; allow time for the other person to respond to questions or complete observations before you speak; validate their experience by matching the intensity of their expression rather than trying to appear calm; use openhanded gestures; signal nondominance by shrugging shoulders when uncertain; maintain a musical tone of voice).

  - *If your valued goal is to not be arrogant, then signal humility* (for example, maintain eye contact, slightly bow your head and shrug your shoulders, use openhanded gestures and a compassionate voice tone).

(Required) Class Exercise

Examining How Valued Goals Are Expressed Without Ever Saying a Word

Instruct. Refer to worksheet 10.A (Flexible Mind Is DEEP: Identifying Valued Goals) and ask participants to pick other examples of valued goals they hold.

Solicit examples of valued goals from the class, and then use the following questions to help understand how they are nonverbally signaled. Encourage the class to act out or practice displaying the overt behaviors that the class identifies for each valued goal.

✓ **Ask:** *How would an objective observer know (or at least be able to guess) that someone might be living according to this valued goal without ever speaking to them? What actions, facial expressions, voice tones, and gestures are most often associated with this valued goal? What types of emotion(s) are most often experienced or expressed when a person lives by this valued goal? Which channel of emotion expression—body, face, or touch—do you think may be most representative of it?*

✓ **Ask:** *Are there any valued goal examples listed that can only be expressed via the use of language—that is, not actions? If so, what might this mean? How is it expressed?*

✓ **Ask:** *Are there any valued goals listed that you would be reluctant to reveal to others? What might this tell you?*

✓ **Ask:** *Are there any valued goals listed that you strongly dislike or consider immoral? What might this tell you about yourself? How might your reaction to these particular valued goals impact your relationships or your behavior?*

More fun: Randomly select several examples from the valued goals handout that none of the class endorsed. Most often these are non-OC valued goals. Encourage the class to use self-enquiry if they have strong reactions or judgments about these other valued goals. What is it they might need to learn?

Now, back to Flexible Mind Is DEEP!

After the Interaction

E Use self-**Enquiry** to **Examine the outcome** *and learn.*

- *Take responsibility for your emotional reactions* rather than blaming them on the other person because the interaction was not perfect or did not go exactly as you had hoped or expected.

- *Use self-enquiry to examine your experience* and record your observations in your self-enquiry journal.

  ➤ *Did your openness appear to change the other person's openness during the interaction? If so, how did they express it? What might this tell you?*

> ➤ *Did the interaction go as you might have hoped or expected? If not, then what is it you might need to learn?*

> ➤ *Do you feel closer or further away from them after the interaction? What might this tell you?*

> ➤ *Is there a part of you purposefully trying to make this difficult? For yourself? For the other person? What might this mean? What is it that you need to learn?*

- **Practice celebrating diversity.** Let go of expecting others to think or behave like you.

- **Appreciate your own unique style of expression, without assuming your way is better.** For example, appreciate your dry sense of humor or soft-spoken manner, yet be willing to go beyond your comfort zone of expression in order to match the expressive level of your interacting partner. Use Match + 1 principles to guide your level of disclosure (see Flexible Mind ALLOWs, lesson 21).

- **Celebrate expression success** when you achieve your relationship goal or live according to your values after open expression. Make sure you take the time to highlight this and reward yourself. This makes it easier to remember the benefits of expression the next time you practice.

P Practice *open expression, again and again.*

- *Make a commitment to practice open expression again and again.*

- *If the relationship is highly conflictual but also highly important...*

  - **Once is not enough.** That is, one instance of openness is unlikely to repair years of damage or distrust.

  - **Commit to open expression, no matter what the outcome.**

  - **Patience, persistence, and forbearance are in your favor.**

  - **Seek feedback from a neutral person to help evaluate and challenge your progress and perceptions.** Encourage your helper to question your description of events rather than automatically validating or attempting to soothe you (recall the core RO principle "We don't see the world as it is, we see it as we are"). Explain to them that part of radical openness living is to actively search for our edge, or our personal unknown, in order to learn.

  - **Consistency and willingness to go all the way are essential for reestablishment of trust in a damaged relationship,** meaning once you start the process of open expression, you cannot simply stop because you are tired, find it difficult, believe them too dependent, and/or because your efforts have worked out the way you had planned. Genuinely close relationships are hard work, and when they have been damaged, the work is even harder, yet the payoff for reestablishing trust can be well worth the effort. Open expression with another person means going all the way, especially when the relationship is highly important and highly damaged.

- **People worth getting to know like and trust you for who you are.** Use Flexible Mind SAGE skills to evaluate whether the relationship may be toxic (see lesson 8). Avoid quick decisions. Seek advice from someone you know will be able to remain neutral before you decide anything.

- **Look for opportunities to stretch your expressive limits.** For example, instead of sitting silently in church while everyone else is singing, join in; rather than avoiding a person you are attracted to, ask them to join you for coffee; rather than begrudging others for not caring, practice expressing how you care, without expecting anything in return.

Lesson 10 Homework

1. **(Required) Worksheet 10.B (Flexible Mind Is DEEP).**

2. **(Required) Instruct participants to practice eyebrow wags** in the mirror when they are tired, stressed, or in pain, and during interactions with others. Encourage them to try using eyebrow wags when they are interacting with a person who appears grumpy. Ask them to combine a closed-mouth smile with an eyebrow wag and then notice what happens to their breathing. Participants should record their observations in their self-enquiry journal.

Radical Openness Handout 10.1

The Three Channels of Emotion Expression

- Emotions have three broad channels of expression: *status, survival,* and *intimacy.*

  - The *body channel* promotes social status emotions (for example, embarrassment, humiliation, shame, and pride).

  - The *face channel* supports survival emotions (for example, anger, disgust, fear, enjoyment-happiness, and sadness).

  - The *touch channel* supports intimate emotions (for example, love, sympathy, empathy, compassion).

Radical Openness Handout 10.2

Face in the Crowd

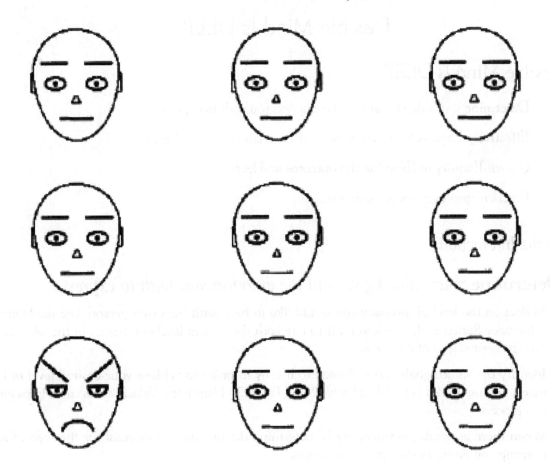

Adapted from Öhman, Lundqvist, & Esteves (2001), fig. 2, p. 384.

Radical Openness Handout 10.3

Using Social Signaling to Live by Your Values

Flexible Mind Is DEEP

Flexible Mind Is DEEP

D **Determine** your valued goal and the emotion you wish to express

E **Effectively Express** by matching nonverbal signals with valued goals

E Use self-**Enquiry** to **Examine the outcome** and learn

P **Practice** open expression, again and again

Before the Interaction

D **Determine** *your valued goal and the emotion you wish to express.*

- **Reflect on the level of intimacy you would like to have with the other person.** Use the Match + 1 Intimacy Rating Scale (see lesson 21) to rate both the current level of intimacy in the relationship and the desired level of intimacy.

- **Identify the valued goals you will need to live by in order to achieve your desired level of intimacy,** and use worksheet 10.A (Flexible Mind Is DEEP: Identifying Valued Goals) to help facilitate this process.

- **When there are multiple valued goals, determine the one most important for the type of relationship you desire in the current situation.**

- **Determine the emotion linked to your most important valued goal** (for example, guilt linked to a valued goal to behave ethically, sadness linked to a valued goal to admit when I am wrong, embarrassment linked to a valued goal to not violate social norms needlessly).

- **Identify the primary channel linked to the emotion you wish to express** (status, survival, or intimacy).

  - **Social status emotions are expressed through the *body*** (for example, embarrassment, humiliation, shame, and pride).

  - **Survival emotions are expressed through the *face*** (that is, anger, disgust, fear, enjoyment-happiness, and sadness).

  - **Intimacy emotions are expressed through *touch*** (for example, love, sympathy).

During the Interaction

E Effectively Express *by matching nonverbal signals with valued goals.*

- **Practice expressing without expecting anything in return.** Give the other person time to react—don't assume that a lack of response means they didn't notice, they don't care, or they disliked what you did. They may be happily astounded by your change in behavior, may struggle with open expression themselves, and/or may simply have not known how to respond.

- **Give the other person the benefit of the doubt,** especially if you have had conflict in the past with the person you are being open with.

- **Use the primary expressive channel—***body, face,* **or** *touch***—linked with the emotion you wish to convey during the interaction** to maximize the likelihood that what is transmitted is what is actually received.

- **Match your nonverbal signals with your valued goals.**

  - **If your valued goal is to be taken seriously, signal gravity and confidence** (for example, by looking the other person in the eye, speaking calmly but firmly, keeping your shoulders back and chin up).

  - **If your valued goal is to establish a close social bond with someone, signal friendliness** (for example, via eyebrow wags, warm smiles, openhanded gestures, adopting a musical tone of voice, head nodding, taking turns when conversing, and/or gently touching them on the arm).

  - **If your valued goal is to be forthright and honest, then when the situation calls for it, express what you are feeling inside on the outside** (for example, when sad after a loss, cry; when uncertain about something, shrug; when you like what you hear, nod your head; when praised, smile warmly and express thanks).

  - **If your valued goal is to be fair-minded, signal openness** (for example, while listening to feedback, use an eyebrow wag; if sitting, lean back in your chair; slow the pace of the conversation by taking a deep breath; allow time for the other person to respond to questions or complete observations before you speak; validate their experience by matching the intensity of their expression rather than trying to appear calm; use openhanded gestures; signal nondominance by shrugging shoulders when uncertain; maintain a musical tone of voice).

  - **If your valued goal is to not be arrogant, then signal humility** (for example, while maintaining eye contact, slightly bow your head and shrug your shoulders, use openhanded gestures and a compassionate voice tone).

After the Interaction

E Use self-Enquiry *to* Examine the outcome *and learn.*

- **Take responsibility for your emotional reactions** rather than blaming them on the other person because the interaction was not perfect or did not go exactly as you had hoped or expected.

- **Use self-enquiry to examine your experience** and record your observations in your self-enquiry journal.

  - *Did your openness appear to change the other person's openness during the interaction? If so, how did they express it? What might this tell you?*

- *Did the interaction go as you might have hoped or expected? If not, then what is it you might need to learn?*

- *Do you feel closer or further away from them after the interaction? What might this tell you?*

- *Is there a part of you purposefully trying to make this difficult? For yourself? For the other person? What might this mean? What is it that you need to learn?*

- **Practice celebrating diversity.** Let go of expecting others to think or behave like you.

- **Appreciate your own unique style of expression without assuming your way is better.** For example, appreciate your dry sense of humor or soft-spoken manner, yet be willing to go beyond your comfort zone of expression in order to match the expressive level of your interacting partner. Use Match + 1 principles to guide your level of disclosure (see Flexible Mind ALLOWs, lesson 21).

- **Celebrate expression success** when you achieve your relationship goal or live according to your values after open expression. Make sure you take the time to highlight this and reward yourself. This makes it easier to remember the benefits of expression the next time you practice.

P Practice *open expression, again and again.*

- **Make a commitment to practice open expression again and again.**

- **If the relationship is highly conflictual but also highly important...**

  - **Once is not enough;** that is, one instance of openness is unlikely to repair years of damage or distrust.

  - **Commit to open expression again and again,** no matter what the outcome.

  - **Patience, persistence, and forbearance are in your favor.**

  - **Seek feedback from a neutral person to help evaluate and challenge your progress and perceptions.** Encourage your helper to question your description of events rather than automatically validating or attempting to soothe you (recall the core RO principle "We don't see the world as it is, we see it as we are"). Explain to them that part of radical openness living is to actively search for our edge, or our personal unknown, in order to learn.

  - **Consistency and willingness to go all the way are essential for reestablishment of trust in a damaged relationship,** meaning once you start to openly express, you cannot stop if you truly wish to improve a damaged relationship.

- **People worth getting to know like and trust you for who you are.** Use Flexible Mind SAGE skills to evaluate whether the relationship may be toxic (see lesson 8). Avoid quick decisions. Seek advice from someone you know will be able to remain neutral before you decide anything.

- **Look for opportunities to stretch your expressive limits.** For example, instead of sitting silently in church while everyone else is singing, join in; rather than avoiding a person you are attracted to, ask them to join you for coffee; rather than begrudging others for not caring, practice expressing how you care, without expecting anything in return.

Radical Openness Handout 10.4

Main Points for Lesson 10: Using Social Signaling to Live by Your Values

Flexible Mind Is DEEP

1. Emotional expressions in humans can be grouped into three broad functional domains: *status*, *survival*, and *intimacy*.

2. Use the primary expressive channel—*body*, *face*, or *touch*—linked with the emotion you wish to convey during the interaction to maximize the likelihood that what is transmitted is what is actually received.

3. Use Flexible Mind Is DEEP to improve relationships and live by your values.

Radical Openness Worksheet 10.A

Flexible Mind Is DEEP

Identifying Valued Goals

- Identify the relationship you wish to improve.

- Reflect on the level of intimacy you would like to have with the other person. Use the Match + 1 Intimacy Rating Scale as a guide (see lesson 21).

- Identify your valued goals linked with your desired level of intimacy, using the following checklist.

- When there are multiple valued goals, determine the one most important for the type of relationship you desire in the current situation.

Place a checkmark in the boxes next to any valued goals that you think are important to live by during the upcoming interaction in order to achieve the type of relationship you desire.

- ☐ To be candid and forthright
- ☐ To be honest and truthful
- ☐ To be ethical and fair-minded
- ☐ To respect myself and others
- ☐ To be taken seriously
- ☐ To have an easy manner
- ☐ To be kind to myself and others
- ☐ To treat other people as I would like to be treated
- ☐ To do the right thing, even if it causes distress in others
- ☐ To be seen as a loving parent, spouse, partner, or friend
- ☐ To attend to relationships
- ☐ To be faithful to my vows and prior commitments
- ☐ To be willing to break a promise when warranted
- ☐ To apologize to those I have harmed and repair the damage if possible
- ☐ To forgive those who have harmed me
- ☐ To acknowledge fallibility without falling apart

- ☐ To acknowledge when I succeed, without arrogance
- ☐ To care about the well-being of others
- ☐ To care about my own well-being
- ☐ To contribute to my tribe, my family, my community, and my society, without always expecting something in return
- ☐ To be self-directed
- ☐ To appreciate direction from others
- ☐ To take responsibility for my actions, emotions, and reactions to the world rather than blaming them on others or getting down on myself
- ☐ To accept those things that I cannot change
- ☐ To seek change when it is within my power
- ☐ To stand up for what I believe
- ☐ To admit when I fail but not let it stop me
- ☐ To not always assume I am right
- ☐ To not always assume I am wrong
- ☐ To be able to play, laugh, and relax
- ☐ To be open-minded
- ☐ To be willing to question everything, including myself
- ☐ To trust myself and others

- ☐ To let others know when I admire them, love them, or feel happy in their presence
- ☐ To be disciplined and orderly
- ☐ To be undisciplined and disorderly
- ☐ To think before I act
- ☐ To act before I think
- ☐ To be self-controlled when the situation calls for it
- ☐ To have the capacity to relinquish control
- ☐ To fight tyranny
- ☐ To be able to stand up against powerful others, with humility, in order to prevent unwarranted harm or unethical behavior
- ☐ To be able to express vulnerability and accept help from others when I need it
- ☐ To seek what may be uncomfortable in order to learn
- ☐ To avoid what I dislike, with awareness
- ☐ To cultivate healthy self-doubt
- ☐ To cultivate healthy self-confidence
- ☐ To celebrate my successes without becoming arrogant
- ☐ To revel in the success of others without resentment
- ☐ To allow others to win when winning or losing doesn't matter to me
- ☐ To not allow others to take advantage of me
- ☐ To appreciate the efforts of others who have contributed to my well-being
- ☐ To relinquish control when the situation calls for it
- ☐ To trust my intuitions without assuming they are true
- ☐ To be open to new experience and value the unexpected
- ☐ To passionately participate in life
- ☐ To be content with my life
- ☐ To appreciate knowledge, education, and learning

- ☐ To see all humans as equal
- ☐ To signal humility, nonarrogance and openness to those who are different from me
- ☐ To experience compassionate love toward myself and others
- ☐ To celebrate problems as opportunities for growth
- ☐ To live here and now
- ☐ To be humble and nonarrogant
- ☐ To make self-sacrifices in order to benefit the lives of others, without expecting anything in return
- ☐ To challenge authority
- ☐ To respect authority
- ☐ To be considerate of other people's feelings or way of thinking
- ☐ To be nonreactive and calm
- ☐ To be reactive and disinhibited when the situation calls for it
- ☐ To understand myself, others, and the world
- ☐ To be dutiful
- ☐ To delight in the pleasure of the moment
- ☐ To plan ahead
- ☐ To act on impulse
- ☐ To appreciate the importance of rules
- ☐ To live without rules
- ☐ To be peaceful, calm, and composed
- ☐ To be excited, enthusiastic, and expressive
- ☐ To feel socially connected with others
- ☐ To value diversity
- ☐ To do what is needed in the moment
- ☐ To be able to question myself without falling apart
- ☐ To behave responsibly
- ☐ To admit when I have been wrong or harmed someone, without expecting anything in return or resorting to harsh self-blame

227

□ To express love to those I care about

□ To not expect others to solve my problems

□ To help others without expecting anything in return

□ To live with integrity

□ To continually strive to improve myself

□ To be physically healthy

□ To be financially stable

□ To live in a safe environment

□ To care for nature and the natural environment

□ To love and be loved

□ To avoid harming others

□ To be spiritually minded

□ To be a leader

□ To be productive

□ To be powerful and influence others

□ To contribute to society

□ To achieve something important

□ To enjoy the work I do

□ To raise a family

□ To establish a long-term romantic relationship or partnership

□ To raise children

□ To experience true romantic love

□ To be creative

□ To seek personal growth and self-discovery

□ To be willing to try new things

Record other valued goals that were not included in the preceding list.

_____

_____

_____

Decide which valued goal best represents how you would like to behave with the other person in order to achieve the relationship and level of intimacy you desire. Take into account how you want to behave with the other person in general, as well as how you might have to adjust your valued goals to flexibly respond to circumstances in the current moment.

What valued goals, globally, are most important for the relationship with this other person?

_____

_____

_____

What valued goal is most important to live by in the upcoming interaction?

_____

_____

_____

Notice when your valued goals appear to be in opposition. For example, a parent might value being peaceful, calm, and composed when interacting with their daughter yet also value being excited, enthusiastic, and expressive when around them.

Opposite valued goals usually mean that the context or situation of the moment will most likely be the deciding factor about how to behave effectively. Thus, being calm and composed with your daughter may matter most when she is relating a personal crisis or when you are with her in a potentially dangerous situation (for example, walking down a dark tunnel late at night on the way to the subway), whereas excitement, enthusiasm, and expressiveness may be called for when she wins a race, receives an honor, or shares her latest interest with you.

> ➤ *What valued goals do I hold that are exact opposites?*

> ➤ *To what extent am I able to flexibly take into account the situation or circumstances of the moment when deciding which valued goal may be most important?*

> ➤ *To what extent do these opposites impact other areas of my life or other relationships? What is it that I might need to learn?*

Record questions and observations that emerged from your practice.

_____

_____

_____

_____

_____

_____

_____

Radical Openness Worksheet 10.B

Flexible Mind Is DEEP

Be alert in the coming week for opportunities to practice Flexible Mind Is DEEP during your everyday interactions.

Purposefully seek out an interaction with someone with whom you would like to have a better relationship or would like to become closer, and practice Flexible Mind Is DEEP.

Describe the situation in which you practiced Flexible Mind Is DEEP (for example, who was present, what their relationship is with you, and what the primary purpose of the interaction was).

_____

_____

_____

_____

_____

Before the Interaction

D Determine *your valued goal and the emotion you wish to express.*

Place a checkmark in the boxes next to the skills you practiced.

☐ Identified the emotion(s) I desired to express during the interaction.

    ☐ *Describe the emotion(s) and sentiment(s) you desired to express, and rank-order them according to importance if there was more than one emotion or sentiment.*

_____

_____

☐ Identified the primary channel of expression linked to the emotion that I wanted to express (or the channel for the highest priority emotion). *Place a checkmark in the box next to the channel you identified.*

    ☐ The *body channel,* linked to social status and self-conscious emotions (for example, embarrassment, humiliation, shame, and pride)

    ☐ The *face channel,* linked to survival emotions (for example, anger, disgust, fear, enjoyment-happiness, and sadness)

    ☐ The *touch channel,* linked to intimate emotions (for example, love, sympathy, compassion, empathy)

During the Interaction

E Effectively Express *by matching nonverbal signals with valued goals.*

Place a checkmark in the boxes next to the skills you practiced.

- ☐ **Practiced expressing without expecting anything in return.**
- ☐ **Gave the other person the benefit of the doubt.**
- ☐ **Used the primary expressive channel**—*body, face,* or *touch*—during the interaction.
- ☐ **Matched my nonverbal expressions with my valued goals.** *Place a checkmark in the boxes next to the skills you practiced.*

  - ☐ **Signaled gravity and confidence** in order to live according to my valued goal to be taken seriously.

  - ☐ **Signaled friendliness** in order to live according to my valued goal for intimate social bonds and cooperative relationships.

  - ☐ **Expressed what I was feeling inside on the outside** in order to live according to my valued goal to be forthright and honest in situations that call for it. *Describe what you expressed.*

  _____

  _____

  - ☐ **Signaled openness** in order to live according to my valued goal to be fair-minded.

  - ☐ **Signaled humility** in order to be live according to my valued goal to not be arrogant.

  - ☐ **Expressed other valued goals.** *Describe.*

  _____

  _____

After the Interaction

E *Use self-*Enquiry *to* Examine the outcome *and learn.*

Place a checkmark in the boxes next to the skills you practiced.

- ☐ **Practiced taking responsibility for my emotional reactions** rather than blaming them on others.
- ☐ **Used self-enquiry to examine my experience** and recorded my observations in my self-enquiry journal. *Write the self-enquiry question you found most likely to elicit your edge and/or you found most helpful.*

  _____

  _____

□ **Practiced celebrating diversity** by letting go of expectations that others should think or behave like I do.

□ **Appreciated my style of expression, without assuming it was better.**

□ **Celebrated expression success.** *Record how you rewarded yourself.*

_____

_____

Other skills used.

_____

_____

P Practice *open expression, again and again.*

Place a checkmark in the boxes next to the skills you practiced.

□ Made a commitment to practice open expression again and again.

□ Remembered that one instance (or even several instances) of open and vulnerable expression of emotion on my part may not result in similar displays of openness or vulnerability by the other person, especially when the relationship has been highly conflictual in the past.

□ Encouraged feedback from neutral others to help evaluate my progress and challenge my perceptions.

□ Sought independent and nonbiased advice when I believed the relationship might be toxic and/ or used Flexible Mind SAGE skills to evaluate the level of toxicity (see lesson 8). *Record what you did.*

_____

_____

□ Looked for opportunities to stretch my expressive limits.

Record what you did or plan to do.

_____

_____

_____

LESSON 11

Mindfulness Training, Part 1

Overcontrolled States of Mind

NOTE TO INSTRUCTORS: Lesson 11 is the first of four RO mindfulness lessons. Today's lesson (part 1) will review the RO mindfulness states of mind targeting overcontrolled problems—that is, *Fixed, Flexible,* and *Fatalistic Mind.* Part 2 (lesson 12) covers the "what" mindfulness skills: *observe openly, describe with integrity,* and *participate without planning.* Parts 3 and 4 teach the four mindfulness "how" skills, essential attitudes or mind-sets that RO encourages practitioners to adopt when practicing the "what" skills. Part 3 (lesson 13) teaches the first of the four mindfulness "how" skills, *with self-enquiry.* Part 4 (lesson 14) teaches the remaining three "how" skills: *with awareness of harsh judgments, with one-mindful awareness,* and *effectively and with humility.* The four parts of RO mindfulness are repeated later in the RO skills training course, for a total of eight lessons focused on mindfulness concepts that are embedded within the thirty-lesson structure.

Main Points for Lesson 11

1. Problematic states of mind for overcontrolled individuals are most often closed-minded.

2. These states function to block learning from new information or disconfirming feedback and can negatively impact interpersonal relationships.

3. A closed mind is a threatened mind. Though frequently triggered by nonemotional predispositions for detail-focused processing and inhibitory control, OC problematic states of mind are emotionally driven.

4. Fixed Mind signals that change is unnecessary because I already know the answer. Fixed Mind is like the captain of the *Titanic,* who, despite repeated warnings, insists, "Full speed ahead, and icebergs be damned."

5. Fatalistic Mind says change is unnecessary because there is no answer. Fatalistic Mind is like the captain of the *Titanic,* who, after hitting the fatal iceberg, retreats to his cabin, locks the door, and refuses to help passengers abandon ship.

6. Flexible Mind represents a more open, receptive, and flexible means of responding. It is like a ship captain who is willing to forgo previous plans and change course or reduce speed when icebergs are sighted. There is no abandoning ship or turning completely around at the first sign of trouble.

Materials Needed

- Handout 11.1 (Overcontrolled States of Mind)
- Handout 11.2 (Being Kind to Fixed Mind)
- Handout 11.3 (Learning from Fatalistic Mind)
- (Optional) Handout 11.4 (Main Points for Lesson 11: Mindfulness Training, Part 1: Overcontrolled States of Mind)
- Worksheet 11.A (Being Kind to Fixed Mind)
- Worksheet 11.B (Going Opposite to Fatalistic Mind)
- Whiteboard or flipchart with marker

(Required) Teaching Point
Learning to Be Open About Being Closed

Refer participants to handout 11.1 (Overcontrolled States of Mind).

> NOTE TO INSTRUCTORS: The OC states of mind known as Fixed Mind and Fatalistic Mind metaphorically represent the two most common OC behavioral patterns that occur when disconfirming feedback or uncertainty is encountered. Mindful awareness of these two "stuck points" serves as a memory cue for skills usage.

- *For overcontrolled individuals, problematic states of mind most often occur when in novel or uncertain situations and/or when feeling challenged, criticized, or the center of attention.*

- *They are problematic because they block new learning and can negatively impact interpersonal relationships.*

- *A closed mind is almost always a threatened mind.*
  - ✓ **Ask:** *What is it that I am afraid I might learn or have to give up if I were to be more open-minded? What am I defending against? What is it that I might need to learn?*

- *Closed-minded thinking can become a habit.* See worksheet 7.B (Finding Our Habitual Ways of Coping). For example, a person may learn to cope with unwanted feedback by pretending not to hear it (reinforced when the other person stops providing feedback), compulsively fixing or controlling (reinforced when a solution works), or shutting down and relinquishing all responsibility (reinforced when another person assumes responsibility).

- *Perhaps the most common OC response when challenged is to immediately deny, dismiss, or dispute the feedback.* This may reduce anxiety but doesn't stop to consider that something could be learned from the situation and the feedback. This state of mind in RO DBT is referred to as Fixed Mind.

(Required) Teaching Point
Learning About Fixed Mind

> NOTE TO INSTRUCTORS: Instructors should point out that everyone not only has a Fixed Mind but we all may be in it more often than we care to admit. We can even be in Fixed Mind about *not* being in Fixed Mind or believing that Fixed Mind doesn't exist. Instructors should have examples ready of Fixed Mind from their own lives to share with participants. Note that Fixed Mind and Fatalistic Mind are not necessarily always problematic; indeed, sometimes a rigid or fixed way of responding can be essential (for example, a soldier in combat may need to obey orders rigidly in order to survive), or wild abandonment of self-control is needed (for example, yelling to stop a mugger). Difficulties emerge when closed-minded, rule-governed, and/or passive responses are mindlessly enacted and negative consequences ignored.

- *Fixed Mind is like the captain of the Titanic who, despite repeated warnings, insists: "Full speed ahead, and icebergs be damned."* Fixed Mind says: *Change is unnecessary, because I already know the answer.*

- *Most of us avoid acknowledging Fixed Mind or deny its existence.* We often are not even aware of times we are acting from Fixed Mind. It is important for us to become mindful of the times we are operating from Fixed Mind because it influences our choices, narrows our field of awareness, and limits our ability to be spontaneous or learn from the environment.

- *When in Fixed Mind, our reactions are based on rules or past experience, and we may react defensively and aggressively to criticism, challenges, questions, or feedback.* We may quickly try to explain, defend, or justify our behavior or quickly turn the tables by questioning or attacking the other person's perspective.

- *Fixed Mind can damage relationships because we are less likely to consider another person's point of view.* It is usually accompanied by bodily tension, frustration, or feelings of pressure. It involves a willful refusal to question one's inner beliefs, convictions, or intuitions. Emotional and mood states associated with Fixed Mind include arrogance, pride, self-righteousness, antagonism, overconfidence, bitterness, and stubbornness. Action urges and behaviors associated with Fixed Mind include dominance, denial, overt actions to block or obstruct another, defiance, noncompliance, noncooperation, revenge, and intolerance. We often deny or avoid acknowledging the existence of Fixed Mind because our position or opinion feels right, or we may secretly know that the feedback we wish to reject bears a grain of truth but we may be ashamed or fearful to admit this possibility.

- *Fixed Mind can feel like a suit of armor that protects us.* We avoid the pain of feeling indecisive, making a mistake, or feeling incompetent by rejecting anything that makes us feel uncomfortable. Unfortunately, this armor often prevents new information from being received and thereby keeps us stuck in old patterns that may no longer be effective in our current situation.

(Optional) Discussion Point
Selfishness

- **Ask participants:** *Imagine someone tells you that you are selfish. How might you respond to this? Would responses vary depending on who gave you this feedback? Now imagine you are the person telling another he is selfish and he reacts to this feedback with an immediate response of outrage and anger.*

235

Instructors should point out that there are two possible ways of interpreting the preceding scenario and how the person reacted: (1) The anger is justified; you are misinformed, and it is important for the accused person to immediately defend himself because he has been inappropriately slandered. (2) The person is actually being selfish in some manner but finds it difficult or threatening to acknowledge this.

Use the following points to facilitate the discussion and teach.

- *Whether we like it or not, we are all selfish some of the time; and moreover, being selfish, at least some of the time, is healthy* (that is, not taking that phone call on Saturday afternoon in order to take a well-deserved nap). Instructors should use this statement as means for discussion.

- *Immediate rejection of feedback may block the opportunity to learn something new or correct a problem.* I might learn, for example, via self-enquiry, that selfishness meant pouring water for myself while neglecting my partner's empty glass at dinner, but without a willingness to acknowledge selfish behavior on my part, I may miss opportunities to care for my partner in a way that is important for me and/or in line with my values.

- *Automatic anger or rejection of feedback may signal Fixed Mind.* Instead of immediately blaming others, we might first want to find out what we may need to learn.

(Required) Class Exercise
Finding My Fixed Mind

NOTE TO INSTRUCTORS: Instructors should use the following questions to encourage discussion and as a means for participants to discover their Fixed Mind. Instructors should review each question, ask for examples from the class, and share examples from their own lives to facilitate understanding. Remind participants that having a strong preference does not always mean that someone is operating from Fixed Mind. Sometimes a person simply does not like the taste of cottage cheese. That said, practicing radical openness involves a willingness to reexamine this preference (to avoid cottage cheese) as circumstances change over time.

- *Have you ever noticed that the very things we don't want to hear about are the very things we are also most resistant to change?*

  ✓ **Ask:** *What have caring others suggested in the past that you change but you have resisted? Do you find yourself wanting to automatically explain, defend, or discount the other person's feedback? Do you immediately respond when this occurs? Is it possible that there is something to learn from this feedback that you just don't want to hear? If you answer yes to some of these questions, then it is possible that you are in Fixed Mind about this issue.*

- *Fixed Mind often has to do with parts of our personality that we are not proud of or wish not to acknowledge.*

- **Miniexercise:** Instruct participants to write down adjectives to describe themselves (for example, thoughtful, determined, intelligent, caring) on a piece of paper. **Next,** instruct them to place an opposite adjective (opposite descriptor) next to each word on their list, without thinking too much about it. **Next,** instruct the class to examine their adjective word pairs and notice if their opposite word is disliked and/or they would feel terrible or horrified if they discovered that they possessed this characteristic.

  Say: *For example, if someone described themselves as a caring person and its opposite for them was the word "selfish"—something terrible to be—how open do you think they would be to feedback suggesting that they were behaving in a selfish manner? Yet the truth is that all of us are selfish at least some of the time. Plus, sometimes being selfish is part of healthy living—for example, to get needed rest, to get what is deserved, or to reward oneself for hard work. Plus, rigidly insisting that one must always be caring makes it less likely for this person to change their behavior and live according to their values, because they are unwilling to entertain any suggestion from someone that they were behaving in a manner that was experienced as selfish by another person. Avoidance of feedback can be a sign of Fixed Mind.* Instructors should remind participants that openness to feedback does not mean automatically agreeing with it; for accepting and declining feedback, see handout 22.1 (Being Open to Feedback from Others: Flexible Mind ADOPTS).

- **Sometimes we can easily notice in others those very things that we need to change in ourselves.** The things we dislike in others may help alert us to the areas in our life we are less open about and might trigger Fixed Mind when feedback suggests we are behaving similarly.

  - ✓ **Ask:** *What characteristic in others do you find very annoying, distasteful, distressing, or intolerable? For example: Do you abhor people who change their opinion? Do you believe it morally wrong for a person to not always behave in a conscientious manner? Do you ever find very opinionated people annoying? Do you detest people who manipulate others? Do you find people who believe they are superior to others intolerable? Do you dislike people who don't listen? Do you believe it morally wrong to behave in a rash, impulsive, or reckless manner?*

  - ✓ **Use self-enquiry:** *What happens when you imagine yourself behaving similarly? Is there a chance that you may have done things similar to those you detest in others? What might this mean? What does this tell you about your personal values? What is it you might need to learn?*

- **In what area do you find it difficult to let go, at least temporarily, of your perspective and consider another point of view?** For example, "There is a right and wrong way of doing things, compliments are phony and manipulative, no one really cares about another person." Those things we find difficult or distressing to think about differently may signal Fixed Mind thinking.

  - ✓ **Use self-enquiry:** *What might this tell me about myself? What might my insistence or resistance to thinking differently mean? What makes it so difficult for me to see a differing perspective? Is there a chance this makes me less open to feedback or new information about this area or perspective? What type of problems in my life has rigidly holding on to this perspective solved? What is it I need to learn?*

- **Have you ever noticed that the things we are most rigid about are often the things that make us most angry?** Anger can sometimes block awareness of things that we need to learn or change.

✓ **Ask:** *What are your hot buttons? What can someone say to you that will make you angry? What do you ruminate or brood about? As the old saying goes, "The truth hurts." What new information might your anger sometimes prevent you from hearing?*

Encourage participants to write down the questions they find most helpful for locating their Fixed Mind and use them as reminders of possible "stuck points."

End by reminding participants that having a strong preference does not always mean that someone is operating from Fixed Mind. Sometimes a person simply does not like the taste of cottage cheese. Yet practicing radical openness involves a willingness to reexamine this preference (to avoid cottage cheese) as circumstances change over time.

(Required) Teaching Point
Being Kind to Fixed Mind

Refer participants to handout 11.2 (Being Kind to Fixed Mind).

- *To let go of trying to fix your Fixed Mind, be kind instead. Use the steps outlined here.*

Step 1. When challenged, look for signs of Fixed Mind.

- For example, bodily tension, annoyance, desire to defend oneself or confront/attack the other person, thinking that the other person or the feedback is wrong.

Step 2. Acknowledge the possibility of being in Fixed Mind.

- Physical tension in the body means we are feeling threatened. When threatened, we either fight or flee. Fixed Mind is our "fighter"—it can help keep us protected but it can keep us stuck. Use self-enquiry to facilitate self-awareness; see worksheet 11.A (Being Kind to Fixed Mind) for examples.

Step 3. Don't try to fix Fixed Mind; be kind instead.

- *Don't fight your Fixed Mind!* Remember that Fixed Mind is there for a reason. Open and soften to your Fixed Mind and allow yourself time to discover what your Fixed Mind might be trying to tell you. You never know what you might learn. Trying to fix or control Fixed Mind is like criticizing yourself for being too self-critical—it just doesn't work.

- *Change physiology:* Closed-mouth smile while breathing deeply, use eyebrow wags, sit back in one's chair (see the Big Three + 1, lesson 3).

- *Use Fixed Mind as a reminder to practice self-enquiry by asking* **What is it that I might need to learn from this experience?** Be open to what is happening in the moment and let go of assuming you have the correct answer. Use handout 22.1 (Being Open to Feedback from Others: Flexible Mind ADOPTS) to evaluate whether you should remain fixed or be more flexible (that is, adopt or decline the feedback).

- *Use a loving kindness practice to loosen the powerful grip of Fixed Mind* by repeating silently to yourself: *May my Fixed Mind find peace, may my Fixed Mind be content, may my Fixed Mind be safe and secure.*

- *Go opposite to Fixed Mind by laughing at one's shortcomings.* Fixed Mind takes life seriously! Research shows that those who can laugh at their personal shortcomings or personality quirks are more likely to experience positive mood states more broadly, be more playful with others, and have a healthy sense of self.

- *Forgive yourself for being in Fixed Mind.* Remember that we all have a Fixed Mind. Remember that Fixed Mind is not always problematic; sometimes a rigid or fixed way of responding is needed (for example, refusing to comply with a mugger may save one's life).

NOTE TO INSTRUCTORS: Some participants may comment that cherishing or loving your Fixed Mind implies approval. Instructors can point out that the reasoning behind this is that OC clients need to learn how to chill out; thus, learning to love your Fixed Mind rather than automatically attempting to fix it can unexpectedly free an OC client from the compulsion of always doing better or trying harder. The major teaching point is to encourage participants to practice radical openness when in Fixed Mind. This does not mean mindless approval or agreement, thoughtless acquiescing, giving up, or becoming fatalistic. It means cultivating a willingness to be open to new information while honoring one's prior learning. Finally, instructors should be prepared to point out the benefits of Fixed Mind. For example, the feelings of tension and resistance that are part of Fixed Mind can alert us to areas of life where we need to learn from and grow. Sometimes being fixed or rigid is what is needed (for example, rigid refusal to engage in unethical behavior despite pressure to do so).

(Required) Teaching Point
Learning About Fatalistic Mind

- *The opposite of Fixed Mind is Fatalistic Mind.* Where Fixed Mind involves vigorous resistance and energetic opposition to challenging feedback, *Fatalistic Mind involves giving up, appeasing, abandoning, or shutting down* when one does not get what one wants or is overwhelmed by life circumstances.

- *Fatalistic Mind is like the captain of the Titanic who, after hitting the fatal iceberg, retreats to his cabin, locks the door, and refuses to help passengers abandon ship.* Fatalistic Mind says: *Change is unnecessary, because there is no answer.*

- *Fatalistic Mind may appear submissive, yet it functions as disguised resistance, indirectly expressed.* Action urges and behaviors associated with Fatalistic Mind include pouty silence, passive-aggressive responses, stonewalling, quietly delaying progress, evading participation, pretending to go along, giving up, shutting down, numbing out, bitter resignation, secretly planning revenge, sudden acquiescence, compliance, or submission. Other examples of Fatalistic Mind include withdrawing or escaping a potentially threatening situation by lying or pretending that all is well, changing the topic to a less emotional one, excusing oneself during a highly exciting or distressing emotional situation, calling in sick prior to a big meeting, minimizing the importance of a problem, limiting vulnerable self-disclosure, or implying that the feedback being given is deeply wounding or that the other person needs to be more understanding (that is, "don't hurt me").

- *Fatalistic Mind can also involve shutdown and the cessation of goal-directed behavior when attempts at resisting unwelcome feedback are frustrated or experienced as overwhelming.* A sense of numbness or immobilization may occur.

NOTE TO INSTRUCTORS: Self-critical thoughts are common after periods of shutdown for OC clients because they feel embarrassed or ashamed that they were unable to control the situation or solve the problem and/or they may fear that others may see them as incompetent. Sometimes OC clients will flip from Fixed Mind (fighting or resisting change) to Fatalistic Mind (shutting down or giving up). For example, one OC client, when pressured to justify her Fixed Mind perspective, would often flip from rigid resistance to sudden agreement—"Okay, fine, I agree with you"—but when queried about this sudden shift would refuse to explain or discuss the issue further. She might reply by saying, "There is no need to discuss this further. I have decided you are right." The problem for the client and her interpersonal relationships was that she was often holding on to her prior convictions. This resulted in continued brooding, rumination, and sometimes desires for revenge. Thus, both Fixed Mind and Fatalistic Mind *often share similar functions or motivations*—for example, a desire for control or to achieve a personal objective. These shared functions are reasons that these states of mind are particularly relevant for OC clients.

(Required) Class Exercise
Finding My Fatalistic Mind

NOTE TO INSTRUCTORS: Instructors should use the following questions to encourage discussion and as a means for participants to discover their Fatalistic Mind. Instructors should review each question, ask for examples from the class, and share examples from their own lives to facilitate understanding. Remind participants that agreeing with someone or giving in does not necessarily mean that you are in Fatalistic Mind.

- *When have you had thoughts that others must be right, that you are to blame, that everything is your fault, or that nothing you ever do is right?*

  - ✓ **Ask:** *Do you ever find yourself thinking that others should change first or at least admit they may have made a mistake before you might be willing to do the same? Do you ever find yourself secretly relishing despair or melancholic emotions? What might this type of thinking signal to others? Is there a chance that you might be secretly hoping that by blaming yourself, the other person will stop giving you feedback?*

- *How often do you say to yourself, "Why bother? Nothing will ever change" or "Nothing really matters"?*

  - ✓ **Ask:** *Do you consider yourself a cynic? Do you ever find yourself feeling like a martyr in an unjust world, a victim of unfair circumstances? Does change appear hopeless because you are powerless or because nothing anyone does ever makes a difference? Do you sometimes believe that other people are users or out to get you?*

- *How often do you shut down, numb out, or lose all of your energy?*

  ✓ **Ask:** *When this happens, what do you do (for example, go to bed and sleep all day)? Have there been times when you find yourself having fantasies about not participating in the world or that your problem will somehow magically disappear? What are the things that you believe are impossible or useless to change in your life?*

- *Do you pout or deliberately go quiet (silent treatment) when things don't go your way?*

  ✓ **Ask:** *When asked, do you ever deny pouting or being silent (even though inwardly you know that you are deliberately pouting or being silent)? How often do you pretend that everything is okay ("I'm fine") when you really know it is not? How often do you simply walk away when things don't go the way you want?*

- *Do you ever disagree with someone and then suddenly agree ("Okay, fine, you're right"), without explanation?*

  ✓ **Ask:** *Are there times that you acquiesce to avoid conflict or avoid feedback that you antici-pate may be unwanted? Have you ever noticed being secretly pleased that someone has given you advice because deep down you know you can blame them if things go wrong?*

- *When have you found yourself thinking that everything will be fine, despite repeated feedback that there is a serious problem that needs attending to?*

Encourage participants to write down the questions they find most helpful for locating their **Fatalistic Mind** and use them as reminders of possible "stuck points."

End by reminding participants that agreeing with someone or giving in does not necessarily mean that you are in Fatalistic Mind. Use self-enquiry instead to find out.

(Optional) Discussion Point
Fatalistic Mind

  ✓ **Ask** participants for times they may have been in Fatalistic Mind. Instructors should share examples from their own life. *What are the major downsides of operating from Fatalistic Mind? How does Fatalistic Mind impact relationships? What are we signaling to others when we operate from Fatalistic Mind?*

  ✓ **Ask** participants which is most problematic for them, Fixed Mind or Fatalistic Mind? Discuss how both extremes can be problematic; some people have a tendency to live in one extreme, whereas others tend to jump from one extreme to the other. Such jumping to another extreme may represent a desperate attempt to solve or avoid a problem. Ask for examples of events or times when participants have noticed themselves jumping from one extreme to another.

(Required) Teaching Point
Challenging Fatalistic Mind

Refer participants to handout 11.3 (Learning from Fatalistic Mind).

Step 1. When challenged, look for possible signs of Fatalistic Mind.

- For example, feeling unappreciated, invalidated, misunderstood, helpless, like a martyr, or like a victim. Feeling resentful, bitter, or cynical about change. Feeling numb or shut down.

Step 2. Acknowledge the possibility of being in Fatalistic Mind.

- *Fatalistic Mind is our "escape artist." Rather than openly resisting or fighting, abandonment is its solution.* It thrives on denial and self-deception; it allows us to avoid admitting avoidance and feel justified in walking away and/or virtuous for giving up.

- *Fatalistic Mind alerts us to those things in our life we may need to change.*

- *Fatalistic Mind can sometimes signal we are overworked or overwhelmed.* The change needed most is rest.

Step 3. Listen and learn from Fatalistic Mind.

- *Take the first step to change Fatalistic Mind by acknowledging you don't want to change it.* Admit that you are choosing to operate from Fatalistic Mind. *No one can force you to behave fatalistically.*

- *Loosen Fatalistic Mind by admitting it. Say:* I am in Fatalistic Mind and this is not how I want to live.

- *Practice self-enquiry by asking* What is it that I might need to learn from my Fatalistic Mind?

- *Take the power away from Fatalistic Mind by publicly revealing it.* Fatalistic Mind thrives on secrecy. Practice nonjudgmentally outing yourself when you find yourself intentionally pouting, stonewalling, or pretending to comply in order to get what you want. Let the other person know that this way of behaving goes against your valued goals. Allow yourself to nonjudgmentally experience any embarrassment that may arise. Observe the impact your disclosure has on your relationships (recall that revealing inner feelings to others increases trust and desires for affiliation by recipients).

- *Stop blaming others for making you miserable.* Go all the way opposite action to Fatalistic Mind by admitting to yourself (and others) how you contributed to the problem, and then actively take steps to solve it.

- *Welcome despair, anxiety, and hopelessness as teachers, not enemies.* Greet them as helpful guides who are preparing you for new learning. Go opposite to desires to numb out or give up. Open your mind to what your pain might be trying to tell you.

- *Let go of longing for the world to change or secretly hoping that the problem will go away.* Accept responsibility for creating your own reality. Practice recognizing the possibility of growth in each moment.

- *Remember, Fatalistic Mind does not necessarily mean that you are doing anything wrong.* You may be working too hard and need a rest and/or you may need to grieve a loss. However,

Fatalistic Mind may also be alerting you to something important that needs to change in your life, something you don't want to acknowledge. Take the time to listen to your Fatalistic Mind. What is its message?

- **Turn your mind toward your predicament.** Closed-mouth smile with eyebrows raised, and breathe deeply while thinking about the problem or feedback your Fatalistic Mind has labeled unsolvable.

- **Turn your mind to the possibility of change and listen fully to the feedback,** using handout 22.1 (Being Open to Feedback from Others: Flexible Mind ADOPTS).

- **Clarify the steps needed to solve the problem and then take the first step.** Focus on mindfully taking one step at a time and block worries about the future. Remember past successes.

- **Remember that rejecting help from others keeps you stuck in Fatalistic Mind.** Practice allowing others to assist you, thank them for their help, and look for ways to actively reciprocate.

- **Forgive yourself** for operating from Fatalistic Mind (see Flexible Mind Has HEART skills, lesson 29).

(Required) Teaching Points
Understanding Flexible Mind

- *Flexible Mind is a synthesis between Fixed Mind and Fatalistic Mind. It involves purposeful self-enquiry, exploration, and discovery and is the essence of radical openness.* See worksheet 1.B (Flexible Mind DEFinitely: Three Steps to Radically Open Living).

- *Flexible Mind is like a ship captain who doesn't abandon ship or turn completely around at the first sign of trouble. Instead, he is willing to change course or reduce speed when icebergs are sighted.*

- *Flexible Mind involves being able to listen openly to criticism or feedback, without immediate denial (or agreement).* It involves a willingness to experience new things with an open heart, without losing track of one's values.

- *Flexible Mind is not about being balanced (that is, always calm, stable, or in the middle). Flexible Mind values both disinhibition* (for example, dancing with abandon, trusting one's intuitions, yelling wildly to stop a mugger, enjoying the present moment) *and inhibition* (for example, delaying gratification, questioning intuitive knowing, refraining from sharing a silly joke during a serious meeting or conversation).

(Required) Class Exercise
Finding My Flexible Mind

NOTE TO INSTRUCTORS: Instructors should use the following statements to encourage discussion and as a means for participants to discover their Flexible Mind. Instructors should review each statement, ask for examples from the class, or share examples from their own life to facilitate understanding.

- *Flexible Mind is turning one's mind to the possibility of change* and changing if that is what is needed.

- *Flexible Mind is doing what is needed in the moment.* For example, strive for perfection, but stop when feedback suggests that striving is counterproductive or damaging a relationship; be rule-governed except when breaking the rules is required (for example, to save someone's life); be polite and cooperative, yet be bad-tempered if the situation calls for it (for example, when safety concerns are overriding).

- *Flexible Mind acknowledges that we don't see the world as it is but instead see it as we are,* meaning that we carry with us perceptual and regulatory biases wherever we go as a function of our differing brains and differing life experiences.

- *Flexible Mind takes responsibility for our personal reactions to the world rather than automatically blaming others or expecting the world to change.* It means taking responsibility for how we may have contributed to a problem, without harsh self-blame or falling apart.

- *Flexible Mind acknowledges that I choose my emotional responses and recognizes that other people cannot force me to feel a particular way; for example, no one can compel me to feel anger or sadness.* Although things outside of our control can trigger emotions, and many people have had traumatic experiences occur outside of their control (for example, abuse as a child), Flexible Mind recognizes that how we respond to life events almost invariably involves some sort of choice on our part.

- *Flexible Mind celebrates diversity by recognizing that there are many ways to live, behave, or think.*

- *Flexible Mind recognizes that one secret to healthy living is the cultivation of healthy self-doubt.*

- *Flexible Mind values negative emotions and judgmental thoughts as opportunities for growth and self-enquiry.*

Lesson 11 Homework

Participants should look for times during the next week they may be in Fixed Mind, Flexible Mind, and Fatalistic Mind.

1. **(Required) Worksheet 11.A (Being Kind to Fixed Mind)**
2. **(Required) Worksheet 11.B (Going Opposite to Fatalistic Mind)**

Radical Openness Handout 11.1

Overcontrolled States of Mind

When one is challenged, OC states of mind emerge

Fixed Mind
Change is unnecessary, because I already know the answer.

It is like being the captain of the *Titanic* and your motto is "Full speed ahead, icebergs be damned!"

Fatalistic Mind
Change is unnecessary, because there is no answer.

The captain of the *Titanic*, after hitting the first iceberg, retreats to his cabin, locks the door, and refuses to help steer the ship to safety, determine the next course of action, or, if necessary, help passengers safely abandon ship.

Flexible-Mind

Synthesis is Flexible Mind

The captain of the ship is open to feedback and willing to change course or reduce speed when icebergs are sighted, without abandoning ship or turning completely around at the first sign of trouble.

Radical Openness Handout 11.2

Being Kind to Fixed Mind

Step 1. When challenged, observe emotions, action urges, and thoughts that may be linked to Fixed Mind.

- Feeling irritated, resentful, indignant, spiteful, paranoid, frustrated, anxious, nervous, angry, numb, frozen, or empty; urges to quickly explain, justify oneself, or discount what is happening

- Thinking that it would be morally wrong for others to question your point of view, confident you know the answer or that the other person is mistaken, unethical, misguided, or wrong

Step 2. Acknowledge the possibility of being in Fixed Mind.

- **Physical tension in the body means feeling threatened.** When threatened, we either fight or flee. Fixed Mind is our "fighter"—it can help keep us protected but it can keep us stuck.

- **Use self-enquiry to facilitate self-awareness;** see worksheet 11.A (Being Kind to Fixed Mind) for examples.

- **Acknowledge that you are fighting or resisting something,** without mindlessly letting go of your point of view.

- **Gently remember that when in Fixed Mind,** your thoughts, emotions, urges, and sensations are determined by your past learning.

- **Remind yourself that Fixed Mind alerts us to those things in our life we need to be more open to in order to improve ourselves or learn.**

Step 3. Don't try to fix Fixed Mind; be kind instead.

- **Practice being open to what is happening in this moment.** Let go of assuming you have the correct answer while encouraging yourself to be more open. Use handout 22.1 (Being Open to Feedback from Others: Flexible Mind ADOPTS) to help yourself be more open to the feedback and determine if you should adopt it.

- **Change physiology:** Closed-mouth smile while breathing deeply; use eyebrow wags.

- **Rather than resisting, fixing, or defending your Fixed Mind, allow it to be.** Open and soften to the experience of Fixed Mind and give yourself time to discover what your Fixed Mind might be saying. You never know what you might learn. Trying to fix or control Fixed Mind is like criticizing yourself for being too self-critical—it just doesn't work.

- **Use a loving kindness practice** by repeating silently to yourself: *May my Fixed Mind find peace, may my Fixed Mind be content, may my Fixed Mind be safe and secure.*

- **Forgive yourself for being in Fixed Mind;** remember that we all have a Fixed Mind.

Radical Openness Handout 11.3

Learning from Fatalistic Mind

Step 1. When challenged, observe emotions, action urges, and thoughts that may be linked to Fatalistic Mind.

- Feeling unappreciated, invalidated, misunderstood, helpless like a small child, like a martyr, or like a victim AND/OR resentful, bitter, or cynical about change AND/OR numbed out or shut down

- Thinking that everything will be fine, despite repeated feedback that there is a serious problem needing your attention. Believing that change is impossible ("Why bother?"), that others must change first before you can, or magically hoping problems will disappear

- Having secret urges to punish the person suggesting change; a desire to pout, cry, walk away, deny, or to make unrealistic promises for self-improvement in order to stop the feedback

Step 2. Acknowledge the possibility of being in Fatalistic Mind by remembering that Fatalistic Mind is the opposite of resisting or fighting.

- **Fatalistic Mind is our "escape artist." Rather than openly resisting or fighting, abandonment is its solution.** It thrives on denial and self-deception; it allows us to feel justified when we walk away, virtuous for giving up, or to avoid admitting we are avoiding something.

- **Fatalistic Mind is not bad.** Nonjudgmental awareness of Fatalistic Mind can help us recognize times when we are pushing ourselves too hard or may need to grieve a loss, as well as alert us to areas in our life that require change.

Step 3. Listen and learn from Fatalistic Mind by using the following skills.

- **Take the first step by acknowledging you don't want to** (take the first step). Admit that you are choosing to operate from Fatalistic Mind—no one can force you to behave fatalistically.

- **Welcome despair, anxiety, and hopelessness as teachers, not enemies.** Greet them as helpful guides who are preparing you for new learning. Go opposite to desires to numb out or give up. Open your mind to what your pain might be trying to tell you.

- **Let go of longing for the world to change or secretly hoping that the problem will go away.** Accept responsibility for creating your own reality. Practice recognizing the possibility of growth in each moment.

- **Remember, Fatalistic Mind does not mean that you are necessarily doing anything wrong**—you may be working too hard and need a rest and/or you may need to grieve a loss. Alternatively, Fatalistic Mind may also be alerting you to something important that needs to change in your life, something you don't want to acknowledge. Take the time to listen to your Fatalistic Mind. What is its message?

- **Turn your mind toward your predicament. Closed-mouth smile, eyebrow wag, and breathe deeply while thinking about the problem or feedback** your Fatalistic Mind has labeled unsolvable.

- **Turn your mind to the possibility of change** and listen fully to the feedback using handout 22.1 (Being Open to Feedback from Others: Flexible Mind ADOPTS).

- **Clarify the steps needed to solve the problem and then take the first step.** Focus on mindfully taking one step at a time and block worries about the future. Remember past successes.

- **Fatalistic Mind thrives on secrecy.** Take the power away from Fatalistic Mind by revealing to the other person your urges to pout, stonewall, or give up. Stop blaming others for "making" you miserable. Go all the way opposite action to Fatalistic Mind by admitting to yourself (and others) how you contributed to the problem, and then actively take steps to solve it.

- **Remember that rejecting help from others keeps you stuck in Fatalistic Mind.** Practice allowing others to assist you, thank them for their help, and look for ways to actively reciprocate.

- **Forgive yourself** for operating from Fatalistic Mind (see lesson 29).

Radical Openness Handout 11.4

Main Points for Lesson 11: Mindfulness Training, Part 1

Overcontrolled States of Mind

1. Problematic states of mind for overcontrolled individuals are most often closed-minded.

2. These states function to block learning from new information or disconfirming feedback and can negatively impact interpersonal relationships.

3. A closed mind is a threatened mind. Though frequently triggered by nonemotional predispositions for detail-focused processing and inhibitory control, OC problematic states of mind are emotionally driven.

4. Fixed Mind signals that change is unnecessary because I already know the answer. Fixed Mind is like the captain of the *Titanic*, who, despite repeated warnings, insists, "Full speed ahead, and icebergs be damned."

5. Fatalistic Mind says change is unnecessary because there is no answer. Fatalistic Mind is like the captain of the *Titanic*, who, after hitting the fatal iceberg, retreats to his cabin, locks the door, and refuses to help passengers abandon ship.

6. Flexible Mind represents a more open, receptive, and flexible means of responding. It is like a ship captain who is willing to forgo previous plans and change course or reduce speed when icebergs are sighted. There is no abandoning ship or turning completely around at the first sign of trouble.

Radical Openness Worksheet 11.A

Being Kind to Fixed Mind

Step 1. Describe a challenging situation linked to Fixed Mind behaviors.

What behaviors, thoughts, action urges, and emotions did you notice?

_____

_____

_____

_____

Step 2. Acknowledge Fixed Mind via self-enquiry.

Check the box next to the items you found helpful, and record your answers or other questions you used in the space provided.

- ☐ *Am I finding it hard to question my point of view or even engage in self-enquiry?*
- ☐ *Do I find myself wanting to automatically explain, defend, or discount the other person's feedback or what is happening?*
- ☐ *Has my rate of speech changed? What is driving me to respond so quickly or to pick my words so carefully?*
- ☐ *Am I discounting the feedback to purposefully displease or punish someone? If so, what does this tell me about my level of openness?*
- ☐ *Am I resisting being open to this feedback because part of me believes that doing so will change an essential part of who I am?*
- ☐ *Am I able to truly pause and consider the possibility that I may be wrong or may need to change?*
- ☐ *Am I saying to myself, "I know I am right," no matter what they say or how things seem?*
- ☐ *Do I believe that further self-examination is unnecessary, because I have already worked out the problem, know the answer, or have done the necessary self-work about the issue being discussed?*
- ☐ *What am I afraid might happen if I were to momentarily drop my perspective?*

_____

_____

_____

Step 3. Go opposite to Fixed Mind.

Place a checkmark in the boxes next to the skills you practiced.

- ☐ Practiced mindful awareness of bodily sensations linked to Fixed Mind (for example, muscle tension, numbness, flushed face, heart racing) rather than automatically discounting, ignoring, or denying their potential significance.

- ☐ Opened and softened to emotions linked to Fixed Mind (such as embarrassment, irritability, anger, indignation) rather than immediately trying to fix them or pretend they were not there.

- ☐ Allowed myself to fully consider the possibility that I was incorrect or misinformed, and/or that "my way" might not work, without harsh self-blame or immediate abandonment of my prior beliefs.

- ☐ Allowed myself time (for example, a day) to mindfully examine my responses, emotions, and urges to correct, improve, plan, or fix the situation before actually doing anything.

- ☐ Reminded myself that there is always something new to learn because the world is in constant change.

- ☐ Went opposite to Fixed Mind rigidity by relaxing my body and face, using half smiles, eyebrow wags, slow breathing, and sitting back.

- ☐ Tried out something small that was related to the new behavior or way of thinking.

- ☐ Reminded myself that you have to crack an egg to make an omelet—that new learning requires breaking down old ways of thinking or doing.

- ☐ Reminded myself that exhibiting a strong preference does not mean that one is necessarily closed-minded or operating from Fixed Mind.

- ☐ Practiced loving my Fixed Mind instead of judging or fixing it. For example, repeated silently three times to myself: *May my Fixed Mind find peace. May my Fixed Mind be happy. May my Fixed Mind be safe and secure.*

- ☐ Forgave myself for being in Fixed Mind while resolving to be more open and flexible.

Other skills and comments.

_____

_____

_____

_____

Radical Openness Worksheet 11.B

Going Opposite to Fatalistic Mind

Step 1. Describe a challenging situation linked to Fatalistic Mind behaviors.

What behaviors, thoughts, action urges, and emotions did you notice?

_____

_____

_____

_____

Step 2. Acknowledge Fatalistic Mind via self-enquiry.

Check the boxes next to the items you found helpful, and record your answers or other questions you used in the space provided.

- ☐ *Do I feel like shutting down, quitting, or giving up?*
- ☐ *Do I feel invalidated, unappreciated, or treated as not "special" by the person giving me feedback, yet choose not to tell them?*
- ☐ *Do I secretly believe that the other person must change, rather than me?*
- ☐ *Do I secretly hope that any change efforts will fail because it will prove that I was right in believing that change is impossible, because there is no answer?*
- ☐ *Do I feel strong urges to acquiesce simply to avoid conflict rather than because I actually agree?*
- ☐ *Do I fantasize that the problem will somehow magically go away if I do nothing?*
- ☐ *Do I secretly want to punish the other person by pouting, being silent, or withdrawing?*
- ☐ *Am I acting like I am hurt or fragile in order to stop the feedback and avoid dealing with the situation?*
- ☐ *Do I think that everything will be fine, despite repeated feedback that there is a serious problem needing my attention?*

_____

_____

_____

Step 3. Go opposite to Fatalistic Mind.

Place a checkmark in the boxes next to the skills you practiced.

- ☐ Practiced mindful awareness of bodily sensations linked to Fatalistic Mind (for example, muscle tension, numbness, flushed face, heart racing) rather than automatically discounting, ignoring, or denying their potential significance.

- ☐ Gently reminded myself that Fatalistic Mind is a learned behavior.

- ☐ Closed-mouth smiled, eyebrow wagged, and took slow deep breaths while thinking about the problem that Fatalistic Mind wanted to avoid.

- ☐ Turned my mind toward the problem while opening and softening to the uncomfortable sensations in my body.

- ☐ Remembered that when I reject help from others, I may keep myself stuck in Fatalistic Mind

- ☐ Turned my mind away from thoughts telling me that I couldn't do it or that the problem was insolvable. Reminded myself that I am competent and have solved many problems in the past.

- ☐ Let go of rigid beliefs that I must do everything myself. Remembered that asking for help doesn't mean I am incompetent.

- ☐ Blocked self-invalidation or self-blame and turned to work on the problem in a flexible and easy manner.

- ☐ Took responsibility by acknowledging that I am choosing to behave fatalistically rather than blaming Fatalistic Mind on others or the world.

- ☐ Let go of desires for the world to change or for the problem to go away and instead looked for ways I might change.

- ☐ Went opposite to urges to pout, shut down, stonewall, sabotage, or take revenge and directly communicated my concern to the other person and took responsibility for how I was feeling.

- ☐ Clarified what I needed to attend to in order to solve the problem.

- ☐ Determined the steps that needed to be taken to solve the problem.

- ☐ Took the first step toward solving the problem and practiced one thing at a time.

- ☐ Forgave myself for operating from Fatalistic Mind.

Other skills and comments.

_____

_____

_____

_____

Mindfulness Training, Part 2

The "What" Skills

> NOTE TO INSTRUCTORS: Lesson 12 is part 2 of RO mindfulness skills training. Its primary focus is teaching mindfulness "what" skills (from an RO perspective).

Main Points for Lesson 12

1. In RO DBT, there are three mindfulness "what" skills, each of which represents a differing aspect or way to practice mindfulness. They are *observe openly, describe with integrity,* and *participate without planning.*

2. "Urge-surfing" mindfulness practices facilitate learning how to not respond to every urge, impulse, and desire, such as urges to fix, control, reject, or avoid.

3. The Awareness Continuum is the core RO "describe with integrity" practice and can also be used as an "outing oneself" practice. It helps the practitioner take responsibility for their inner experiences, block habitual desires to explain or justify oneself, and learn how to differentiate between thoughts, emotions, sensations, and images. It is a core means for learning how to step off the path of blame (habitual blaming of self or others).

4. Participating without planning means learning how to passionately participate in one's life and in one's community and let go of compulsive planning, rehearsal, and/or obsessive needs to get it right.

Materials Needed

- Handout 12.1 ("Describe with Integrity" Skills: The Awareness Continuum)

- Handout 12.2 (Main Points for Lesson 12: Mindfulness Training, Part 2: The "What" Skills)

- Worksheet 12.A ("Observe Openly" Skills)

- Worksheet 12.B (Making Participating Without Planning a Daily Habit)

- Worksheet 12.C (The Three "What" Skills: Daily Practice Log for the "Observe Openly," "Describe with Integrity," and "Participate Without Planning" Skills)

- Whiteboard or flipchart with marker

(Recommended) Mindfulness Practice

Urge-Surfing

NOTE TO INSTRUCTORS: Each RO class normally begins with a brief mindfulness exercise or practice prior to reviewing homework. The required urge-surfing mindfulness practice that follows most often would be done at the beginning of the class, just before reviewing the homework assigned from the previous lesson's class. For this practice, it is important to teach the following required teaching points before starting the practice. Plus, instructors should use the script provided here and read it aloud, verbatim (see "Additional Instructions for Using the Skills Manual," in chapter 4, for a rationale).

- *By definition, overcontrolled individuals are masters of inhibitory control.* That is, they are good at delaying gratification, inhibiting an emotional action urge or an urge to eat, controlling facial expressions, and high persistence.

- Say: *Our mindfulness practice today will capitalize on your already existing superior inhibitory control capacities—the practice is known as* urge-surfing.

- *Mindful urge-surfing means consciously choosing to not respond to every urging sensation or impulse* in order to more fully live according to one's valued goals.

- *Urge-surfing is the same skill used by jet fighter pilots when first learning how to manage the extreme G-forces associated with high speeds at high altitudes.* Novice fighter pilots commonly experience nausea and urges to vomit, but throwing up clogs the face mask and breathing apparatus needed to survive at high altitudes. They are taught to mindfully observe the sensations of nausea, dizziness, and bloating and the urge to vomit as simply sensations rather than a crisis requiring immediate attention, or "truths" suggesting that they have been poisoned and need to expel a dangerous substance, and so forth. They are taught to simply watch the sensations and recognize that they are transitory in nature—nauseous sensations will come, and then they will go, then they may come again later, but they always go away of their own accord. Over time, these sensations are no longer experienced as signals that something is wrong or dangerous. It is not so much that the nausea fully goes away, but with repeated practice, over time, the pilot's relationship to the sensations of nausea changes; they are seen as simply slightly uncomfortable bodily reactions. Responding to them (that is, throwing up) not only is dangerous but makes it more likely for them to experience nausea the next time they fly (assuming they survived). Similarly, urge-surfing is used to overcome a wide range of other uncomfortable, yet not dangerous, bodily sensations (for example, overcoming seasickness, quitting cigarettes, not giving in to an urge to scratch a rash).

  ✓ **Ask:** *When do you think knowing how to urge-surf might be useful?* Solicit ideas from the class and augment this discussion with examples of your own (for example, urges to smoke a cigarette after deciding to quit, urges to honk one's horn when caught in traffic, urges to quickly write an angry response via email, urges to eat too much or not enough).

Instructors should emphasize that the goal of urge-surfing is not to eliminate desires, urges, or impulses (an impossible task) but to learn that not all desires, urges, or impulses *must be satisfied* (that is, responded to).

Begin the practice by reading aloud the following script.

So, as just discussed, our mindfulness practice today will be one that is designed to help us become better at noticing and not responding to urges to do something that we inwardly know will create more suffering for us. The practice is known as urge-surfing—a way of becoming more mindfully aware of urges by seeing them as waves; they crest and then pass away. This practice involves learning to appreciate urges as transitory experiences, not mandates for action. Most of us already have experience in not responding to urges—for example, quitting cigarettes or not scratching an itch. Today's practice is designed to help us become better at using this skill. And so, to start, I would like you to sit in a comfortable yet alert position and take a breath with awareness in order to center yourself into this moment. Notice the rise and fall of your breathing, not trying to change or do anything about it, just being fully present with the full duration of your inbreath and the full duration of your outbreath. [Slight pause.] Now, as best you can, allow your attention to focus on any urges that might arise during your practice of mindful breathing. For example, you might notice an urge to move, an urge to scratch an itch, or perhaps even an urge to giggle. As best you can, observe these urges without giving in to them—not trying to make them go away, but simply allowing them to crest and fall like a wave, knowing that they are transitory experiences that don't require an immediate response. If you find your mind wandering, notice that, and without giving yourself a hard time, gently guide your attention back to the sensations of your breath and your awareness of any urges that may arise. Urges can involve many things…for example, you might notice an urge to stop this practice, or an urge to fall asleep, or an urge to think about other things….you might notice an urge to stand up or walk out of this room…all kinds of experiences might emerge during the practice…including not being able to notice any urges whatsoever. Either way, the practice today is to get better at noticing urges rather than automatically giving in to them…by simply observing them like waves and then turning our attention back to our breath. [Slight pause.] Finally, if you have an urge that you decide to respond to…do so with awareness. Now let's take a few minutes to silently practice urge-surfing, with the understanding that doing so will help us become better at not responding to every impulse or desire that may arise.

Allow the practice to continue silently for about three to four more minutes, and then end the practice.

Solicit observations from the class and teach additional information as needed. Use the following questions and teaching points to facilitate this.

- ✓ **Ask:** *What did you observe? What type of urges arose for you? Were you able to mindfully observe them?*

- ✓ **Ask:** *If you were able to resist giving in to the urge, what happened to it over time?*

- **When urges are not responded to immediately (for example, you don't scratch that itch), most often the intensity of the urge increases.** That is, urges don't immediately just go away after you decide not to respond to them.

   - ✓ **Ask:** *Did anyone notice this during our practice today?*

- **Interestingly, if a person responds to an urge when the intensity is high (for example, you can't stand it anymore, and you scratch that itch!), your brain learns that intense urges (for example, itchy sensations) will eventually be responded to if it just waits you out!** This makes it harder to not give in again the next time you urge-surf.

- **Essentially, responding to an urge (for example, having that cigarette) reinforces the response.**

- **All urges are transitory.**

- **The good news is that with repeated practice (that is, consciously nonresponding to the urge), the urging sensations become less intense over time.** Your brain acquires new learning—for example, nausea or bloating after eating a meal is no longer a crisis, the urge to recheck the lock on one's door is simply another sensation, urges to fix or control are not imperatives, and urges for a cigarette will eventually pass.

- **With practice, you can learn to urge-surf almost anything—remember those jet fighter pilots!**

(Required) Teaching Point

Mindfulness "What" Skill: Observe Openly

- *Observing openly—that is, with an open mind—means attending to what is happening in the current moment, even when it is distressing.*

- *It involves conscious awareness at the level of pure sensation, without added words* (for example, visceral awareness of bodily sensations, emotions, thoughts, and urges, or of the sights, sounds, textures, and smells emerging from the external environment).

- *The mere act of observing oneself with conscious awareness alters what is observed, which means that it alters perception,* even when the act of observing involves observing oneself observing oneself. For example, anger observed mindfully is qualitatively different from anger experienced mindlessly.

- *Open-minded observing means attending to unwanted emotions or events with open curiosity rather than automatically regulating or attempting to exit the situation.*

  - It means observing without categorizing the situation or experience as good or bad.

  - It means observing without assuming that what is observed represents truth or reality.

- *It is the first step in new learning because it means being in the place where we are most likely to become aware of our edge, or personal unknown.*

Examples of "Observe Openly" Practices for Overcontrol

- Go to an art museum and practice observing various paintings close up and then far away. *What do you observe?* Notice which you prefer and whether this depends on the type of painting.

- Practice observing when you are open- versus closed-minded. *What are the differences between these two states?*

- Mindfully observe the thoughts, images (for example, memories), emotions, and sensations that arise when you are detail-focused. Do the same when you are globally focused. *Are there differences between the two?*

- Observe how detail-focused versus globally focused processing influences your perception and interpretations of an event. *For example, do you use more or less emotional words when detail-focused? Are you more or less judgmental when detail-focused? Are you more or less emotional when globally focused?*

- Practice seeing the forest, not just the trees.

- Go to a park or a shopping mall and mindfully observe facial expressions, gestures, body movements, voice tone, rate of speech, and so on, of other people, without getting caught up into analyzing them. Notice the types of gestures, facial expressions, and movements associated with people who are interacting or together. Observe which ones result in people moving closer together or touching, and which ones result in people moving away, averting their gaze, or breaking contact.

- Mindfully observe how your tone of voice impacts those around you.

- Mindfully observe what happens when you raise your eyebrows and smile when interacting with others.

- Mindfully observe who talks more when interacting with someone. Observe what happens when you go opposite to what you were doing (that is, talk more or listen more).

- **Observe what happens when you practice taking a break, relaxing, or rewarding yourself**—for example, curl up for half an hour with a nonserious book, have a glass of wine, eat one of your favorite chocolates, take a long hot bath with aromatic candles, take a nap, listen to your favorite music while enjoying your favorite beverage, watch your favorite TV show, sit out in your garden and enjoy the sunshine.

- **Mindfully observe what happens when you closed-mouth smile and raise your eyebrows when interacting with someone.**

- **Practice observing sensations that may be linked with emotion**—for example, suddenly feeling hot or sweaty.

- **Practice urge-surfing** by mindfully observing urges, impulses, and desires, without getting caught up in the thoughts or giving in to the urges. When an urge occurs, practice noticing the urge and, instead of automatically responding to it, turn your mind to something else. Be aware of the urge, without getting caught up in it—ride it like a wave. Repeat frequently and observe how your relationship with the urging sensation you have chosen changes over time (for example, practice surfing the same urge for several weeks in a row). Here are some examples of common OC urges or impulses—pick one and start practicing!

  - **Urges to control or correct.** Observe what happens when you don't immediately attempt to fix or control a situation.

  - **Urges to walk away during a conflict.** Notice the urge to abandon or walk away during a disagreement; practice remaining engaged instead. Use worksheet 1.B (Flexible Mind DEFinitely: Three Steps for Radically Open Living) to facilitate open-minded engagement.

  - **Urges to tidy or clean.** Notice these urges and consciously choose to not clean or tidy; turn your mind instead to something pleasant or distracting and keep turning you mind back to the pleasant event when the urge to clean returns. After the intensity of the urge to clean or tidy up has passed, use Flexible Mind to decide whether to clean up or not. Make sure you don't clean or tidy when the urges are high, because this will only reinforce them (that is, make this habit harder to break).

  - **Urges to correct, improve, or tell another person what to do or how to do it.** For example, when riding in the car with your son, observe urges to tell him how to drive better; when reading a neighborhood pamphlet, observe urges to correct grammar. Rather than automatically giving in to the urge, turn your mind to something neutral or pleasant (for example, notice the beautiful colors on the pamphlet, observe your breath, think of the dinner you will be having with your neighbor) or, if appropriate, ask for their opinion. Wait until your urge has passed completely (this may take minutes) before you decide to respond. Use self-enquiry and Flexible Mind to determine whether expressing your urge might still be effective. Remember that correcting and telling can always wait but, once done, can never be taken back. Watch how this practice impacts relationships over time. Ask: *Does less correcting and telling on my part result in better or worse interpersonal closeness with others? What might this mean?* Use stall tactics from worksheet 1.B (Flexible Mind DEFinitely: Three Steps for Radically Open Living) to further facilitate this.

  - **Urges to change the topic when you don't like what is being discussed.** Practice watching the urge and staying with the unwanted or disliked topic. Use self-enquiry to deepen your understanding by asking *What is it that I might need to learn?* rather than automatically blaming the other or avoiding.

  - **Urges to redo someone's work** (for example, restacking a dishwasher because it wasn't done according to your standards, or rewriting the minutes of a meeting). Watch the urge; see how long it takes for it to dissipate on its own. Notice what you do or think to keep the urge fired up. Use self-enquiry to deepen your practice—for example, by asking *How might redoing others' work impact my relationships? What am I afraid might happen if I didn't redo this work? What is it I need to learn?*

- **Urges to check** (for example, whether a door is locked, a light is switched off, hands are clean). Practice seeing urges and thoughts linked to checking behaviors as painful experiences only—they are not crises, they are not lethal, they are simply thoughts, sensations, images, and emotions that are reinforced every time you give in to an urge to check. Pick one checking behavior at a time to change, and practice urge-surfing automatic responses. Give yourself weeks or months to lay down new learning about the behavior. Remember that intermittent reinforcement (that is, giving in occasionally) makes it harder for an urge to fade away (remember, giving up checking behavior is as hard as or harder than giving up cigarettes).

- **Urges to gossip about a rival.** Practice watching urges to socially compare, gossip, or negatively fantasize about a rival or competitor and, rather than giving in to them, use self-enquiry by asking yourself *What is it that I might need to learn from this?*

- **Urges to restrict food intake, vomit, or expel food after eating** (ideal for clients with anorexia nervosa). Observe urges to restrict food intake, emotions (for example, disgust, fear, anger), sensations of bloating and nausea, and/or catastrophizing thoughts (for example, *This is horrible, I am going to throw up, I have to get out of here*) that arise while eating or immediately following eating. Practice seeing them as just thoughts, just emotions, just sensations—not literal truth, a crisis, or a problem that must be solved.

(Required) Teaching Point
Describe with Integrity

- **Describe with integrity *is the RO mindfulness "what" skill of putting into words what one has observed, with humility.***
- *You can only describe what you have already observed.*
- *The "describe with integrity" skill emphasizes the importance of labeling a thought or feeling as just a thought or emotion; they are mental events, no more and no less.* They are not inherent, truthful, or accurate reflections of reality.
- *In RO DBT, "describe with integrity" practices are founded on three core RO principles:*
  1. *"We don't see the world as it is, we see it as we are." Thus, anything we describe is biased, even when we try to stick to the facts,* because our perceptions are always limited by our personal biology, our past experience, and current context.
  2. *The importance of acknowledging our descriptions as limited in order to be more open and receptive to differing perspectives.*
  3. *The importance of describing what we perceive to other members of our tribe* in order for them to reflect back our blind spots—a process in RO DBT known as "outing oneself."
- *The core "describe with integrity" practice in RO DBT is known as the Awareness Continuum.* It encompasses all three of the preceding principles, plus it has several other advantages:

- ***The structure of the Awareness Continuum makes it obvious that the perception originates from the describer,*** thereby facilitating a person to take responsibility for how they see the world.

- ***It provides a coherent means to practice labeling and differentiating between thoughts, emotions, sensations, and images.***

- ***It provides a structured means to practice revealing one's inner experience to another person without rehearsal or planning in advance what one might say.*** Thus, the Awareness Continuum is an RO "outing oneself" practice and going opposite to automatic tendencies to mask inner feelings is an essential skill that OC clients need to learn in order to rejoin the tribe.

- ***The practice can be used during interpersonal interactions, including those involving conflict,*** to slow down the pace of the exchange, increase awareness of what one is experiencing moment by moment, and signal that you are taking responsibility for your emotions, thoughts, sensations, and images, rather than blaming the other person.

NOTE TO INSTRUCTORS: The Awareness Continuum has its roots in Malâmati Sufism (see chapter 7 of the RO DBT textbook for more on Malâmati Sufism and its links to RO DBT).

(Required) Class Exercise
The Awareness Continuum

Teach the Awareness Continuum step by step.

Step 1. Start by saying the word "I."

- This signals to yourself and others that you are the source of the observation.

Step 2. Clarify that you are mindfully observing by adding the words "am aware of."

Step 3. Label what is being observed by classifying it as one of four different forms: sensation, emotion, image, or thought.

- A *sensation* includes any experience involving the five senses (sound, taste, touch, hearing, or sight). *Emotions* include emotional experiences, mood states, (for example, fear or anxiety), urges, impulses, and desires (for example, a *feeling of desire* to walk out of a room). *Images* generally fall into observations about the past (for example, a memory), the future (for example, what might happen), or mind reading of others (for example, imagining what another is thinking or feeling). *Thoughts* are cognitive experiences of the current moment.

Step 4. Describe the content of the experience, without further explanation, rationalization, or justification.

- For example, "I am aware of a thought about being precise." The words "being precise" reflect the *content* of the thought, without *explaining why it occurred*. Not explaining or justifying our experience helps us recognize how we automatically assume criticism from others and defend ourselves. Labeling without justifying can provide a powerful means for self-discovery.

- **Avoid clumping, meaning long statements that combine two or more forms of experience into one statement.** For instance, "I am aware of an emotion of sadness" consists of one form—an emotion—whereas "I am aware of an emotion of sadness because I just thought about my lost dog that ran away three weeks ago" is an explanation about the initial experience of sadness that clumps several forms together. Keeping statements to one form helps prevent justification or rationalization of one's experience. Instructors should demonstrate clumping and contrast it with nonclumping.

- **The practice ideally involves describing, moment by moment, what one is aware of, without long pauses between statements.** The idea is to not think too much before one describes.

- **"Editing" is okay when using the Awareness Continuum as part of an "outing oneself" practice.** Feeling free to not report every experience is not only okay but also reflects what we do all of the time in real life, since there are many more thoughts, emotions, sensations, and images occurring moment by moment than are possible to describe.

The instructor can then demonstrate a brief Awareness Continuum practice aloud in front of the class. Remember, you cannot rehearse what you will say beforehand—it requires moment-by-moment awareness of your ever-changing conscious experience and then picking from your field of awareness what is described aloud. See the following example.

I am aware of the sensation of looking at my coffee cup. I am aware of imagining that the class finds this odd. I am aware of an emotion of anxiety. I am aware of an image of my wife making breakfast this morning. I am aware of a sensation of a slight smile.

Note how each phrase reflects the structure described—for example, I (self) am aware of (observing) an image (form) of my wife making breakfast (content).

The good news is that the Awareness Continuum can be used almost anytime or anywhere. Encourage class members to establish a daily or regular five-minute "spoken aloud" practice.

Awareness Continuum practice at home (this can be done alone): Watch to see if over time it influences how you reveal inner feelings to others. Record your observations in your self-enquiry journal and watch how your practice evolves over time.

NOTE TO INSTRUCTORS: "Outing oneself" practices in RO DBT are generally done in pairs in RO skills training classes (that is, the entire class practices together at the same time, but each class member only works with their partner in a dyadic pair). A core aim of "outing oneself" practices is to provide a structured venue to help OC clients get better at revealing their inner feelings to another person, not to become a better public speaker, a toastmaster, or able to speak extemporaneously in front of a group.

NOTE TO INSTRUCTORS: When someone finds themselves speechless during an Awareness Continuum "outing oneself" practice, they can be instructed to say, "I am aware of a thought that I have nothing to say" or "I am aware of a thought that I have no thoughts" (the humor in this quickly becomes apparent).

Practice: The Awareness Continuum

Split the class into pairs. Instructors may need to pair up with someone if there is an odd number of people in the class, and/or sometimes it is useful for an instructor to work with a very reluctant client.

Explain that partners in each dyad will be taking turns speaking aloud their Awareness Continuum (while the other mindfully listens; eyes can be closed).

Prior to the start of the practice, the instructor and coinstructor should model an Awareness Continuum practice in front of the class and demonstrate how to pass the practice on to the other person.

Read aloud the following script to guide the practice.

(Optional) Script for an Awareness Continuum "Outing Oneself" Practice

As we have just discussed, the Awareness Continuum is a mindfulness "describe with integrity" practice in RO DBT that helps us become more aware of and take responsibility for our experiences and perceptions. It is also best practiced aloud and with a partner, which is why we have asked each of you to work in pairs. The practice will involve both describing and listening to your partner's experience—with awareness. The practice of the Awareness Continuum involves a way of describing inner experience that begins with "I am aware of…" Each statement of awareness uses this introductory phrase as the starting point, followed by a description that labels the experience as a thought, emotion, image, or sensation. Images can be memories, thoughts of the future, or even what you may imagine your partner is thinking, whereas sensations involve our sensory perceptions that may involve sight, sound, taste, touch, or hearing.

For example, if I were sitting in a room where I could see trees outside the window, I might start my practice of the Awareness Continuum by saying, "I am aware of the sensation of the sight of trees." You may then wonder what kind of tree it is, and so you would say out loud, "I am aware of a thought wondering what kind of tree it is." You may feel embarrassed at not knowing what kind of tree it is, and so you would say, "I am aware of an emotion of embarrassment at not knowing what kind of tree it is." You may then guess it is a chestnut tree, and so you would say, "I am aware of a thought that it may be a chestnut tree." You may then have an image of eating chestnuts around an open fire at Christmastime, and so you would say, "I am aware of an image of eating chestnuts around an open fire at Christmas." This may provoke feelings of happiness, and so you would say, "I am aware of an emotion of happiness." You may then feel the breeze on your skin, and you would say, "I am aware of the sensation of the breeze touching my skin."

You may notice that your awareness is disjointed, jumping about from subject to subject. This observation becomes part of the practice: "I am aware of a thought that my awareness is jumping about all over the place." And remember, if you suddenly realize you have not been aware because you spaced out, that too can become part of the practice: "I am aware of a thought that I was spaced out." And then simply carry on observing and describing aloud whatever arises next into your awareness, without explanation or justification. If you find yourself judging, you can label that, too: "I am aware of a judgmental thought about not doing this perfectly." Remember, one of the reasons this can be so helpful is that you cannot rehearse what you are going to say beforehand, because the practice involves describing what you are experiencing right here and now. Thus, if you find yourself wanting to rehearse, you could say, "I am aware of a desire to rehearse what I am going to say." Are there any questions about what I have just said? [Pause and allow time for questions.]

Now let's get ready to begin your practice, just like we demonstrated. One person goes first, while the other mindfully listens, without commenting, questioning, soothing, or validating, and then switch roles when the speaker says, "Pass." Each turn should only last a minute, or even less, making it likely for each person in each pair to have two turns before I call an end to the practice. Eye contact is not required during the practice. Sometimes it makes it easier to listen to the other person and to speak aloud your Awareness Continuum when you direct your gaze elsewhere—for example, at your partner's shoes—or even close your eyes. Finally, remember that the goal is to listen fully to your partner while they are practicing and to let go of trying to rehearse what you might say when it is your turn. Okay…now begin!

End the practice after about four to five minutes, and then solicit observations.

Use the following questions to facilitate discussion.

- *What was it like to practice revealing inner experiences to another person this way? What did you notice?*

- *Were you able to silently listen with full awareness when your partner was speaking? If not, what got in your way?*

- *To what extent were you able to let go of rehearsing what you were going to say?*

- *How difficult was it to not want to jump in and dialogue, validate, ask a question, or soothe your partner during the practice? What might this tell you about yourself?*

- *Of the four forms—thoughts, emotions, sensations, and images—did you tend to notice only certain ones (for example, thoughts and sensations, but not emotions and images)? What might this tell you about yourself? What is it that you might need to learn?*

- *Did this practice impact how you now see your partner? Do you know your partner more or less after this practice? What does this tell you about relationships?*

(Recommended) Teaching Point

Examples of "Describe with Integrity" Practices for Overcontrol

- *Use the Awareness Continuum during an argument or conflict with someone* (for example, spouse, family member, friend). Doing so automatically makes it clear to both the practitioner and recipient that the practitioner is taking responsibility for their perceptions while slowing the pace of the conversation, allowing space for more reflection. For example, instead of saying, "You make me angry," use the Awareness Continuum, saying, "I am aware of a feeling of anger" or "I am aware of imagining that you are purposefully trying to make me angry."

- *Practice describing (silently) the facial expressions of someone you are interacting with.* Label what you observe without making interpretations. For example, say "I am aware of the corners of their mouth turning upward and slight creases at the edges of their eyes" rather than "They are happy" or "They are smiling."

- *Institute a five-minute Awareness Continuum practice that becomes part of your daily routine.* This can be done alone (yet, ideally, spoken aloud).

- *Use the Awareness Continuum when you are feeling a strong emotion to describe your thoughts, sensations, and images that arise.*

(Required) Class Exercise
"I Am NOT Pouting!"

NOTE TO INSTRUCTORS: Mindfulness practices that involve silent sitting or deliberate slowing of body movements (for example, redirecting one's attention back to one's breath when it wanders, or walking slowly while mindfully attending to body sensations) may be iatrogenic for some OC clients *if not* interspersed with practices involving disinhibited expression, passionate participation in community, and publicly revealing inner experience. RO DBT dialectically balances this by emphasizing practices that involve both *dispassionate awareness* and *passionate "participate without planning" practices* (T. R. Lynch, Lazarus, & Cheavens, 2015). Plus, in RO DBT it is important for instructors to model what they teach because OC clients are unlikely to believe it is socially acceptable for an adult to play, relax, or openly express emotions unless they see their therapist model it first.

Begin this section with a mini–"participate without planning" exercise known as "I am NOT pouting!" (aka "Let's Have a Temper Tantrum").

Remember, it is essential to *not* orient or forewarn OC clients about a "participate without planning" practice. Instructors should familiarize themselves thoroughly with the guidelines for "participate without planning" practices (outlined later in this section) before conducting this exercise. Keep the practice brief (about sixty seconds) in order to reduce social comparisons and self-consciousness (see rationale later in this section).

Start the exercise by saying to the class with a smile and eyebrows raised: *Okay…EVERYONE STAND UP! Since we're all going to JUST HATE this next part of our lesson, LET'S START POUTING ABOUT IT FIRST! Follow my lead, do what I do!* Warm smile with eyebrows raised: *OH NO…NOT pouting again! I DON'T WANT TO!* Make a sad face and stamp feet: *Why do I have to? It's not fair!* Stamping feet: *You need to be nice to me!* Pause slightly: *Okay, now, place the back of your hand over your forehead and moan: OHHHH, WOE IS ME! Again…OHHHHH, WOE IS ME! Now STAMP YOUR FEET! Again…I'm SO WRETCHED! WOE IS ME! STAMP OUR FEET! LOUDER! One more time…I'm SO WRETCHED! WOE IS ME! STAMP OUR FEET! Okay, that's enough—what a great temper tantrum! Well done!* Begin clapping, and encourage a round of applause: *Okay, let's all sit back down now. Nicely done!*

Say to the class: *I think our little temper tantrum was a perfect introduction to our next topic.*

- ✓ **Ask:** *To what extent did you feel self-conscious during this practice?*
- ✓ **Ask:** *How does self-consciousness feel? How do you define self-consciousness?*

(Required) Teaching Points
Participate Without Planning

- *Self-consciousness is a social phenomenon, meaning that when we are alone we are less likely to feel self-conscious.* For example, Robinson Crusoe most likely rarely experienced self-consciousness until his "man Friday" (that is, his native companion and helper) came along.

- *When we are self-conscious, we are checking our tribal status: Are we in or out of the tribe? Are we safe?* This necessitates stepping outside of what our experience is in the present moment in order to evaluate our actions and the reactions (or imagined reactions) of nearby others.

- *Thus, when we feel self-conscious, we experience a sense of separation from both our tribe and the present moment.* SNS defensive arousal is triggered and PNS-VVC social safety responses are deactivated; see handout 2.1 (The RO DBT Neuroregulatory Model of Emotions). Our body becomes tense, our breathing fast and shallow; our heart rate increases; we feel embarrassed, ashamed, or afraid; we may begin to sweat, and our facial expressions and body gestures feel constrained. We lose our easy manner and are less able to genuinely signal friendly or cooperative intentions.

- *Defining self-consciousness: It arises whenever…*

  - **We become aware** *that others are observing our actions.* For example, an Olympic gymnast may suddenly become self-conscious during their performance if they catch a glimpse of the judge scoring their routine.

  - **We imagine** *that others are critically observing our actions.* For example, a criminal may suddenly feel self-conscious when they spot a CCTV camera pointed directly at them when they are about to steal someone's purse.

  - **We imagine** *that we will be critically evaluated by others in the future.* For example, we catch a glimpse of ourselves in a mirror on the way to an important job interview and notice that we spilled red wine on our white shirt the night before.

- *The very presence of self-consciousness is proof of our caring about tribal status* (that is, if we didn't care, we wouldn't feel self-conscious). Yowzers! ☺ For those of us who pride ourselves on not caring about social status, this can feel a little mind-blowing. Encourage self-enquiry, using the following questions.

  - ➤ *To what extent do you find yourself resisting this definition of self-conscious behavior?*

  - ➤ *Do you like or dislike the words "social status"? What might this tell you about yourself? How do you socially signal your self-consciousness?*

  - ➤ *To what extent do you try to hide self-consciousness from others? What is it that you might need to learn?*

★ **Fun Facts:** *The Attraction of Nonparticipation*

Choosing not to participate in a shared tribal experience—that is, a community or group activity, event, or custom—is frequently (but not always) motivated by a desire to avoid self-conscious emotions (for example, shame, embarrassment, humiliation) and/or to escape real or imagined public scrutiny, disapproval, and/or social exclusion [see "(Not So) Fun (but Interesting) Facts: The Use of Shaming Rituals," in lesson 8]. Declining an offer to join in with a tribal activity or community experience is attractive because it promises relief from critical scrutiny yet paradoxically is noteworthy. All tribes expect members to participate in tribal activities (to some extent) and contribute to the common good if they are to remain in the tribe (think sports teams, clubs, work groups, families, marital partners, and so on). Thus, rather than avoiding public scrutiny, nonparticipation can make us stand out in a crowd! For example, refusing to dance or sing at a party may feel like independence or the right thing to do, but it can feel isolating when we realize we are the only one not participating.

✓ **Ask:** *To what extent do you think you refuse to participate in a group activity or community event because you desire to avoid public scrutiny and/or self-conscious emotions? What is it you might need to learn?*

• ***The good news is that to feel less self-conscious, all you have to do is join with your tribe!*** When we feel part of a tribe, we feel safe and secure. Self-consciousness naturally diminishes because our status in our tribe is secure. We can let go of hypervigilant scanning for potential signs of social disapproval. *We can relax, 'cause we got tribe! Oh yeah!* ☺ See handout 8.1 (Tribe Matters: Understanding Rejection and Self-Conscious Emotions).

✓ **Ask:** *What are the types of tribes you would like to be part of? What tribes do you currently belong to (for example, sports clubs, work teams, family units, and so on)?*

✓ **Ask:** *To what extent do you choose to sit on the sidelines versus passionately participate in the tribes you belong to? How do you feel about this? What might you need to learn?*

✓ **Ask:** *Is our skills class a type of tribe? Would you like it to be?*

★ **Fun Facts:** *Tribes Are Built Around Shared Values and Goals*

From an RO DBT perspective, a tribe can consist of just two people. Tribal bonds begin when two people (or the members of a group) commit to make self-sacrifices to benefit the well-being of other tribal members or the tribe itself, without always expecting anything in return. [See lesson 8, "Tribe Matters: Understanding Rejection and Self-Conscious Emotions," for more details.] Tribes are usually founded upon shared values and goals, although some tribes we are born into (for example, our family, our nation), and others may be forced upon us (for example, an inmate in a prison). However, most of the time, we choose our tribes. The motto of a healthy tribe may be best represented by the motto of the lead characters in the 1844 book The Three Musketeers, by Alexandre Dumas: "All for one, one for all!" Interestingly, according to this definition, our RO DBT skills class is a type of tribe; we share a common goal of learning new skills, and we strive to support each other in achieving this. Wow! ☺

- *When we choose to participate with our tribe, we send a powerful social signal to other members.* Translated loosely, the signal says: *I am part of my tribe. I care about my fellow tribal members. I am not just concerned about my own needs. I am willing to make self-sacrifices to contribute to the well-being of my tribe* (see Flexible Mind SAGE, in lesson 8).

- *Participating without planning helps us loosen the evolutionarily hardwired grip of self-conscious checking and concerns about tribal status.* Each time we throw ourselves in, without self-consciousness, we begin to build a powerful store of positive memories associated with socializing and joining with others.

- *It is not something that can be grasped solely via intellectual means. Participating without planning is experiential.* It's something you do, not something you think about.

- *Participating without planning is the opposite of trying, performing, or pretending. It is freeing.*

Instructor Guidelines for "Participate Without Planning" Practices

"Participate without planning" practices share three core features.

FIRST, a "participate without planning" practice is something you do, not something you talk about doing.

- **The practice is unannounced. "Participate without planning" practices with OC clients should NOT begin with an orientation or forewarning of the upcoming practice** (if possible). Any form of prewarning, orientation, or forewarning prior to a "participate without planning" practice (at least for most OC clients) frequently triggers intense anxiety, shutdown responses, and/or frantic attempts to plan ahead and mentally rehearse how they will behave. Plus, in the meantime, no one is really listening to what you are saying anymore, and since they are OC clients, you may never know about it (at least directly). Lack of forewarning, combined with an unexpected command by an instructor to mimic, or "do what I do," almost always elicits automatic compliance because it doesn't allow any time to consider doing anything else. Plus, the brief nature of the practice makes it less likely for self-consciousness to arise and more likely for individual members to experience a sense of positive connection or cohesion with the class as a whole. Frequent and unpredictable "participate without planning" practices create a store of positive memories associated with joining in with others. With repeated practice, these associations begin to generalize to social situations outside of the classroom. Attendance at social events is no longer motivated solely by obligation. Instead, often for the first time in their life, clients begin to experience anticipatory reward or pleasure prior to social interactions, making it more likely for them to willingly desire to approach and engage with others.

- **The practice involves mimicking the instructor's movements. The easiest way to accomplish this is for the instructor to simply instruct the class to mimic whatever they do and then begin the practice without further explanation.** For example, if the practice is to make funny facial expressions, the instructor would begin by making a silly face while saying, "Okay, everyone, do what I do! Make a funny face, like this! And this!" Change expression. "Now try this one!" Mimicking the instructors' movements or sounds makes self-consciousness less likely. The reason is that it reduces the necessity of planning or thinking about how to behave in advance. Instead, all one needs to do is follow the leader. This usually translates into instructors both showing and telling participants what to do moment by moment during the practice (like the instructor for an aerobic workout). This keeps the attention focused on the instructor, not on what other classmates might be doing, thereby maximizing the likelihood for genuine non-self-conscious pleasure to be linked with participating with the tribe. This means avoiding practices that are competitive and/or require a certain type of attentional focus, dexterity, speed of processing, or memory to perform well. For example, in general, avoid the temptation to simply pick some music and encourage free-range dancing. Although most OC clients will comply, they are likely to feel highly self-conscious doing so, making the point of the practice moot. Recall the goal of "participate without planning" exercises is to slowly build a bank of positive experiences linked to participating with others.

SECOND, "participate without planning" practices should be brief.

- **Practices should be very short—ideally, no longer than thirty seconds to one minute.** Long-lasting participation practices (for example, lasting more then one or two minutes), or practices that require very slow and deliberate body movements or sitting still without moving, can quickly become a contest (Who's the stillest of them all?) or trigger painful emotions and/or shutdown responses. Long practices are analogous to someone telling you to smile before they take your photograph and then fumbling about with their camera, leaving you with a frozen expression that quickly feels phony (which is why we ask the fumbling friend to hurry up and take the picture).

- **Long practices can also inadvertently smuggle the idea that the practice is trying to fix or correct a problem.** Recall that OC clients already take life very seriously.

- **End the practice with applause all around** and then tell everyone to sit down (if they are standing). Celebrating "participate without planning" exercises is essential when working with OC clients. OC individuals are overly serious. They don't know how join in with others and often feel awkward in groups. Applause signals social approval and liking. Thus, whenever a group practice has been completed, rather than behaving somberly, instructors should congratulate everyone for joining in (including themselves) by giving each other a round of applause (ideally, instructors should look in the eyes of each class member as they clap, smiling warmly with eyebrows raised). Importantly, instructors should NOT set a class precedent by applauding *individual* class member participation (for example, applauding a reluctant client who finally joins in). Providing applause to one (rather than the entire group) results in expectations (unspoken) that every individual accomplishment should be recognized (that is, applauded). This can trigger unhelpful social comparisons and resentment (that is unlikely to be spoken aloud) if the applause is ever forgotten.

THIRD, talking about the practice, if done at all, occurs only after the practice is over.

- **Importantly, minipractices are usually best not to discuss whatsoever after they are done.** They do not have to be discussed afterward when conducted spontaneously (that is, the practice was not the formally scheduled mindfulness practice for that day's class; see "Structuring RO Skills Training Classes," in chapter 1).

- **However, if you do want to discuss it, do it after the practice. Ask for observations about the practice, provide the rationale for the mindfulness practice** (for example, making funny faces helps break down inhibitory barriers), **and teach important concepts** (for example, help clients recognize that they were able to participate even though they might have not believed it possible if they had been forewarned).

- **Link the practice to everyday life, and solicit examples of how class members can bring a "participate without planning" practice more into their life.**

- **Instructors should get into the habit of introducing brief (thirty seconds) mini–"participate without planning" practices whenever tension is in the room.** For example, during a homework review, or while teaching new material, if the class suddenly appears to be subdued, shut down, or less talkative and responsive, the instructors can, without any orientation or preamble, conduct a spontaneous "participate without planning" practice—for example, by saying: *Okay, everybody—let's stand up. Now raise your arms above your head.* The intructors raise their arms. *Now shake your arms all about.*

The instructors shake their arms. *Now wiggle your body.* And so on. The instructors should end the practice as abruptly as they began it by asking everyone to sit down: *Okay, well done. Now let's all sit down!* And then, with a big smile, the instructors sit down, and the lead instructor says: *Well done! Applause all around.* Then, without further discussion, the instructors return to the lesson plan. See the following examples of differing practice ideas.

Examples of "Participate Without Planning" Practices for Overcontrol

Remember, each example is done without forewarning or orientation and should not be long-lasting (that is, about thirty to sixty seconds). The idea is to end the practice slightly before participants begin to feel too self-conscious, thereby making it more likely for them to experience joining in with others as rewarding.

- **Practice "Yippee, I'm a Puppet!"** Say to the class: *Wow, look at me… I'm a puppet! And so are YOU! Move your head to the side, now to the other, raise your arm and dangle it about… flop and flop them all about… make your knee go up and down of its own accord…MY OH MY OH MY OH MY, we're OUT OF CONTROL! And that's okay! Ha ha ho ho ho ha ha tee hee hee…jiggle your body and make your arms go here…make your arms go there…MY OH MY someone's pulling our strings…someone else has control… and that's okay…Ha ha ho ho ho ha ha ha tee hee hee HO HO hee hee HAAA!* Instructors should end by clapping their hands in celebration and encouraging the class to give themselves a round of applause: *Well done! OK, now sit down and let's share our observations about our mindfulness practice.*

- **Practice "Sailing the Seven Seas."** Say to the class: *Okay…EVERYONE STAND UP! GREAT! NOW, DO WHAT I DO!* Instructors should keep their feet stationary while leaning their body to one side…and then back the other way. Then say: *WOW, WE'RE SAILORS OF THE SEVEN SEAS! SEE HOW THE BOAT ROCKS AND SWAYS,* while encouraging the class to mimic the rocking and swaying movements of a ship out at sea, rocking slowly back and forth with the waves. Then say: *WHOA… THIS ONE'S REALLY BIG…WHEE…LOOK OUT, IT'S GOING THE OTHER WAY…. and back again…WHOA…WE ARE NOT IN CONTROL! And that's okay! We're not in control, and that's okay…WHEE…Ha ha ho ho ho ha ha ho ho ho…Tee hee…hee hee hee!* Instructors should end by clapping their hands in celebration and encouraging the class to give themselves a round of applause: *Well done! Okay, now sit down and let's share our observations about our mindfulness practice.*

- **Practice the "Chicken Little."** Say to the class: *Okay… EVERYONE STAND UP! GREAT! NOW, DO WHAT I DO!* Instructors start by pointing at the ceiling and shouting for everyone to quickly mimic what they say and do: *Look up! The sky is falling! EEK! YIKES!* Instructors should begin flapping their arms like a chicken while encouraging the entire class to join in. Have everyone flap their arms and run around in a circle while making clucking sounds. Instructors can shout *There's nobody here but us chickens! The sky is falling! THE SKY IS FALLING! Run away…RUN AWAY!* Instructors should end by clapping their hands in celebration and encouraging the class to give themselves a round of applause: *Well done! OK, now sit down and let's share our observations about our mindfulness practice.*

- **Practice "I am NOT pouting!"** (aka "Let's Have a Temper Tantrum"). Say to the class: *Okay… EVERYONE STAND UP! GREAT! Now, do what I do! LET'S START POUTING!* Warm smile with eyebrows raised: *OH NO…not pouting again! I DON'T WANT TO!* Make a sad face and stamp feet: *Why do I have to? It's not fair!* Stamping feet: *You need to be nice to me!* Slight pause: *Okay, now everyone sit down and hide your head! Quickly now!* The instructor sits and places their head on table and covers their face: *Now everyone get up and stamp your feet! Now place the back of your hand over your forehead and moan: OHHHH, WOE IS ME! Again…OHHHHH, WOE IS ME! Again…one more time: I'm SO WRETCHED! WOE IS ME!* Instructors should end by clapping their hands in celebration and encouraging the class to give themselves a round of applause. *Well done! Okay, now sit down and let's share our observations about our mindfulness practice.*

- **Practice the "WE ARE OC AND WE ARE TOUGH" marching song** (this chant or dirge should mimic the style and rhythm of military marching songs employed by soldiers to establish camaraderie and teamwork during basic training exercises). Say to the class: *OKAY...EVERYONE STAND UP! GREAT!* Warm smile, eyebrows raised, and shouting: *OKAY, LET'S MARCH TOGETHER!* Instructor should begin rhythmically marching in place while vigorously swinging their arms: *NOW REPEAT AFTER ME AND DO WHAT I DO! WE ARE OC AND WE ARE PROUD, 'CAUSE WE'RE EFFICIENT YET NEVER LOUD!* Continue marching in place with arms vigorously moving back and forth: *WE ARE OC AND THAT'S OKAY! WE SEE DETAILS IN EVERY WAY!* Keep marching in place and swinging arms in time with the chant: *WE ARE OC AND WE ARE TOUGH, 'CAUSE WE RUN AROUND IN THE BUFF! HURRAH! HURRAH! HURRAH!* Instructors should feel free to make up their own lines for the chant or extend this chant creatively. The exercise should end with applause all around, with instructor saying *Well done! Okay, now sit down and let's share our observations about our mindfulness practice.*

- **Practice "Yelling TOMATO."** Say to the class: *Okay...EVERYONE STAND UP! GREAT! NOW DO WHAT I DO! Let's all yell TOMATO! Reach for the sky! Yell...TOMATO! Now with gusto: TOMATO! Now with an Italian accent! MAMMA MIA, TOMATO! ITSA TOMATO, AH MAMMA MIA!* Instructors then switch and shout *Oh no! I meant to say POTATO! Quick, everyone, hurry... reach to the ground and whisper POTATO! Again...but softer! POTATO! One more time, just to make sure...but really quiet now...POTATO!* Instructors should end by clapping their hands in celebration and encouraging the class to give themselves a round of applause: *Well done! Okay, now sit down and let's share our observations about our mindfulness practice.*

- **Practice "Big Gestures."** Say to the class: *Okay...everyone stand up! Now do what I do!* The instructor should then begin to exaggerate facial expressions and body movements while simultaneously describing whatever they are doing and encouraging the class to mimic their movements. For example: *Okay, let's all raise our eyebrows...let's make them go up and make them go down...now scrunch your eyes together and pucker out your mouth. Now let's stretch our lips and open our mouth as wide as it can go...let's open our eyes too, as wide as we can! Stick out your tongue as far as it can go, raise your eyebrows again and stretch all of your facial muscles as much as you can at the same time! Now close your eyes as hard as you can and scrunch up all of the muscles in your face. Tense them, tense them as hard as you can...now release the tension...slowly, slowly, and slower still. Okay, now...rotate your head from side to side, up and down, stretching and tensing each muscle. Use your hands to massage the muscles in your face. Stretch your arms up to the ceiling and open your hands to the sky!* Instructors should end by clapping their hands in celebration and encouraging the class to give themselves a round of applause: *Well done! Okay, now sit down and let's share our observations about our mindfulness practice.*

- **Practice "Speaking Nonsense."** Say to the class: *OKAY...EVERYONE STAND UP! NOW DO WHAT I DO! Say BLAH. Now say it again: BLAH. Say BLOO-BLIP AND BLIPPTY-BLOOP! OK, now say BLIPPITY-BE-BA-BLIPTY BLOO!* Pause with warm smile, eye contact all around, and eyebrows raised: *Getting better. LET'S GO LOUDER! Say OHRAW! Say OHRAWWW! Say it again: OOOHHHRAWWWW! Okay, all together now...let's start speaking GOBBLEDYGOOK! IT'S A NEW LANGUAGE! Haven't you heard? BOO...BOO...BLICKETY-BLOCK AND FLOPPITY-FLOW WITH DON-DON-ROW! FLIPPTY-HEY-HO AND MIGHTY SO-SO! FORMITY-BEE AND FRANKLY-SEE WHILE COMPILY-FRAW AND MOCKINGLY-MAW!* Instructors should end by clapping their hands in celebration and encouraging the class to give themselves a round of applause: *Well done! Okay, now sit down and let's share our observations about our mindfulness practice.*

- **Practice "Going Tribal."** Instructors should bring differing musical instruments (which don't require any experience to use) into class and ask participants to pick one. The instructor begins the practice by saying *Okay…everyone stand up! Take up your instrument and repeat after me.* The instructor should start rhythmically beating the drum or bell they have chosen, with a smile and eyebrows raised, to encourage class members to join in similarly. Instructors should encourage participants to throw themselves into the practice by beating their drum or ringing their bell with abandon. Instructors should end by clapping their hands in celebration and encouraging the class to give themselves a round of applause: *Well done! Okay, now sit down and let's share our observations about our mindfulness practice.*

- **Practice "Silly Walking and Talking."** Say to the class: *Okay…EVERYONE STAND UP! Now do what I do!* The instructor should then begin to walk and talk in a silly manner, smiling and making eye contact to all and changing repeatedly. For example, practice goose-stepping (raising straightened legs high with each step) or duckwalking (squat low and with each step make a squawking sound) or the "Chicken Little" (walk in a circle while flapping one's arms and clucking) or the "doo-rab" (slinking along while sneering, sometimes accompanied by clicking one's fingers). Instructors should feel free to make up their own silly walks and encourage participants to do the same. Instructors should end by clapping their hands in celebration and encouraging the class to give themselves a round of applause: *Well done! Okay, now sit down and let's share our observations about our mindfulness practice.*

- **Practice "I'm NOT Arrogant, I'm Just Better Than You!"** Say to the class: *Okay…EVERYONE STAND UP! NOW DO WHAT I DO! Put your chin up in the air, shoulders back and hold your head high! Put a swagger in your gait!* Instructors should start swaggering about: *Now shout OUT OF MY WAY! DON'T YOU KNOW WHO I AM? I AM A VERY IMPORTANT PERSON! JUST WHO DO YOU THINK YOU ARE? HRRMMPH!* Keep marching about and *hrrmmph*ing for another ten to fifteen seconds. Instructors should end by clapping their hands in celebration and encouraging the class to give themselves a round of applause: *Well done! Okay, now sit down and let's share our observations about our mindfulness practice.*

- **Practice "Loving Public Humiliation."** Have the entire class stand up, raise their arms above their head, and yell in unison: *PUBLIC HUMILIATION, I LOVE YOU! Again: PUBLIC HUMILIATION, I LOVE YOU! Raise your arms higher…louder now! PUBLIC HUMILIATION, I LOVE YOU! Again: PUBLIC HUMILIATION, I LOVE YOU! Again, only this time with a smile! PUBLIC HUMILIATION, I LOVE YOU! One more time, but this time let's see if we can rock the building! Raise those arms high! PUBLIC HUMILIATION, I LOVE YOU!* Instructors should end by clapping their hands in celebration and encouraging the class to give themselves a round of applause: *Well done! Okay, now sit down and let's share our observations about our mindfulness practice.*

(Required) Class Exercise
Mini–"Participate Without Planning" Practice

End the class with an impromptu mini–"participate without planning" practice. Pick one of the examples provided earlier (for example "Yippee, I'm a Puppet!" or "Silly Walking and Talking" or "I'm NOT Arrogant—I'm Just Better Than You!"), and without any forewarning, conduct a short (thirty to sixty seconds) practice. End the practice with applause for all and then, without further discussion, assign lesson 12 homework.

Lesson 12 Homework

1. **(Required) Participants should be instructed to pick one practice example from the "observe openly," "describe with integrity," and "participate without planning" mindfulness handouts and worksheets. Thus, they should use...**

   - Worksheet 12.A ("Observe Openly" Skills), or

   - Handout 12.1 ("Describe with Integrity" Skills: The Awareness Continuum), or

   - Worksheet 12.B (Making Participating Without Planning a Daily Habit).

2. **(Required) Worksheet 12.C (The Three "What" Skills: Daily Practice Log for the "Observe Openly," "Describe with Integrity," and "Participate Without Planning" Skills).** Participants should use this worksheet to record how things went.

3. **(Optional)** Instruct participants to practice speaking the Awareness Continuum aloud, either alone or with someone else. Encourage them to use the Awareness Continuum during a conflict with someone, and to observe how this impacts the interaction. This more advanced practice is a useful supplementary practice for those who have already participated at least once in RO DBT mindfulness training.

Radical Openness Handout 12.1

"Describe with Integrity" Skills: The Awareness Continuum

- The *Awareness Continuum* is a mindfulness "describe with integrity" practice in RO DBT.

- An Awareness Continuum practice can be done…

  - Alone, with each step spoken silently

  - Alone, and spoken aloud

  - With another person, and spoken aloud

  - With a small group, taking turns, and spoken aloud

- **It is useful because it helps us take responsibility for our perceptions about ourselves, others, and the world,** rather than blaming our experience on other people or the world.

- **It teaches us to notice and label differing forms of inner experience** (thoughts, sensations, emotions, and images).

- **It provides an opportunity for us to practice describing our perceptions, without needing to explain, justify, or defend ourselves.** This frees up energy to notice other things in our life and helps us create a nondefensive sense of self.

- **It provides a structured means to practice revealing our inner experience to another person in a manner that is both self-effacing and self-respecting.**

  - It is *self-effacing* because an Awareness Continuum practice signals to the other person that our perceptions are potentially fallible; they are not absolute truths.

  - It is *self-respecting* because an Awareness Continuum practice signals to others that we are taking responsibility for our own perceptions rather than blaming them on others or the world. It helps us remember that we choose our reality; no one can force us to perceive, think, or feel in a particular way.

Four Steps for an Awareness Continuum Practice

Step 1. Begin by saying the word "I."

- This signals to yourself and others that you are the source of the observation.

Step 2. Clarify that you are mindfully observing by adding the words "am aware of."

Step 3. Label what is being observed by classifying it as one of four different forms: sensation, emotion, image, or thought.

- **Sensations** include any experience involving the five senses (sound, taste, touch, hearing, or sight).

- **Emotions** include emotional experiences, mood states (for example, fear or anxiety), urges, impulses, and/or desires (for example, a feeling of desire to walk out of a room).

- **Images** generally fall into observations about the past (for example, a memory), the future (for example, what might happen), or mind reading of others (for example, imagining what another is thinking or feeling).

- **Thoughts** are cognitive experiences of the current moment (for example, thinking about learning the Awareness Continuum, thinking about a math problem).

Step 4. Describe the content of your experience, without explanation, rationalization, or justification.

- **Avoid clumping,** or combining two or more forms into one statement. For example…

  - **Nonclumping:** "I am aware of an emotion of sadness" consists of one form—an emotion.

  - **Clumping:** "I am aware of an emotion of sadness because I just thought about my lost dog that ran away three weeks ago" is an explanation about the initial experience of sadness that clumps several forms together (the emotion of sadness is clumped with thoughts and memories about a lost dog).

- **"Editing" is okay.** Feel free to choose what you label or reveal. The choice to keep certain parts of our life private is an important part of independent living.

- **Use the Awareness Continuum during an argument or conflict.** Instead of saying "You make me angry," use the Awareness Continuum to take responsibility for your perceptions by saying, "I am aware of a feeling of anger" or "I am aware of imagining that you are purposefully trying to make me angry."

Radical Openness Handout 12.2

Main Points for Lesson 12: Mindfulness Training, Part 2

The "What" Skills

1. In RO DBT, there are three mindfulness "what" skills, each of which represents a differing aspect or way to practice mindfulness. They are *observe openly, describe with integrity,* and *participate without planning.*

2. "Urge-surfing" mindfulness practices facilitate learning how to not respond to every urge, impulse, and desire, such as urges to fix, control, reject, or avoid.

3. The Awareness Continuum is the core RO "describe with integrity" practice and can also be used as an "outing oneself" practice. It helps the practitioner take responsibility for their inner experiences, block habitual desires to explain or justify oneself, and learn how to differentiate between thoughts, emotions, sensations, and images. It is a core means for learning how to step off the path of blame (habitual blaming of self or others).

4. Learning the "participate without planning" skill means learning how to passionately participate in one's life and in one's community and let go of compulsive planning, rehearsal, and/or obsessive needs to get it right.

Radical Openness Worksheet 12.A

"Observe Openly" Skills

Aware and Focused on the Present Moment

THE PAST IS GONE... You are here now ...THE FUTURE IS YET TO BE

Look for opportunities to practice mindful observing.

Place a checkmark in the box next to the statement that best describes your experience.

- ☐ Remembered that our lives are lived *now*—all we have is the present moment.

- ☐ Practiced being aware of each and every moment, without trying to change or label it.

Examples of "Observe Openly" Practices

Place a checkmark in the boxes next to the statements that best describe your experience.

- ☐ **Practiced mindful awareness, using one or more of my five senses.** Smell (light an aromatic candle), touch (stroke a rough surface), sight (gaze at the horizon), hearing (listen to sounds around you), taste (notice different flavors).

- ☐ **Practiced sitting quietly for five minutes each day and observing my breath.** *Turn your attention to the sensations of your breathing, not trying to do anything with it or change it in any way, just being fully present, as best you can, with the full duration of your inbreath and the full duration of your outbreath. When you notice your mind wandering, gently guide your attention back to your breath, again and again. Use this practice to help remember that you can choose where you focus your attention.*

- ☐ **Went to an art museum. Practiced observing various paintings close up and then far away.** Notice how each viewpoint impacts what you see.

- ☐ **Practiced observing times when I was naturally more open-minded.** Record what you notice in your RO self-enquiry journal.

- ☐ **Mindfully observed how my tone of voice impacted those around me.** Record what you notice in your RO self-enquiry journal.

- ☐ Mindfully observed what happened when I raised my eyebrows and smiled during interactions.

- ☐ Mindfully observed who talked more when interacting with someone. Observe what happens when you go opposite to what you were doing (that is, talk more or listen more).

- ☐ Observed how other people responded when they realized I was allowing myself some time for relaxation.

- ☐ Mindfully observed how closed-mouth smiling combined with eyebrow wags influenced the person I was interacting with.

- ☐ Observed my bodily sensations (for example, suddenly feeling hot or sweaty) and then used self-enquiry to deepen my practice.

- ☐ Practiced urge-surfing by mindfully observing urges, impulses, and desires, without getting caught up in the thoughts or giving in to the urges. Notice how the urge rises and falls and eventually passes with time.

  - ☐ Urges to control or correct: Observe what happens when you don't immediately attempt to fix or control a situation.

  - ☐ Urges to walk away during a conflict: Notice the urge to abandon or walk away during a disagreement. Practice remaining engaged instead.

  - ☐ Urges to tidy or clean.

  - ☐ Urges to correct, improve, or tell another person what to do or how to do it.

  - ☐ Urges to change the topic when you don't like what is being discussed.

  - ☐ Urges to redo someone's work (for example, restack a dishwasher because it wasn't done according to your standards, or rewrite the minutes from a meeting).

  - ☐ Urges to check (for example, whether a door is locked, a light is switched off, hands are clean).

  - ☐ Urges to gossip about a rival.

  - ☐ Urges to restrict food intake, retch, or expel food after eating.

Record other skills practiced.

_____

_____

_____

_____

Radical Openness Worksheet 12.B

Making Participating Without Planning a Daily Habit

- **When we feel self-conscious, we experience a sense of separation from both our tribe and the present moment.** We lose our easy manner and are less able to genuinely signal friendly or cooperative intentions.

- **Participating without planning sends a powerful cooperative social signal that helps facilitate genuine social engagement** and helps us to regain our sense of belonging and connection to our tribe.

- **Participating without planning is not something that can be grasped solely via intellectual means; it is experiential,** and for most adults it requires direct and repeated practice.

- **Practice participating without planning daily** and use worksheet 12.C (The Three "What" Skills: Daily Practice Log for the "Observe Openly," "Describe with Integrity," and "Participate Without Planning" Skills) to record your observations.

- **Record other observations.**

_____

_____

_____

_____

Radical Openness Worksheet 12.C

The Three "What" Skills: Daily Practice Log for the "Observe Openly," "Describe with Integrity," and "Participate Without Planning" Skills

- **Practice one "observe openly" skill every other day,** and record your observations in the space provided.

- **Practice the Awareness Continuum on the other days.** Record in the space provided how difficult it was to not explain, justify, or rationalize what you labeled. (That is, how much did you clump?) What functions did you tend to use the most (for example, thoughts, sensations, images, or emotions)?

- **To minimize planning,** practice "participate without planning" skills on any day you wish (tee hee ☺).

- **Record in the following daily practice log** what you practiced each day, and your observations (even if it was "The Art of Practicing Without Practicing"—tee hee ☺).

Day	Observation
Sunday	
Monday	
Tuesday	
Wednesday	
Thursday	
Friday	
Saturday	

Mindfulness Training, Part 3

The Core Mindfulness "How" Skill: With Self-Enquiry

> NOTE TO INSTRUCTORS: Lesson 13 focuses on teaching the core mindfulness "how" skill, *with self-enquiry*. The other three "how" skills—*with awareness of harsh judgments, with one-mindful awareness,* and *effectively and with humility*—will be taught in lesson 14.

Main Points for Lesson 13

1. In RO DBT, there are four mindfulness "how" skills that represent the kind of attitude or state of mind to bring to a practice of mindfulness. They are *with self-enquiry, with awareness of harsh judgments, with one-mindful awareness,* and *effectively and with humility.* Lesson 13 focuses on the first of these four skills, *with self-enquiry.*

2. *With self-enquiry* is the core RO DBT mindfulness "how" skill. It is the key to radically open living. It means actively seeking the things one wants to avoid or may find uncomfortable in order to learn, and cultivating a willingness to be wrong, with an intention to change, if needed.

3. Self-enquiry involves both willingness for self-examination and willingness to reveal to others what self-examination has uncovered. This process is known as *outing oneself* in RO DBT.

Materials Needed

- Handout 13.1 (The Core Mindfulness "How" Skill: With Self-Enquiry)

- Handout 13.2 (Cultivating Healthy Self-Doubt)

- Handout 13.3 (Practicing Self-Enquiry and Outing Oneself)

- (Optional) Handout 13.4 (Main Points for Lesson 13: Mindfulness Training, Part 3: The Core Mindfulness "How" Skill: With Self-Enquiry)

- Handout 1.3 (Learning from Self-Enquiry)

- Worksheet 13.A (Practicing the Core Mindfulness "How" Skill: With Self-Enquiry)

- Whiteboard or flipchart with marker

(Required) Teaching Point

Introducing the "With Self-Enquiry" Skill

NOTE TO INSTRUCTORS: Instructors should practice what they preach by using self-enquiry whenever an OC client struggles, criticizes, or demonstrates an atypical response. Instead of automatically assuming the problem lies solely within the client, ask instead *Who am I to assume that there is only one way to learn this skill? Is it possible that this skill makes no sense for a person with an OC style of coping? What is that I might learn from this experience?*

- *Last lesson, we learned three mindfulness "what" skills.* "What" skills are what one does when practicing mindfulness—that is, *observe openly, describe with integrity,* or *participate without planning.*

- *Today we focus on one of the four RO "how" skills, with self-enquiry.*

- *"How" skills refer to the stance or attitude a person takes when practicing the differing "what" skills.* The four "how" skills in RO DBT are *with self-enquiry, with awareness of harsh judgments, with one-mindful awareness,* and *effectively and with humility.*

- *Self-enquiry is the core RO mindfulness "how" skill.*

(Required) Teaching Point
What Is Self-Enquiry?

Refer participants to handout 13.1 (The Core Mindfulness "How" Skill: With Self-Enquiry).

What Is Self-Enquiry?

- *In RO DBT, self-enquiry represents the core stance or attitude a person takes when practicing the mindfulness "what" skills* (that is, *observe openly, describe with integrity,* and *participate without planning*).

- *Self-enquiry involves a willingness to challenge our core beliefs,* things we might normally consider facts or truths. It means courageously facing what we don't want to admit or change about ourselves, in order to grow.

- *Self-enquiry means taking responsibility for our personal perceptions, beliefs, and/or choices we have made in our life,* rather than automatically blaming others or the world.

- *Self-enquiry celebrates the pursuit of truth, not the attainment of truth.* Self-enquiry recognizes that each new insight or understanding we achieve is always fallible, limited, and potentially biased.

- *Self-enquiry actively turns toward the very experiences we want to avoid, discount, and/or are challenged by, in order to learn.*

- *Self-enquiry facilitates the creation of new meanings, new insights, and novel behaviors.* Consequently, it represents a core means for personal self-growth.

What Self-Enquiry Is Not

- *The goal of self-enquiry is to find a good question, NOT a good answer.*

- *Self-enquiry is NOT ruminating about a problem* because it is not looking to *solve the problem or avoid discomfort.*

- *Self-enquiry is NOT regulation, distraction, denial, rationalization, opposite action, soothing, cheerleading, problem solving, or acceptance.*

- *Self-enquiry does NOT mean that truth does not exist, or that we should never trust our intuitions.* For example, when in a room with a hungry tiger, believing in what is true (that is, I see a tiger) is more effective than believing in what is false (that is, I see a bunny), especially if one does not want to be dinner.

- *Self-enquiry does NOT mean getting down on oneself,* yet it can be painful, at least temporarily, because it often requires surrendering long-held convictions or cherished beliefs.

- *Self-enquiry is NOT expecting the world to change or blaming others.* For example, instead of saying *You need to validate me because what you said hurt me,* self-enquiry asks *Is it possible that my hurt feelings represent an opportunity for me to learn something important about myself? What is it that I don't want to hear from this other person? What is it that I need to learn?*

NOTE TO INSTRUCTORS: Harsh self-blame often functions to regulate a person (that is, move them away from their edge) because it provides an answer for the self-enquiry dilemma (that is, "It's entirely my fault" or "This just proves I am worthless"). Harsh self-blame is a strong social signal (see the required teaching point "'Don't Hurt Me' Responses," in lesson 16) that can function to block feedback from others, allow people to avoid taking responsibility for change, or block further self-enquiry. Instructors must be alert for this when it occurs and help clients discover the function of the behavior (see also Fatalistic Mind, in lesson 11).

NOTE TO INSTRUCTORS: Rumination about self-enquiry represents an attempt to find a solution to a problem and/or unexpected information that allows us to stay the same because it justifies our way of thinking. Instructors should encourage clients caught in this to practice self-enquiry about their practice of self-enquiry. Examples of possible self-enquiry questions include *Why do I feel it is so important to engage in long self-enquiry practices? What am I trying to socially signal to other people by behaving this way? Is it possible that I am trying to control the outcome of my self-enquiry practice? What might this mean? Could this represent another way to keep myself stuck or prove to myself (or others) that change is not possible? Is there something I need to learn?* Long practices can also be motivated by a sense of social obligation (that is, the client may think this is what the therapist expects), desires for self-verification (for example, finding flaws proves I am a bad person), or competition (for example, desires to be the best at self-enquiry). Thus, rather than immediately assuming that obsessive thinking or rumination about a self-enquiry practice is the problem, therapists should encourage OC clients to view this as an opportunity for further self-growth and encourage the client to further explore what this new dilemma may be telling them (with a warm smile and eyebrows raised).

(Required) Teaching Point

How Does Self-Enquiry Facilitate Mindful Living?

- *Self-enquiry alerts us to areas of our life that may need to change and helps us be more open and receptive to an ever-changing environment.* It helps us learn because it doesn't assume we already know the answer.

- *Practicing self-enquiry is particularly useful whenever we find ourselves strongly rejecting, defending against, or agreeing with feedback that we find challenging or unexpected.*

- *Self-enquiry celebrates problems as opportunities for growth rather than obstacles preventing us from living fully.* The core premise underlying self-enquiry stems from two observations: (1) we do not know everything; therefore, we will make mistakes, and (2) in order to learn from our mistakes, we must attend to our error.

- *Self-enquiry can enhance relationships because it models humility and willingness to learn from what the world has to offer when we share our self-enquiry practices with others* (see the required practice "Outing Oneself," later in this chapter).

  ✓ **Ask:** *How many of you like to spend time with people who communicate that they know it all or are closed-minded? What might this tell us about the utility of self-enquiry?*

  ✓ **Ask:** *If you have been using self-enquiry already, what self-enquiry question have you found most helpful for your personal growth?*

(Required) Teaching Point

Deepening Our Understanding of Self-Enquiry

- *Self-enquiry is the key to radically open living.* It means actively seeking the things one wants to avoid or may find uncomfortable in order to learn, and cultivating a willingness to be wrong, with an intention to change, if needed.

- *Self-enquiry challenges our perceptions of reality. It says, "We don't see things as they are, we see things as we are."*

- *It involves a willingness to question ourselves when we feel threatened or challenged* rather than automatically defending ourselves.

- *Self-enquiry means finding a good question in order to elicit one's edge* and then allowing an answer (if there is one) to be self-discovered by the practitioner. This is why self-enquiry practices should be expected to last over days or weeks.

- *It begins by asking* **What is it that I might need to learn [from this painful experience]?** This simple question can help us develop a healthy habit of recognizing that our tension and/or negative reaction to something may have more to say about ourselves than it does another person or the world. It helps break down automatic avoidance, denial, or regulation. It helps us be more open to the world, in order to learn.

- *The best self-enquiry question brings us face to face with our edge—our personal unknown, our shameful secret, our arrogance.* When we locate our edge, we are likely to uncover our dark side, that is, something we prefer not to admit about ourselves or may work hard to keep secret or deny. That said, our edge doesn't always have to be so heavy; sometimes it is the little things in life that matter, and/or it may not be something we are so ashamed of; it is simply something we were unaware of. Recall: we don't know what we don't know.

NOTE TO INSTRUCTORS: Recall that RO DBT considers defensive arousal helpful because it can alert us to areas in our lives where we may need to change or grow. Rather than automatically assuming that the world needs to change (for example, "You need to validate me because I felt misunderstood by what you said") or automatically prioritizing regulation or acceptance strategies, RO DBT posits that we often learn the most from those areas of our life that we find most challenging. Thus, RO DBT considers an unwanted emotion, thought, or sensation in the body a reminder to practice self-enquiry by redirecting one's attention toward the challenging or threatening experience by asking *Is there something to learn here?* Self-enquiry might eventually lead a person to the conclusion that there is nothing for them to learn, or that being closed is what is needed at this time and place. However, radical openness means retaining a willingness to revisit the issue and practice self-enquiry again—for example, when circumstances change, or tension in the body keeps reemerging.

- **Self-enquiry is able to question self-enquiry.** It recognizes that every query (or answer) emerging from a practice of self-enquiry, regardless of how seemingly profound, wise, or discerning it may appear, is subject to error.

- **Self-enquiry means having the courage to admit our faults to others** and/or how we may have contributed to a problem, without getting down on ourselves.

- **Self-enquiry seeks self-discovery and yet is suspicious of quick answers.** Quick answers to self-enquiry questions often reflect old learning and/or desires to avoid distress by coming up with an explanation or solution.

- **Self-enquiry acknowledges that, on some level, we are responsible for our perceptions and actions, in a manner that avoids harsh blame of self, others, or the world.**

- **Self-enquiry means purposefully cultivating a sense of healthy self-doubt, without falling apart, harsh self-blame, or simply giving in.**

NOTE TO INSTRUCTORS: From an RO DBT perspective, facts or truth can often be misleading, partly because we don't know what we don't know, things are constantly changing, and there is a great deal of experience occurring outside of our conscious awareness. For OC individuals, encouraging the *pursuit of truth* is important because when in Fixed Mind or Fatalistic Mind we are less open to learning from new information and may be mistakenly convinced that we know what the facts are.

(Optional) Teaching Point
Cultivating Healthy Self-Doubt

Refer participants to handout 13.2 (Cultivating Healthy Self-Doubt).

- *One secret of healthy living is the cultivation of healthy self-doubt.*

> NOTE TO INSTRUCTORS: To facilitate class involvement, randomly pick a class member to read aloud one of the points in handout 13.2 (Cultivating Healthy Self-Doubt), briefly discuss what the point may mean, and then move on to the next point by picking a different person to read it aloud. Continue in this manner until all points have been covered. Use the minipractice to deepen the learning.

What Is Healthy Self-Doubt?

- Healthy self-doubt is able to consider that one may be wrong or incorrect, without falling apart or harshly blaming others.

- Healthy self-doubt doesn't take itself too seriously—it has a sense of humor. It can laugh at its own foibles, strange habits, and/or unique quirks with a sense of kindness. It acknowledges that all humans are fallible.

- Healthy self-doubt takes responsibility for one's actions and emotions by not giving up when challenged.

- Healthy self-doubt is relationship-enhancing because it signals a willingness to learn from the world.

- It is neither Fixed nor Fatalistic Mind thinking.

What Is Unhealthy Self-Doubt?

- Unhealthy self-doubt fears self-examination.

- Unhealthy self-doubt may appear on the surface to be willing to question oneself and/or admit a mistake in order to grow.

- Unhealthy self-doubt often implies that the doubter has been wrongly accused and/or unjustly forced to reexamine themselves (for example, by implying that further self-examination would be damaging because it would automatically undermine their newly earned sense of self-confidence and/or would trigger hidden memories of abuse that they are unprepared to deal with, leading to shutdown, collapse, or relapse).

- Unhealthy self-doubt is characterized by a secret desire to not change or be challenged. It is a social signal that often functions to block further feedback (see the required teaching point "'Don't Hurt Me' Responses," in lesson 16).

- Unhealthy self-doubt often involves secret anger or resentment directed toward the persons or events that the doubter believes are responsible for triggering uncertainty or unhelpful self-examination.

- Unhealthy self-doubt powerfully impacts social relationships despite being passively expressed (for example, via sulking, pouting, walking away, giving up, or behaving helplessly).

- If unhealthy self-doubt could speak, it might say, "See? I am admitting that I am a bad person, so you can now stop expecting me to change, because I have already told you I am no good."

- OR it might say, "See what you've made me do? Your questioning has now made me question myself. I'm now miserable. Are you happy?"

- Thus, unhealthy self-doubt represents Fatalistic Mind thinking.

(Optional) Mini–Class Exercise
Fun with Self-Doubt

When conducting this minipractice, instructors should feel free simply to read aloud the following script. Make sure you have extra pens and blank sheets of paper available for participants who may be without.

Instruct (preferably in what you imagine to be a Texas cowpoke accent—tee hee ☺). *Okeydoke, now, ever'body, git a good tight grip on them pens 'n' pencils, an' buckle up yer seat belts real tight, 'cause here comes a big ol' passel o' questions that's gonna ROCK, RUMBLE, 'n' ROLL ya! Ohhh YEAH!* Raise arms high in celebration, then pause in perplexed contemplation.

Continue (now preferably with a posh British accent—tee hee ☺). *Okay, perhaps that was a bit over the top. What I really meant to say is that in a few moments I will be asking you a number of questions. In preparation, please ensure that you have your writing utensils poised and paper available, in order to record any thoughts that may arise. I am confident that you will find it a smashing experience!*

Continue (back to your regular voice—and if that's posh British-speak, that's cool). *Sorry, an overcorrection on my part. Let's start again. What I really, really meant to say is that I am going to read some questions aloud soon, and your job will be to write down the very first thought that pops into your mind on the blank sheet of paper in front of you. We will not be sharing what we write down afterward, so whatever you write is yours and yours alone. You can keep it, throw it away, or use it as part of a self-enquiry practice—the choice is entirely yours. So we can all relax. Are you ready? Here are the questions.*

- *Ask yourself:* **What do I think about self-doubt?** *Record the very first thought that comes into your mind.*

- *Ask yourself:* **Is there a part of me that is afraid that if I question myself, I will fall apart? What do I fear discovering that I don't already know?** *Record the very first thought that comes into your mind.*

- *Ask yourself:* **Is there a part of me thinking this is a waste of time because I already know the answer? How open am I to what's happening right now?** *Record the very first thought that comes into your mind.*

- *Ask yourself:* **To what extent am I genuinely able to laugh at my own foibles or mistakes in a kindhearted way? How often do I show this side of me to others? What is it that I might need to learn?** *Record the very first thought that comes into your mind.*

- *Ask yourself:* **Where did I ever get the idea that questioning myself or self-examination is dangerous?** *Record the very first thought that comes into your mind.*

- *Ask yourself:* **What is it that I might need to learn?** *Record the very first thought that comes into your mind.*

(Optional) Self-Enquiry Practice
"Who Makes These Changes?"

The Rumi poem "Who Makes These Changes" can be used to introduce the concept of self-enquiry or further facilitate it. Outlined here is a script that can be used to incorporate this poem into a brief mindfulness practice. (*Note:* The use of a mindfulness bell is optional.)

> *The practice we are about to do will involve listening to a poem I am about to read, and noticing the images, memories, thoughts, sensations, or emotions that might arise, without getting caught up with them. Simply observing what arises and then turning your mind back to listening, again and again. If your mind wanders, notice that, and, without judgment, turn back again to the words being read aloud. I will be reading the poem three times in a row and will ring the mindfulness bell at the end of each repetition. Now sit in a comfortable yet alert position, and take a breath, with awareness, in order to center yourself into this moment. Notice the rise and fall of your breathing, not trying to change or do anything about it, just being fully present with the full duration of your inbreath and the full duration of your outbreath. [Slight pause.] I will now ring the bell and begin. As best you can, turn your mind now to the words of the poem, noticing what arises and bringing yourself back to the task of listening.*

Who Makes These Changes?

I shoot an arrow right.
It lands left.
I ride after a deer and find myself
chased by a hog.
I plot to get what I want
and end up in prison.
I dig pits to trap others
and fall in.

I should be suspicious
of what I want.

—Mewlana Jalaluddin Rumi, 1230/2004 (translated by Coleman Barks)

After the mindfulness practice, the instructor can ask participants to share observations and use them as a basis to teach from or for further discussion of the key points described earlier. This poem is also extremely useful in prompting discussion about the pros and cons of controlling the world, other people, or ourselves, and the implications these may have for how a person may choose to live.

NOTE TO INSTRUCTORS: The Rumi poem provides additional opportunities for self-enquiry because it can occasionally trigger defensive arousal or resistance from an OC client. For example, some clients have a strong reaction to the last two lines in the poem, "I should be suspicious / of what I want." Rather than soothing or validating a client when this occurs, instructors should encourage them to use this experience as an opportunity to practice self-enquiry—that is, is there something here to learn? Instructors can help a client begin this process by suggesting a few potentially useful self-enquiry questions (delivered with a warm smile and eyebrows raised): *Is it possible that my bodily tension means that I am not fully open to the concept of healthy self-doubt? If yes or possibly, then what am I afraid of? Or do I find myself wanting to automatically explain or defend myself? What might this mean? Or is it possible that I believe further self-examination would be harmful or unnecessary because I have already completed the necessary self-work? If yes or maybe, then what is it that I fear I may lose?*

> NOTE TO INSTRUCTORS: Instructors should encourage participants to silently use self-enquiry whenever possible, including during skills training classes. When instructors invite someone in the class to consider using self-enquiry in the moment, it is important that the invitation is not seen as a demand or coercive (instructors should use nondominant nonverbal signaling combined with cooperative-friendly signals—that is, prolonged shoulder shrug, slight smile, eyebrow wag, and warm eye contact; see Flexible Mind SAGE and Flexible Mind Is DEEP skills for more about nonverbal signaling). Examples of self-enquiry questions that can be smuggled into a lesson plan or modified as needed to fit a given context include *When I am tense, is it possible that the class or the instructors are giving me feedback that I am resisting or trying to avoid? Is it possible that my feelings of defensiveness or resistance signal that I do not want to listen to what is being said, recommended, or instructed? Am I secretly blaming the instructors or someone else for not being supportive or validating? If so, what is it that I need to learn? Am I quickly jumping to self-blame, shutting down, or wanting to give up? What might this tell me about how open I am in this moment? Is it possible I may be operating from Fixed Mind or Fatalistic Mind?*

(Required) Practice

Outing Oneself

Refer participants to handout 13.3 (Practicing Self-Enquiry and Outing Oneself).

- ***Self-enquiry involves both willingness for self-examination and willingness to reveal to others what self-examination uncovered. This process is known as outing oneself in RO DBT.***

- ***Outing oneself means practicing self-enquiry in the presence of another person,*** by disclosing the outcomes of a self-enquiry practice to someone or by using mindfulness "describe with integrity" practices that involve self-disclosure (for example, the Awareness Continuum; see lesson 12).

- ***Outing oneself is important because we need other people to reflect back our blind spots.*** This is because we carry perceptual and regulatory biases with us no matter where we go or what we do, including our practice of mindfulness.

- ***Outing oneself helps us take responsibility for our perceptions and actions.*** It blocks habitual avoidance and denial. For OC clients, this can be an important process in self-discovery. Many OC clients avoid revealing personal feelings or opinions because it means they could be criticized and/or that they may then be expected to change (see "The Enigma Predicament," in chapter 10 of the RO DBT textbook).

- ***Outing oneself goes opposite to unwarranted shame or embarrassment that may arise when self-enquiry reveals parts of our personality we are not proud of or might wish to deny.*** Shame is unwarranted because acknowledging fallibility, after resisting doing so or being afraid of others' reactions, is a courageous and noble pursuit. It is the opposite of complacency, passivity, or resignation, and it brings people closer together (see lesson 8). By outing yourself, you are telling your brain that there is nothing to be ashamed of, whereas hiding signals is telling your brain that you must be doing something wrong.

- ***Outing oneself enhances relationships because it models humility and willingness to learn from what the world has to offer.*** When we reveal vulnerability, we signal to others that we are the same as them (not superior), and that we are open to new learning.

- ***Self-enquiry "outing oneself" practices grant permission to the practitioner to speak candidly.*** The person outing themselves should feel free to say almost anything, regardless of how silly, inarticulate, or judgmental it may seem, in order to locate their edge. Personal growth often involves acknowledgment of parts of us that are not necessarily nice, politically correct, or well mannered. Although elsewhere there are limits to what might be said, RO DBT "outing oneself" practices share similarities with the concept known as *parrhesia*, first defined by the ancient Greeks (such as Plato, Socrates, and Diogenes of Sinope, around 400 BCE) as the practice of speaking the truth for the common good, or speaking boldly and candidly.

NOTE TO INSTRUCTORS: Importantly, "outing oneself" practice DOES NOT mean expressing emotions or judgments without awareness or consideration. On the contrary, just as practitioners are encouraged to speak freely, they are equally encouraged to feel free to edit what is spoken. "Outing oneself" practices are not opportunities to practice self-castigation, or contests of who can reveal the most.

NOTE TO INSTRUCTORS: Self-enquiry requires one to actively look for one's faults, not one's successes. Thus, self-enquiry practice often results in embarrassment or feelings of shame (though not always). Instructors must be prepared to share personal experiences from their own practice of self-enquiry in order to encourage clients to use self-enquiry more deeply. Outing one's personality quirks or weaknesses publicly goes opposite to OC tendencies to mask inner feelings. Therefore, the importance of this when treating OC cannot be overemphasized. Importantly, since expressing vulnerability to another enhances rather than detracts from desires by others to affiliate with the self-disclosing person, the practice of outing oneself can become a powerful means for OC clients to rejoin the tribe.

(Required) Practice
A Step-by-Step Self-Enquiry and "Outing Oneself" Practice

Allow about twenty minutes for teaching, practice, and discussion.

NOTE TO INSTRUCTORS: This exercise DOES NOT involve participants outing themselves in front of the entire class. The exercise is done in pairs and discussed by the entire class afterward. Only the instructors will practice in front of the class when they are demonstrating what the practice will consist of; that is, one instructor practices outing themselves while the other instructor uses the four steps outlined later in this section to facilitate self-enquiry. This demonstration should be brief (as all self-enquiry practices are), yet the instructor modeling self-enquiry should make it real. Instructors should feel free to pick a relatively minor emotional incident to self-enquire about, as this encourages class members to get into the habit of self-examination about both small and big things in life.

Orient: Explain that the primary aim of this brief practice will be to learn how to make self-enquiry and "outing oneself" practices come alive! (☺)

Instruct: Divide the class up into pairs (instructors may need to pair up with reluctant class members or if there is an odd number of participants in the class). Then ask participants to take a moment to silently recall a recent time when they experienced an unwanted private experience and the events surrounding it.

Remind participants that our edge almost always pertains to actions, thoughts, feelings, images, or sensations that are associated with something we want to avoid, are embarrassed about, and/or don't want to think about or admit to. Importantly, self-enquiry practices do not have to be about big issues or big emotions. In fact, sometimes we learn more about ourselves when we enquire into a relatively small event.

Provide examples: For example, getting lost while walking in your home city and feeling embarrassed about needing to ask for directions; feeling irritated by a look given to you by another customer in a restaurant; feeling unappreciated when your boss doesn't acknowledge your hard work during a meeting; having strong urges to restack how a family member stacked the dishwasher; feeling irritated when you discover the gym in a hotel you are staying at is not open; feeling irritated by someone cutting in front of you on the highway. Instructors should be prepared to share one or two examples from their own life.

Encourage participants to practice speaking candidly yet to feel free to edit what is spoken during the practice.

Say: *So you can relax. You only have to say to the other person what you want to say, which is probably what you would do anyway (☺), but at least it's nice to be given permission, eh? So take a deep breath, everyone, and raise those eyebrows, because we are in complete control. How deep or shallow we go is entirely up to us—it's our choice and there is no right or wrong way to practice self-enquiry. So, enjoy yourself…and see what happens when you approach something that you might normally avoid.*

Teach the importance of blocking anti-self-enquiry behaviors that function to move the practitioner away from their edge. Examples include soothing or desires for soothing (for example, "Don't worry, everything will work out"), validating or desires for validation (for example, "I would have found that hard, too"), regulating (for example, "I think you should take a deep breath"), assessing (for example, "You must have learned this somewhere—do you know where?"), cheerleading (for example, "Remember, you are a really caring person"), problem solving or urges to fix (for example, "You need to confront this person about this"), or encouraging acceptance (for example, "You need to accept that you cannot fix this problem").

Practice, using the steps that follow.

1. **The person outing themselves attempts to locate their edge by briefly telling their partner about the emotional event,** without justifying, defending, or rationalizing what happened (about one to two minutes).

2. **The listener listens without problem solving, assessing, soothing, validating, cheerleading, or encouraging acceptance,** and then, after one to two minutes, stops the person outing themselves and asks, "Are you at your edge?" If not, "What do you need to do to get there?" **The listener writes down their response on a blank sheet of paper.** Then, whether they have found their edge or not, the listener asks, "What is it that you might need to learn from this situation?" AND/OR "What question might you need to ask yourself in order to learn?" **The listener records the practitioner's responses on a piece of paper.** These last two questions represent the core queries of self-enquiry; they are useful because they can be just as helpful when a person is struggling to find their edge, resisting self-enquiry, or when they have found their edge.

3. **The listener helps the practitioner stay in contact with their edge** by asking occasionally (about every thirty seconds), "Are you still at your edge, or have you regulated? If you've regulated, then what question do you need to ask to get back there?"

4. **The listener then asks the practitioner to identify the question(s) that most strongly elicited their edge** and writes down what they say.

After about five minutes, end the practice and allow one to two minutes of feedback/discussion within each pair. Encourage participants to consider in their discussions (1) *To what extent did the practitioner attempt to justify, explain, or defend themselves? (2) To what extent did the listener attempt to (or desire to) soothe, validate, reassure, or problem solve during the practice?*

NOTE TO INSTRUCTORS: If someone reports that they didn't think they had enough time, then gently remind them that the goal is not to find a good answer but a good question. This is one of the reasons self-enquiry practices are always brief—to allow practitioners time (days) to practice self-enquiry around the same issue. If they feel unsatisfied, were unable to find their edge, or found themselves resisting self-enquiry, instruct them to record what happened on their worksheet and commit to using handout 1.3 (Learning from Self-Enquiry) to explore what this might mean for them and/or discover how they might learn from this experience rather than giving up, blaming the practice, or blaming themselves.

Then switch roles. The listener becomes the practitioner, and vice versa, repeating the same steps, including the discussion in pairs after the five-minute practice.

Solicit observations from the entire class, and teach accordingly. Encourage the class to commit to a daily three-to-five-minute self-enquiry practice for the next week that uses their experience today to deepen their practice: *Each day, gently reask the self-enquiry question you discovered that brought you closest to your edge, and record what arises each time you ask.* Remind participants to...

- *Remember that self-enquiry means finding a good question that brings you closer to your edge (that is, your unknown), not a good answer.* Allow yourself time to discover what you might need to learn rather than quickly searching for a way to explain things away or regulate.

- *Practice being suspicious of quick answers or urges to regulate, as they may be masquerading as avoidance.* Keep your self-enquiry practices short (for example, five minutes in duration). Short and frequent (for example, daily) practices, using the same question or a new question that has emerged from the previous day, are usually more effective. Longer practices can sometimes be secretly motivated by desires to find an answer or a solution.

- *Get into the habit of frequent practices and recording observations in your self-enquiry journal.* Watch how questions and their practice evolve over time.

NOTE TO INSTRUCTORS: Instructors should block attempts by themselves or class members to summarize, make interpretations, validate, regulate, cheerlead, provide advice, assess, problem solve, soothe, or encourage acceptance after a class self-enquiry practice because it almost inevitably functions as a type of answer or resolution to the self-enquiry dilemma. This is why self-enquiry practices are encouraged to last over days or weeks. This allows an answer (if there is one) to be self-discovered by the practitioner and then later, at some point, ideally shared with the class or individual therapist. **Importantly, a resolution or answer that emerges can be anticipated to become the next area of self-growth.** Instructors can feel free to share copies of what a self-enquiry journal looks like or distribute photocopies of the RO self-enquiry journal entries found in the textbook (Chapter 7).

(Optional) Class Exercises

Examples of Self-Enquiry and "Outing Oneself" Exercises That Can Be Practiced in Class

- **Ask participants to identify a recent time when they experienced envy, resentment, embarrassment, shame, anger, or desires for revenge.** Class members should get into pairs and then take turns practicing self-enquiry about these emotional experiences (see the preceding four-step "outing oneself" protocol). Instructors should allow approximately two to three minutes for each self-enquiry practice period before signaling for partners to switch roles (that is, the listener becomes the practitioner, and vice versa). Instructors can use handout 1.3 (Learning from Self-Enquiry) for examples of potential questions.

- **Ask participants to get into pairs and conduct an Awareness Continuum practice** (see lesson 12) where their focus of awareness is on their partner's shoes. The practice is to observe and describe aloud the emotions, thoughts, sensations, and images that occur while examining their partner's shoes (and then to pass the practice to their partner; see instructions for passing on the Awareness Continuum in lesson 12).

- **At the start of a skills class, ask participants to share one self-enquiry discovery they had in the past week.** Instructors should join in this practice by sharing their personal experiences in self-enquiry as well.

- **Conduct a mindfulness practice in which participants are instructed to ask themselves silently** *What is it that I need to learn?* Following this, instructors should encourage participants to out themselves to a partner or to the class by revealing what they may have discovered (even if it was nothing) and use this as a means to deepen teaching of self-enquiry principles.

Lesson 13 Homework

1. **(Required) Handout 13.1 (The Core Mindfulness "How" Skill: With Self-Enquiry).**

2. **(Required) Worksheet 13.A (Practicing the Core Mindfulness "How" Skill: With Self-Enquiry).**

3. **(Required) Assign self-enquiry journaling.** Instructors should encourage participants to deepen their practice of self-enquiry by committing to a three-to-five-minute self-enquiry practice in the coming week(s) during which they ask the self-enquiry question(s) that emerged from the class practice and then record in their self-enquiry journal any memories, sensations, emotions, and thoughts triggered by the question(s). What they record should include any new self-enquiry questions that emerged during additional practice, and/or descriptions of how they attempted to regulate or to avoid the practice.

Radical Openness Handout 13.1

The Core Mindfulness "How" Skill: With Self-Enquiry

What Is Self-Enquiry?

- **Self-enquiry involves a willingness to challenge our core beliefs**—things we might normally consider facts or truths.

- **Self-enquiry recognizes that…**

    1. *We don't know what we don't know.*

    2. *We don't see things as they are but instead we see things as we are.*

- **Self-enquiry alerts us to areas of our life that may need to change and helps us be more open and receptive to an ever-changing environment.**

- **Practicing self-enquiry is particularly useful whenever we find ourselves strongly rejecting, defending against, or agreeing with feedback that we find challenging or unexpected.** Self-enquiry begins with asking *Is there something to learn here?*

- **Self-enquiry seeks self-discovery and yet is suspicious of quick answers.** Quick answers to self-enquiry questions often reflect old learning and/or desires to avoid distress by coming up with an explanation or solution.

- **Self-enquiry acknowledges that, on some level, we are responsible for our perceptions and actions,** in a manner that avoids harsh blame of self, others, or the world.

- **Self-enquiry involves questioning our habits and a willingness to reveal to others what we discover** so that they can reflect back our blind spots.

- **Self-enquiry is able to question self-enquiry.** It recognizes that every query (or answer) emerging from a practice of self-enquiry, regardless of how seemingly profound, wise, or insightful it may appear, is subject to error.

What Self-Enquiry Is Not

- **Self-enquiry is NOT about finding a good answer; it is about finding a good question** that helps bring us to our edge—our personal unknown—in order to learn.

- **Self-enquiry is NOT ruminating about a problem** because it is not looking to solve it or avoid discomfort.

- **Self-enquiry is NOT regulation, acceptance, distraction, denial, rationalization, or resignation.**

- **Self-enquiry does NOT mean that truth does not exist, or that we should never trust our intuitions.** For example, when in a room with a hungry tiger, believing in what is true (that is, I see a tiger) is more effective than believing in what is false (that is, I see a bunny), especially if you don't want to be dinner!

- **Self-enquiry does NOT mean getting down on oneself,** yet it can be painful, at least temporarily, because it often requires surrendering long-held convictions or cherished beliefs.

Radical Openness Handout 13.2

Cultivating Healthy Self-Doubt

- One secret of healthy living is the cultivation of healthy self-doubt.

What Is Healthy Self-Doubt?

- Healthy self-doubt is able to consider that one may be wrong or incorrect, without falling apart or harshly blaming others.

- Healthy self-doubt doesn't take itself too seriously—it has a sense of humor. It can laugh at its own foibles, strange habits, and/or unique quirks with a sense of kindness. It acknowledges that all humans are fallible.

- Healthy self-doubt takes responsibility for one's actions and emotions by not giving up when challenged.

- Healthy self-doubt is relationship-enhancing because it signals a willingness to learn from the world.

- It is neither Fixed nor Fatalistic Mind thinking.

What Is Unhealthy Self-Doubt?

- Unhealthy self-doubt fears self-examination.

- Unhealthy self-doubt may appear on the surface to be willing to question oneself and/or admit a mistake in order to grow.

- Unhealthy self-doubt often implies that the doubter has been wrongly accused and/or unjustly forced to reexamine themselves (for example, by implying that further self-examination would be damaging because it would automatically undermine their newly earned sense of self-confidence and/or would trigger hidden memories of abuse that they are unprepared to deal with, leading to shutdown, collapse, or relapse).

- Unhealthy self-doubt is characterized by a secret desire to "not change or be challenged." It is a social signal that often functions to block further feedback (see the information about "don't hurt me" responses in lesson 16).

- Unhealthy self-doubt often involves secret anger or resentment directed toward the persons or events that the doubter believes are responsible for triggering uncertainty or unhelpful self-examination.

- Unhealthy self-doubt powerfully impacts social relationships despite being passively expressed (for example, via sulking, pouting, walking away, giving up, or behaving helplessly).

- If unhealthy self-doubt could speak, it might say, "See? I am admitting that I am a bad person, so you can now stop expecting me to change, because I have already told you I am no good."

- OR it might say, "See what you've made me do? Your questioning has now made me question myself. I'm now miserable. Are you happy?"

- Thus, unhealthy self-doubt represents Fatalistic Mind thinking.

Radical Openness Handout 13.3

Practicing Self-Enquiry and Outing Oneself

- **Get in the habit of sharing your self-enquiry practices with other people**—a process known in RO DBT as *outing oneself*. Outing oneself means practicing self-enquiry in the presence of another person.

- **We need other people to reflect back our blind spots** because we don't know what we don't know, things are constantly changing, and there is a great deal of experience occurring outside of our conscious awareness.

- **Outing oneself enhances relationships because it models humility and willingness to learn from what the world has to offer.** When we reveal vulnerability, we signal to others that we are the same as them (not superior), and that we are open to new learning.

- **Outing oneself helps us take responsibility for our perceptions and actions.** It blocks habitual avoidance and denial.

- **Outing oneself goes opposite to unwarranted shame or embarrassment that may arise when self-enquiry reveals parts of our personality we are not proud of or might wish to deny.**

  - Shame is unwarranted because acknowledging fallibility after resisting doing so, or because of being afraid of others' reactions, is a courageous and noble pursuit. It is the opposite of complacency, passivity, or resignation, and it brings people closer together.

  - By outing yourself, you are telling your brain that there is nothing to be ashamed of, whereas hiding signals tells your brain that you must be doing something wrong.

- **Self-enquiry "outing oneself" practices grant permission to the practitioner to speak candidly.**

Radical Openness Handout 13.4

Main Points for Lesson 13: Mindfulness Training, Part 3

The Core Mindfulness "How" Skill: With Self-Enquiry

1. In RO DBT, there are four mindfulness "how" skills that represent the kind of attitude or state of mind to bring to a practice of mindfulness. They are *with self-enquiry*, *with awareness of harsh judgments*, *with one-mindful awareness*, and *effectively and with humility*. Lesson 13 focuses on the first of these four skills, *with self-enquiry*.

2. *With self-enquiry* is the core RO DBT mindfulness "how" skill. It is the key to radically open living. It means actively seeking the things one wants to avoid or may find uncomfortable in order to learn, and cultivating a willingness to be wrong, with an intention to change, if needed.

3. Self-enquiry involves both willingness for self-examination and willingness to reveal to others what self-examination has uncovered. This process is known as *outing oneself* in RO DBT.

Radical Openness Worksheet 13.A

Practicing the Core Mindfulness "How" Skill: With Self-Enquiry

Use the "with self-enquiry" skill to enhance how you practice mindfulness.

Place a checkmark in the boxes next to the skills you practiced.

- ☐ **Practiced purposefully cultivating a sense of healthy self-doubt,** without falling apart or automatically giving in.

- ☐ **Acknowledged that I don't know what I don't know.**

- ☐ **Remembered that self-enquiry means finding a good question** that brings me closer to my personal edge, rather than being obsessed about finding a good answer.

- ☐ **Practiced being suspicious of quick answers** to my self-enquiry questions.

- ☐ **Kept my self-enquiry practices short** (for example, five minutes in duration).

- ☐ **Recorded what arose from my self-enquiry practices** in my self-enquiry journal.

- ☐ **Practiced outing myself** to another person in order to learn from their feedback.

- ☐ **Used the self-enquiry questions from handout 1.3 (Learning from Self-Enquiry)** to facilitate my self-enquiry practice.

Mindfulness Training, Part 4

The "How" Skills

> NOTE TO INSTRUCTORS: Lesson 14 is the fourth part of RO mindfulness training. Part 1 covered common OC states of mind (*Fixed, Flexible,* and *Fatalistic Mind*; see lesson 11). Part 2 covered the "what" mindfulness skills (*observe openly, describe with integrity,* and *participate without planning*; see lesson 12). Part 3 covered the first of the four mindfulness "how" skills, *with self-enquiry* (see lesson 13). Part 4 pertains to the remaining three "how" skills, the mind-sets one should work to cultivate when practicing mindfulness.

Main Points for Lesson 14

1. In RO DBT, there are four mindfulness "how" skills that represent the kind of attitude or state of mind to bring to a practice of mindfulness. They are *with self-enquiry, with awareness of harsh judgments, with one-mindful awareness,* and *effectively and with humility.* The core mindfulness "how" skill, *with self-enquiry,* was taught in lesson 13. Lesson 14 focuses on the other three "how" skills.

2. The second "how" skill is *with awareness of harsh judgments.* Judgments become harsh and/or problematic when they are rigidly believed as accurate perceptions of reality; they lead to unhelpful rumination, they make us less open to feedback or new information, and/or they negatively impact how we socially signal or express our intentions and experience to others.

3. *With one-mindful awareness* is the third mindfulness "how" skill. It means doing one thing at a time by purposefully and repeatedly turning one's attention toward the present moment. In RO, *one-mindfulness* means practicing awareness, with humility. We need humility because what we are aware of in any given moment is an edited version of the present moment, not a true representation of it.

4. *Effectively and with humility* is the fourth RO DBT mindfulness "how" skill and means being able to adapt one's behavior to ever-changing circumstances in order to achieve a goal or live according to one's values, in a manner that accounts for the needs of others. For OC clients, it can mean learning how to *not* always play by the rules, to be less political, to not always base decisions on winning or achievement, to let go of compulsive striving and obsessive self-improvement, and to learn how to celebrate ineffective moments as opportunities for growth.

Materials Needed

- Handout 14.1 (The Four RO "How" Skills)
- Handout 14.2 (Using Self-Enquiry to Examine Harsh Judgments)
- (Optional) Handout 14.3 (Main Points for Lesson 14: Mindfulness Training, Part 4: The "How" Skills)
- Worksheet 14.A (Practicing the "How" of RO Mindfulness)
- Whiteboard or flipchart with marker

(Required) Teaching Point

With Awareness of Harsh Judgments

> NOTE TO INSTRUCTORS: Linehan (1993a, 2015a) identifies two types of judgments: those that discriminate and those that evaluate. Evaluative judgments are considered problematic because they are "based on opinions, personal values, and ideas in our minds," meaning they add something to the facts (Linehan, 2015a, p. 200). Judgments that discriminate are considered helpful because they describe "reality" as "what is," without adding evaluations of "good" and "bad" (Linehan, 2015a, p. 201). RO DBT considers these two forms of judgment more similar than different. They both represent emotionally driven evaluative processes that differ primarily according to the extent to which the incoming stimuli are appraised as personally relevant (helpful or harmful) or intense (a high number of sensory neurons is activated). RO DBT posits that we only notice things that matter to us personally. Broadly defined, emotions arise when an individual attends to a stimulus that is relevant to his or her goals—they function to motivate actions (for example, flight/fight) and organize behavior toward salient goals (Davidson & Irwin, 1999; Gross, 2007). Thus, the reason we notice a swimming pool is because it has some personal relevance to us (however minor that relevance may be). For example, we are more likely to notice whether a pool is empty or full if we don't know how to swim and fear falling in. A judge might be motivated to determine (discern, discriminate) whether a particular action violates the US Constitution because they find it satisfying to perform their job well. Discriminative judgments appear nonemotional simply because they involve less personally relevant and/or less intense stimulus evaluations.

- *The second "how" skill in RO DBT mindfulness is* **with awareness of harsh judgments.**

- *Our brain is constantly scanning for changes or inconsistencies in the environment that may be relevant to our well-being.*

- *Our brains are hardwired to evaluate the extent to which we like or dislike what is happening each and every moment.* When we detect an inconsistency (something unexpected), we quickly evaluate or judge it as safe, potentially helpful, or potentially harmful. This process happens so fast that we rarely know it is happening—that is, in milliseconds, beginning at the preconscious or sensory receptor level of awareness.

- *Thus, we are always judging and always feeling something,* though oftentimes at low, barely noticeable levels of intensity. It is impossible for us not to judge!

(Optional) Discussion Point

Emotions

Refer participants to handout 2.1 (The RO DBT Neuroregulatory Model of Emotions).

- *Even when it appears that nothing is happening, we are feeling something.*

  ✓ **Ask:** *In this moment—right here, right now—what do you feel? For example, to what extent are you content, happy, sad, fearful, angry, or numb? Do you like or dislike your current mood? What might this mean?*

✓ **Ask:** *Are you interested or intrigued by our discussion? Recall that curiosity is part of the PNS social safety system.*

✓ **Ask:** *Do you feel excited and animated? Recall that urges to approach and pursue are part of our SNS reward system.*

✓ **Ask:** *Or do you dislike my questions or yearn for me to change the topic? Recall that SNS defensive arousal triggers escape or attack behaviors.*

✓ **Ask:** *If you don't feel anything, where on the RO DBT model of emotion might you be? Are you feeling safe? Is your body relaxed? Is your breathing slow and deep? Are you finding it easy to make eye contact? All of these represent features of the social safety system.*

✓ **Ask:** *If you are feeling numb, what might happen if I walked over and pinched you? Would you feel it? (Recall that when the PNS shutdown system is activated, not only do we feel numb but we also feel less pain.)*

✓ **Ask:** *Does my suggestion of a pinch change how you feel? Are you still numb? If not, then notice how quickly your brain-body changes to incoming stimuli. What emotion system might you be in now?*

NOTE TO INSTRUCTORS: Unlike models that focus on emotions as temporary phenomena, RO DBT posits affective experience to be ever present, albeit oftentimes at low, barely noticeable intensity levels. Thus, we are always feeling something and can become conscious of the extent to which we are content, happy, sad, fearful, or angry at any given moment. Valence (degree of pleasantness versus unpleasantness) and arousal/intensity (degree of excitation that stimuli elicit) differentiate among affective states, together yielding four poles of affective experience: aroused versus unaroused positive affect (for example, joy/excitement versus calm/contentment) and aroused versus unaroused negative affect (for example, fear/anxiety/anger versus indifference) that wax and wane continuously (Pettersson, Boker, Watson, Clark, & Tellegen, 2013). Consequently, emotions and mood states stem from the same neuroreceptive evaluative process.

(Required) Teaching Point

Judgmental Thinking

Judgments Become Problematic When…

- **They are rigidly believed as accurate perceptions of reality or literal truth.** Recall that RO DBT posits that we bring perceptual and regulatory biases with us wherever we go; that is, *we don't see things as they are, we see things as we are.*

- **They lead to unhelpful rumination.** Rumination and brooding almost invariably arise when our expectations about the world fail to materialize. **When we ruminate, we are not trying to learn; we are trying to find a solution that allows us to stay the same** (for example, to prove to ourselves that we are right, and they are wrong).

- **They make us less open to feedback or new information.** When we harshly judge ourselves or others, we almost always operate from our threat system. We feel tense. Recall that tension in the body suggests that our brain has evaluated a situation as a potential threat, making us less open. Our social safety system has been disengaged, and our empathic and prosocial signaling becomes impaired.

- *They negatively impact how we socially signal or express our intentions and experience to others.* For example, they trigger pouting, walking away, phony smiling, sabotaging, harsh gossip, sarcastic comments, insincere praise, pretending to agree, not talking, and so on.

Judgmental Thinking Impacts Our Social Signaling

- *Judgmental thinking influences how we behave around others, even when we try hard not to show it.* When we are uptight, we are most often harshly judging other people, the world, the situation we are in, or ourselves. Research shows that we can often tell when another person is uptight or feeling safe; that is, we are good social safety detectors.

  - ✓ **Ask:** *Have you ever noticed that you can often tell whether a person is uptight just by hearing their voice over the telephone?*

- *Notice how harsh self-judgments impact your behavior, both verbally and nonverbally.* Use the following self-enquiry questions to facilitate this.

  - ➤ *When I am self-critical or self-judgmental, how do I behave around others? For example, do I hide my face, avoid eye contact, slump my shoulders, and/or lower my head? Do I speak with a lower volume or slower pace? Or do I tell others that I am overwhelmed, unable to cope, or that this is "too much"?*

  - ➤ *What am I trying to communicate when I behave in this way? What might my self-judgmental social signals tell me about my desires or aspirations?*

  - ➤ *To what extent does my self-critical social signaling fit my valued goals? Do I ever secretly hope that my harsh self-blame will stop someone from giving me feedback I don't want to hear and/or do I ever use harsh self-blame in order to avoid taking responsibility, achieve a desired goal, or get another person to take care of me?*

  - ➤ *What prevents me from directly asking the other person for what I need or want? What might this tell me about my relationship with this person or how I perceive myself? What is it that I might need to do differently, change, or learn?*

  - ➤ *To what extent does my self-judgmental social signaling communicate to others that I am competent versus incompetent? Do I like this? What might this tell me about my personal values? What do I need to learn?*

- *Notice how harsh other-judgment or blaming others impacts your verbal and nonverbal behavior.* Use the following examples and questions to facilitate self-enquiry.

  - ➤ *How do I express harsh judgmental thoughts about others? For example, do I exhibit a flat face, scowl, look away, laugh or chuckle, seek agreement from others, tell them it is for their own good, stare, puff out my chest, talk faster, adopt a commanding voice, roll my eyes, pout, go silent, act disgusted, behave as if I am not bothered or they are unimportant, begin planning revenge, or smile while giving backhanded praise? How do I feel when others behave similarly toward me? Would I encourage or teach a young child to behave in the same way? What might this tell me about my behavior?*

  - ➤ *How does my harsh judgment of others influence my relationship(s)? What am I trying to communicate when I harshly blame others or the world? To what extent do I directly reveal to others my judgmental thoughts? What might this tell me about myself?*

  - ➤ *Do I ever secretly enjoy judging others? Have I ever been secretly proud that I can appear nonjudgmental when in fact I am highly judgmental? Do I ever purposefully use judgmental behavior to control or dominate others, block unwanted feedback, or achieve a goal? What might this tell me about myself and how I think about the world? Would I encourage a young child to think similarly? What might I need to learn?*

> ➤ How would I feel if I were to suddenly discover that others actually knew my true intentions or secret thoughts about them? What might my response to this question tell me about my core values or how I may truly feel about the way I behave toward others? What is it that I might need to learn?

- **Rather than keeping judgments a secret, use the Awareness Continuum to practice outing them to a friend.** The Awareness Continuum automatically blocks harsh gossip because it acknowledges that our perceptions and interpretations are our personal creations, not literal truths. For example…

  - I am aware of imagining that this other person is purposefully trying to hurt me, not I know they want to hurt me.

  - I am aware of a thought that I am right and they are wrong, not I know I'm right and they are wrong.

  - I am aware of a feeling of desire for you to agree with my judgmental thinking (for example, how bad the other person is or how bad I am) rather than Don't you think I'm right?

- **Practice humility by revealing to your friend why you are outing yourself.** For example, explain to your friend that you are choosing to out yourself to them because you trust them or desire to get closer to them. Or explain that the purpose of RO "outing oneself" practices is to learn how to be more open to differing perspectives and practice self-enquiry rather than seek reassurance, validation, or soothing from the listener. Thank them for their willingness to listen.

- **Notice any judgmental thoughts about your friend when you practice outing yourself.** Observe your reactions when…

  - **Your friend** responds in a way that you don't like or did not expect.

  - **Your friend** responds in a way that you like, approve of, or expected.

- **Celebrate feedback from your friend as opportunities for self-enquiry,** using the following questions.

  > ➤ What does my reaction to my friend's feedback tell me about my relationship with my friend? How might another person view their feedback? Did I feel closer or more distant after outing myself to my friend? What is it that I might need to learn?

  > ➤ Does my reaction to my friend's feedback suggest that I am still trying to control the world, despite my attempts to signal otherwise? What is it that I might need to learn?

  > ➤ Is it possible that I was I secretly hoping my friend would validate or agree with my perspective, despite telling them that I did not want this? Or is it possible that I was using this practice to signal superiority—for example, that I am more courageous, more open, or better at self-improvement than my friend? What is it that I might need to learn?

- **Take responsibility for your unhelpful judgments by recognizing that harsh judgments are freely chosen.** No one can force you to harshly judge yourself or another person.

- **Notice how your judgmental thinking is reinforced** (for example, harsh self-criticism can elicit caregiving from others; automatically blaming others when things go wrong can avoid self-doubt; harsh gossip can feel pleasurable). Practice self-enquiry by asking…

  > ➤ To what extent do I enjoy judging others or myself? What is it that I find enjoyable? Do I believe the pleasure I feel when I harshly judge is deserved or the right way to live? Would I advise a small child to behave similarly? What might this tell me about my values? What is it I might need to learn?

  > ➤ Is there a part of me that believes harsh judgments are necessary in order to punish others (or myself), protect myself, and/or be effective? If so, or maybe, then what might this tell me about how I respond to the world? What is it I might need to learn?

- *Judge a little, and then get over it; harsh judgmental thinking is not always maladaptive.* RO DBT considers harsh judgments as signposts pointing us to our personal unknown, or our edge. Our edge is where self-enquiry is most likely to result in the acquisition of new learning, new insight, or entirely new ways of responding (that is, free operant behavior). Yet new learning can be painful because it often requires sacrificing firmly held convictions or self-constructs.

- *Notice when you are judging your judging.* Judging is something humans do (it is not good or bad). Judgmental thinking is our way of life; even when we think we are being nonjudgmental, we are judging.

- *Rather than trying to stop judging your judging, practice self-enquiry by asking…*

  - *What am I trying to tell myself or signal to others by judging my judging? Is there a possibility that my harsh self-judgment represents another way for me to punish myself, stay depressed, or avoid taking responsibility? To what extent is my judging my judging leading me to Fatalistic Mind? What is it that I need to learn?*

- *Turn on your social safety system to help loosen the grip of harsh judgments.* For example, use the skills in handout 3.1 Changing Social Interactions by Changing Physiology or practice a brief loving kindness meditation; see worksheet 4.A (Daily Practice of Loving Kindness Meditation).

- *Practice giving people the benefit of the doubt. Look for benign explanations for another person's behavior before assuming the worst.*

- *Practice grieving the loss of an expectation or belief about how things should or ought to be when events don't go as planned, or when other people don't behave as expected.* Allow yourself to experience the sadness associated with not being in control rather than automatically trying to regain control, persuading others you are right, or moving to Fatalistic Mind.

NOTE TO INSTRUCTORS: OC individuals almost always value the idea of living a relatively nonemotional life. Equanimity, nonreactivity, and/or nonattachment are highly valued and sought after. They may exhibit strong opinions about themselves, others, and the world that they insist are unemotional statements of fact or observations of "what is." Thus, the preceding points cannot be overstated when it comes to treating OC clients. Their desire for certainty is their blessing and curse. The realization that they are always feeling something—that is, we are emotional by nature—represents an essential element for change when treating overcontrol.

Awareness of Unhelpful Judgments: Practice Examples for Overcontrolled Clients

- **Write down all of the words you can think of that begin with the letter C,** and notice judgmental thoughts or desires to be the best at this.

- **Deal an emotion.** Have group members pick a number between one and ten, and then assign them an emotion (for example, if you picked number one, you have the emotion of humiliation; if you picked number two, you have fear; if you picked three, you have envy; and so on). Ask participants to repeat their emotion word silently to themselves while observing bodily sensations. Have participants notice judgmental thoughts about the emotion they were dealt, or desires for one of the other emotions.

- **Observe disordered or chaotic environments,** and mindfully observe judgmental thoughts that arise.

- **Observe clouds or inkblots.** Notice differing patterns or shapes that emerge (for example, a bunny rabbit) and any judgmental thoughts.

- **Complete a task without looking back over the details** or double-checking your work. For example, draw a cow with your nondominant hand; observe judgmental or competitive thoughts. Share them with someone.

- **Practice revealing your judgmental thoughts to others.** Let go of sugarcoating or trying to make your opinion sound cooperative or nice.

- **Practice being bold and confrontational.** For example, say aloud to your therapist three judgmental thoughts you have about therapy during your individual therapy session; block attempts to minimize or downplay your judgment.

- **Practice being self-interested or decadent twice per day, and observe judgmental thoughts that may arise.** For example, watch the TV program you like, for a change; turn off your telephone for an evening; go to a restaurant and order everything that you might secretly desire but normally avoid because it is unhealthy; eat as much as you can; or tell your boss about a recent success.

- **Practice being lazy while being aware of any judgmental thoughts.** For example, leave work at the same time as others; take a nap on Saturday afternoon; read a book that is not designed to make you a better person.

- **Practice playing and developing hobbies or leisure activities that don't require a lot of planning or preparation;** notice judgmental thoughts.

- **Spend only a set amount of time to complete a task. Purposefully try to not get it completed.** Watch for judgmental thoughts; plus, notice how difficult it is to choose not to get the task done.

- **Practice engaging in positive judgments about oneself.** For example, develop a sense of pride for being capable of letting go of rigid desires to work and not always having to be *right*.

- **Practice making minor mistakes and watching the outcome.** Notice that a mistake does NOT always mean that something bad will happen. Observe judgmental thinking, and use self-enquiry to deepen your practice. For example, mistakes often lead to new learning or unexpected and beneficial outcomes.

- **Practice interacting with individuals who are different, less serious, or less work-focused** (for example, go to a fair where hippies hang out). Notice judgmental thoughts; practice celebrating diversity.

- **Prepare a meal without following a recipe,** and then eat it with a close friend and observe judgmental thinking about how it turned out.

- **Practice grieving the loss of expectations about how the world should be.** For example, when we are judgmental of a friend who behaved rudely, we might need to practice grieving our expectation that people will treat us nicely or that others will play fair; see also handout 29.3 (Strengthening Forgiveness Through Grief Work: Examples of Common Beliefs or Expectations).

(Required) Teaching Point
With One-Mindful Awareness

✳ *The interesting thing about boredom is that if you actively seek it, you no longer find it.* ✳

- **With one-mindful awareness *is the mindfulness "how" skill of doing one thing at a time.***

- **With one-mindful awareness *means purposefully turning one's attention toward the present moment,*** without getting caught up in thoughts, emotions, images, or sensations that are unrelated to what is happening. It requires repeated practice.

- **With one-mindful awareness *in RO DBT means practicing awareness with humility.***

- **We need humility because it is impossible for someone to ever be fully or completely aware of the multitude of factors that influence our present-moment experience.** For example, our brain is capable of being consciously aware of a thought, emotion, sensation, or image approximately every fifty milliseconds, making it theoretically possible for us to be consciously aware of eighty distinct moments *in the span of one breath.* Yet if we attempted to attend to each and every one of these experiential moments, not only would we likely be overwhelmed but we might fail to remember that we have not yet made our morning coffee.

- **What we are aware of in any given moment is an edited version of the present moment, not a true representation of it.**

Read the following text aloud.

> *Imagine that your brain is a TV with simultaneous access to ten thousand different channels, yet it can only truly receive one channel at a time. Plus, the channel your brain chooses to receive, and that you are thus aware of, is determined by the extent to which the show being broadcast might impact your well-being, a decision that is influenced by your past experiences, your brain's unique biological makeup, and/or the intensity of the incoming signal. Sometimes, especially if you haven't eaten recently, your brain seems to prefer the food channel, whereas at other times you find your brain tuned in to the nature channel, especially after you remember how you loved to take walks with your grandmother. Yet at other times both the food and the nature channel are ignored; for example, your brain is riveted to the weather channel—the forecast is for a tornado!*

> NOTE TO INSTRUCTORS: According to the RO DBT neuroregulatory model (see lesson 2), perceptual gating parameters most often occur at the preconscious or subcortical level (for example, brain stem, reticular activating system), which functions to quickly assign potential relevance to continuing, new, or changing stimuli, specifically as either safe, novel, threatening, rewarding, or overwhelming. Thus, a great deal is happening inside of us all of the time that is outside of conscious awareness.

- ***Thus, our conscious awareness of the present moment is selected from a vast array of potentially relevant or evocative stimuli,*** albeit most often without conscious awareness or intention.

  - ✓ **Ask:** *What are you aware of right now? Right now? What about now? Notice that each moment is different.*

  - ✓ **Ask:** *What channel do you tend to watch the most (that is, which one are you mostly aware of)?*

  - ✓ **Ask:** *To what extent are you awake to your present moment? For example, when you take a shower, are you feeling the water or are you already planning your day? When you eat a meal, do you taste your food or are you thinking of something else? When you are talking with someone, are you truly listening or are you rehearsing what you will say? When you are worrying, are you worrying with awareness?*

- ***A heightened sense of urgency characterizes overcontrolled coping,*** most often manifested by compulsive attempts to quickly resolve problems (or potential problems) and then just as quickly move on to the next one (or imagined next one) without a rest in between. **Let's return to our TV/ brain metaphor.**

Read the following text aloud.

Imagine now not only that your brain has simultaneous access to ten thousand different channels but also that your quick detail-focused processing and superior pattern recognition allow you to channel-surf faster than most people. You can quickly evaluate the importance of any given channel and then move on to the next channel. And then the next channel. And the next. How might this impact a person's way of living or experience of life? Is there a chance that they might miss out on something? What might that be?

  - ✓ **Ask:** *To what extent do you multitask? How might this relate to our story?*

- ***"I'm late! I'm late! For a very important date! No time to say hello, goodbye! I'm late! I'm late! I'm late!" Compulsive striving can start to feel like the White Rabbit character*** in Walt Disney's 1951 animated film *Alice in Wonderland,* based on Lewis Carroll's book *Alice's Adventures in Wonderland.*

  - ✓ **Ask:** *To what extent do you experience a heightened sense of urgency or a sense that there is never enough time?*

  - ✓ **Ask:** *Do you ever feel like there is always something more to do (or something more important to do)?*

  - ✓ **Ask:** *To what extent do you find yourself trying to quickly resolve problems (or potential problems) and then just as quickly moving on to the next one (or imagined next one) without a rest in between?*

  - ✓ **Ask:** *How do you think this might impact a person's experience of the present moment?*

- **With one-mindful awareness means allowing oneself to slow down and relish the moment.** It is learning how to let go of compulsive goal-focused coping and self-improvement.

  - ✓ **Ask:** *To what extent do you allow yourself to relish your present moments?*

(Optional) Class Exercise
Everything Is Relative

Read the following phrases aloud.

- *The past is gone, the future has yet to be.*

- *The notes in a musical composition depend on the spaces between.*

- *The interesting thing about boredom is that if you actively seek it, you no longer find it.*

  ✓ **Ask:** *What might these phrases mean?*

  ✓ **Ask:** *How do they relate to one-mindfulness? How might they help us know how to practice one-mindfulness?*

With One-Mindful Awareness: Practice Examples for Overcontrolled Clients

- **After accomplishing a goal, one-mindfully allow yourself to feel the pleasure of your success** rather than automatically moving on to the next task.

- **One-mindfully multitask;** that is, be aware of your actions, thoughts, desires, emotions, and sensations linked to your goal or intention in the current moment (for example, replying to a friend's email) as well as your unrelated actions, thoughts, desires, emotions, and sensations (for example, thinking about your cat).

- **One-mindfully ruminate.** When worrying, do so with awareness. Consciously set aside time to brood or ruminate. Notice how this impacts your worry or rumination.

- **Practice disobeying urgency by one-mindfully experiencing it.** When a sense of urgency arises—for example to go faster, to work harder, or to do more—allow yourself to experience the feeling sense of urgency without giving in to it.

- **Practice slowing down when you find yourself speeding up.** One-mindfully take a deep breath and lean back in your chair, raise your eyebrows, and closed-mouth smile. Notice what happens.

- **Practice one-mindfully seeking boredom, and notice what happens.** Use self-enquiry if you find yourself resisting or disliking this. What is it that you might need to learn?

- **Practice living fully by doing one thing at a time.** For example, when in the shower, experience the water flowing down your back rather than automatically planning your day; when walking, experience your feet on the ground and the feel of your body moving rather than thinking about your destination; when in conversation, one-mindfully listen rather than rehearsing what you might say.

(Required) Teaching Point
Effectively and with Humility

- **Individuals characterized by overcontrol often pride themselves on being effective.** For example, they are good at delaying gratification rather than giving in to temptation in order to achieve a goal or persisting in the face of adversity regardless of the odds.

- ✓ **Ask:** *What does being effective mean to you?*

- ✓ **Ask:** *To what extent do you believe that being effective means striving, achieving results, doing the right thing, or working hard? What might this mean about how you see the world?*

- ✓ **Ask:** *To what extent do you believe being effective means cooperating, being humble, being able to change your mind, or admitting to fault? What might this tell you about yourself?*

- **Effectively and with humility** *means being able to adapt one's behavior to ever-changing circumstances in order to achieve a goal or live according to one's values, in a manner that accounts for the needs of others.*

- **No one is an island.** RO DBT effectiveness remembers our tribal nature; our well-being is dependent on other people.

- **Be savvy about people, but not arrogant.** Flexible Mind is humble. It acknowledges our essential fallibility and is willing to practice healthy self-doubt. It celebrates diversity by recognizing there are many ways to reach Chicago; that is, people have different ways of solving problems or perceiving the world, and rarely is there only one correct way.

- **Context matters! Celebrate both disinhibition and inhibition.** For example, delaying gratification *and* dancing with abandon; questioning intuitive knowing *and* trusting one's intuitions; whispering in church *and* yelling wildly to stop a mugger—all can be effective, depending on the context.

- **What is effective in one moment may not be in the next.** It is *turning one's mind to the possibility of change* and changing if new information suggests that change is needed.

- **Break a rule when necessary.** Overcontrolled individuals often compulsively play by the rules. Flexible Mind recognizes that sometimes effectiveness can involve playing by the rules, whereas at other times it means breaking the rules. This can include looking for compromise or synthesis.

Effectively and with Humility: Practice Examples for Overcontrolled Clients

- **Practice breaking rules—especially your own—when the situation suggests a prior rule is no longer effective.**

- **Practice going opposite to what you would normally do in a situation—for the fun of it—and see what happens.** For example, rather than pointing out the downsides of a new proposal, point out its advantages and then observe what happens. *How does changing what you normally do impact others or your environment?*

- **Practice acknowledging dependence as a fundamental part of human success** rather than seeing it as a sign of weakness, bad, or cowardly. For example, notice how you depend on your grocer to provide you with fresh milk, your friend to tell you the truth, or your mechanic to properly repair your car.

- **Practice acknowledging your arrogance rather than defending yourself or pretending you are being nonjudgmental.** Being able to admit one's weakness to another is a core part of behaving effectively.

Lesson 14 Homework

1. **(Required) Handout 14.1 (The Four RO "How" Skills)**
2. **(Required) Handout 14.2 (Using Self-Enquiry to Examine Harsh Judgments)**
3. **(Required) Worksheet 14.A (Practicing the "How" of RO Mindfulness)**

Radical Openness Handout 14.1

The Four RO "How" Skills

1. With self-enquiry
2. With awareness of harsh judgments
3. With one-mindful awareness
4. Effectively and with humility

Use the following skills to enhance how you practice mindfulness.

With Self-Enquiry

- *With self-enquiry* means actively seeking the things one wants to avoid or may find uncomfortable in order to learn, and cultivating a willingness to be wrong, with an intention to change, if needed.

- Self-enquiry involves both willingness for self-examination and willingness to reveal to others what self-examination uncovered. This process is known as *outing oneself* in RO DBT.

- See handout 13.1 (The Core Mindfulness "How" Skill: With Self-Enquiry) for more details about *with self-enquiry*.

With Awareness of Harsh Judgments

Judgments are a problem when...

- **They are rigidly believed as accurate perceptions of reality or literal truth.**

- **They lead to unhelpful rumination.** When we ruminate, we are not trying to learn; we are trying to find a solution that allows us to stay the same (for example, to prove to ourselves that we are right, and they are wrong).

- **They make us less open to feedback or new information.** When we harshly judge ourselves or others, our brain has already evaluated a situation as a potential threat, making us less open. Our social safety system has been disengaged, and our empathic and prosocial signaling becomes impaired.

- **They negatively impact how we socially signal or express our intentions and experience to others.** For example, they trigger pouting, walking away, phony smiling, sabotaging, harsh gossip, sarcastic comments, insincere praise, pretending to agree, not talking, and so on.

With One-Mindful Awareness

- *With one-mindful awareness* means purposefully turning one's attention toward the present moment, without getting caught up in unrelated thoughts, emotions, images, or sensations. It requires repeated practice.

- *With one-mindful awareness* recognizes that we can never be fully or completely aware.

- *With one-mindful awareness* means allowing oneself to slow down and relish the moment. It is learning how to let go of compulsive goal-focused coping and self-improvement.

Effectively and with Humility

- **Adapt to changing circumstances, in a manner that accounts for the needs of others.**

- **No one is an island.** Our personal well-being is dependent on other people.

- **Be savvy about people, but not arrogant.** There are many ways to solve a problem or perceive the world; rarely is there only one correct way.

- **Flexible Mind is humble.** It acknowledges our essential fallibility and is willing to practice healthy self-doubt.

- **Celebrate both disinhibition and inhibition.**

- **Recognize that what is effective in one moment may not be in the next.**

- **Break a rule when necessary.**

Radical Openness Handout 14.2

Using Self-Enquiry to Examine Harsh Judgments

➤ *Am I secretly pretending that I am not judgmental? Am I hoping that if I don't challenge others or put myself down first that they won't challenge me? What is it I need to learn?*

➤ *Is there a possibility that I may not really want to change a harsh judgment?*

➤ *What am I trying to communicate when I harshly blame myself, others, or the world?*

➤ *To what extent does my harsh self-blame fit my valued goals? Do I ever secretly hope that my harsh self-blame will stop someone from giving me feedback I don't want to hear? Do I ever use harsh self-blame in order to avoid taking responsibility, achieve a desired goal, or get another person to take care of me?*

➤ *What prevents me from directly telling another person that I am blaming them (or blaming myself)?*

➤ *To what extent do I directly reveal my judgmental thoughts to others? When revealing my judgments to others, to what extent do I acknowledge to the other person that my judgment may be wrong or inaccurate?*

➤ *How does my harsh judgment of myself or others impact my relationships?*

➤ *Where did I ever get the idea that hiding my judgments or pretending that I was not judging others was the way to live?*

➤ *Do I ever secretly enjoy judging others?*

➤ *Have I ever been secretly proud that I can appear nonjudgmental when in fact I am highly judgmental?*

➤ *Do I ever purposefully use judgmental behavior to control or dominate others, block unwanted feedback, or achieve a goal? What might this tell me about myself and how I think about the world? Would I encourage a young child to think similarly? What might I need to learn?*

➤ *How would I feel if I were to suddenly discover that others actually knew my true intentions or secret thoughts about them? What is it that I might need to learn?*

When I am judging my judging, use self-enquiry by asking…

➤ *What am I trying to tell myself or signal to others by judging my judging?*

➤ *Is there a possibility that my harsh self-judgment represents another way for me to punish myself, stay depressed, or avoid taking responsibility?*

➤ *To what extent is my judging my judging leading me to Fatalistic Mind?*

Radical Openness Handout 14.3

Main Points for Lesson 14: Mindfulness Training, Part 4

The "How" Skills

1. In RO DBT, there are four mindfulness "how" skills that represent the kind of attitude or state of mind to bring to a practice of mindfulness. They are *with self-enquiry, with awareness of harsh judgments, with one-mindful awareness,* and *effectively and with humility.* The core mindfulness "how" skill, *with self-enquiry,* was taught in lesson 13. Lesson 14 focuses on the other three "how" skills.

2. The second "how" skill is *with awareness of harsh judgments.* Judgments become harsh and/or problematic when they are rigidly believed as accurate perceptions of reality; they lead to unhelpful rumination, they make us less open to feedback or new information, and/or they negatively impact how we socially signal or express our intentions and experience to others.

3. *With one-mindful awareness* is the third mindfulness "how" skill. It means doing one thing at a time by purposefully and repeatedly turning one's attention toward the present moment. In RO, *one-mindfulness* means practicing awareness, with humility. We need humility because what we are aware of in any given moment is an edited version of the present moment, not a true representation of it.

4. *Effectively and with humility* is the fourth RO DBT mindfulness "how" skill and means being able to adapt one's behavior to ever-changing circumstances in order to achieve a goal or live according to one's values, in a manner that accounts for the needs of others. For OC clients, it can mean learning how to *not* always play by the rules, to be less political, to not always base decisions on winning or achievement, to let go of compulsive striving and obsessive self-improvement, and to learn how to celebrate ineffective moments as opportunities for growth.

Radical Openness Worksheet 14.A

Practicing the "How" of RO Mindfulness

Instructions: Use the following prompts to practice RO mindfulness "how" skills.

With Awareness of Harsh Judgments

Place a checkmark in the boxes next to the skills you practiced.

☐ I noticed times when I behaved as if my judgments were better or more accurate than those made by other people.

☐ I noticed times when my body was tense (headache, upset stomach, constipation) and used them as a reminder to look for hidden judgments.

☐ I practiced observing how harsh other-blame impacted my social signaling. Write in the following space what you discovered (for example, *I displayed a flat face, scowled, looked away, laughed or chuckled, sought agreement from others, told the other person it was for their own good, stared, puffed out my chest, talked faster, adopted a commanding voice, rolled my eyes, pouted, went silent, acted disgusted, or smiled while giving backhanded praise*).

_____

_____

_____

☐ I practiced observing how harsh self-blame impacted my social signaling, without getting down on myself. Write in the following space what you discovered (for example, *I hid my face, avoided eye contact, slumped my shoulders, lowered my head*). Did you speak with a lower volume or slower pace? Or did you tell others that you were overwhelmed, unable to cope, or that it was "too much"?

_____

_____

_____

☐ I used the Awareness Continuum to take responsibility for my harsh judgments by labeling them. For example, *I am aware of a judgmental thought about my neighbor* or *I am aware of a feeling of resentment about my neighbor*.

☐ Rather than keeping judgments a secret, I used the Awareness Continuum to practice outing them to a friend. The Awareness Continuum automatically blocks harsh gossip because it acknowledges that our perceptions and interpretations are our personal creations, not literal truths. Place a checkmark next to the examples that best represent what you did.

☐ *I am aware of imagining that this other person is purposefully trying to hurt me, not I know they want to hurt me.*

☐ *I am aware of a thought that I am right and they are wrong, not I know I'm right and they are wrong.*

☐ *I am aware of a feeling of desire for you to agree with my judgmental thinking (for example, how bad the other person is or how bad I am), rather than Don't you think I'm right?*

☐ **I practiced self-enquiry about my harsh judgments and used handout 14.2 (Using Self-Enquiry to Examine Harsh Judgments) to deepen my practice.** Record the self-enquiry questions or new learning that emerged from your self-enquiry practices.

_____

_____

_____

☐ **I practiced activating my social safety system to help loosen the grip of harsh judgments**—for example, by using the skills in handout 3.1 (Changing Social Interactions by Changing Physiology) or via a brief loving kindness meditation with worksheet 4.A (Daily Practice of Loving Kindness Meditation).

☐ **I practiced giving people the benefit of the doubt and actively looked for benign, reasonable, and valid explanations for another person's behavior before assuming the worst.**

☐ **I practiced grieving my harsh judgments rather than seeing them as truth.** Place a checkmark next to the skills that you used.

  ☐ **I identified and labeled the expectation or belief that I needed to grieve.**
  - **Examples of beliefs or expectations:** a belief that other people will treat you with respect; a belief that the world should be stable or orderly; a conviction that one is able to accurately predict what will happen in the future; an expectation that people will always be honest; a belief that you will always do the right thing; a belief that others will be polite. Record the unmet expectation or belief.

_____

_____

_____

  ☐ **I allowed myself to experience the sadness or disappointment associated with my harsh judgment, and then let it go, without falling apart.**

  ☐ **I remembered that sadness helps me let go of harsh judgmental thinking because it acknowledges that I am not always right.**

  ☐ **I repeated my grief work over multiple days (or weeks).**

  ☐ **I purposefully kept my grief practices brief, recognizing that longer practices often represent disguised attempts to regain control or fix the problem.**

☐ I used self-enquiry when I found myself ruminating or brooding about my grief practices (for example, by asking *What is it that I might need to learn?* rather than using this as another opportunity to get down on myself or blame others).

☐ I remembered that grief work is a process, not an end point, and that it requires ongoing commitment and practice.

☐ I used the following script to facilitate my grief work.

I am learning to face the pain of my loss of expectations or beliefs about how things should or ought to be when events don't go as planned or when other people don't behave as expected, without getting down on myself, falling apart, or automatically blaming others. I am learning to recognize that my harsh judgments often stem from a desire to avoid self-examination, take responsibility, or accept that I cannot control the world. For today's practice, I need to grieve the loss of my expectations that…[insert your unmet expectation or belief here]. My sadness helps me recognize that the world is not always as I expect it to be. By allowing myself to experience the sadness of this loss, I am learning to let go of my unhelpful judgments.

☐ I forgave myself for having a harsh judgment—for example, by using the forgiveness skills in worksheet 29.A (Flexible Mind Has HEART).

☐ I practiced noticing whether I was operating from Fixed Mind or Fatalistic Mind when harshly judging, and then I used handout 11.2 (Being Kind to Fixed Mind) or handout 11.3 (Learning from Fatalistic Mind) to help loosen their grip.

☐ I used handout 22.1 (Being Open to Feedback from Others: Flexible Mind ADOPTS) when I noticed my harsh judgments were triggered by critical feedback.

☐ I practiced Flexible Mind DARES skills, using worksheet 27.A (Opposite Action to Unhelpful Envy: Flexible Mind DARES [to Let Go]), to let go of unhelpful envy when I recognized that my harsh judgments pertained to feeling that another person had unjustly received a reward that I believed should have been mine or that the person had an advantage over me.

☐ Rather than trying to stop judging my judging, I practiced self-enquiry by using the questions in handout 14.2.

Judging is something humans do (it is not good or bad). Judgmental thinking is our way of life; even when we think we are being nonjudgmental, we are judging. Record the self-enquiry questions or new learning that emerged from your self-enquiry practices.

_____

_____

_____

With One-Mindful Awareness

Place a checkmark in the boxes next to the skills you practiced.

☐ After accomplishing a goal, I one-mindfully allowed myself to feel the pleasure of my success rather than automatically moving on to the next task.

☐ I purposefully let go of compulsive multitasking by allowing myself to relish my present moment.

☐ I used self-enquiry to explore the differences between multitasking and one-mindful attention to my present experience. For example, you asked yourself…

> *How did multitasking impact my emotional well-being? How did one-mindful attention impact my emotional well-being? Were there any differences? What might this tell me?*

☐ I practiced one-mindful rumination by purposefully setting aside time each day (twenty minutes) to one-mindfully brood or ruminate. Record what you noticed or learned.

_____

_____

_____

☐ I practiced urge-surfing compulsive desires to go faster, work harder, or do more by slowing down rather than speeding up. For example, you one-mindfully took a deep breath and leaned back in your chair, raised your eyebrows and closed-mouth smiled, and then observed what happened next rather than quickly trying to move on. Record what you noticed or learned.

_____

_____

_____

☐ I practiced doing one thing at a time. For example, when making your bed, you focused on making your bed rather than ruminating about the past or planning for the future.

☐ I practiced one-mindful multitasking by attending fully to each task in the current moment and watching how and when my attention shifted to another task.

☐ I practiced one-mindfully seeking boredom and noticed what happened. I used self-enquiry when I found this difficult. For example, if you found yourself resisting or disliking even the idea of seeking boredom, you asked yourself what this might mean about who you are or how you see the world, and what it was that you might need to learn.

☐ I practiced remembering that all I have is now—the past is gone, and the future has yet to be—in order to experience my life more fully.

Effectively and with Humility

Place a checkmark in the boxes next to the skills you practiced.

☐ I practiced being flexible when encountering something new or unexpected.

☐ When doing what I believed was effective, I did so with humility by remembering that what is effective for one person or one situation might not be effective for all people or all situations.

☐ **I practiced embracing my dependence on others rather than seeing it as a sign of weakness.** For example, you reminded yourself that our species' success depended on our learning how to work together and live in tribes, or you noticed the multitude of everyday experiences (such as your TV working properly, your car starting, your bank keeping your money safe, and so on) when you depend on the goodwill or work of other people. Record what you did.

_____

_____

_____

☐ **I celebrated diversity by remembering that there are many ways to solve a problem or perceive the world, and that rarely is there only one correct way.**

☐ **I practiced acknowledging fallibility and healthy self-doubt when challenged,** in order to more effectively adapt to changing conditions or live by my values.

☐ **I practiced celebrating both disinhibition and inhibition.** For example, you were candid when asked for an opinion by a friend rather than being political, you persisted in a task when your goal was in reach rather than giving up, you danced with abandon when out with friends rather than watching from the sidelines, or you whispered in church but yelled wildly to stop a mugger after the service. Record what you actually did.

_____

_____

_____

☐ **I practiced breaking a rule—especially my own—when necessary,** and when the situation I was in suggested that the rule would no longer be effective.

☐ **I practiced going opposite to what I would normally do in a situation, for the fun of it,** and then observed how this impacted my personal well-being and my relationships with others. For example, rather than always looking for the potential errors or mistakes in a new idea, you practiced looking for potential advantages. Record what you actually did—and feel free to be creative!

_____

_____

_____

Interpersonal Integrity, Part 1

Saying What We Really Mean

Main Points for Lesson 15

1. How we say something matters more than what we say.

2. When apparently innocent questions become disguised demands, relationship problems often follow.

Materials Needed

-   (Optional) Handout 15.1 (Main Points for Lesson 15: Interpersonal Integrity, Part 1: Saying What We Really Mean)

-   Worksheet 15.A (Recognizing Indirect Communication)

-   Flipchart or whiteboard and markers

(Required) Teaching Point

Why Do We Dislike Deception?

-   *All humans desire to be treated fairly, and we believe in equity.*

-   *We also desire to be perceived by others as impartial* (Shaw & Olson, 2012). For example, unlike most species, humans do not automatically side with their allies or kin (DeScioli & Kurzban, 2009).

-   *Yet we frequently communicate our intentions indirectly—we are economical with the truth* by omitting, pretending, or misleading, even when there is no apparent risk or reward.

-   *Indirect speech is powerful: it allows a person to make requests of others and yet deny ever doing so.* A recipient positively inclined to the request can simply agree to it, whereas an antagonistic recipient is unable to argue against it (Lee & Pinker, 2010).

-   *We tend to be indirect with people who are indirect with us.* Unfortunately, indirect speech often leads to misunderstanding and distrust because it is hard to know the true meaning or intentions of the sender.

-   *When indirect speech is purposefully used to gain advantage or cause harm, it transforms into a particularly damaging form of deception.*

- *But everyone lies, right? Except me, of course! Okay, that's a lie (tee hee ☺).*

- *It is true, however: we all lie, and some people lie more than others*—but all people lie, at least occasionally.

  ✓ **Ask:** *Why do you think people lie?*

- *People lie to save face and avoid punishment*—that is, to avoid social disapproval, social sanctions, and social ostracism (see Flexible Mind SAGE, in lesson 8).

- *People also lie to gain advantage, to cause harm, or obstruct others* (these are the lies we fear the most).

(Required) Class Exercise
Mindful Awareness of Lies

Instructors should read aloud the following script.

Unlike many other RO mindfulness practices, this practice will be done in silence and without discussion afterward, meaning we will not share what we thought, felt, or observed at the end of the practice. So we can all relax. This moment of silent reflection is for us alone. What we discover or do not discover is for us alone to learn from or to not learn from. We alone can decide how deep or shallow we go, including the extent to which we participate at all. There is no right way to respond. The choice is ours. We are completely in charge.

So, to begin...let's take a slow deep breath and turn our attention to the sensations of our breath, not trying to do anything or go anywhere, just simply being fully present with the full duration of the inbreath and the full duration of the outbreath. If you like, it sometimes can be helpful to gently close your eyes for this type of practice.

Now let's direct our attention inward, allowing ourselves a moment of self-enquiry about the types of lies we tell...to ourselves...to other people. Notice the sensations, emotions, images, memories, or thoughts that arise. Observe any desires to avoid the practice, refuse to participate, justify ourselves, or harshly get down on ourselves. Gently ask: **What might my response to this practice tell me about myself, or what I might need to learn?** *Remind yourself that we are not sharing what we observe today...that for this moment, we can feel free to examine our own unique pattern of lying, without fear of exposure. As you do so, gently ask yourself:* **What is it that I may need to learn?** *[Allow thirty seconds of silence.]*

Okay, we are done...[Smile.] You can bring your attention back to the room and open your eyes. Notice whether you desired more time or less time for this practice. Take whatever happened and use it to deepen your self-enquiry work in the coming week. Don't forget to keep your practices short—self-enquiry is not about fixing or finding the perfect solutions. Allow yourself the grace to grow at your own pace.

Well done, all! Now, without further ado, let's get back to work!

NOTE TO INSTRUCTORS: As noted, instructors should avoid discussing personal reactions at the end of the preceding practice, although this should not be taken as a rigid rule. Moving directly onward to the next teaching point smuggles several important RO principles: (1) when you say you will do or not do something, you will follow through; (2) you see them as capable people—that is, you trust them to regulate or manage their own experience, without outside intervention; (3) you do not consider negative, painful, or aversive emotions dangerous—feeling distressed is part of life; (4) it is okay to "edit" in life. By not allowing sharing to occur afterward, you reinforce an important RO dialectical principle—that is, both openness and privacy have utility. In addition, since this exercise addresses something none of us really care to talk about, it can be experienced as heavy. Thus, it is essential for instructors to keep the practice short by sticking to the script (recall that all RO self-enquiry practices are designed to be purposefully short in order to build a store of positive associations linked with self-examination). Plus, when moving on to the next teaching points, it is essential for instructors to use their nonverbal behavior to signal joy, happiness, and pride, for both themselves and the class, to celebrate their willingness to courageously approach something normally feared in order to learn (that is, keep your chin up, shoulders back, eyebrows raised, warm smiling, and attempt to engage eye contact with each member of the class). The eye contact and smiling are particularly important; they communicate to the recipient that they have done nothing wrong and that they are still in your tribe (that is, it blocks unwarranted shame). Instructors should also feel free to acknowledge angst or distress expressed by class members (or yourself and your coinstructor) after the exercise, but avoid trying to make everyone feel better by overtly attempting to soothe, validate, or apologize for how difficult the practice was (recall that self-enquiry is by definition painful). If the class starts sharing observations spontaneously, remind them of your promise to not discuss afterward (this takes the heat off those not wanting to share) and encourage individuals to share their observations with each other if they would like after the class is over. But be flexible in how you respond. Some classes simply get so excited about some constructs that they cannot restrain themselves—and, frankly, this is one of the primary goals of the treatment. On the very rare occasion when a particular class member reports feeling highly distressed, shut down, and/or has something really important to share, in general instructors should acknowledge the reasonableness of response and then gently ask if they would like to discuss their experience with you in private after the class has ended.

- *Research suggests that people tell an average of one or two lies a day* (DePaulo & Kashy, 1998; Kashy & DePaulo, 1996). People lie most frequently about their feelings, their references, and their attitudes and opinions. Less often, they lie about their actions, plans, and whereabouts. Lies about achievements and failures are also commonplace.

- *We also lie to ourselves to avoid acknowledging the truth. However, the truth is that lying to ourselves is a lie.* You cannot lie to yourself, because deep down you know that you are avoiding. We cannot hide from ourselves—we can only pretend ignorance. Your self knows you are attempting to deceive your self.

> ★ **Fun Facts:** *Culture Matters!*
>
> *Display rules, or how one habitually expresses their emotions, are learned early in life and vary according to one's culture. For example, in nonstressful situations, both Japanese and American research participants exhibit the same facial expressions when viewing emotional films [Ekman, 1972]. However, this changed when the same films were viewed a second time in the presence of a higher-status individual—the Japanese tended to cover up or mask their expressions of disgust by smiling, whereas the Americans tended to display the same emotions, albeit somewhat downregulated than what had been shown earlier. Thus, when it comes to how certain emotions are expressed, cultural experience matters. Although all cultures downregulate certain emotions when around high-status individuals—disgust, for example—the means by which this is achieved appears to vary according to culture.*

(Required) Teaching Point
Not All Lies Are Bad

- **Lies can be altruistic** (aka "white lies"). For example, telling a friend who is dying of cancer that they look great may represent kindness.

- **Lying can de-escalate conflict** (for example, making up a silly story about oneself to lighten the mood during a tense negotiation).

- **Being economical with the truth can function as an act of kindness** (for example, tactfully turning a person's attention to a blunder or error they have made, without rubbing their nose in it or publicly making a big deal out of it).

- **The good news is, we are less likely to lie to people with whom we feel intimately connected.** When we are emotionally connected with someone, we feel distressed both before and after telling a lie (DePaulo & Kashy, 1998).

- **Plus, acknowledging moments of self- and other-deception can help repair damaged relationships (see Flexible Mind SAGE skills)** and also alerts us to areas of personal growth.

(Required) Teaching Point
Saying What We Really Mean

"I do what I do because that's the way I am." (Hidden message: "Don't expect me to change.")

"I am not like other people." (Hidden message: "I am better than other people.")

"No, really, it's okay. I'm fine with the decision. Let's do it your way." (Hidden message: "I disagree totally and will make you pay.")

- **Indirect speech may be so popular because it allows us to save face** (for example, avoid shame, humiliation, or embarrassment; see lesson 8). It allows both speaker and listener, if they choose, to pretend that they are both behaving impartially and ethically.

- **Plus, sometimes we don't say what we mean out of politeness.**

- **Research shows that we are most likely to be polite when we want something** (not just because we are nice).

  ✓ **Ask:** *How often are you polite without expecting anything in return, or as an act of kindness or genuine respect? To what extent do you think you may use polite behavior as a way to get something you want?*

NOTE TO INSTRUCTORS: Remind participants that polite behavior serves many useful functions in communities, which is why it is so often discussed, commented on, and has books written about it (that is, social etiquette manuals). Although it has some downsides, it functions as an important prosocial lubricant that can ease awkward moments and provide structure for how to behave. It is also an important signal of equality, deference, and respect, and it can help mitigate potentially damaging escalations of conflict (see "Fun Facts: We Are Not Always So Polite!" later in this lesson).

(Required) Mini–Class Exercise
Phony Polite Versus Impolite: What's the Social Signal?

- **Instruct:** Split the class up into pairs, and ask them to share with their partner what type of social signals a person displays when they are being too polite or phony polite versus the types of behaviors that characterize impoliteness or rudeness. *What types of facial expressions, voice tones, gestures, and body movements characterize each type? Which type would you prefer to spend time with? Which type do you believe to be a more honest reflection of the person's inner state? Is the type you prefer to spend time with the same as the type you see as more genuine? What might your answer tell you about your own style?*

- **Discuss:** Allow five to eight minutes for discussion among pairs, and then bring the class back together and solicit observations.

★ **Fun Facts:** *We Are Not Always So Polite!*

Our use of polite language varies, depending on how well we know the other person, the degree of imposition in our request, and the degree of power or authority the speaker has over the recipient. The feeling of being polite is similar to feeling self-conscious—we are likely to feel slightly inhibited, modest, self-deprecating, or deferential. Polite behavior and modesty are more common in situations where the potential for conflict or aggression is more likely. For example, consuming food is a potential area of conflict among most animal species, and humans have developed a wide range of elaborate rules or table manners involving restraint of impulses and signals of deference to the needs of others. Interestingly, research suggests that being blunt or direct (that is, impolite) about one's intentions is actually needed to prompt a skeptical or antagonistic individual to act on what was communicated, whereas a more cooperative listener will respond to more indirect communication [see Lee & Pinker, 2010].

(Required) Teaching Point

Hiding Intentions and Disguising Demands

- **How we say something matters more than what we say.** This is why email communications can be so difficult. People often misread the sender's intentions in an email, based simply on the length of the message, the use of punctuation or capitalization, or the words used in the message—precisely why text emoticon symbols emerged (☺).

- **Most overcontrolled individuals signal discreetly; for example, they tend to mask, hide, or deamplify their inner feelings, making it harder for others to know their true intentions.**

- **For example, which of the following questions is more direct?** *Have you put the garbage out?* or *Will you please take the garbage out?*

- **When apparently innocent questions become disguised demands, relationship problems often follow. Particularly when...**

  - **The apparently innocent question is not genuine,** either because the sender already knows the answer or they believe they do (for example, the sender already knows that the garbage has not been taken out).

  - **The sender conceals their true intentions or desires** in the guise of a question (for example, they actually want their spouse to take the garbage out).

  - **The question is designed to punish noncompliance** or imagined noncompliance (for example, my spouse should have already taken the garbage out, without me having to ask).

- **Hidden intentions and disguised demands erode goodwill.**

  - For example, research has shown that indirect communication of expectations, disappointments, or disagreement by one or both members of a couple relationship, despite its initial apparent non-conflictual nature, frequently results in greater dissatisfaction, distrust, resentment, and relationship dissolution (for example, divorce).

  - The negative social impact of disguised demands is even greater when the receiver can see the facial expressions of the sender (for example, a disgust eye roll).

- **Disguised demands are difficult to challenge: they have plausible deniability.**

  - For example, when the meaning or intention behind an apparently innocent question (such as *Have you put the garbage out?*) is challenged by the recipient to really mean *You have really screwed up—the garbage should have been taken out long ago*, the sender can refute the challenge by simply saying: *Who, me? No, I wasn't trying to tell you what to do or order you around—I was simply asking a question.*

- **Plus, when disguised demands are challenged, their covert nature makes it easy for the sender to turn the tables on the challenger by blaming the problem on them.**

  - For example: *Who me? No, I was simply asking a question. The very fact that you are getting all worked up about this suggests that you're the one with the problem, not me. Maybe you're feeling guilty.*

(Recommended) Mini–Class Exercise

Curiosity Versus Sarcasm

Instructors should split the class up into pairs.

Say to the class…

- *First, using a voice tone that signals genuine and open curiosity, ask your partner:* **Have you put the garbage out?**

- *Now repeat the same question, this time using a sarcastic, disgusted, or contemptuous voice tone when you ask:* **Have you put the garbage out?** *Did you or your partner notice a difference between the two? What did you notice?*

- *Now switch roles and repeat the practice. The person asking now becomes the person listening, and the listener now becomes the asker.*

Mix it up. Have participants say, "I love you" or even a one-word sentence, such as "Hi," in a manner that signals genuine caring, and then with sarcasm.

End by soliciting observations and discussing what was learned.

NOTE TO INSTRUCTORS: You can expand the preceding exercise by adding a mixture of nonverbal components or phrases. An additional twist on this exercise is to have participants ask their partner "Have you put the garbage out?" using a flat facial expression, compared to asking the same question with eyebrows raised. Alternatively, instructors can experiment with this exercise by keeping the tone of voice the same throughout (for example, a positive tone of voice or sarcastic tone of voice) but change what is said—for example, by first asking, "Have you put the garbage out?" followed by "Will you please take the garbage out?"

(Required) Mini–Class Exercise

"What's the Real Meaning Behind This?"

Say to the class: *Let's have some fun exploring OC verbal communication. Let's play "What's the Real Meaning Behind This?" As we have been discussing, most OC individuals tend to mask their inner feelings. Masking inner feelings influences how a person talks. Habitual use of words or phrases that are vague, indirect, obscure, or perplexing makes it harder for others to know what a person might be trying to say, or what they want. Indirect communication is a major factor in relationship dissatisfaction. HERE IS HOW THE GAME IS PLAYED. First, I will be reading aloud a statement or phrase that an overcontrolled person actually made. The game is to see how fast all of us can figure out what they actually meant, and then see if we can figure out what most other people might actually hear. OKAY—LET'S PLAY!*

What an OC Person Said	What the OC Person Actually Meant	What Other People Heard
Hmmm	I don't agree	They are interested in our discussion
Probably	No OR Not likely	A very good chance
I'm fine	I don't agree OR I am unhappy	They agree OR They are satisfied
Not exactly	You're wrong OR You're an idiot	They think I nearly understand
Yes, but…	No, and here is how you are wrong…	They agree in principle but may have a few minor concerns
I was a bit disappointed	I was really annoyed OR I was really distressed	It doesn't really matter
Maybe	No	Possibly yes
I'm sure it is my fault	It's your fault	Why are they blaming themselves?
I'll try	I plan on doing nothing	They are committed to doing something different
I guess so…	No, what you suggest is ridiculous	They are in agreement
I don't know	I know, but I'm not going to tell you	They don't know
Let's do it your way	I plan on sabotaging things if this continues	They are finally in agreement.
Not bad	It's good OR I liked it	Barely tolerable OR Awful

Game Instructions

1. **Read aloud the phrase in column 1,** prefacing it by saying: *This is what the OC person said.*

2. **Ask:** *What is the OC person actually saying? For example, what does "Hmmm" mean in OC language?* Encourage the class to go wild with guesses (for about ten seconds), then quickly read aloud the answer provided in column 2. Applaud and celebrate participation as a tribe, not individual efforts or success. (*Note:* Most often OC clients are very good at identifying column 2.)

3. **Without further discussion, ask:** *What do other people hear? For example, when the OC person says "Hmmm," what do non-OC people hear?* Encourage the class go wild again with guesses (for about ten seconds), then quickly read aloud the answer provided in column 3. Applaud and celebrate participation.

4. **Quickly move to the next round in the game** by reading aloud the next phrase in column 1 and repeating the preceding steps.

NOTE TO INSTRUCTORS: Don't feel obligated to cover all of the phrases in the table. Plus, the class can make up new OC phrases of their own. The idea is to make this a quick and fun exercise, with little discussion during the actual game itself.

5. **End the game by soliciting observations and discussing what was learned. For example...**

   ✓ **Ask:** *What does this game tell us about OC communication habits?*

   ✓ **Ask:** *To what extent do you use some of the OC phrases in the game?*

   ✓ **Ask:** *To what extent do you purposefully use vagueness or indirect communication as a way to avoid something, control something, or get what you want?*

   ✓ **Ask:** *What is it that we might need to learn from this?*

Lesson 15 Homework

1. **(Required) Worksheet 15.A (Recognizing Indirect Communication).** Ask the class to look out for any disguised demands they may exhibit over the next week and record what the disguised demand was, what they desired to signal to the other person, what they think the other person may have understood, and what the consequence was (similar to the miniexercise conducted in class). Next week's teaching will continue with this topic.

Radical Openness Handout 15.1

Main Points for Lesson 15: Interpersonal Integrity, Part 1

Saying What We Really Mean

1. How we say something matters more than what we say.
2. When apparently innocent questions become disguised demands, relationship problems often follow.

Radical Openness Worksheet 15.A

Recognizing Indirect Communication

Look for three times you communicated indirectly in the coming week, and record them in the following table.

What was the disguised demand or indirect communication?	What did you intend to communicate?	How did the other person react to the indirect communication? Describe what they said and did.	How could you have communicated your intentions more directly?
1	1	1	1
2	2	2	2
3	3	3	3

Interpersonal Integrity, Part 2

Flexible Mind REVEALs

Main Points for Lesson 16

1. There are two common OC disguised demands, referred to as *"pushback"* and *"don't hurt me"* responses.

2. Both are disguised demands, or maladaptive social signals, that negatively impact relationships.

3. Both function to block unwanted feedback or requests to join with others; they are nonengagement signals.

4. Both function to control others, yet the indirect manner by which they are expressed makes it plausible for the sender to deny this.

5. Both function to allow one to avoid taking responsibility for how one may have contributed to a problem or difficulty by implying that the fault lies with the other person or elsewhere.

6. Both are experienced as aversive or punishing by those on the receiving end.

7. Use Flexible Mind REVEALs to let go of habitual "pushback" and "don't hurt me" responses.

Materials Needed

- Handout 16.1 (Identifying "Pushbacks" and "Don't Hurt Me" Responses)
- Handout 16.2 (Using Self-Enquiry to Explore "Don't Hurt Me" and "Pushback" Behaviors)
- (Optional) Handout 16.3 (Main Points for Lesson 16: Interpersonal Integrity, Part 2: Flexible Mind REVEALs)
- Worksheet 16.A (Flexible Mind REVEALs)
- Worksheet 16.B (Identifying Secret Desires for Control)
- Flipchart or whiteboard and markers

(Required) Role Play

"Pushbacks" and "Don't Hurt Me" Responses

> NOTE TO INSTRUCTORS: This role play viscerally demonstrates all the teaching points to come and smuggles fun at the same time. By now, most class participants will recognize the apparently perplexing interchange between their previously friendly instructors as a deliberate and clever way to make a teaching point (and will be grinning with delight). Instructors should feel free to ham it up or make up their own lines.

- *There are two common disguised demands, known as "pushbacks" and "don't hurt me" responses.*

Immediately after communicating the preceding teaching point, start the role play.

The instructor turns toward the coinstructor, and they have the following exchange.

Instructor: (*matter-of-fact friendly voice tone*) Can you please demonstrate to the class what a "pushback" might look like?

Coinstructor: (*cool and aloof voice tone, flat facial expression*) What do you want me to do that for?

Instructor: (*pleading voice tone*) Well, I think it would be really nice if we could show the class what they look like rather than just talk about them.

Coinstructor: (*unsympathetic voice tone with slightly disgusted facial expression*) Where did you ever get that idea?

Instructor: (*placating and beseeching voice tone*) Well, you know, we have done these types of demonstrations together before, and they have really helped our teaching. Couldn't you just help me out this one time by showing the class a "pushback"—please?

Coinstructor: (*contemptuous or sarcastic voice tone and hostile stare*) It sounds to me like you've really got a problem here. Maybe you need to rethink what you're doing.

End the role play here, with the instructor applauding the performance of the coinstructor, who can take a bow.

Immediately teach the following points.

- *That was what is known as a "pushback."*
- *"Pushbacks" block unwanted requests or feedback from others. In this case, the "pushback" functioned to allow my coinstructor to block a request for help on my part, without having to admit it.*
- *Thus, "pushbacks" always have plausible deniability.*
  - *For example, if I had tried to challenge my coinstructor's apparent lack of helpfulness, my challenge could be easily dismissed.*
  - *The "pushback" implies that the request is inappropriate, stupid, or would be demeaning to comply with, despite the fact that their job is to help teach!*
  - *My coinstructor could simply claim that they were trying to ascertain the rationale behind my request before they complied with it* (that is, there is no definitive proof of deliberate sabotaging).

Without further discussion, the instructor turns toward the coinstructor, and they have the following exchange.

Instructor: (*matter-of-fact friendly voice tone*) Can you please demonstrate to the class what a "don't hurt me" might look like?

Coinstructor: (*overly friendly or syrupy voice tone, smiling and nodding*) Wow, thanks for asking—but, you know, I really think you are much better than me at demonstrating these types of things.

Instructor: (*inquisitive voice tone*) Well, I think it would be really nice if you could show the class what a "don't hurt me" looks like, especially since it has really helped our teaching when you have done so in the past.

Coinstructor: (*distraught voice tone, chin tilted slightly downward, loss of eye contact, slight frown*) You know, I really try hard to help you out whenever you ask me to do things, but I am really tired today, and I just don't think I can help you with this one.

Instructor: (*perplexed voice tone*) I'm a bit confused—you have helped me out in the past with something like this. All I am asking is for you to show the class what a "don't hurt me" might look like. Don't you think you could at least try?

Coinstructor: (*wounded or persecuted voice tone with slumped shoulders, bowed or lowered head, no eye contact, and feigned tearfulness*) I'm starting to get a headache. If you really cared about me, you would understand that I just can't do what you want—it's just too much. If you were really my friend, you would know this already.

End the role play here, with the instructor again applauding the performance of the coinstructor, who can take another bow.

Then teach the following points.

- *That was what is known as a "don't hurt me."*
  - ✓ **Ask:** *How is it different from a "pushback"? How is it similar?*
- *A "don't hurt me" functions to block unwanted requests or feedback from others.*
  - *It allowed my coinstructor to avoid or control the situation, without having to admit to it.*
  - *It also simultaneously implied that my request for help was inappropriate or mean-spirited, despite the fact that their job is to help teach!*
- *Thus, just like a "pushback," a "don't hurt me" has plausible deniability.*
  - ✓ **Ask:** *What do you think might have happened if I had challenged my coinstructor's behavior as being feigned or irresponsible?*

(Required) Teaching Point
"Don't Hurt Me" Responses

- *A "don't hurt me" response contains two disguised social signals:*
  1. **You don't understand me.**
  2. **You are hurting me.**

- *Essentially, it says:* **If you were a nice person you would stop asking me to change, or stop giving me feedback, because you would recognize the inappropriateness of what you are doing.**

- *"Don't hurt me" responses are signaled nonverbally. Examples include* pouting, sulking, moping, pursed lips, frowning, head down, hiding face, downcast eyes, brooding, sighing, whining, whimpering, moaning, beseeching, and begging.

- *We react emotionally to "don't hurt me" social signals whether we like it or not* (for example, recall that facial expressions trigger unconditioned emotional responses).

- *Despite their apparently compliant or submissive nature, "don't hurt me" responses function to covertly control the behavior of others,* most often by blocking unwanted feedback and/or by disrupting requests for change.

- *"Don't hurt me" responses are extremely effective because they function to elicit caregiving responses from the tribe rather than confrontation*—for example, desires to soothe, help, or apologetically reassure. Plus, their covert nature makes it difficult for someone to challenge their authenticity.

- *People tend to avoid individuals who habitually use "don't hurt me" responses and may perceive them as incompetent, unwell, or fragile* (for example, walking on eggshells whenever around them, for fear of upsetting them).

  ✓ **Ask:** *To what extent do you think you engage in "don't hurt me" responses? How and when do they show up?*

  ✓ **Ask:** *Have you ever purposefully used a "don't hurt me" response to get someone to do what you wanted or stop them from doing something you didn't want? What might this tell you?*

  ✓ **Ask:** *Is a "don't hurt me" social signal more vague and ambiguous OR more candid and up-front? Which way of social signaling do you prefer to be seen doing? What might this tell you about your values?*

  ✓ **Ask:** *What are you trying to say to others when you engage in a "don't hurt me" response? What prevents you from being more direct?*

  ✓ **Ask:** *What type of message does a "don't hurt me" response send to others? For example, does a "don't hurt me" response signal competence or incompetence to another person? How confident would you feel about flying with an airline captain who signaled a "don't hurt me" response just before takeoff? Or putting yourself in the hands of a surgeon who signaled a "don't hurt me" response just before performing heart surgery?*

  ✓ **Ask:** *If a person frequently engages in "don't hurt me" behaviors—for example, head down, shoulders slumped, eyes downcast, dejected facial expressions—what type of message are they sending to themselves? How might this impact their sense of well-being?*

  ✓ **Ask:** *How do you feel when another person engages in a "don't hurt me" response around you? Do you like it? Do you feel sorry for them? Do you ever feel manipulated?*

  ✓ **Ask:** *How might "don't hurt me" responses impact relationships? What are the advantages of "don't hurt me" responses?*

  ✓ **Ask:** *To what extent are you resisting, avoiding, or disliking this discussion about "don't hurt me" responses? Does your resistance signal that there is something important for you to acknowledge or recognize about yourself? What might your resistance say if it could speak? Is it possible that you are numbing out or shutting down in order to avoid taking responsibility or make important changes? What is it that needs to be learned?*

(Required) Teaching Point

"Pushback" Responses

- *A "pushback" response contains two disguised social signals:*

  1. **I'm not telling you what to do.**

  2. **But you'd better do what I want.**

- *Essentially, it says:* If you were wise, you would immediately stop challenging me, asking me questions, or giving me feedback, because I will make your life miserable if you don't comply with my wishes, in a way that no one can ever prove.

- *"Pushback" responses are signaled nonverbally.* Examples include flat and stony facial expressions, the silent treatment; scowling; hostile stares; walking away; contemptuous expressions; eye rolls; disgust reactions; cold, sharp, sarcastic, patronizing, and monotonic voice tones; callous smiles; burglar smiles; dismissive gestures; sneering, snickering, mockery, scornful giggling, laughing disdainfully.

- *"Pushback" responses trigger the threat system and defensive arousal in the other person* (that is, they are likely to want to flee or fight; run away or punch them).

NOTE TO INSTRUCTORS: A burglar smile is an expression of secret pleasure. It is signaled by a quick upturn of the mouth into a slight smile that is not easily controlled and most often occurs without conscious awareness. It appears whenever a secretly held belief, desire, or behavior has been uncovered, highlighted, or exposed that would normally be considered improper, bad-mannered, or inappropriate to publicly reveal pleasure or boast about. For example, a burglar smile is likely following praise of superior capacities for self-control by a person who values self-control, whereas a person valuing intelligence is likely to exhibit a burglar smile following praise concerning their superior intellectual abilities. Burglar smiles also emerge whenever a person experiences secret pleasure at having gotten away with something socially inappropriate, after feeling vindicated that one was right or correct, or upon hearing about a failure of a rival (see lesson 27, on envy).

- *"Pushbacks" are social dominance signals stemming from Fixed Mind thinking.* They function to control others and/or block unwanted feedback, without the sender having to take responsibility for doing so. They are designed to elicit compliance, capitulation, submission, obedience, and/or apologies from others.

- *Most people tend to avoid individuals who frequently use "pushback" responses to get what they want because they fear reprisal* (for example, they may walk on eggshells in order to avoid annoying, upsetting, or appearing to oppose them).

  ✓ **Ask:** *To what extent do you think you engage in "pushback" responses? How and when do they show up?*

  ✓ **Ask:** *Have you ever purposefully used a "pushback" response to get someone to do what you wanted or stop them from doing something you didn't want? What might this tell you?*

  ✓ **Ask:** *Is a "pushback" social signal direct and forthright, or evasive and indirect? Which type of social signaling do you prefer or value? What might this tell you about your values?*

✓ **Ask:** *What are you trying to say to others when you engage in a "pushback" response? What prevents you from being more open and direct about your intentions, needs, or wants?*

✓ **Ask:** *What type of message does a "pushback" response send to others? How does it feel when another person uses a "pushback" on you? Is it a pleasurable experience? Do you feel warmhearted toward them? Do you want to spend more time with them? Does it lead to greater trust? What might this tell you about how "pushbacks" impact relationships?*

✓ **Ask:** *How might habitual use of "pushback" responses impact a person's sense of self or their emotional well-being? To what extent do you think "pushback" behaviors could lead to a self-fulfilling prophecy (for example, a person believes that others are out to get them, so they attack first, thereby making it less likely for others to behave kindly toward them).*

✓ **Ask:** *What are the advantages of engaging in "pushback" behaviors? What do you fear might happen if you stopped engaging in "pushback" behaviors? Is there something here to learn?*

✓ **Ask:** *To what extent are you resisting, avoiding, or disliking this discussion about "pushback" responses? What might this tell you? Does your resistance suggest that there is something important for you to acknowledge or recognize about yourself? What are you afraid might happen if you let your guard down? What is it that you need to learn?*

NOTE TO INSTRUCTORS: The silent treatment represents another good example of a powerful yet indirect social signal. It most often occurs following a disagreement with someone, or when a person fails to conform to expectations. It signals disagreement or anger without overtly disclosing it, involving a sudden reduction in verbal behavior, a flattened facial expression, and avoidance of eye contact. If asked by the recipient about the sudden change in social signaling, the sender will usually deny the change and with a blank face and unemotional tone of voice say, "No, I'm fine" or "Everything's okay." The sudden nature of the silent treatment and its plausible deniability is what makes it so infuriating to those on the receiving end and so damaging to interpersonal relationships.

In summary, both "pushback" and "don't hurt me" responses…

- *Represent hidden intentions or disguised demands* that negatively impact relationships

- *Function to block unwanted feedback* or requests to join with others; they are nonengagement signals

- *Function to secretly control others,* yet the indirect manner in which they are expressed makes it plausible for the sender to deny this

- *Function to allow one to avoid taking responsibility* for how one may have contributed to a problem or difficulty by implying that the fault lies with the other person or elsewhere

- *Are experienced as aversive* or punishing by those on the receiving end

(Required) Teaching Point
Letting Go of Habitual "Pushback" and "Don't Hurt Me" Responses: Flexible Mind REVEALs

Refer participants to worksheet 16.A (Flexible Mind REVEALs).

NOTE TO INSTRUCTORS: Write out the acronym (REVEAL) on a flipchart or whiteboard with each letter arranged vertically in a column, but *without* teaching or naming the specific skills that each letter signifies. Next, starting with the first letter in the acronym (R in REVEAL), teach the skills associated with each letter in the acronym, using the key points outlined in the following sections, until you have covered all of the skills associated with each individual letter. Importantly, only write out on the whiteboard or flipchart the global description of what each letter actually stands for when you are teaching the skills associated with its corresponding letter. This teaching method avoids long explanations about the use of certain words in the acronym and/or premature teaching of concepts, since the meaning of each letter is only revealed during the formal teaching of the skills associated with it.

Flexible Mind REVEALs

R   **Recognize** secret desires for control

E   **Examine** your social signaling and label what you find

V   Remember your core **Values**

E   **Engage** with integrity by outing yourself

A   Practice Flexible Mind **ADOPTS**

L   **Learn** through self-enquiry

R **Recognize** *secret desires for control.*

- *Use the following self-enquiry questions to help identify when you may be hiding your intentions from others or secretly hoping to control or manipulate them.*

    - *To what extent am I proud of the way I am behaving? Would I encourage another person or a young child to behave similarly when they interact with me? What might this tell me about my values and/or how I feel about the way I am behaving or thinking? What is it that I might need to learn?*

    - *If I am proud of how I am behaving or thinking, then what is preventing me from more openly revealing my true intentions to the other person or persons?*

    - *Would I feel embarrassed, distressed, or annoyed if my intentions or desires were to be revealed to others or made public?*

- *Practice acknowledging your desires for control* rather than denying, pretending, or telling yourself that you will fall apart if you were to ever admit their existence.

- *Use the following examples to help identify secret desires for control.*

    ➢ Desires for someone to stop giving you feedback (for example, criticism or praise) or expressing how they feel (for example, how angry they are with you).

    ➢ Desires to punish someone for not behaving according to your standards or for failing to complete a task in the manner or time frame you believe appropriate.

    ➢ Desires for someone to help you and/or your expectations that they should either already be helping or know when you need it.

    ➢ Desires for someone to acknowledge how hard your life has been and as a consequence not push you to make needed changes or expect much from you.

335

➤ Desires for the world or others to change in order to suit how you think things should be or enable you to get what you want.

➤ Desires for the other person to be nice to you, soothing, or validating.

➤ Desires to walk away or for another person to walk away or leave you alone.

➤ Desires for someone to behave or think like you do.

➤ Desires to get what you want, prove another wrong, and/or dominate a situation or another person.

➤ Desires to sabotage the efforts of others in order to prove a point or win.

➤ Desires to change the topic in order to avoid a potential conflict.

➤ Desires for others to recognize your good intentions, acknowledge your hard work, and appreciate your self-sacrifices.

➤ Desires for vengeance and/or to pay back another person for what you perceive to be wrongdoings and/or moral failings on their part.

➤ Desires for someone to stop talking.

E Examine *your social signaling and label what you find.*

- *Secret desires thrive on secrecy. (Shhhh…that's why they're a secret. ☺)* Labeling brings them into the limelight.

- *Identify the type of disguised demand you are using via the following steps;* see also handout 16.1 (Identifying "Pushbacks" and "Don't Hurt Me" Responses) for additional clues.

- *You are likely signaling a "don't hurt me" if…*

  - You are secretly hoping the other person will acknowledge how hard your life has been and/or recognize that your prior traumas, struggles, or hard work entitle you to special treatment.

  - You secretly believe that it is unfair for others to challenge, question, or provide you with unwanted feedback, unless it is delivered in just the right way and/or it is agreed beforehand that expectations for change are either minimal or fully in your control.

  - Your head is hanging low, your shoulders are slumped, and you avoid eye contact; you are sighing and/or are tearful; you are pouting; you feel like things are hopeless and/or that you are being unfairly picked on.

- *You are likely signaling a "pushback" if…*

  - You are secretly hoping to prove the other person wrong, sabotage their efforts, and/or dominate what is happening in order to win, prove a point, or punish them for not behaving according to your standards.

  - You feel superior to them and are offended by what you perceive as an inappropriate challenge of your authority over them, your superior knowledge or experience, and/or your better character. You desire to make them pay for their lack of respect.

  - You desire to correct them. You are secretly annoyed by what you imagine is the other person's lack of awareness, lack of intelligence, selfishness, and/or inability to apply the effort needed to behave in a manner that you believe to be proper or correct. You desire to ridicule them.

  - Your facial expression is flat and unexpressive; you stare at them intensely; you sneer, curl your lips, or roll your eyes whenever they speak; your voice tone is clipped, cold, flat, or sarcastic, and/or when you laugh it feels false or derisive.

NOTE TO INSTRUCTORS: Knowing whether you are using a "pushback" or a "don't hurt me" response is important because it can help a person recognize how they might habitually perceive the world and/or themselves. It can help a person begin to identify areas in their life that may require self-work. For example, if someone tends to display "don't hurt me" responses when under stress, this often suggests that they need to work on signaling competence; standing up for what they believe; expressing anger, dislike, and/or their opinions more directly; and taking a more active role in solving their own problems rather than expecting others to. If someone tends to use "pushbacks" under stress, this usually means they need to focus on revealing vulnerability or weakness, admitting mistakes, and/or being more open to differing points of view. "Don't hurt me" responses are more common among the overly agreeable OC subtype, whereas "pushback" responses are more common among the overly disagreeable OC subtype (see chapter 3 of the RO DBT textbook).

V *Remember your core* **Values**.

- *Identify core values that are inconsistent with secret desires to manipulate or control others, in order to help loosen their grip.* Use the following questions to facilitate values clarification.

  - ✓ **Ask:** *To what extent do I believe it important for a person to do the right thing, be honest, have integrity, and/or be fair and straight with others? What might this tell me about my core values?*

  - ✓ **Ask:** *Do I believe deceiving, manipulating, and/or concealing one's true intentions from another the best way to live? If not, then what might this tell me about my values?*

  - ✓ **Ask:** *Would I teach a young child to cheat, lie, or manipulate others? What might this say about what I believe important?*

- *Stop assuming that no one knows you are pretending or hiding something from them.* Research shows that others are able to detect when a person is deliberately attempting to suppress an emotion (Gross & John, 2003). Although imperfect, humans are good social safety detectors (that is, we are able to know when a person is feeling safe and/or when they like us). Our species' and tribal survival depended on our ability to recognize whether another person intended us harm. This is why we are so good at detecting a fake smile, an uptight tone of voice, and/or a phony laugh.

- *Practice living by your values by going opposite to your manipulative social signal.*

  - *When signaling a "don't hurt me," go opposite to desires to appear weak, submissive, or helpless by being direct, candid, and open.*

    1. **Go opposite to urges to hide your face or slump your shoulders** by puffing your chest out, standing or sitting upright, putting your shoulders back, and keeping your chin up when speaking.

    2. **Activate your social safety system** (for example, Big Three + 1, LKM practice; see lessons 3 and 4) prior to social interactions that may trigger habitual "don't hurt me" responses.

    3. **Remember your superior capacity for inhibitory control when you find yourself wanting to slip back into "don't hurt me" social signaling** (for example, recall times when you made self-sacrifices or persisted in difficult tasks in order to help others or benefit society, and/or recall people who have thrived despite terrible odds against them).

  - *When using a "pushback," go opposite to desires to appear dominant, unflappable, or invulnerable by signaling vulnerability, openness, and humility.*

1. **Activate your social safety system** (for example, Big Three + 1, LKM practice; see lessons 3 and 4) prior to social interactions that may trigger habitual "pushback" responses.

2. **Go opposite to urges to stand tall and stare them down** (like Clint Eastwood before he shoots the bad guy) by rounding your shoulders, using openhanded gestures, and raising your eyebrows when you speak.

3. **Remember your core values for fair-mindedness and truthfulness** when you find yourself speaking in riddles, purposefully answering questions with a question, and/or deliberating, making things difficult for the other person.

E Engage *with integrity by outing yourself.*

- *"Pushback" and "don't hurt me" responses thrive on secrecy.* They tend to immediately shrivel up or disappear when publicly revealed or admitted.

- *Practice outing yourself whenever you find yourself conspiring to control another person or a situation you are in.* Take responsibility for your emotional reactions rather than blaming them on others or expecting the world to change. Explain that outing oneself to another person is a core part of RO mindfulness training and a core means by which overcontrolled individuals learn how to go opposite to automatic tendencies to mask inner feelings. Outing oneself means taking responsibility for one's own perceptions rather than expecting the world to change.

- *Block automatic attempts by the listener to reassure, validate, or soothe when you practice outing yourself* by reminding them that part of your practice is to learn to be more forthright and open to critical feedback. Let go of assuming that outing yourself to another person will get you what you want.

- *Disclose your desire to either push back or signal a "don't hurt me" to the person you are interacting with* instead of keeping it secret. For example, tell the other person that you are working on being more candid and open about your inner experience rather than hiding or pretending that everything is okay.

- *Use Flexible Mind Is DEEP skills to practice openly expressing your needs,* wants, and desires in order to live by your valued goals (see lesson 10).

- *Encourage those you care for to be more open with you,* and reinforce them when they are (for example, say "Thank you").

- *Practice being more candid with people in general;* for example, if you want someone to take the garbage out, ask them to do so directly rather than hinting at it or assuming they should already have done it or known about it.

- *Practice revealing dislike or disagreement without expecting the other person to change.* For example, openly reveal your discomfort to the person who is giving you feedback, but make it clear that you are not implying they should stop or change what they are doing. Or explain how you are working to see discomfort as an opportunity for growth via a practice of self-enquiry.

- *Practice revealing desires for the other person to be soothing, validating, or give you what you want.* For example, if you are pouting, rather than pretending otherwise, tell the other person that you are purposefully trying to punish them by pouting because you are angry about not getting your way and/or you want them to recognize how hard you are working or trying to do the right thing.

A *Practice Flexible Mind* **ADOPTS***.*

- *Use handout 22.1 (Being Open to Feedback from Others: Flexible Mind ADOPTS) to enhance open listening after revealing your secret intentions, in order to learn and/ or enhance social connectedness.*

- *Use the twelve steps for evaluating feedback in Flexible Mind ADOPTS to determine whether to accept or decline any feedback you might receive.*

L **Learn** *through self-enquiry.*

- **Practice self-enquiry in order to strengthen your learning.**

- **Remember, self-enquiry involves a willingness to question ourselves when we feel threatened or challenged** rather than automatically defending ourselves.

- **It means finding a good question, in order to learn,** and then allowing an answer (if there is one) to be self-discovered by the practitioner. This is why self-enquiry practices should be expected to last over days or weeks.

- *It begins by asking:* **What is it that I might need to learn [from this painful experience]?**

- *Keep your practices short, and be suspicious of quick answers. Record what emerges from your practice in your self-enquiry journal.*

- *Use the following questions to help guide your practice and/or the questions in handout 16.2 (Using Self-Enquiry to Explore "Don't Hurt Me" and "Pushback" Behaviors).*

  ➢ *What is it that I need to learn from how I communicate my needs, wants, and desires to others? To what extent am I willing to truly examine my social signaling behaviors? What might this tell me?*

  ➢ *What am I trying to say or signal to others when I engage in a "pushback" or "don't hurt me" response? What is preventing me from being more open and direct about my intentions, needs, or wants? What is it that I might need to learn?*

  ➢ *Where did I ever get the idea that being direct or open about one's inner experience is wrong, inappropriate, ineffective, or dangerous?*

  ➢ *Is it possible that my automatic distrust or suspicion of others creates a self-fulfilling prophecy? What am I afraid of?*

  ➢ *To what extent do I expect others to treat me as special? What might this tell me about my social signaling?*

  ➢ *How often do I feel that my efforts or self-sacrifices go unrecognized by others? What prevents me from telling others about my disappointment or desires for appreciation? How might my lack of disclosure impact my personal well-being and my relationships with others? What is it that I might need to learn?*

  ➢ *To what extent do I believe others should know what I am thinking, wanting, or expecting to happen, without me having to tell them? How often do I assume that I have been direct with someone about what I wanted, only to find out later that the other person did not actually know what it was that I wanted? What might this tell me about my assumptions about the world? What might this tell me about my style of communication? Is there something to learn here?*

339

Lesson 16 Homework

1. (Required) Worksheet 16.A (Flexible Mind REVEALs)
2. (Required) Handout 16.2 (Using Self-Enquiry to Explore "Pushback" and "Don't Hurt Me" Behaviors) to augment the skills in Flexible Mind REVEALs
3. (Optional) Worksheet 16.B (Identifying Secret Desires for Control)

Radical Openness Handout 16.1

Identifying "Pushbacks" and "Don't Hurt Me" Responses

Both "pushback" and "don't hurt me" responses...

- *Represent hidden intentions or disguised demands* that negatively impact relationships

- *Function to block unwanted feedback* or requests to join with others; they are nonengagement signals

- *Function to secretly control others,* yet the indirect manner in which they are expressed makes it plausible for the sender to deny this

- *Function to allow one to avoid taking responsibility* for how one may have contributed to a problem or difficulty by implying that the fault lies with the other person or elsewhere

- *Are experienced as aversive* or punishing by those on the receiving end

- A "don't hurt me" response contains two disguised social signals:

  1. *You don't understand me.*

  2. *You are hurting me.*

- **"Don't hurt me" responses are signaled nonverbally** via pouting, sulking, moping, pursed lips, frowning, head down, hiding face, downcast eyes, brooding, sighing, whining, whimpering, moaning, beseeching, and begging.

- Despite their apparently compliant or submissive nature, "don't hurt me" responses function to **covertly control the behavior of others,** most often by blocking unwanted feedback and/or by disrupting requests for change.

- They are extremely effective because they function to elicit caregiving responses from the tribe rather than confrontation—for example, desires to soothe, help, or apologetically reassure.

- Their secret or covert nature makes it difficult for someone to challenge their authenticity.

- Most people tend to avoid individuals who habitually use "don't hurt me" responses (for example, walking on eggshells whenever around them, for fear of upsetting them) **and/or may perceive them as incompetent, unwell, or fragile.**

- A "pushback" response contains two disguised social signals:

  1. *I'm not telling you what to do.*

  2. *But you'd better do what I want.*

- **"Pushback" responses are signaled nonverbally** via flat and stony facial expressions, the silent treatment; scowling; hostile stares; walking away; contemptuous expressions; eye rolls; disgust reactions; cold, sharp, sarcastic, patronizing, and monotonic voice tones; callous smiles, burglar smiles; dismissive gestures; sneering, snickering, mockery, scornful giggling, laughing disdainfully.

- **"Pushback" responses are likely to elicit "pushback" responses from the recipient.** Most people don't like being pushed, and the most common reaction is retaliation or hostility, triggering "pushback" wars or feuds. The end result can be a severely damaged relationship. Ask yourself: *Is this the type of reaction I want to elicit?*

341

- **"Pushbacks" are social dominance signals stemming from Fixed Mind thinking.** They function to control others and/or block unwanted feedback, without the sender having to take responsibility for doing so. They are designed to elicit compliance, capitulation, submission, obedience, and/or apologies from others.

- **Most people tend to avoid individuals who frequently use "pushback" responses to get what they want because they fear reprisal** (for example, they may walk on eggshells in order to avoid annoying, upsetting, or appearing to oppose them).

Describe other social signaling habits that you have developed over the years.

_____

_____

_____

_____

Radical Openness Handout 16.2

Using Self-Enquiry to Explore "Pushback" and "Don't Hurt Me" Behaviors

- **Remember, self-enquiry involves a willingness to question ourselves when we feel threatened or challenged** rather than automatically defending ourselves.

- **It means finding a good question, in order to learn,** and then allowing an answer (if there is one) to be self-discovered by the practitioner. This is why self-enquiry practices should be expected to last over days or weeks.

- **It begins by asking:** *What is it that I might need to learn [from this painful experience]?*

- **Remember to keep your practices short and to be suspicious of quick answers.** Record what emerges from your practice in your self-enquiry journal. Use the following questions to help guide your practice.

  ➢ *To what extent am I proud of the way I am behaving? Would I encourage another person or a young child to behave similarly when they interact with me? What might this tell me about my values and/or how I feel about the way I am behaving or thinking? What is it that I might need to learn?*

  ➢ *If I am proud of how I am behaving or thinking, then what is preventing me from more openly revealing my true intentions to the other person or persons?*

  ➢ *Would I feel embarrassed, distressed, or annoyed if my intentions or desires were to be revealed to others or made public?*

  ➢ *To what extent do I engage in "don't hurt me" responses? How and when do they show up?*

  ➢ *To what extent do I engage in "pushback" responses? How and when do they show up?*

  ➢ *Have I ever purposefully used a "don't hurt me" response to get someone to do what I wanted or stop them from doing something I didn't want? What might this tell me about my style of social signaling?*

  ➢ *Have I ever purposefully used a "pushback" response to get someone to do what I wanted or stop them from doing something I didn't want? What might this tell me about myself?*

  ➢ *Is a "don't hurt me" social signal more vague and ambiguous OR more candid and up-front? Is a "pushback" social signal direct and forthright OR evasive and indirect? Which type of social signaling do I prefer or value? What might this tell me about my values or my style of social signaling?*

  ➢ *What am I trying to say to others when I engage in a "don't hurt me" response? What prevents me from being more direct?*

  ➢ *What am I trying to say to others when I engage in a "pushback" response? What prevents me from being more open and direct about my intentions?*

  ➢ *What type of message does a "don't hurt me" response send to others? Does a "don't hurt me" signal competence or incompetence to another person? How confident would I feel about flying with an airline captain who signaled a "don't hurt me" response just before takeoff? Or putting myself in the hands of a surgeon who signaled a "don't hurt me" response just before performing heart surgery? What might this tell me about how "don't hurt me" responses impact relationships?*

  ➢ *What type of message does a "pushback" response send to others? How does it feel when another person uses a "pushback" on me? Is it a pleasurable experience? Do I feel warmhearted toward them? Do I want*

343

to spend more time with them? Does it lead to greater trust between us? What might this tell me about how pushbacks impact relationships?

➤ *If a person frequently engages in "don't hurt me" behaviors—for example, head down, shoulders slumped, eyes downcast, dejected facial expressions—what type of message are they sending to themselves? How might this impact their sense of well-being?*

➤ *How might habitual use of "pushback" responses impact a person's sense of self or their emotional well-being?*

➤ *How do I feel when another person engages in a "don't hurt me" response around me? Do I like it? Do I feel sorry for them? Do I ever feel manipulated?*

➤ *How might "don't hurt me" responses impact relationships?*

➤ *What are the advantages of "don't hurt me" responses? What do I fear might happen if I stopped engaging in "don't hurt me" behaviors? Is there something here for me to learn?*

➤ *How do I feel when another person engages in a "pushback" response around me? Do I like it? Do I feel bullied or belittled? Do I ever feel manipulated?*

➤ *How might "pushback" responses impact relationships?*

➤ *What are the advantages of "pushback" responses? What do I fear might happen if I stopped engaging in "pushback" behaviors? Is there something here for me to learn?*

➤ *To what extent am I resisting, avoiding, or disliking self-enquiry about "don't hurt me" and "pushback" responses? Does my resistance signal that there is something important for me to acknowledge or recognize about myself?*

➤ *What might my resistance say to me if it could speak? Is it possible that I am numbing out or shutting down in order to avoid taking responsibility or make important changes in my life? What am I afraid might happen if I let my guard down? What is it that I might need to learn?*

➤ *What is it that I need to learn from how I communicate my needs, wants, and desires to others? To what extent am I willing to truly examine my social signaling behaviors? What might this tell me?*

➤ *What am I trying to say or signal to others when I engage in a "pushback" or "don't hurt me" response? What is preventing me from being more open and direct about my intentions, needs, or wants? What is it that I might need to learn?*

➤ *Where did I ever get the idea that being direct or open about one's inner experience is wrong, inappropriate, ineffective, or dangerous?*

➤ *Is it possible that my automatic distrust or suspicion of others creates a self-fulfilling prophecy? What am I afraid of?*

➤ *To what extent do I expect others to treat me as special? What might this tell me about my social signaling?*

➤ *How often do I feel that my efforts or self-sacrifices go unrecognized by others? What prevents me from telling others about my disappointment or desires for appreciation? How might my lack of disclosure impact my personal well-being and my relationships with others? What is it that I might need to learn?*

➤ *To what extent do I believe others should know what I am thinking, wanting, or expecting to happen, without me having to tell them? How often do I assume that I have been direct with someone about what I wanted, only to find out later that the other person did not actually know what it was that I wanted? What might this tell me about my assumptions about the world? What might this tell me about my style of communication? Is there something to learn here?*

Other self-enquiry questions.

Radical Openness Handout 16.3

Main Points for Lesson 16: Interpersonal Integrity, Part 2

Flexible Mind REVEALs

1. There are two common OC disguised demands, referred to as *"pushback"* and *"don't hurt me"* responses.

2. Both are disguised demands, or maladaptive social signals, that negatively impact relationships.

3. Both function to block unwanted feedback or requests to join with others; they are nonengagement signals.

4. Both function to control others, yet the indirect manner by which they are expressed makes it plausible for the sender to deny this.

5. Both function to avoid taking responsibility for how one may have contributed to a problem or difficulty by implying that the fault lies with the other person or elsewhere.

6. Both are experienced as aversive or punishing by those on the receiving end.

7. Use Flexible Mind REVEALs to let go of habitual "pushback" and "don't hurt me" responses.

Radical Openness Worksheet 16.A

Flexible Mind REVEALs

Flexible Mind REVEALs

R   **R**ecognize secret desires for control

E   **E**xamine your social signaling and label what you find

V   Remember your core **V**alues

E   **E**ngage with integrity by outing yourself

A   Practice Flexible Mind **ADOPTS**

L   **L**earn through self-enquiry

R   **R**ecognize *secret desires for control.*

Place a checkmark in the boxes next to the skills you practiced.

☐   Noticed times when I wanted to control a social interaction but did not want the other person to know about my secret intentions (for example, to influence, direct, stop, or change their behavior or the outcome of a social event).

     Describe an example of a secret desire for control.

_____

_____

_____

☐   Used self-enquiry to help identify times when I might want to hide my intentions from others or secretly control or manipulate the situation or behavior of others.

     Record the self-enquiry question you found most helpful.

_____

_____

_____

E **Examine** *your social signaling and label what you find.*

"Don't Hurt Me" Responses

Place a checkmark in the boxes next to the skills you practiced.

☐ Noticed desires to be treated as special.

☐ Noticed hidden beliefs that it is unfair for others to challenge, question, or criticize me without my approval, or unless it is delivered in just the right way.

☐ Recognized nonverbal signals linked to "don't hurt me" responses: head hanging, shoulders slumped, lack of eye contact, sighing, tearfulness, pouting.

Write in the space provided how your "don't hurt me" response was nonverbally signaled.

_____

_____

_____

"Pushback" Responses

Place a checkmark in the boxes next to the skills you practiced.

☐ Noticed secret desires to prove the other person wrong, sabotage their efforts, and/or dominate what is happening.

☐ Noticed times I felt offended by what I imagined to be an inappropriate challenge.

☐ Recognized times I strongly desired to correct or punish others for perceived wrongdoing.

☐ Recognized nonverbal signals linked to "pushback" responses: flat facial expression, intense stare, curling my lips, or rolling my eyes whenever the other person spoke; voice tone clipped, cold, or sarcastic.

Write in the space provided how your "pushback" response was nonverbally signaled.

_____

_____

_____

V *Remember your core* **Values**.

Place a checkmark in the boxes next to the skills you practiced.

- ☐ Used self-enquiry to identify my core values that conflict with desires to manipulate or control other people.

    Write in the space provided the self-enquiry questions you found most helpful.

    _____

    _____

    _____

- ☐ Stopped pretending to myself that others didn't already know most or many of my secrets.
- ☐ Practiced living by my values by going opposite to my manipulative social signal.

When Signaling a "Don't Hurt Me"…

Place a checkmark in the boxes next to the skills you practiced.

- ☐ **Went opposite to desires to appear weak, submissive, or helpless** by being direct, candid, and open.
- ☐ **Went opposite to urges to hide my face or slump my shoulders** by puffing out my chest, standing tall, sitting upright, and holding my head and chin high.
- ☐ **Activated my social safety system.**
- ☐ **Remembered that I am competent** (for example, recalled times when I made self-sacrifices or persisted in difficult tasks in order to help others or benefit society).

When Using a "Pushback"…

Place a checkmark in the boxes next to the skills you practiced.

- ☐ **Went opposite to desires to appear dominant, unflappable, or invulnerable** by signaling vulnerability, openness, and humility.
- ☐ **Activated my social safety system.**
- ☐ **Went opposite to urges to stand tall and stare them down** by rounding my shoulders, using open-handed gestures, and/or raising my eyebrows with a slight smile when I spoke.
- ☐ **Remembered my core values for fair-mindedness and truthfulness.**

E Engage *with integrity by outing yourself.*

Place a checkmark in the boxes next to the skills you practiced.

☐ Practiced outing myself rather than hiding my true intentions.

☐ Blocked attempts by the listener to reassure, validate, or soothe me when I outed myself.

☐ Disclosed my desire to either push back or signal a "don't hurt me" to the person I was interacting with instead of keeping it secret.

☐ Practiced taking responsibility for my personal reactions by revealing them.

☐ Practiced noticing what happened when I was more forthcoming with people.

☐ Took responsibility for my emotional reactions rather than blaming them on others or expecting the world to change.

☐ Practiced being more direct and candid with people in general.

☐ Used Flexible Mind Is DEEP skills in order to link my open expression with my valued goals.

☐ Practiced revealing dislike or disagreement, without expecting the other person to change.

☐ Encouraged others to feel free to reveal their inner feelings or reactions when interacting with me.

☐ Practiced revealing my desires for the other person to be soothing, validating, or give me what I wanted.

A *Practice Flexible Mind* ADOPTS.

Place a checkmark in the boxes next to the skills you practiced.

☐ Used handout 22.1 (Being Open to Feedback from Others: Flexible Mind ADOPTS) to enhance my receptivity to feedback.

☐ Used the twelve steps for evaluating feedback in Flexible Mind ADOPTS to determine whether to accept or decline feedback.

L Learn *through self-enquiry.*

Place a checkmark in the boxes next to the skills you practiced.

☐ Remembered that self-enquiry involves a willingness to question my intentions, beliefs, or behavior, without falling apart.

☐ Used the questions in handout 16.2 (Using Self-Enquiry to Explore "Don't Hurt Me" and "Pushback" Behaviors) to facilitate my self-enquiry practice.

Write in the space provided the self-enquiry questions you found most helpful.

_____

_____

_____

Radical Openness Worksheet 16.B

Identifying Secret Desires for Control

Use the following examples to help identify secret desires for control.

Place a checkmark in the boxes next to the desires that you have or have had and have struggled to reveal or disclose to others directly.

- ☐ Desires for someone to stop giving you feedback (for example, criticism or praise) or expressing how they feel (for example, how angry they are with you)

- ☐ Desires to punish someone for not behaving according to your standards or for failing to complete a task in the manner or time frame you believe appropriate

- ☐ Desires for someone to help you and/or expectations that they should either already be helping or know when you need it

- ☐ Desires for someone to acknowledge how hard your life has been and as a consequence not push you to make needed changes or expect much from you

- ☐ Desires for the world or others to change in order to suit how you think things should be or enable you to get what you want

- ☐ Desires for the other person to be nice to you, soothing, or validating

- ☐ Desires to walk away or for another person to walk away or leave you alone

- ☐ Desires for someone to behave or think like you do

- ☐ Desires to get what you want, prove another wrong, and/or dominate a situation or another person

- ☐ Desires to sabotage the efforts of others in order to prove a point or win

- ☐ Desires to change the topic in order to avoid a potential conflict

- ☐ Desires for others to recognize your good intentions, acknowledge your hard work, and appreciate your self-sacrifices

- ☐ Desires for vengeance and/or to pay back another person for what you perceive to be wrongdoings and/or moral failings on their part

Interpersonal Effectiveness

Kindness First and Foremost

Main Points for Lesson 17

1. Prior to an interaction, clarify your goals and objectives, and determine which one takes priority—that is, your personal objective, your relationship objective, or your self-respect objective.

2. Block excessive rehearsal of what you will say or how you will act, particularly when the interaction is purely social (for example, a picnic, a party).

3. Identify the valued goals you will need to live by when interacting with others. Use worksheet 10.A (Flexible Mind Is DEEP: Identifying Valued Goals) to help facilitate this process.

4. During the Interaction, practice kindness first and foremost.

5. Kindness signals affection and openness—it involves contributing to the well-being of others, without expecting anything in return.

6. Use Flexible Mind ROCKs ON to enhance interpersonal kindness, effectiveness, and connectedness.

Materials Needed

*   Handout 17.1 (Enhancing Interpersonal Kindness, Effectiveness, and Connectedness, Using Flexible Mind ROCKs ON)

*   Handout 17.2 (New Year's Resolutions)

*   Handout 17.3 (Signaling an Easy Manner)

*   (Optional) Handout 17.4 (Main Points for Lesson 17: Interpersonal Effectiveness: Kindness First and Foremost)

*   Handout 21.2 (Match + 1 Intimacy Rating Scale)

*   Worksheet 17.A (Overcontrolled Myths About Interpersonal Relationships)

*   Worksheet 17.B (Kindness First and Foremost)

*   Worksheet 17.C (Using Flexible Mind ROCKs ON to Enhance Interpersonal Effectiveness)

*   Flipchart or whiteboard and markers

(Recommended) Class Exercise
OC Myths About Interpersonal Relationships

NOTE TO INSTRUCTORS: The teaching for this lesson is recommended to start with a class exercise that involves identifying interpersonal myths and then using self-enquiry to learn more. Since time is always limited when teaching new material, instructors should keep this exercise short (ideally ten minutes). To help facilitate this, encourage participants to let go of doing it perfectly. Their goal for the exercise today is to find just one myth on the list that they want to practice self-enquiry with. It's about having fun exploring ourselves, not to get too heavy about it. Instructors may need to briefly demonstrate to the class how to use the recommended self-enquiry questions. You can also remind the class that this worksheet will be assigned as homework, so they will have more time over the coming week to go into greater depth with the material (at their leisure).

Refer participants to Worksheet 17.A (Overcontrolled Myths About Interpersonal Relationships).

Instruct the class to place a checkmark in the box next to each myth about interpersonal relationships that they believe to be true or somewhat true.

Divide participants into pairs. Have each member of the pair choose a myth that they believe in strongly and then take turns practicing self-enquiry and outing themselves about their respective myths. **Use the following steps to structure how to accomplish this.**

- The revealing partner—that is, the person who is outing themselves—begins by reading aloud their myth three times in a row to their partner.

- The listening partner then reads aloud several of the self-enquiry questions found in handout 1.3 (Learning from Self-Enquiry)—for example, *What is it that you need to learn from this myth? What might this myth be telling you about yourself and your life? Does the thought of reexamining this myth elicit tension? If so, then what might this mean? How open are you to thinking differently about this myth? If you are not open or only partly open, then what might this mean?*

- Pairs should then switch roles with the listener now taking the role of outing themselves by speaking aloud the images, thoughts, and memories linked to the myth they have chosen for their practice.

- After each pair has played both roles at least once, instructors should encourage participants to share their observations about the exercise with the entire class.

- Participants should incorporate the questions they found most provocative into their daily practice of self-enquiry and record their observations that result from this in the self-enquiry journal.

(Required) Teaching Point

Enhancing Interpersonal Kindness, Effectiveness, and Connectedness

- *Our previous lessons have focused on how to use social signaling to repair or improve damaged relationships (SAGE skills), openly express our emotions (DEEP skills), and live with integrity by saying what we really mean (REVEAL skills).*

- *Today's lesson will focus on how to prioritize our interpersonal objectives and use them to guide our behavior, and be able to go about it in a kind and easygoing manner.*

- *So just to be wicked—har har ☺—we call these new skills "Flexible Mind ROCKs ON!"*

- *To help remember them all, simply repeat the phrase "SAGE DEEP(ly) REVEALs—and ROCKs ON!" (tee hee ☺)*

(Required) Class Exercise

Making Flexible Mind ROCKs ON Come Alive

Instructors should look for creative ways to introduce Flexible Mind ROCKs ON. Use RO "participating without planning" principles to guide what you might do (that is, the exercise should be unannounced, should involve mimicking the instructor's movements, and should last no more than one minute; see lesson 12 for guidelines).

Example 1: Immediately after saying the preceding teaching point ("So just to be wicked—har har ☺—we call these new skills 'Flexible Mind ROCKs ON!'"), say to the class…

OKAY, EVERYBODY, STAND UP! GREAT! Now repeat after me, and do what I do! RAISE YOUR ARMS HIGH AND REACH FOR THE SKY—STICK YOUR CHIN OUT! We can remember our skills by repeating this phrase "SAGE DEEP(ly) REVEALs—and ROCKs ON!" Again! "SAGE DEEP(ly) REVEALs—and ROCKs ON!" One more time! "SAGE DEEP(ly) REVEALs—and ROCKs ON!" Okay, that's enough fun for now—everybody can sit back down. [Smile warmly.]

Instructors should then immediately move to the next teaching point (without discussion) and behave as if the practice you have just engaged in is a normal part of everyday life (that is, resume your normal voice tone and style of teaching). This smuggles not taking life too seriously and playful irreverence, without making it a big deal. A formal discussion of the preceding practice makes having fun or acting silly a serious affair. (See also "Fun Facts: Teasing and Being Teased," lesson 22).

Example 2: Prepare ahead of time a rock 'n' roll sound clip (one of our favorites is Huey Lewis and the News singing "The Power of Love"), and use the protocol already outlined to guide the exercise. Immediately after saying the preceding teaching point ("So just to be wicked—har har ☺—we call these new skills 'Flexible Mind ROCKs ON!'"), press the "play" button on your audioplayer and say to the class…

EVERYONE STAND UP! GREAT! OKAY, DO WHAT I DO. RAISE YOUR ARMS UP HIGH AND LET'S ROCK A LITTLE. MAKE YOUR ARMS GO LOW. NOW WIGGLE THEM ABOUT AND SHAKE YOUR HIPS! GROOVY, BABY! LET'S ROCK ON. OH YEAH—REACH TO THE SKY LIKE A BUTTERFLY! OH YEAH!

Instructors will need to shout their instructions over the music. Try to match your movements to the beat of the music, and keep the practice short—that is, turn off the music after about forty to sixty seconds, and stop the practice by saying: *Okay, that's great! Let's all sit back down.* **(Smile warmly; applause all around.)**

Without further discussion, immediately move on to the next teaching point, behaving as if the musical interlude is a normal part of everyday life.

Importantly, instructors both show and tell participants what to do moment by moment during this exercise (like the instructor for an aerobic workout). This keeps the attention focused on the instructor, not on what other classmates might be doing, thereby maximizing the likelihood for genuine non-self-conscious pleasure to be linked with participating with the tribe. Thus, despite it being tempting, avoid just playing the music and encouraging free-range dancing. Although most OC clients will comply, they are likely to feel highly self-conscious doing so, making the point of the practice moot. Recall that the goal of "participating without planning" exercises is to slowly build a bank of positive experiences linked to participating with others.

(Required) Teaching Point
Flexible Mind ROCKs ON

Refer participants to handout 17.1 (Enhancing Interpersonal Kindness, Effectiveness, and Connectedness, Using Flexible Mind ROCKs ON).

NOTE TO INSTRUCTORS: Write out the acronym (ROCKs ON) on a flipchart or whiteboard, with each letter arranged vertically in a column, but *without* teaching or naming the specific skill that each letter signifies. Next, starting with the first letter in the acronym (R in ROCKs ON), teach the skills associated with each letter in the acronym, using the key points outlined in the following sections, until you have covered all of the skills associated with each individual letter. Importantly, only write out on the whiteboard or flipchart the global description of what each letter actually stands for when you are teaching the skills associated with its corresponding letter. This teaching method avoids long explanations about the use of certain words in the acronym and/or premature teaching of concepts, since the meaning of each letter is only revealed during the formal teaching of the skills associated with it.

R	**Resist** the urge to control other people
O	Identify your interpersonal effectiveness goals and degree of **Openness**
C	**Clarify** the interpersonal effectiveness goal that is your priority
K	Practice **Kindness** first and foremost
ON	Take into account the **Other** person's **Needs**

Prior to the Interaction

R Resist *the urge to control other people.*

- **When it comes to relationships, control is like plutonium—it only takes a little for a major disaster to occur.** For example...

  - Attempts to force compliance result in the other person hating us.

  - Rigid insistence that our way is more efficient gets three more bowls in the dishwasher but fractures a relationship.

  - Refusing to dance or sing at a party may feel like independence or doing what one thinks is best, but it can feel isolating when you are the only one and/or can result in others seeing you as uptight.

  - Trying to buy someone's love or force someone to love you almost always fails in the long run.

NOTE TO INSTRUCTORS: Refer participants to handout 17.2 (New Year's Resolutions), and randomly ask a class member to read aloud the cartoon text and then to pick someone else to read aloud one of the three sentences underneath the cartoon. The new reader then picks a different person to read the next sentence aloud, and so on. Briefly discuss the meaning of the cartoon text and the three sentences, and then move on to the next teaching point.

  ✓ **Ask:** *To what extent do you think you try to control other people, either overtly or covertly?*

  ✓ **Ask:** *What are the downsides of controlling people we are close to? What are the advantages? Which way gets you closer to how you want to live?*

- **Plan a little, then let it go. Block excessive rehearsal of what you will say or how you will act, particularly when the interaction is purely social** (for example, a picnic, a party). Remember, part of learning how to break the habit of overcontrol is to practice relinquishing it. Remind yourself of your RO "participating without planning" skills (see lesson 12).

- *Stop expecting the other person to think, feel, or act like you do. Let go of rigid convictions that there is only one way of doing things.* Remember, there are many ways to cook potatoes (for example, a french-fried potato is just as edible as a boiled potato; the primary difference is one of preferred taste).

- *If urges to plan, check, or rehearse what you will say or do during the interaction begin to interfere with everyday living (for example, by impeding sleep, work, or leisure) then...*

- *Practice self-enquiry in order to learn.*

> ➢ *What are my desires to plan, rehearse, or check trying to tell me? If they could speak, what would they say? Am I down on myself for wanting to check, rehearse, or plan?*

> ➢ *Where did I ever get the idea that planning, rehearsing, or checking is the only way to behave? Where did I ever get the idea that planning, checking, or rehearsing is bad? What am I afraid would happen if I were to let go of my planning, checking, or rehearsal? What is it I might need to learn?*

> ➢ *To what extent am I willing to take responsibility for my thoughts and behaviors around planning, rehearsing, and checking? Is there a part of me not wanting to stop or change? Is it possible that I am more controlling of other people than I would care to admit? What might this tell me?*

- **Explain your situation to a neutral person,** and ask them how much preparation they might recommend. Use Flexible Mind ADOPTS skills to enhance openness to feedback.

- **You will have pain if you plan and pain if you don't.** Which pain gets you closer to how you want to live?

- **Activate your social safety system prior to the interaction, especially if the relationship has been difficult in the past, in order to maximize openness and flexible responding** (for example, conduct a short loving kindness meditation; see lesson 4).

⭘ *Identify your interpersonal effectiveness goals and degree of Openness.*

(*Note:* The first three interpersonal effectiveness factors that follow are adapted from Linehan, 2015a, pp. 243–244).

- *Identify interpersonal effectiveness goals and degree of openness, using the following steps.*

  1. **Objective effectiveness pertains to what you hope to achieve during the interaction.**

     - ✓ **Ask:** *What results or changes do I want to occur during or after the interaction?*

  2. **Relationship effectiveness pertains to the type of relationship you desire with the other person.**

     - ✓ **Ask:** *How do I want the other person to feel about me after the interaction is over (independent of achieving or not achieving my personal objective)?*

  3. **Self-respect effectiveness pertains to the core valued goals you will need to attend to during the interaction.**

     - ✓ **Ask:** *How do I want to feel about myself after the interaction is over (independent of achieving or not achieving my personal objective)?*

Identify the valued goals you will need to live by in order to maintain your self-respect during the interaction. Use worksheet 10.A (Flexible Mind Is DEEP: Identifying Valued Goals) to help facilitate this process.

  4. **Self-enquiry effectiveness pertains to the extent to which you are willing to question your beliefs, convictions, or perceptions about the other person.** Use the following questions to facilitate awareness and self-enquiry.

     - ➢ *What do I imagine the other person's needs, wants, or desires will be during the interaction? What do I imagine will be their primary objective? How might my beliefs impact my perceptions or behavior during the interaction?*

➢ *How open am I to considering the possibility that I may be wrong about how I perceive the other person?*

➢ *Am I discounting or minimizing positive things about the person or situation in order to obtain what I want or punish them for prior wrongs? Is it possible that I am not really giving them a chance?*

➢ *Am I refusing to consider alternative explanations for the other person's behavior? Is it possible that I am neglecting potential factors or causes outside of the other person's control that may have led to the painful event? What am I afraid might happen if I were to momentarily drop my perspective?*

➢ *Do I have evidence that the relationship may be toxic? Have I evaluated the potential toxicity of the relationship? (See Flexible Mind SAGE skills.)*

➢ *To what extent am I resisting, avoiding, or disliking self-enquiry about my beliefs, judgments, or appraisals of the other person? What might my resistance say to me if it could speak? What is it that I might need to learn?*

C **Clarify** *the interpersonal effectiveness goal that is your priority.*

- *Determine the interpersonal effectiveness factor you consider most important in the upcoming interaction, and then use that to guide your behavior.*

   1. **Objective effectiveness is your priority if you believe that achieving your goal or the changes you desire is most important** (for example, getting the raise, saying no to a request), even if doing so might cause some damage to the relationship, could undermine self-respect, and/or could prevent you from learning from the interaction.

   2. **Relationship effectiveness is your priority if you consider your relationship with the other person most important** (for example, establishing or maintaining intimacy, proving your commitment to the other person), even if it might mean not achieving your objective, losing some self-respect, or disregarding an opportunity for self-growth.

   3. **Self-respect effectiveness is your priority if you believe that living by your valued goals and doing what you believe morally correct are most important** (for example, to protect those in need, to fight tyranny), even if it might mean not achieving your objective, damaging your relationship, and being seen as arrogant.

   4. **Self-enquiry effectiveness is your priority if you believe self-examination is most important** (for example, to challenge oneself, to stretch one's limits, to discover new things) even if it might mean not achieving your goal, damaging your relationship, or experiencing embarrassment as a result of losing your sense of mastery.

During the Interaction

K *Practice* **Kindness** *first and foremost.*

✳ *Welcome home—we've been eagerly awaiting your return.* ✳

✳ *Kindness is humility in action.* ✳

✓ **Ask:** *What do you think about when you hear the word "kind"?*

- *Practice kindness toward self and others* as your first response, and as your go-to response when unsure about how to respond. Use the following concepts to help remind yourself of core principles.

NOTE TO INSTRUCTORS: To maximize class involvement, randomly select a member of the class to read aloud the first point listed on the worksheet 17.B (Kindness First and Foremost), and discuss briefly. Then randomly select someone else to read the next point aloud, briefly discuss, and then move on to the next point, in a similar manner, until all have been covered and each person in the class has had a chance to participate in reading at least one of the points.

- *Kindness first and foremost* means treating other people as we would like to be treated.

- *Kindness first and foremost* means giving the other person the benefit of the doubt. It acknowledges that our perceptions, beliefs, and convictions can be (and often are) invalid.

- *Kindness first and foremost* recognizes that we are better when together; it celebrates our tribal nature.

- *Kindness first and foremost* is willing to suffer pain or make self-sacrifices for another person, without always expecting something in return.

- *Kindness first and foremost* recognizes that all humans have personality quirks and loves them for this rather than expecting perfection or harmony.

- *Kindness first and foremost* recognizes it is arrogant to expect the world or others to conform to our personal beliefs or bend to our needs.

- *Kindness first and foremost* is able to stand up against powerful others, with humility, in order to prevent unwarranted harm or unethical behavior.

- *Kindness first and foremost* means being kind to oneself by blocking automatic self-blame or self-hatred while retaining an ability to question oneself in order to learn from what the world has to offer.

- *Kindness first and foremost* means admitting when one is wrong or has harmed another.

- *Kindness first and foremost* means telling a good friend (or close other) a painful truth in order to help them achieve their valued goals, in a manner that acknowledges one's own potential for fallibility.

- *Kindness first and foremost* means hoping that the best will come to others and, when it does, celebrating their success, without resenting their advantage.

- *Kindness first and foremost* is willing to let another person win (and never tell them), simply because it matters more to them than it does to you.

- *Kindness first and foremost* recognizes that when I lend a hand, it is because I choose to, not because I have been forced. My self-sacrifices are freely chosen; thus, those I help don't owe me. I alone am responsible for my decisions to help or not help.

(Required) Discussion Points

Kindness First and Foremost

✓ **Ask:** *Were there any points about kindness that created tension in your body? What might this mean?*

✓ **Ask:** *Were there any concepts that you didn't believe? What might this tell you when it comes to your interactions with others?*

✓ **Ask:** *Which of the points did you like the most or feel easily drawn toward? What does this tell you?*

✓ **Ask:** *Who are your kindness heroes? Who do you admire for behaving in a kind manner? Why do we admire kindness?*

NOTE TO INSTRUCTORS: **The difference between kindness and compassion:** Kindness and compassion are often used interchangeably to mean the same thing. Yet, from an RO DBT perspective, there are some important differences worth noting. Broadly speaking, compassion is a response to suffering: "It has but one direction, which is to heal suffering" (Feldman & Kuyken, 2011). Compassion involves a feeling state of sympathetic understanding that can be directed either outward (for example, empathy regarding another person's suffering) or inward (self-compassion). Interestingly, kindness entails affection or love, whereas compassion entails empathy, mercy, and sympathy; for example, judges reduce punishments because they feel merciful toward the accused, not affectionate. Compassion emerges as a response to pain, whereas kindness can occur independent of pain. The emphasis on differences here is not intended to minimize or ignore shared features; the focus instead is on helping OC clients recognize that—for them, at least—compassion is probably not enough. RO DBT contends that emotional loneliness is the core problem underlying maladaptive overcontrol secondary to social signaling deficits. Therefore, for OC clients, learning how to behave kindly toward others is a core component of regaining or improving social connectedness. The following table provides an overview of some other differences between kindness and compassion in RO DBT.

Kindness	Compassion
Social signal	Inner experience
Affection, warmth, playfulness	Sympathy, empathy, concern
Priorities are humility, openness, and willingness to publicly admit fault or wrongdoing	Priorities are acceptance, nonjudgmental thinking, distress tolerance, and validation
Orientation is toward questioning oneself and signaling openness to others in order to learn and socially connect with others	Orientation is toward healing oneself and others via empathetic understanding, validation, and nonjudgmental awareness
Emphasis is on celebrating our differences as well as our tribal nature and on contributing to others' well-being without expecting anything in return	Emphasis is on alleviating suffering and acknowledging the universality of human suffering with tolerance, equanimity, acceptance, and generosity

(Required) Teaching Point

Using Valued Goals to Guide Behavior

- **During the interaction, use valued goals to guide behavior.** For example, a parent who arrives home after a hard day's work, only to find their teenage daughter in desperate need for help completing homework, is likely to experience a conflict between their valued goals for rest and their valued goals for good parenting. Assuming they value their daughter's success at school over their desire for rest, living according to their values would mean that they will be helping with homework that evening.

- **When valued goals conflict, prioritize.** For example, a parent who values being seen as a trusting and approving parent by their teenage daughter may need to reprioritize this valued goal in order to effectively provide corrective feedback to her after she is caught stealing from her classmates. Their valued goal related to doing the right thing, even if it causes distress in others in this circumstance, takes priority over other valued goals. Thus, the situation matters when deciding which valued goal to live by, moment by moment.

- **Use the Match + 1 skills** in Flexible Mind ALLOWs to establish or deepen intimacy (see lesson 21).

- **Use Flexible Mind SAGE DEEP(ly) REVEALS skills** to improve trust and social closeness, and to signal nondominant friendliness (see lessons 8, 10, and 16).

- **Cultivate an easy manner by letting go of rigid desires to control the outcome.** *Attempting to control other people is like mixing lemon juice and milk in a cup of tea—it spoils the appetite.*

> ★ **Fun Facts:** *"But What's an Easy Manner?"*
>
> Refer participants to handout 17.3 (Signaling an Easy Manner).
>
> *Easygoing people seem to roll with what life throws at them, even when it is their turn to scrub the toilet. So what is it all about? It's certainly not just about being calm. When my foot is on fire, equanimity will not put the fire out. This situation calls for immediate action and a raucous distress call to my tribe (that is, screaming for help ☺). Plus, you don't need an easy manner when living in complete isolation. Thus, Robinson Crusoe could afford to be pigheaded until his "man Friday" came around. Thus, an easy manner pertains to how we behave in relationships. What might this tell us about the habits of a person who has lived alone (like a hermit) for long periods of time? How might the social signals of a hermit differ from the signals of those living in the tribe? How might hermit behavior and/or thinking benefit a tribe? How might our hermit appear to other tribal members when he returns to the tribe? What might a hermit need to learn or remember to do when they return to a tribe? To what extent do you behave like a hermit? Importantly, an easy manner may not always be easy or appear nice; sometimes being tough with someone is the most caring thing a person can do, and sometimes harshness is needed to stop harmful behavior. Plus, an easy manner does not mean being irresponsible and just hanging out. If anything, from an RO DBT perspective, it requires hard work, persistence, and a willingness to make self-sacrifices for one's tribe.*

ON *Take into account the* **Other** *person's* **Needs.**

- **Remember that getting what you want is more likely to happen if you recognize that others may want something different.** Rather than assuming you already know, ask the other person directly about their goals and objectives—and then, if possible, help them achieve them, without undermining your own.

NOTE TO INSTRUCTORS: In the short term, a person is more likely to give you what you want if you acknowledge what they want (as legitimate). In the long term, getting what one wants is more likely when one helps others achieve or meet their needs, without expecting anything in return, in a consistent manner.

- **Use Flexible Mind ADOPTS** to facilitate open listening and learning from the other person (see lesson 22).

- *In the heat of the moment, be alert for bodily tension, uncomfortable emotions, or strong action urges, and when they arise, practice self-enquiry by asking yourself "What is it that I might need to learn?"* before you attempt to change the situation, feel better, accept what is happening, or abandon the relationship. Use the following self-enquiry questions to help facilitate this.

    > *Is it possible that my bodily tension means that I am not fully open to what's happening right now? What is it that I need to learn?*

    > *Do I find myself wanting to automatically explain, defend, or discount the other person's feedback or what is happening? If yes or maybe, then is this a sign that I may not be truly open?*

    > *Am I talking more quickly, or immediately responding to the other person's feedback or questions?*

    > *Am I holding my breath or breathing more quickly? Has my heart rate changed? If yes or maybe, then what does this mean? What is driving me to respond so quickly? Is it possible I am feeling threatened?*

- *When tension is present, use nonverbal social signaling to slow the pace, and chill out* by leaning back in your chair (if you are sitting), taking a deep breath, raising your eyebrows, and engaging a warm closed-mouth smile (that is, the Big Three + 1). See lesson 3; see also handout 17.3 (Signaling an Easy Manner).

NOTE TO INSTRUCTORS: Refer participants to the illustration in handout 17.1 (Enhancing Interpersonal Kindness, Effectiveness, and Connectedness, Using Flexible Mind ROCKs ON). These universal social safety signals communicate that you are open and receptive to the other person's viewpoint while simultaneously triggering your social safety system (that is, it's safe to relax because if it was unsafe, you wouldn't be leaning back or engaging in eyebrow wags) and the social safety system in the other person (that is, via the mirror neuron system; see lesson 6).

★ **Fun Facts:** *When a Crisis Is Not a Crisis*

The only crisis, from an RO DBT point of view, is when a person stops breathing (Okay, perhaps a slight exaggeration ☺). Of course there other types of crises, like your heart stopping (oops, another medical reference—tee hee ☺). Seriously, now, the major point is that most obstacles in life may often feel like a crisis, but very few are actually genuine emergencies (for example, life-or-death scenarios). Thus, most of the time we can afford to slow down and allow ourselves (and the other person) time to think through what might be most important to do next.

> ✓ **Ask:** *What types of problems are actual emergencies requiring immediate attention and problem solving? To what extent do you think you tend to treat minor problems as a crises by immediately trying to fix or resolve them?*

- *Take the heat off when things seem extremely tense by allowing the other person (and yourself) the grace of not having to understand, resolve, or fix a problem or issue immediately.* Use stall tactics—ask if it would be okay to get back together and discuss again in the future. Use self-enquiry during the break to seek out your blind spots, and make sure you reengage with the person again in the near future to resolve the apparent conflict. Don't let resentments build.

Lesson 17 Homework

1. **(Required) Worksheet 17.B (Kindness First and Foremost).** Instruct participants to pick two or three kindness principles to practice this week.

2. **(Required) Worksheet 17.C (Using Flexible Mind ROCKs ON to Enhance Interpersonal Effectiveness).**

3. **(Optional) Worksheet 17.A (Overcontrolled Myths About Interpersonal Relationships).** Encourage participants to use this worksheet to facilitate the practice of self-enquiry during the coming week.

Radical Openness Handout 17.1

Enhancing Interpersonal Kindness, Effectiveness, and Connectedness, Using Flexible Mind ROCKs ON

Flexible Mind ROCKs ON

R **Resist** the urge to control other people

O Identify your interpersonal effectiveness goals and degree of **O**penness

C **C**larify the interpersonal effectiveness goal that is your priority

K Practice **K**indness first and foremost

ON Take into account the **O**ther person's **N**eeds

Prior to the Interaction

R **Resist** *the urge to control other people.*

- Plan a little, then let it go.

- Stop expecting the other person to think, feel, or act like you do.

- When urges to plan, check, or rehearse are high, practice self-enquiry in order to learn.

  ➤ *What are my desires to plan, rehearse, or check trying to tell me? If they could speak, what would they say? Am I down on myself for wanting to check, rehearse, or plan?*

  ➤ *Where did I ever get the idea that planning, rehearsing, or checking is the only way to behave? Where did I ever get the idea that planning, checking, or rehearsing is bad? What am I afraid would happen if I were to let go of my planning, checking, or rehearsal? What is it I might need to learn?*

  ➤ *To what extent am I willing to take responsibility for my thoughts and behaviors around planning, rehearsing, and checking? Is there a part of me not wanting to stop or change? Is it possible that I am more controlling of other people than I would care to admit? What might this tell me?*

- **Explain your situation to a neutral person,** and ask them how much preparation they might recommend. Use Flexible Mind ADOPTS skills to enhance openness to feedback.

- **You will have pain if you plan and pain if you don't.** *Which pain gets you closer to how you want to live?*

O *Identify your interpersonal effectiveness goals and degree of* **O**penness.

- Identify interpersonal effectiveness goals and degree of openness, using the following steps.

  1. *Objective effectiveness* pertains to what you hope to achieve during the interaction.

     ✓ **Ask:** *What results or changes do I want to occur during or after the interaction?*

  2. *Relationship effectiveness* pertains to the type of relationship you desire with the other person.

    ✓ **Ask:** *How do I want the other person to feel about me after the interaction is over (independent of achieving or not achieving my personal objective)?*

3. *Self-respect effectiveness* **pertains to the core valued goals you will need to attend to during the interaction.**

    ✓ **Ask:** *How do I want to feel about myself after the interaction is over (independent of achieving or not achieving my personal objective)?*

- Identify the valued goals you will need to live by in order to maintain your self-respect during the interaction. Use worksheet 10.A (Flexible MIND Is Deep: Identifying Valued Goals) to help facilitate this process.

4. *Self-enquiry effectiveness* **pertains to the extent to which you are willing to question your beliefs, convictions, or perceptions about the other person.** Use the following questions to facilitate awareness and self-enquiry.

    ➤ *What do I imagine the other person's needs, wants, or desires will be during the interaction? What do I imagine will be their primary objective? How might my beliefs impact my perceptions or behavior during the interaction?*

    ➤ *How open am I to considering the possibility that I may be wrong about how I perceive the other person?*

    ➤ *Am I discounting or minimizing positive things about the person or situation in order to obtain what I want, or am I punishing them for prior wrongs? Is it possible that I am not really giving them a chance?*

    ➤ *Am I refusing to consider alternative explanations for the other person's behavior? Is it possible I am neglecting potential factors or causes outside of the other person's control that may have led to the painful event? What am I afraid might happen if I were to momentarily drop my perspective?*

    ➤ *Do I have evidence that the relationship may be toxic? Have I evaluated the potential toxicity of the relationship? (See Flexible Mind SAGE skills.)*

    ➤ *To what extent am I resisting, avoiding, or disliking self-enquiry about my beliefs, judgments, or appraisals of the other person? What might my resistance say to me if it could speak? What is it that I might need to learn?*

C Clarify *the interpersonal effectiveness goal that is your priority.*

- Determine the interpersonal effectiveness factor you consider most important in the upcoming interaction, and then use that to guide your behavior.

1. *Objective effectiveness* **is your priority if you believe that achieving your goal or the changes you desire is most important** (for example, getting the raise, saying no to a request), even if doing so might cause some damage to the relationship, could undermine self-respect, and/or could prevent you from learning from the interaction.

2. *Relationship effectiveness* **is your priority if you consider your relationship with the other person most important** (for example, establishing or maintaining intimacy, proving your commitment to the other person), even if it might mean not achieving your objective, losing some self-respect, or disregarding an opportunity for self-growth.

3. *Self-respect effectiveness* **is your priority if you believe that living by your valued goals and doing what you believe morally correct are most important** (for example, to protect those in

365

need, to fight tyranny), even if it might mean not achieving your objective, damaging your relationship, and being seen as arrogant.

4. *Self-enquiry effectiveness* is your priority if you believe that self-examination is most important (for example, to avoid arrogance, complacency, or self-satisfaction; to learn from what the world has to offer), even if it might mean not achieving your goal, damaging your relationship, or experiencing embarrassment as a result of losing your sense of mastery.

During the Interaction

K Practice **Kindness** *first and foremost.*

- **Practice kindness toward self and others** as your first response, and as your go-to response when unsure about how to respond. Use worksheet 17.B (Kindness First and Foremost) to facilitate this practice.

- **Use valued goals to guide behavior, and when they conflict, decide which value is more important** (for example, a conflict between a valued goal for rest and a valued goal for good parenting).

- **Use the Match + 1 skills** in Flexible Mind ALLOWs to establish or deepen intimacy (see lesson 21).

- **Use Flexible Mind SAGE DEEP(ly) REVEALS skills** to improve trust, social closeness, and signal nondominant friendliness (see lessons 8, 10, and 16).

- **Cultivate an easy manner by letting go of rigid desires to control the outcome.**

ON Take into account the **Other** *person's* **Needs**.

- **Remember that getting what you want is more likely to happen if you recognize that others may want something different.**

- **Use Flexible Mind ADOPTS** to facilitate open listening and learning from the other person (see lesson 22).

- **In the *heat of the moment,* be alert for bodily tension, uncomfortable emotions, or strong action urges,** and when they arise, practice self-enquiry by asking yourself: *What is it that I might need to learn?* Use the following self-enquiry questions to help facilitate this.

  ➤ *Is it possible that my bodily tension means that I am not fully open to what's happening right now? What is it that I need to learn?*

  ➤ *Do I find myself wanting to automatically explain, defend, or discount the other person's feedback or what is happening? If yes or maybe, then is this a sign that I may not be truly open?*

  ➤ *Am I talking more quickly, or immediately responding to the other person's feedback or questions?*

  ➤ *Am I holding my breath or breathing more quickly? Has my heart rate changed? If yes or maybe, then what does this mean? What is driving me to respond so quickly? Is it possible I am feeling threatened?*

- **When tension is present, use nonverbal social signaling to slow the pace, and chill out** by leaning back in your chair (if you are sitting), taking a deep breath, raising your eyebrows, and engaging a warm closed-mouth smile (that is, the Big Three + 1). See lesson 3; see also handout 17.3 (Signaling an Easy Manner).

- **Take the heat off when things seem extremely tense** by allowing the other person (and yourself) the *grace* of not having to understand, resolve, or fix a problem or issue immediately.

Radical Openness Handout 17.2

New Year's Resolutions

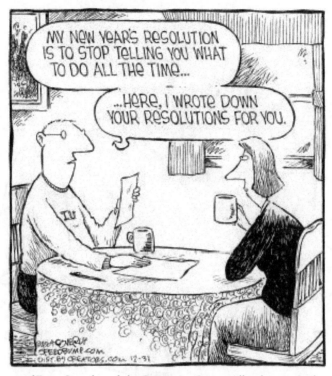

Radical Openness Handout 17.3

Signaling an Easy Manner

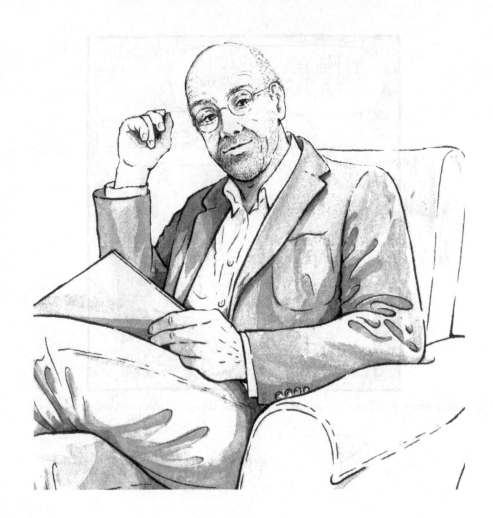

Radical Openness Handout 17.4

Main Points for Lesson 17: Enhancing Interpersonal Effectiveness

Kindness First and Foremost

1. Prior to an interaction, clarify your goals and objectives, and determine which one takes priority—that is, your personal objective, your relationship objective, or your self-respect objective.

2. Block excessive rehearsal of what you will say or how you will act, particularly when the interaction is purely social (for example, a picnic, a party).

3. Identify the valued goals you will need to live by when interacting with others. Use worksheet 10.A (Flexible Mind Is DEEP: Identifying Valued Goals) to help facilitate this process.

4. During the interaction, practice kindness first and foremost.

5. Kindness signals affection and openness—it involves contributing to the well-being of others, without expecting anything in return.

6. Use Flexible Mind ROCKs ON to enhance interpersonal kindness, effectiveness, and connectedness.

Radical Openness Worksheet 17.A

Overcontrolled Myths About Interpersonal Relationships

Place a checkmark in the box next to each myth that you believe is true or somewhat true.

- ☐ If you give someone an inch, they will take a mile.
- ☐ Love is fake, and romance is for fools.
- ☐ Dependence means you are weak.
- ☐ People can't be trusted.
- ☐ Compliments are used to manipulate others.
- ☐ If someone wrongs me, it is important to always pay them back, no matter how long it takes.
- ☐ Feeling detached and alone is normal.
- ☐ No one can ever truly understand another person.
- ☐ Being dependent on another person is foolish.
- ☐ People are nice to others only when they want something.
- ☐ When conflict occurs, it is best to walk away.
- ☐ If you reveal your true feelings to another person, they will use it against you.
- ☐ There is a right and a wrong way to interact with others.
- ☐ People only truly care about themselves.
- ☐ In the long run, people will always let you down.
- ☐ Being correct is more important than being liked.
- ☐ Always smile, even when you are miserable.
- ☐ Talking about inner feelings is a waste of time.
- ☐ If I show vulnerability, others will take advantage of me.
- ☐ I have to sacrifice my time and energy to get it right because others are incompetent.
- ☐ It is a sign of weakness to ask for help.
- ☐ I must be inadequate if I can't get what I want.
- ☐ People are always secretly gossiping about others behind their backs.
- ☐ No one is capable of understanding me.
- ☐ I am not like other people.
- ☐ Holding on to a grudge is necessary because people cannot be trusted.
- ☐ Relationships are not meant to be fun.
- ☐ If I don't do it myself, then it will never get done or done properly.
- ☐ When phone calls or emails are not returned promptly, it is a sign of disrespect or lack of caring.

☐ Keeping experiences to oneself will improve relationships.

☐ Having a friend means being obligated.

☐ People must be punished for mistakes.

☐ When I am wronged by someone, it is a sign of weakness to forgive and forget.

☐ People don't appreciate my self-sacrifices.

☐ Other people do not deserve my help.

☐ I feel that people do not understand me because I am better than they are.

In the space provided, write out any other myths you may have that were not already mentioned.

• **Remember to record the images, thoughts, emotions and sensations that emerge when you practice self-enquiry in your self-enquiry journal.**

_____

_____

_____

_____

Next, pick one of the preceding myths that you believe in strongly, and practice self-enquiry about the myth over the next week.

• **Remember, self-enquiry does not automatically assume that a myth is wrong, bad, or dysfunctional.** Use the following questions to enhance your practice.

  ➤ *What might I need to learn from this myth?*

  ➤ *What might this myth be telling me about myself and my life?*

  ➤ *Am I feeling tense doing this exercise?*

  ➤ *Am I feeling tense right now? If so, then what might this mean? What is it that I might need to learn?*

  ➤ *How open am I to thinking differently about this myth or changing the myth?*

  ➤ *If I am not open or only partly open, then what might this mean?*

  ➤ *How does holding on to this myth help me live more fully?*

  ➤ *How might changing this myth help me live more fully?*

  ➤ *What might my resistance to changing this myth be telling me?*

  ➤ *Is there something to learn from my resistance?*

  ➤ *What does holding on to this myth tell me about myself?*

  ➤ *What do I fear might happen if I momentarily let go of this myth?*

  ➤ *What is it that I need to learn?*

Use the space provided to record additional self-enquiry questions or observations that emerged from your practice.

_____

_____

_____

_____

- **Remember, keep your self-enquiry practices short in duration**—that is, not much longer than five minutes. The goal of self-enquiry is to *find a good question* that brings you closer to your edge, or personal unknown (the place you don't want to go), in order to learn. After a week, move to another myth, and repeat your self-enquiry practice.

- **Remember to record** the images, thoughts, emotions, and sensations that emerge when you practice self-enquiry about your myths about emotions in your self-enquiry journal.

- **Remember to practice being suspicious of quick answers** to self-enquiry questions. Allow any answers to your self-enquiry practice to emerge over time.

Radical Openness Worksheet 17.B

Kindness First and Foremost

- **During interpersonal interactions, practice cultivating a state of being that reflects kindness toward self and others** as your first response, and as your go-to response when unsure about how to respond.

Place a checkmark in the boxes next to the acts of kindness that you practiced.

☐ *Kindness first and foremost* means treating other people as we would like to be treated.

☐ *Kindness first and foremost* means giving the other person the benefit of the doubt. It acknowledges that our perceptions, beliefs, and convictions can be (and often are) invalid.

☐ *Kindness first and foremost* recognizes that we are better when together; it celebrates our tribal nature.

☐ *Kindness first and foremost* is willing to suffer pain or make self-sacrifices for another person, without always expecting something in return.

☐ *Kindness first and foremost* recognizes that all humans have personality quirks and loves them for this rather than expecting perfection or harmony.

☐ *Kindness first and foremost* recognizes it is arrogant to expect the world or others to conform to our personal beliefs or bend to our needs.

☐ *Kindness first and foremost* is able to stand up against powerful others, with humility, in order to prevent unwarranted harm or unethical behavior.

☐ *Kindness first and foremost* means being kind to oneself by blocking automatic self-blame or self-hatred while retaining an ability to question oneself in order to learn from what the world has to offer.

☐ *Kindness first and foremost* means admitting when one is wrong or has harmed another.

☐ *Kindness first and foremost* means telling a good friend (or close other) a painful truth in order to help them achieve their valued goals, in a manner that acknowledges one's own potential for fallibility.

☐ *Kindness first and foremost* means hoping that the best will come to others and, when it does, celebrating their success, without resenting their advantage.

☐ *Kindness first and foremost* is willing to let another person win (and never tell them), simply because it matters more to them than it does to you.

☐ *Kindness first and foremost* recognizes that when I lend a hand, it is because I choose to, not because I have been forced. My self-sacrifices are freely chosen; thus, those I help don't owe me. I alone am responsible for my decisions to help or not help.

Record other acts of kindness.

_____

_____

_____

Radical Openness Worksheet 17.C

Using Flexible Mind ROCKs ON to Enhance Interpersonal Effectiveness

Look for opportunities in the coming week to practice Flexible Mind ROCKs ON.

Pick a relationship with someone you care about or would like to get to know better, if possible. Describe the relationship that you chose.

_____

_____

_____

What is your current level of intimacy? Use handout 21.2 (Match + 1 Intimacy Rating Scale), and write a number from 1 to 9. _____

What is your desired level of intimacy? Use handout 21.2 (Match + 1 Intimacy Rating Scale), and write a number from 1 to 9. _____

Practice Flexible Mind ROCKs ON, using the following skills.

Prior to the Interaction

R Resist *the urge to control other people.*

Place a checkmark in the boxes next to the skills you practiced.

    ☐ **Practiced letting go of obsessive planning or rehearsal,** *and if they became intense...*

        ☐ Practiced self-enquiry. *Record the question you found most helpful.*

_____

_____

    ☐ **Explained my situation to a neutral person,** and asked them how much preparation they might recommend. *Record what you learned.*

_____

_____

☐ **Remembered that I will have pain if I plan and pain if I don't,** and then asked myself which type of pain will get me closer to how I want to live, and used this to guide my actions.

☐ **Remembered to not expect the other person to behave like me,** without judging it as good or bad.

O *Identify your interpersonal effectiveness goals and degree of* **Openness**.

Place a checkmark in the boxes next to the skills you practiced.

☐ **Identified my objective effectiveness by asking:** *What results or changes did I want to occur during or after the interaction?* Record your answer here.

_____

_____

☐ **Identified my relationship effectiveness by asking:** *How do I want the other person to feel about me after the interaction is over (independent of achieving or not achieving my personal objective)?* Record your answer here.

_____

_____

☐ **Identified my self-respect effectiveness by asking:** *How do I want to feel about myself after the interaction is over (independent of achieving or not achieving my personal objective)?* Record your answer here.

_____

_____

☐ **Identified the valued goals I will need to live by** in order to maintain my self-respect during the interaction. *Use handout 10.A (Flexible Mind Is DEEP: Identifying Valued Goals) to help facilitate this process.* Record what you discovered.

_____

_____

☐ **Identified my self-enquiry effectiveness by asking** the self-enquiry questions from handout 17.1 (*Enhancing Interpersonal Kindness, Effectiveness, and Connectedness, Using Flexible Mind ROCKs ON*). Record the self-enquiry question(s) you found most helpful.

_____

_____

C **Clarify** *the interpersonal effectiveness goal that is your priority.*

☐ **Determined the interpersonal effectiveness factor I consider most important to guide my behavior during the upcoming interaction.** *Use the questions in handout 17.1 (Enhancing Interpersonal Kindness, Effectiveness, and Connectedness, Using Flexible Mind ROCKs ON) to facilitate this. Record the interpersonal factor you decided is most important.*

_____

_____

During the Interaction

K *Practice **Kindness** first and foremost.*

Place a checkmark in the boxes next to the skills you practiced.

☐ **Practiced kindness toward self and others,** and observed the effect it had on others. *Write out what you noticed.*

_____

_____

☐ **Examined valued goals to guide behavior, and when they were in conflict, decided which value was more important** (for example, a conflict between your valued goals for rest and your valued goals for good parenting). *Record a conflict between valued goals.*

_____

_____

☐ **Practiced MATCH + 1 skills** in Flexible Mind ALLOWs to establish or deepen intimacy (see lesson 21).

☐ **Cultivated an easy manner** by letting go of rigid desires to control the outcome.

☐ **Used Flexible Mind SAGE DEEP(ly) REVEALS skills** to improve trust, social closeness, and signal nondominant friendliness. *Record what you discovered.*

_____

_____

ON *Take into account the* **Other** *person's* **Needs.**

Place a checkmark in the boxes next to the skills you practiced.

☐ **Remembered that getting what I want is more likely when I am able to acknowledge the validity of the other person's needs or expectations.**

☐ **Used Flexible Mind ADOPTS to facilitate open listening and learning** from the other person (see lesson 22).

☐ **Used self-enquiry when I experienced tension during the interaction.** *Record the question you found most useful.*

_____

_____

☐ **When tension was present, used nonverbal social signaling to slow the pace, and chilled out** by leaning back in my chair (if I was sitting), taking a deep breath, raising my eyebrows, and engaging a warm closed-mouth smile.

☐ **Took the heat off both myself and the other person** by allowing myself and the other person to not have to solve the problem immediately. *Describe how you made this happen.*

_____

_____

Being Assertive with an Open Mind

Main Points for Lesson 18

1. When making requests or turning down requests, use Flexible Mind PROVEs skills to assert your needs with an open mind and maximize success.

2. Describe the circumstances triggering asking or saying no, and use qualifiers to signal open-mindedness.

3. Openly reveal emotions and perceptions about the circumstances or the other person.

4. Identify what might reinforce the other person to give you what you want or respond positively to your assertion, and then seek a means to provide it.

5. Assert with humility if you desire a close relationship with the other person by combining nondominance and cooperative-friendly signals.

6. Assert with confidence, *or even urgency*, if getting what you want is your most important objective and/or the situation is an emergency.

7. When the relationship is important, you are more likely to get what you want if you signal openness and social safety.

8. When the relationship is important, try not to repeat yourself too much—it can start to be experienced as coercive and/or that you are uninterested in the other person's needs.

9. Don't ignore personal criticism or attacks. Respond with kindness and self-enquiry instead.

10. Negotiate collaboratively by putting yourself in the other person's shoes.

11. Use self-enquiry after the interaction to learn, and use RO skills (for example, Flexible Mind SAGE or Flexible Mind Has HEART) to assess and manage self-conscious emotions, determine if the relationship is toxic, and/or practice forgiveness.

Materials Needed

- Handout 18.1 (Self-Enquiry About Rumination After a Social Interaction)
- (Optional) Handout 18.2 (Main Points for Lesson 18: Being Assertive with an Open Mind)
- Worksheet 18.A (Being Assertive with an Open Mind: Flexible Mind PROVEs)
- Flipchart or whiteboard and markers

NOTE TO INSTRUCTORS: The aim of this lesson is to learn how to ask for what we want, or say no to what we do not want, in a manner that combines openness, kindness, humility, and assertiveness.

(Required) Teaching Points
Flexible Mind PROVEs

- *You can assert with humility and still get what you want.*
- *Use Flexible Mind PROVEs skills to maximize success.*

Refer participants to worksheet 18.A (Being Assertive with an Open Mind: Flexible Mind PROVEs).

NOTE TO INSTRUCTORS: Write out the acronym (PROVE) on a flipchart or whiteboard, with each letter arranged vertically in a column, but *without* teaching or naming the specific skill that each letter signifies. Next, starting with the first letter in the acronym (*P* in PROVE) teach the skill(s) associated with each letter in the acronym, using the key points outlined in the following sections, until you have covered all of the skills associated with each individual letter. Importantly, only write out on the whiteboard or flipchart the global description of what each letter actually stands for when you are teaching the skill(s) associated with its corresponding letter. This teaching method avoids long explanations about the use of certain words in the acronym and/or premature teaching of concepts, since the meaning of each letter is only revealed during the formal teaching of the skills associated with it.

Flexible Mind PROVEs

P   **Provide** a brief description of the underlying circumstances

R   **Reveal** your emotions about the circumstances, without blaming

O   Acknowledge the **Other Person's** needs, wants, and desires

V   Use your **Valued Goals** to guide how you socially signal your needs

E   Practice self-**Enquiry** to decide whether (or not) to repeat your assertion

P **Provide** *a brief description of the underlying circumstances motivating your request or refusal.*

- *Briefly describe the underlying circumstances prompting you to make a request or turn down a request, without defending, justifying, or rationalizing your point of view*—for example, *I've noticed that you rarely return my phone calls.*
- *Use qualifiers to signal open-mindedness and humility:*
  - *From what I can tell…*
  - *Is it possible that…?*
  - *I am aware of the thought that…*
  - *I'm not sure if I am correct, but it seems to me that you have…*

R Reveal *your emotions about the underlying circumstances, without blaming.*

- *Openly and directly reveal your emotions about the circumstances, without assuming they represent truth or facts.* Open expression increases trust and social connectedness, making it more likely for you to get what you want.

- *Use "I" statements when revealing inner experience, to signal that you are taking responsibility* for your emotions, thoughts, and beliefs rather than blaming the other person. Instead of saying *You make me annoyed when you…*, practice saying *I feel annoyed when you…*

- *When expressing your inner feelings, use the primary expressive channel (face, body, touch) linked with the emotion you wish to express,* to maximize the likelihood that what is transmitted is what is actually received; see Flexible Mind Is DEEP skills.

  - *For example, say:* When you don't reply to my phone call, I worry about you, and sometimes I am aware of imagining that you might not care.

  - *Nonverbal behavior:* Signal friendliness via a warm smile combined with a gentle touch on the arm (the primary channel for signaling affection; see Flexible Mind Is DEEP skills).

- *Remind yourself that outing oneself means taking responsibility for one's personal perceptions* and actions rather than automatically expecting the world to change or blaming others.

- *Use the Awareness Continuum when expressing opinions about the other person's intentions, in order to take responsibility for your perceptions.*

  - *For example, say:* I am aware of imagining that you have gone quiet because you are annoyed with me, and the thought of this is starting to trigger some worry and sadness in me.

  - *Nonverbal behavior:* Combine a slight downturn of the lips (matching words with facial expression) with direct eye contact (signaling openness) in order to communicate that you are taking responsibility for your feelings and not attempting to control the other person via a "don't hurt me" response (see Flexible Mind REVEALs skills).

O *Acknowledge the* **Other Person's** *needs, wants, and desires.*

- *Let the other person know you want to take their feelings and desires into consideration.* People naturally help those who help them.

- *Don't assume you know with certainty what the other person's inner thoughts, emotions, or motivations are.*

- *Practice being empathically aware of what the other may need or want rather than focusing solely on your own needs and wants.* Silently ask yourself the following questions in order to put yourself in the other person's shoes.

  - ✓ **Ask:** *What might the other person want from me during the interaction? What might be their most desired outcome after the interaction is over?*

  - ✓ **Ask:** *What problems or stressors might they have in their life that could influence how they behave?*

- *Identify what might reinforce the other person to give you what you want or respond positively to your assertion,* and then seek a means to provide it.

  - ✓ **Ask:** *How might I help the other person achieve what they desire or want? To what extent am I able or willing to give them what they want or most desire?*

- *Directly ask the other person what they want in exchange for giving you what you want.* Reciprocal and fair-minded exchanges of valuable resources are the essence of healthy business relations. They signal forthrightness and honesty because you are making it clear to the other person that you recognize that both people involved must be satisfied by the outcome—that is, *if you give me what I want, I will give you what you want.*

- *Prioritize social over arbitrary reinforcers, especially when desiring a close relationship with the other person*—for example, give priority to expressions of warmth and appreciation rather than to thank-you cards, gifts, or money.

  - *For example, say:* For me, at least, being able to ask for something and then have you respond by telling me what's going on inside of you, even if it is not what I imagined it to be, makes me feel really close to you and value our relationship. Thanks.

  - *Nonverbal behavior:* Signal friendly nondominance by combining a slight bowing of the head, a slight shoulder shrug, and openhanded gestures with a warm smile, eyebrow wags, and direct eye contact (see Flexible Mind SAGE skills).

NOTE TO INSTRUCTORS: Remind participants that punishment and aversive contingencies (for example, "If you don't give me what I want, I will take you to court and sue you") are less effective than positive reinforcers (for example, expressing appreciation or promising to return the favor). Punishment (or the threat of punishment) is also less likely to result in long-term changes—when the cat's away, the mice will play (that is, when the punisher is not around old behavior reemerges). Although punishment or threats of punishment can force compliance, among humans punishment often results in resentment, grudges, desires for revenge, and/or passive-aggressive behavior directed at the punisher. The price for punishing behavior in long-term close relationships is rarely worth it.

(Optional) Discussion Point

The Pros and Cons of Punishment

- ✓ **Ask:** *When someone tries to force you to do what they want by threatening or implying punishments if you don't comply with their wishes, are you more likely to feel happy or resentful afterward?*

- ✓ **Ask:** *What might this tell you about how to manage close, intimate relationships? To what extent do you experience resentment in your life? What might this tell you about yourself, your environment, and/or your relationships? What is it that you might need to learn? See Flexible Mind DARES and Flexible Mind Is LIGHT for RO skills pertaining to resentment, bitterness, and revenge (lessons 27 and 28).*

- *Look for secret desires to control the situation or the other person, and practice self-enquiry instead.*

  - ✓ **Ask:** *Why am I keeping my desires for control a secret? Am I proud of my desires for control? Why not give the other person control? What is it I fear will happen? What is it that I might need to learn?*

  - ✓ **Ask:** *To what extent would I feel comfortable revealing my desires for control to the other person? What might this tell me about myself or my relationship with the other person?*

  - ✓ **Ask:** *Am I in a position of authority or in a socially sanctioned role that necessitates control or guidance on my part (for example, am I a parent, boss, teacher, doctor, judge, or police officer)? If so, then what is preventing me from being more direct about my intentions or desires for control?*

> NOTE TO INSTRUCTORS: Although RO DBT emphasizes candid, open, and direct expressions of emotion and intentions as a core means for establishing and maintaining healthy relationships, there are many times when editing is either essential or an act of kindness, and effective emotional expression is always context-dependent.

V Use your **Valued Goals** to guide how you socially signal your needs.

- **Combine nondominance and cooperative-friendly signals when asserting your needs with a friend or close other.**

    - *For example, say:* So instead of imagining what's going on, and being wrong and sad for no reason, I thought it best just to ask directly. Can you tell me what's going on inside of you?

    - *Nonverbal behavior:* Signal nondominance and openness by combining a slight bowing of the head, a slight shoulder shrug, and openhanded gestures with a warm smile, eyebrow wags, and direct eye contact (see Flexible Mind SAGE skills in lesson 8).

    - *Take the heat off* by allowing the other person (and yourself) the grace of not having to understand, resolve, or fix a problem or issue immediately (see Flexible Mind ROCKs ON, in lesson 17, for skills on how to signal an easy manner).

- *Avoid indirect assertions and disguised demands.*

    - **Don't use "pushbacks" or "don't hurt me" responses to say no to something you want to avoid.** Practice being direct instead (see Flexible Mind REVEALs skills in lesson 16).

    - **Avoid temptations to charm, sweet-talk, or flatter the other person in order to get what you want.** Insincere expressions of admiration are experienced as manipulative and off-putting.

    - **Don't ignore personal attacks; respond with kindness instead**—for example, by treating the other person as you would like to be treated, giving the other person the benefit of the doubt, or acknowledging that your perceptions, beliefs, and convictions can be (and often are) invalid (see Flexible Mind Is DEEP, in lesson 10).

- *Be polite, especially if your request or your refusal will place an imposition on the other.*

    - *For example, say:* So I thought I might check in with you and ask a favor—could you please strive to reply in a more timely way to my phone calls?

    - *Nonverbal behavior:* Signal polite respect and affection by combining friendly signals with low-level nondominance signals via a prolonged shoulder shrug along with a warm smile, direct eye contact, and a gentle touch on the arm (see Flexible Mind Is DEEP skills, in lesson 10).

- **When getting what you want is most important, or the situation is an emergency, signal urgency, and repeat your request or refusal again** (and again, if necessary).

    - *For example, say:* I need you to tell me right now—what's going on?

    - *Nonverbal behavior:* Signal confidence by standing or sitting upright with shoulders back and chin up. Maintain eye contact, and speak with a matter-of-fact tone of voice and normal volume of speech (don't whisper; see Flexible Mind SAGE skills, in lesson 8).

E *Practice self-**Enquiry** to decide whether (or not) to repeat or increase the intensity of your assertion.*

- *Use the level of intimacy or closeness you desire with the other person to help guide how intense or repetitive you should be in asserting your needs.* For example, when you are not interested in a close relationship, or when your personal objective is your highest priority, repeat your assertion (again and again, if needed) until you get what you want (or you get so tired that you decide it's nap time ☺).

- *During the interaction—when challenged, or when things appear to not go your way—before responding, ask* **Is there something here for me to learn?** The simple act of asking or questioning oneself automatically changes perceptions and loosens the grip of rigid closed-minded thinking, even in the heat of the moment.

- *Practice self-enquiry more formally.* Use the following questions to further help determine whether or not to repeat or increase the intensity of your assertion.

  ➢ *What might my friend's or colleague's refusal to comply with my request tell me about the request itself? About our relationship? About myself? Is there something here to learn?*

  ➢ *Do I find myself wanting to automatically explain, defend, or discount the other person's feedback or what is happening? If yes or maybe, then is this a sign that I may not be truly open to considering their needs or circumstances?*

  ➢ *Where did I ever get the idea that I should always get what I want? Is there a part of me that desires to blame the other person or punish them for not complying with my request? Would I encourage a child to behave similarly? What might this tell me about my valued goals?*

  ➢ *Do I feel invalidated, hurt, unappreciated, or misunderstood by the person giving me the disconfirming feedback? If yes or maybe, then what is it that I need validated? Is there a chance that my desire for validation, feeling appreciated or understood, may make me less open to the criticism? Why am I expecting them to change rather than myself? Is there something here for me to learn?*

  ➢ *Is it possible that I am not responding to the actual situation but am bringing into the situation past experiences that may be influencing my perception? If so, then can I allow myself time to explore my responses before I push further for what I want?*

- **When the relationship with the other person is more important than getting what you want, then, in general, try not to repeat yourself too much.** I SAID, TRY NOT TO REPEAT YOURSELF! Did I tell you yet that you should try not to repeat yourself too much? Oops, did I just repeat myself? (tee hee ☺)

  - *Repeating the same thing over and over again in a close relationship can start to feel like coercion.* It can imply that you are not accounting for the needs of the other person.

  - *Instead, ask the other person for help in resolving the impasse rather than walking away or escalating your prior stance or mindlessly repeating your assertion or opinion.*

(Recommended) Class Exercise

Having Fun with Asking—and Saying No!

Instructors should encourage the class to come up with some examples of times when they needed to ask for something or say no to someone, and use it as an example to work through each of the Flexible Mind PROVEs steps.

Have participants practice asking for something, using a polite tone of voice and manner (for example, "Could you please pass me the butter?"). Then have them ask for the same thing (that is, the butter) without politeness. Discuss the differences between the two and why it matters (see Flexible Mind REVEALs skills for more about the importance of polite behavior in society).

Instructors should have an example prepared beforehand (ideally from their own life) that they can offer to use as the first practice example. Instructors should feel free to be a little silly (silly is good for OC ☺). For example, show the "Dead Parrot" sketch from the first season of *Monty Python's Flying Circus* (available on YouTube), and then afterward use Flexible Mind PROVEs skills to say no to someone trying to sell the class a dead hamster, with one of the instructors playing the role of the person selling while the other instructor works with the class to play the role of the customer wanting to say no (if you can mimic a British accent, all the better ☺).

Regardless of what type of exercise you come up with, the major point is to provide an opportunity to practice Flexible Mind PROVEs skills together before they are assigned as homework.

(Required) Teaching Point

After the Interaction

- *Use self-enquiry after the interaction, especially if you find yourself ruminating about it or repeatedly replaying the event in your mind.* Use handout 18.1 (Self-Enquiry About Rumination After a Social Interaction) to facilitate finding your edge and to deepen your practice.

- *If you experienced shame, humiliation, guilt, or embarrassment during the interaction,* use handout 8.5 (The RO DBT Self-Conscious Emotions Rating Scale) to determine whether your self-conscious emotion was warranted or unwarranted. Then use Flexible Mind SAGE skills (lesson 8) to know how to respond effectively.

- *If you believe the relationship may be toxic,* use Flexible Mind SAGE skills to identify potential disguised toxic social environments.

- *Practice forgiveness if you find yourself nurturing a grudge,* using Flexible Mind Has HEART skills (see lesson 29).

Lesson 18 Homework

1. **(Required) Worksheet 18.A (Being Assertive with an Open Mind: Flexible Mind PROVEs).** Encourage participants to look for a time in the coming week when they need to ask for something, or say no to a request, for which they can practice Flexible Mind PROVEs skills.

NOTE TO INSTRUCTORS: It is important to highlight to participants that what they choose need not be around an important event or major issue for them (that is, when first learning a new skill, it is best to start with lower-level issues and then build over time to more difficult ones).

Radical Openness Handout 18.1

Self-Enquiry About Rumination After a Social Interaction

Practice self-enquiry if you find yourself ruminating about the interaction after it is over by asking the following sample questions; see also the self-enquiry questions in handout 1.3 (Learning from Self-Enquiry).

Carry a copy of this list with you, and write down in your self-enquiry journal new questions you discover.

> ➤ *What might my rumination be telling me about what I expected to happen that did not happen? What is it I might need to learn?*

> ➤ *Is it possible that I have learned something about the other person that I don't want to admit to myself? What might this mean?*

> ➤ *Is my rumination about being right or correct about an issue that was discussed? Or is my rumination more about being liked or disliked by the other person? What might that tell me about my relationship with this person? What do I need to learn?*

> ➤ *Is it possible that my rumination suggests that there is something important for me to learn about myself that I don't want to hear or acknowledge? What is it that I don't want to hear?*

> ➤ *Do I desire to find a way to discount their perspective? What might this mean about my relationship with them? What might this mean about myself?*

> ➤ *Is there a part of me that wants to get revenge or to hurt the other person? What might this mean?*

> ➤ *Am I able to truly pause and consider the possibility that I may be wrong or may need to change? Is it possible that I am in Fixed Mind?*

> ➤ *Do I feel like shutting down, quitting, or giving up? If yes or maybe, then is it possible that I am operating from Fatalistic Mind?*

> ➤ *Am I blaming the other person for my emotional reactions? If yes or maybe, then why am I finding it difficult to take responsibility for my personal reactions? What might this tell me about myself or the relationship?*

> ➤ *Is it possible that I was not really giving them a chance? What am I afraid might happen if I were to momentarily drop my perspective?*

Write out the questions you found most useful, or other questions that emerged.

_____

_____

_____

Radical Openness Handout 18.2

Main Points for Lesson 18: Being Assertive with an Open Mind

1. When making requests or turning down requests, use Flexible Mind PROVEs skills to assert your needs with an open mind and maximize success.

2. Describe the circumstances triggering asking or saying no, and use qualifiers to signal open-mindedness.

3. Openly reveal emotions and perceptions about the circumstances or the other person.

4. Identify what might reinforce the other person to give you what you want or respond positively to your assertion, and then seek a means to provide it.

5. Assert with humility if you desire a close relationship with the other person by combining nondominance and cooperative-friendly signals.

6. Assert with confidence, *or even urgency*, if getting what you want is your most important objective and/or the situation is an emergency.

7. When the relationship is important, you are more likely to get what you want if you signal openness and social safety.

8. When the relationship is important, try not to repeat yourself too much—it can start to be experienced as coercive and/or that you are uninterested in the other person's needs.

9. Don't ignore personal criticism or attacks. Respond with kindness and self-enquiry instead.

10. Negotiate collaboratively by putting yourself in the other person's shoes.

11. Use self-enquiry after the interaction to learn, and use RO skills (for example, Flexible Mind SAGE or Flexible Mind Has HEART) to assess and manage self-conscious emotions, determine if the relationship is toxic, and/or practice forgiveness.

Radical Openness Worksheet 18.A

Being Assertive with an Open Mind: Flexible Mind PROVEs

Flexible Mind PROVEs

P   **Provide** a brief description of the underlying circumstances

R   **Reveal** emotions about the circumstances, without blaming

O   Acknowledge the **Other person's** needs, wants, and desires

V   Use your **Valued Goals** to guide how you socially signal your needs

E   Practice self-**Enquiry** to decide whether (or not) to repeat your assertion

Practice asking for what you want, or saying no to what you don't want, with someone in the coming week. Provide a brief description of the interaction around which you chose to practice Flexible Mind PROVEs skills.

_____

_____

_____

Place a checkmark in the boxes next to the skills you practiced.

P   **Provide** *a brief description of the underlying circumstances.*

☐ Described to the other person the circumstances leading me to ask for something or say no to their request.

☐ Used qualifiers to signal open-mindedness and respect (for example, *From what I can tell…*or *Is it possible that…?* or *I am aware of the thought that…*)

R   **Reveal** *emotions about the circumstances, without blaming.*

☐ Expressed my feelings and opinions about the circumstances.

☐ Practiced openly revealing feelings and perceptions rather than masking them.

☐ Used the **primary expressive channel (face, body, touch)** linked with the emotion I wished to **express** to maximize the likelihood that what was transmitted was what was actually received.

☐ Used the Awareness Continuum when expressing opinions about the other person's intentions, in order to take responsibility for my perceptions.

O *Acknowledge the* **Other person's** *needs, wants, and desires.*

☐ Practiced seeing the world from the perspective of the other person, in order to understand their needs, wants, desires, and struggles.

☐ Looked for ways to help the other person achieve their valued goals rather than focusing solely on my own.

☐ Directly asked the other person what they wanted in exchange for giving me what I wanted.

☐ Sought a means to reinforce the other person for responding positively to my assertion.

☐ **Prioritized social safety reinforcers over material rewards** (for example, by expressing warmth, appreciation, praise, gratitude, respect, trust, or love). *Record what you actually did and what the outcome was.*

_____

_____

☐ Asked them directly for help in solving the problem or resolving the impasse.

☐ Recognized secret desires to control the situation or the other person indirectly, and used Flexible Mind REVEALs skills to help me be more direct.

V *Use your* **Valued Goals** *to guide how you socially signal your needs.*

☐ Asserted with humility when I desired a close relationship with the other person by combining *nondominance* and *cooperative-friendly* signals when asserting my needs with a friend or close other.

☐ Was mindful of being polite, particularly when my request or refusal might place a burden on the other person.

☐ Asserted with confidence, *or even urgency*, when getting what I wanted was the most important objective or the situation was an emergency.

    ☐ I signaled **confidence** by looking the other person in the eye, speaking calmly but firmly, and keeping my shoulders back and my chin up.

    ☐ I signaled **urgency** by enhancing expressions of concern, using a commanding voice, speaking more rapidly, or pointing and gesturing more expansively.

☐ Signaled social safety and openness to the other person when the relationship was important. I remembered that people are more likely to help those they feel safe around.

    ☐ I signaled **openness** via eyebrow wags, warm smiles, openhanded gestures, adopting a musical tone of voice, head nodding, taking turns when conversing, slowing the pace of the conversation by taking a deep breath, and allowing time for the other person to respond to questions or complete observations before I spoke.

    ☐ I **took the heat off** by allowing the other person (and myself) the grace of not having to understand, resolve, or fix a problem or issue immediately.

    ☐ **In the heat of the moment,** I used nonverbal social signaling to slow the pace of the conversation and practiced signaling an easy manner, using nonverbal signaling (such as the Big Three + 1; see lesson 3).

☐ Avoided temptations to charm, cajole, sweet-talk, or flatter the other person.

☐ Avoided temptations to use disguised demands, such as "pushbacks" or "don't hurt me" responses (see Flexible Mind REVEALs).

E *Practice self-Enquiry to decide whether (or not) to repeat your assertion.*

☐ When challenged in the heat of the moment, practiced self-enquiry before responding, by asking *Is there something here for me to learn? Use the space provided to record your experience.*

_____

_____

☐ Used my desired level of intimacy with the other person to help guide how intense or repetitive I made my assertion.

    ☐ When the relationship did not matter, or when my valued goal was important, I repeated my assertion again and again (if necessary) in order to achieve my goal.

    ☐ When the relationship mattered to me, I blocked repeating my request again and again and practiced listening to the other person's response to my request with an open mind.

☐ Remembered that it is arrogant for me (or anyone else) to assume that other people should conform to my wishes or personal beliefs simply because I believe they are correct or that my needs are a higher priority.

☐ Rather than ignoring personal criticism or attacks, practiced kindness (for example, by treating the other person as I would like to be treated).

☐ Used the following questions to facilitate my self-enquiry work and recorded what I discovered in my self-enquiry journal. *Place a checkmark in the boxes next to the questions you found most helpful.*

    ☐ *What might my friend's or colleague's refusal to comply with my request tell me about the request itself? About our relationship? About myself? Is there something here to learn?*

    ☐ *Do I find myself wanting to automatically explain, defend, or discount the other person's feedback or what is happening? If yes or maybe, then is this a sign that I may not be truly open to considering their needs or circumstances?*

    ☐ *Where did I ever get the idea that I should always get what I want? Is there a part of me that desires to blame the other person or punish them for not complying with my request? Would I encourage a child to behave similarly? What might this tell me about my valued goals?*

    ☐ *Do I feel invalidated, hurt, unappreciated, or misunderstood by the person giving me the disconfirming feedback? If yes or maybe, then what is it that I need validated? Is there a chance that my desire for validation, feeling appreciated or understood, may make me less open to the criticism? Why am I expecting them to change rather than myself? Is there something here for me to learn?*

    ☐ *Is it possible that I am not responding to the actual situation but am bringing into the situation past experiences that may be influencing my perception? If so, then can I allow myself time to explore my responses before I push further for what I want?*

Record in the space provided the questions you found most helpful and/or other questions that arose during your practice.

_____

_____

_____

After the Interaction

Place a checkmark in the boxes next to the skills you practiced.

- ☐ I practiced self-enquiry when I found myself ruminating about what happened or when I was repeatedly replaying the event in my mind.

  - ☐ I used handout 18.1 (Self-Enquiry About Rumination After a Social Interaction) to deepen my practice and help locate my edge.

Record the questions you found most useful and/or others that emerged during your practices.

_____

_____

_____

- ☐ If I felt self-conscious, embarrassed, or ashamed during the interaction, I used handout 8.5 (The RO DBT Self-Conscious Emotions Rating Scale) to determine whether my self-conscious emotion was warranted or unwarranted. I practiced Flexible Mind SAGE skills (see lesson 8).

- ☐ I used Flexible Mind SAGE skills to identify potential disguised toxic social environments if I decided afterward that the relationship might be toxic.

- ☐ I practiced forgiveness when I found myself nurturing a grudge, using Flexible Mind Has HEART skills (see lesson 29).

Record other skills you used.

_____

_____

_____

Using Validation to Signal Social Inclusion

Main Points for Lesson 19

1. We are both transmitters and receivers of information.

2. Ruptures in relationships occur when people feel misunderstood. Ruptures are inevitable in close relationships and can be intimacy-enhancing if repaired. Validation is a core means of achieving this.

3. Validation requires us to understand the other person AND to communicate this understanding.

4. The intended receiver must experience the communication as validating, or it is not actually validating.

5. Not everything requires validation—some behaviors are invalid (for example, stealing from others) and require corrective feedback. Plus, from an RO perspective, the discomfort of invalidation serves as a reminder to practice self-enquiry.

Materials Needed

- (Optional) Handout 19.1 (Main Points for Lesson 19: Using Validation to Signal Social Inclusion)

- Worksheet 19.A (Flexible Mind Validates: The Seven Levels)

- (Optional) Photocopies of the (in)validation cards on page 380 and the newspaper clippings on page 381 for the optional class exercise "The Nonverbal Validation Game." Prepare in advance by cutting along the dotted lines to create enough cards for all participants.

- Whiteboard or flipchart and markers

Level 1 Validation Class Exercise CARDS
To make cards, use scissors to cut along the dotted line.

Validate your partner without using words

- Use eyebrow wags
- Turn your body toward them
- Make eye contact
- Head-nod to show you are listening
- Mimic their facial expression or tone of voice
- Half smile

Invalidate your partner without using words

- Pretend to read a newspaper
- Turn away slightly from them
- Make no eye contact
- No head-nods to show agreement
- Frozen expression
- Act bored--yawn or look at watch

No hamsters involved in Accident

According to the *New York Times* no hamsters were involved in an accident on I-95 today when a tanker truck carrying high-octane fuel collided with a pole mistakenly placed by workmen the night before in the middle of the road. A spokesman for hamsters said he was glad no hamsters were involved.

Man heroically stays quiet throughout entire two-hour meeting

An office worker was lauded as a hero yesterday, after not saying a single word during a two-hour meeting, choosing to slowly eat a bag of Maltesers instead. Word of the man's valiant effort quickly spread around his office, with many of his colleagues paying tribute to his selfless act of silence.

Britain's first pop-up goose café ends in disaster

East London's first pop-up goose-petting café ended in disaster on its launch day today as 17 people reported goose-related injuries within 2 hours of the café's opening. The café opened at 10 a.m. this morning, and by midday 17 phone calls to 999 had been placed, all of which concerning goose-related injuries. Bites were most common, however, one customer is in critical condition after a barrage of goose rage.

Londoners can now live in a cutlery drawer for £500

Prospective tenants are being asked to fork out two thousand pounds a month to live inside a drawer in posh South Kensington. Three other cutlery drawers are also available for rent, creating what the landlord calls "a community feeling... With people seriously struggling to find somewhere to live in the capital we wouldn't expect them to share a drawer with some forks and those corn-on-the-cob holders that never get used. That would be ridiculous. Tenants will have to provide their own cutlery."

National Health Service to replace antibiotics with Gin

The move comes after a number of warnings about the growing threat of resistance to antibiotics that could cast the world "back into the dark ages of medicine." "It's obviously very unsafe to mix medicine with alcohol, so we intend to stop using medicine altogether," said a senior NHS spokesman.

"Not-Turn-Up Fridays" increasingly popular with office workers

"Previously we've tried 'dress down Fridays,' 'cupcake Wednesdays,' and 'pizza Thursdays,' but 'not-turn-up Fridays' has improved staff moraletono end," said the manager of a marketing company. "In fact our employees love it so much they are now asking if it can be rolled out for the rest of the week."

(Required) Teaching Point
"We Are Tribe!"

$*$ *We feel safe when we are part of a tribe.* $*$

- **As we have learned in prior lessons, tribe matters!** The extent to which we are perceived by others as being in or out of our tribe strongly impacts our personal well-being (see Flexible Mind SAGE skills, lesson 8).

- **We are evolutionarily hardwired to be hypersensitive for signs of social exclusion.** Social ostracism hurts, and social inclusion feels good (Eisenberger & Lieberman, 2004; Leary et al., 1998; Murray et al., 2003).

- **Feeling part of a tribe is dependent on feedback from fellow tribal members.** Innately, most of us recognize that simply looking in the mirror and telling ourselves that we are lovable, competent, or a good person doesn't really help much. We depend on our fellow tribal members to verify our worthiness.

- **Social signals that overtly validate our status as a worthy tribal member are strongly desired and vigorously pursued.** We feel safe, secure, and relaxed when part of a tribe (see Flexible Mind SAGE skills, lesson 8).

- **Validation is an antishaming ritual;** see "(Not So) Fun (but Interesting) Facts: The Use of Shaming Rituals," in lesson 8.

- **It involves communicating understanding and acceptance of another's feelings, thoughts, desires, actions, or experience** (Fruzzetti & Worrall, 2010; Linehan, 1993b). It essentially says, "You are part of my tribe."

  ✓ **Ask:** *What does it feel like to be understood? Where do you experience it in your body?*

- **Healthy relationships depend on mutual and frequent validation.** They involve an intention to openly listen, actively self-disclose, signal kindness, and make self-sacrifices, without always expecting anything in return. They are two-way streets that require active participation from both participants.

- **A validating response does not directly seek to change or alter a person's emotional experience.** We signal to the other person that it is safe for them to share their inner experience with us and that we recognize our shared fallibility as humans.

- **Yet what is validating to one person may be experienced as invalidating by another.** Recall: each of us carries perceptual and regulatory biases with us wherever we go that influence how we see the world and other people, as well as how we cope within it.

- **Importantly, when we try to validate someone, the only true judge of our success is the person we are communicating with!** If they *do not* perceive our communication as validating, then—by definition—it was not validating.

- **Thus, good intentions don't matter; what matters is whether our social signals were actually experienced as validating by the other person.** Validation is a dynamic process whereby one person communicates their understanding to another person and the other person then signals in return whether or not these observations were perceived as accurate.

- **Plus, actions often speak louder than words.** For example, saying: *It must be painful when I step on your foot* is nice, but removing your foot is validating (and feels better ☺).

395

(Optional) Discussion Points

Enhancing Intimacy

- ✓ **Ask:** *Have you ever found yourself waiting for the other person to make the first move toward intimacy? What are you waiting for?*

- ✓ **Ask:** *What do you normally do to show others that you love or care about them?*

- ✓ **Ask:** *To what extent do you fully participate in relationships? How well do people know you? What is it that you might need to learn?*

NOTE TO INSTRUCTORS: Validation is often absent in the lives of many OC individuals, especially when they try to communicate problems with an emotional or vulnerable content. OC individuals may have been invalidated, criticized, or punished in the past for their *expression of private experiences* (for example, "You're not sad, you're just tired"), *displays of emotion* (for example, "Only weaklings cry"), *attempts at intimacy* (for example, "You don't need to be understood—you need to get back to your studies"), *self-initiated behaviors* (for example, "Stop acting silly"), and/or *being imprecise or not following rules* (for example, "Only stupid people color outside the lines"). Moreover, control, competency, and performance may have been the expected norm of the culture, family, or environment they were raised in. As such, small achievements may have rarely been highlighted or their pain may have rarely been acknowledged. Consequently, many OC clients may have relatively little personal experience in being validated or validating others. Thus, some class members may struggle with understanding the importance of validation.

(Required) Teaching Point

Using Validation to Signal Social Inclusion

Refer participants to worksheet 19.A (Flexible Mind Validates: The Seven Levels).

NOTE TO INSTRUCTORS: Remind participants that from an RO perspective, validation fundamentally represents a social signal from one person to another, essentially saying: "Not to worry—you are in my tribe." Since overcontrol is posited as a disorder of emotional loneliness, it is essential to learn not only how to rejoin a tribe (for example, using Flexible Mind ALLOWs skills) but also how to signal to other people that you want them in your tribe or consider them in your tribe. The following skills are designed to cover how to do the latter. In addition, higher levels of validation are not necessarily better than lower levels, and what is experienced as most validating varies considerably, depending on the context in which it is delivered.

Level 1. Being Attentive: "You Are a Worthy Tribe Member"

- *Nonverbally signal to the other person that you are attending to them.* Examples include…

  - Use affirmative head nods (up-and-down movement) to signal that you like them, that you are interested in what they are saying, and that they are in your tribe.

  - Use eyebrow wags (raised eyebrows) and a warm smile to signal friendliness and cooperation.

- Turning one's body toward the other person signals interest.

- A prolonged shoulder shrug combined with openhanded gestures signals nondominance and openness.

- Eye contact signals interest, caring, or concern in most cultures.

(Optional) Class Exercise
The Nonverbal Validation Game

Needed: Cut-up photocopies of the (in)validation cards on page 380 and the newspaper clippings on page 381.

Instruct participants to work in pairs, with one person designated A and the other B. Instructors should then provide member A of each dyad a brief newspaper clipping and hand partner B either a validating card or an invaliding card.

Read aloud these game instructions.

Okay, class, here is how the game will go. First, you and your partner are now a tribe. Feel free to give it a name, but not the Know-It-Alls—our experience has repeatedly shown that any group choosing this name somehow is unable to learn anything from the experience. We are still investigating (☺).

Second, teammate A has been provided with a brief news clipping. Their job is to read aloud to their teammate the first paragraph in the news clipping and then make a brief comment about it. In the meantime, teammate B has been provided with a card that contains instructions to either nonverbally validate or invalidate their teammate during the exercise. Teammate B should keep secret (sshhhh…it's a secret ☺) what's written on their card. The aim of the game is to work together—one transmitter, one receiver—and see how long it takes for teammate A to accurately guess whether teammate B was instructed to validate or invalidate them.

The game begins when teammate A reads aloud their news clipping and makes a comment about what they read to their teammate. Teammate A should be alert to the nonverbal behavior of teammate B while they are reading or commenting. Importantly, even if teammate A guesses correctly in two seconds whether teammate B is invalidating or validating (it usually is obvious), don't stop there—keep playing. Teammate A should continue reading aloud and making comments while teammate B nonverbally signals validation or invalidation.

My coinstructor and I will now demonstrate how this might look.

NOTE TO INSTRUCTORS: The coinstructor should pretend their card has instructed them to nonverbally invalidate the other instructor (that is, look away when they are reading or commenting, look bored, yawn, scowl, frown, pout, or huff). The instructor should continue reading the following script—and, for maximum comedic relief, the instructor ideally appears completely oblivious to rather blatant nonverbal invalidation skills by the coinstructor (tee hee ☺).

The instructor reads aloud the following clipping while the coinstructor attempts to get the instructor's attention via invalidating nonverbal gestures and facial expressions. Have fun! ☺

The Associated Press is reporting that a tanker truck carrying high-octane fuel overturned and burst into flames this morning on southbound I-71 after colliding with an abandoned La-Z-Boy recliner blocking the right-hand lane outside Walton, Kentucky. A representative of the American Society for the Prevention of Cruelty to Animals expressed the organization's gratitude that no hamsters were involved in the incident.

Next, the instructor makes a comment about the news clipping as they just read, while their coinstructor continues to nonverbally invalidate. For example, while looking directly at the instructor (for validation), the instructor might say:

I think this hamster story is a little silly. I mean, after all, why would hamsters even be concerned about a tanker truck exploding? It's not like tanker truck drivers are required to drive around with hamsters, are they? And even if they were, what exactly would a hamster's job be in a tanker truck, anyway?

After this demonstration, immediately start the game.

Teammate A should begin to read aloud the first paragraph of the news clipping they have been given and then make a brief comment about what they have just read.

Teammate B should practice nonverbally *validating or invalidating* teammate A (per instructions on card) as they read their news story and make their comments.

Allow approximately two minutes, then stop the role play. Provide sixty seconds for a discussion between partners and then switch roles. Provide a different news clipping to partner B and a new card for partner A. If time permits, switch again. Ideally, both partners get a chance to be on the receiving end of nonverbal validation and nonverbal invalidation. You can mix it up—the goal is to make learning fun and to encourage experimentation!

Discuss.

- ✓ **Ask:** *How easy was it to know whether the partner was assigned to the validating versus invalidating card? What did it feel like to be invalidated? How aware are you of nonverbal validation signals? How often do you use them? How aware are you of nonverbal invalidation signals? How often do you use them? What is it you might need to learn?*

(Required) Teaching Point
Reflecting Back

Level 2. Reflecting Back: "We're in the Same Tribe"

- **Reflecting back *means simply repeating back to the other person what we heard them saying, with humility.*** It signals that you care about understanding who they are, and it allows them an opportunity to correct your reflection (if they experience it as inaccurate).

- *Reflecting back does not assume our reflection is necessarily accurate.* Indeed, one of the core goals of this level is to signal a desire to know who they are and a willingness to be corrected by them until our reflection is perceived by them as accurate. Often our own worldview blocks us from seeing theirs.

(Required) Mini–Role Play by Instructors

Instructors should role-play the following example, with each taking a different part (that is, person A or B). Feel free to read directly from the text—doing so models to OC clients that it is okay to *not* have everything planned out perfectly in advance.

- **Person A** (reflecting back what they believe was said): *So sometimes you listen to people and you don't like it.*

- **Person B** (correcting the feedback): *It's not that I don't like it. It's that if it makes them feel a whole lot better, then it doesn't matter to me all that much.*

- **Person A** (reattempting reflection): *Okay, so what I am hearing is that it fits within your values to help other people, but you don't necessarily find it pleasurable to listen to them. Is that right?*

- **Person B** (agrees): *Yeah, I feel duty-bound to listen to others. I may not be enjoying it, but if it makes them feel better, then that's Okay by me.*

  ✓ **Ask:** *Why did person B correct person A during their first attempt to reflect back what they heard?* (Reread the two statements.)

  Answer: Person A appeared to be operating from a worldview that says, "Human behavior is motivated by emotions." For example, if someone goes to a party, it's because they anticipate feeling pleasure or a sense of connection when they listen to others. Person B is motivated by a differing worldview—they listen to others out of dutifulness or obligation, not because they anticipate pleasure or social safety. Their perceptions and motivation are rule-driven. This is a good example of how fundamentally different worldviews and motivating factors can influence our interactions. Fortunately, in this example, person A was able to quickly recognize that person B was motivated more by valued goals or rules and less by emotion; otherwise, this could have ended up as an argument (for example, imagine person A insisting to person B that a person can only ever be motivated to listen to someone because they are driven by an emotion such as fear or pleasure).

  ✓ **Ask:** *How often do you find yourself confronted by people with very different worldviews from yours? What does the preceding example tell us about the skill of reflecting back?*

> NOTE TO INSTRUCTORS: Sometimes our reflection may be technically accurate (if an audiorecording of the event was played back). However, the other person perceives our reflection as inaccurate and consequently feels invalidated. This can be frustrating when it happens, but the good news is, you can always try again. ☺

(Required) Class Exercise

Practicing Reflection

Split the group into pairs, and ask one member of the dyad (partner A) to start off by describing his or her experiences of traveling to the skills class that day. Partner B practices reflecting back what was said. Instructors should instruct partner A to pause frequently in order to allow partner B a chance to reflect back what was heard. Encourage partner A to provide details about inner thoughts, sensations, images, urges, and emotions. For example: "Today I woke up at 8 a.m. as usual and I took a shower as usual. I felt slightly annoyed when I realized that I was almost out of shampoo but made a note to myself to go to the store later" *(pause)*. Partner B then reflects back what they heard partner A saying, using level 2 validation skills.

Instructors should briefly demonstrate with their coinstructor how the exercise might go, if this isn't clear already from the mini–role play by instructors. Partners should switch roles and allow opportunities for both to practice reflection. The idea is to have fun with this exercise. Instructors should make sure that they are modeling Flexible Mind principles (for example, problems can be solved in a light and easy manner, and learning can be fun).

Discuss.

- ✓ **Ask:** *How accurate were you in being able to reflect back what your partner said?*

- ✓ **Ask:** *To what extent did you feel validated by the other? To what extent do you think you shared similar worldviews? If they were different, were you able to adjust your reflection to more accurately fit with how they see the world?*

(Required) Teaching Point

Empathic Mind Reading

Level 3. Empathic Mind Reading: "Welcome Home!"

- *Empathic mind reading is most usually needed whenever the person you are interacting with signals nonengagement, withdrawal, or appears to be shutting down OR they appear to be struggling to label their internal experience.* At level 3, the listener offers guesses about how he or she thinks the other person might be feeling or thinking, with humility.

- *"I am aware of imagining…"* One way to begin an empathic mind read is to use the Awareness Continuum (see lesson 12) and start by saying, *"I am aware of imagining that you are…"* and then complete this sentence with what you imagine the other person might be thinking, feeling, or wanting. Starting the sentence in this manner sends the message that you are taking responsibility for your personal observations as guesses, not truths.

The instructor can then smuggle a bit of fun into the class while teaching at the same time—for example, by winking at the class and then turning to the coinstructor and saying…

> So, [coinstructor's name], *I am aware of imagining that you are worried that there might not be enough time for you to show the class that little dance and jig you showed me last week. Not to worry—I'm here to help. We'll make time! How did I do? Did I get it right?* [tee hee ☺]

NOTE TO INSTRUCTORS: Recall that playful teasing between instructors is essential. It models a core RO principle—namely, that one can give feedback to others playfully and with warmth. It also shows participants that being silly is okay, that learning can be fun, and to not always take life so seriously (see "Fun Facts: Teasing and Being Teased," lesson 22).

- *Another way to start out an empathic mind read is to begin by saying, "If I were in your shoes…"* and similarly complete the sentence with what you are imagining the person may be experiencing.

  - For example, consider a father discussing whether to allow his teenage son to use the family car to go out with friends. The father notices during the conversation that the son becomes increasingly less responsive. The son's quiet behavior might reflect an emotion (for example, fear) or uncertainty about how to ask for what he wants effectively (or a range of other things, too ☺). Assuming the relationship is important, the father might say something like "If I were in your shoes right now, I might be thinking, 'Dad just doesn't realize how careful I will be—he just doesn't get it.'" The good news is that even if the father is completely off base (maybe the son's flat face was because he had a stomachache), at a very basic level he has communicated caring. Specifically, by trying hard to put himself in his son's shoes, he is signaling that he desires to know his son's worldview. The main point here is that empathic attempts at mind reading, even when inaccurate, often positively impact relationships.

- *"Please join with me."* When empathic mind reading is attempted with someone who appears to be shutting down or refusing to respond (albeit see also the required teaching point "'Don't Hurt Me' responses," in lesson 16), it sends a powerful social signal that essentially says, "I care about you so much that I am going to attempt to speak for you." This represents a variation of kindness first and foremost (see Flexible Mind ROCKs ON, in lesson 17) and is a strong prosocial joining signal.

- *"Wow, thanks for the help."* For someone who is genuinely struggling to label their inner experience (that is, they are not shut down), an accurate empathic mind read is almost always experienced as highly validating. Having another tribal member help us label what we are feeling inside helps us define what we are seeing—that is, is it a bunny rabbit or is it a tiger? See also "Fun Facts: The Story of Oog-Ahh (Sometimes a Cow Is Not a Cow)," later in this lesson.

- *Expect to get it wrong, and then repair, if necessary.* Whenever we are inaccurate in our empathic mind read, there is an easy way to repair the misunderstanding—namely, to apologize (see steps for appeasing in Flexible Mind SAGE, lesson 8).

- *Finally, successful mind reading does not mean approval.* One can understand and still disagree. For example, assuming the original mind read was experienced as validating, the father we met earlier might say to his son, "I understand that from your perspective you will do everything you can to drive safely. I still don't want you to drive the car tonight." In other words, the father can accurately mind read his son yet still stand firm about what he believes important.

Level 4. "Based on Your History…"

- *"Based on your history…"* Level 4 validation involves communicating to the other person that his or her experience is understandable because of what's happened to them in the past (or because of their biology).

- *"Your behavior makes sense."* It says, essentially, that anyone with a similar background (and/or biology) would behave in a similar manner.

- *"You are still in the tribe, but..."* Level 4 signals that one's behavior is understandable, based on history (or biology). Yet when the behavior is potentially harmful (to self or others), it often carries with it a caveat (that is, it doesn't mean approval). For example, a mother's emotional abuse toward her daughter may be understandable if she has had a history of abuse herself or it appears her biology is driving some of her responses, yet only to a certain extent. The relative seriousness of the emotional abuse may necessitate change on the mother's part. If she is unable to accomplish this, then the kindest thing to do (but not necessarily validating) for all involved is for a caring other to intervene and hopefully find a way to block or mitigate the mother's abuse (for example, whistleblowing or reporting her behavior to social services; see also the required teaching point "Despite Being Painful, Shame Is Prosocial," and "(Not So) Fun (but Interesting) Facts: The Use of Shaming Rituals," both in lesson 8.

(Optional) Class Exercise
Validating Based on History

Split the group into pairs. One partner in the pair should play the part of the guilty friend in the following story (let's call them partner A) while the other person in the pair plays the role of the validating friend (partner B). B's task is to practice using level 4 validation with partner A, using the scenario described here. Encourage participants to block urges to solve the problem or offer solutions; focus on validating instead, using level 4 principles. Instructors should read aloud the story and instructions.

Imagine you have a friend who you know to be very concerned about doing the right thing and not making waves. Moreover, you know that when your friend was young, her mother punished her harshly whenever she disagreed or stood up for herself. One day your friend tells you that she is feeling extremely guilty because she made a big mistake. It involved telling a colleague at work how she really felt about the new boss. She thought their new boss didn't seem interested in getting to know people, and she was really worried that her work schedule might change.

Have partner A play the guilty friend—that is, tell the preceding story in the first person. For example, start out by saying, "I wanted to let you know that I am feeling so guilty. The other day, I made a big mistake. I..." (and so on). Partner B should play the validating friend and practice level 4 validation. Instructors may need to demonstrate what a level 4 validation might look and sound like.

After about five minutes of practice, instructors should instruct class members to stop the role play and give each other feedback. Then switch roles (that is, A becomes the validating friend and B the guilty friend) and practice again. Instructors should feel free to make up other scenarios or use examples from participants' real lives. Remind participants to let go of rigid desires to validate perfectly, and encourage experimentation.

Discuss. After both partners have had a chance to experiment with level 4 validation, bring the class back together and solicit discussion. Use the following questions to facilitate this.

- ✓ **Ask:** *How successful were you in being able to validate your guilty friend, using her past history?*

- ✓ **Ask:** *What did you find most difficult about a level 4 validation? Is it possible to use level 4 if you do not know anything about a person's history?*

- ✓ **Ask:** *How hard was it to not offer solutions?*

- ✓ **Ask:** *How often did you find yourself asking questions rather than validating what you heard?*

Level 5. Normalizing: "You Never Left the Tribe"

- **Normalizing behavior:** Validating someone's behavior as normal signals to the recipient that how they behaved or emotionally responded is no different from how other tribe members would have reacted in similar circumstances.

- **"Welcome back to the tribe."** Normalizing says, "You are one of us." It is a powerful social safety signal. Recall that for our very early ancestors living in harsh environments, being in a tribe was essential for personal survival.

(Optional) Class Exercise

Differentiating Validating Based on History from Validating Based on Normalizing

Orient. Instructors should divide the group into pairs and then read aloud the following scenario.

Consider a friend who recently moved to the United States from England. Unfortunately, while learning to drive on the right-hand side of the road (English traffic flow is opposite to American), she sideswiped another car, causing a minor accident. You know about her mishap because you helped her deal with the aftermath. A few days later, you decided to ask your nervous British friend for help with moving. You asked her whether she might be willing to drive her battered but still functional car into midtown Manhattan during rush hour to help transport boxes. Your friend hesitated—she was a bit nervous about driving.

Instruct. Partner A role-plays the British friend in the preceding story, while B practices validating them based on their past history (level 4). Keep the role play short—about two to three minutes. Stop the role play, and ask dyads to evaluate briefly between themselves how the role play went. Next, switch roles, and B should play the British friend and A the validating friend, only this time the person doing the validation should try to validate by normalizing their friend's fear of driving into midtown Manhattan (level 5).

NOTE TO INSTRUCTORS: A level 4 validation (based on history) might be "It makes sense that you are feeling anxious about driving into midtown—you just had an accident learning how to drive in the US." A level 5 validation (normalizing) would be "It makes sense that you are feeling anxious about driving into midtown—everyone gets anxious in rush-hour traffic, and midtown is a nightmare!"

Encourage self-enquiry by asking participants to notice any differences about being on the receiving end of the differing types. Ask participants to evaluate how their role play went with their partner. Then solicit feedback and observations from the entire class, and use the following questions to deepen teaching.

- ✓ **Ask:** *Which level of validation felt more validating to you as the receiver—level 4 or 5? If there were differences, why do you think this may have occurred?*

- ✓ **Ask:** *Which type of validation did you find easier to communicate—that is, validating based on history (level 4), or validating by normalizing (level 5)? If there were differences, why do you think they may have occurred?*

- ✓ **Ask:** *If someone has trouble accepting a validation that suggests their behavior is normal, what might this mean? What are the downsides?*

Level 6. Signaling Trust: "I Believe in You"

- *Level 6 validation signals equality, respect, genuineness, and trust.*

- *It is kind;* it treats the other person as we would like to be treated.

- *It gives the other person the benefit of the doubt.* If level 6 could speak, it would say…

  - *"I trust you to do the right thing."*

  - *"I believe in your competence."*

  - *"I have faith in your ability to follow through with prior commitments."*

- *It does not mean treating the other person as fragile or incompetent by micromanaging or checking up on them* to see if they are doing what was promised.

- *It does not mean walking on eggshells or treating them as fragile by immediately jumping in to solve a problem or telling them how to solve it.*

- *It is often expressed playfully and irreverently—teasing, playing, laughing, and participating with others send a powerful social safety signal of friendship.*

- *It does mean speaking the truth and openly expressing what you feel, with humility.*

- *It does mean trusting in the other person's abilities to find a solution for their problem, without outside interference* (even if that solution might not be what we would have chosen). This allows the other person the opportunity to learn new skills on their own and build confidence in solving problems on their own (the primary exception to this is when it is a genuine emergency—that is, life-or-death scenarios).

- *It can sometimes mean having greater confidence in the other person than they do themselves.* When we are operating from level 6 validation, we are often able to see the other person's underlying goodness and/or competency that they themselves may not always believe is there.

- *When validating at level 6, practice using the Awareness Continuum* to help take ownership and describe your emotions, thoughts, sensations, and images when talking to the other person. For example, "I am aware of a thought that…," "I am aware of an emotion of…," "I am aware of imagining that…," or "I am aware of a sensation of…"

(Optional) Class Exercise

Signaling Trust

Read aloud the following scenario to the class.

Your eighteen-year-old son has gotten a part-time job and has recently opened a bank account. He has just received a letter from the bank informing him he is overdrawn. This was caused by a misunderstanding with his payroll department, which issued a check for his salary instead of paying it directly into his bank account. He has asked you to call the bank on his behalf to explain the problem because he has no experience with this and doesn't want to make a mistake. Plus, he's worried about how he will pay the overdraft fee.

Instruct the class to break into pairs. Partner A is to be the parent, and partner B is to be the son. Ask partner A to validate the son, using level 6 validation (behaving in a manner that communicates that the parent sees him as competent, without masking genuine feelings).

Encourage. If time permits, encourage participants to try to use all of the validation skills that they have learned to date (levels 1 through 6), if an opportunity arises. Remind participants to avoid offering solutions but to focus on validating. To make the exercise more challenging and fun, instructors can encourage participants to overplay or exaggerate the role of the son. For example, he might try to verbally or nonverbally persuade the parent that he is fragile or incompetent by pouting or sighing when the parent explains that he could handle calling the bank by himself. Then switch roles and practice again.

NOTE TO INSTRUCTORS: Although there is a wide range of potentially validating level 6 responses for this scenario, in general a level 6 validation in this situation would involve the parent displaying confidence in their son's abilities to make a telephone call to a bank manager, not calling for him and not telling him what to do. For example, they might say something like "The thing is, son, if I just go and take care of this problem for you, then it implies that I don't think you are capable of handling it on your own—and, frankly, I believe you are. So even though it may feel like I'm not helping, my intention is to treat you like an equal," using a warm yet matter-of-fact voice tone in order to nonverbally signal calm confidence in him.

Discuss.

- ✓ **Ask:** *How successful were you in communicating trust to your partner?*
- ✓ **Ask:** *Were you able to weave in other validation strategies?*
- ✓ **Ask:** *Was it difficult to not jump to solutions?*
- ✓ **Ask:** *How did it feel to be the son?*

Level 7. Reciprocity: "We Are the Same"

- *You cannot rely solely on words to express how you feel or to signal understanding.*

- *Strong, intimate bonds require nonverbally matching the other person's emotions.* The intensity, degree of expressiveness, types of gestures, voice tone, and facial expressions communicate to the other person that we care about what they are experiencing because we are feeling similarly.

- *Practice examples…*

  - **Imagine that your son or daughter has just won a prestigious award. Ask:** *Which scenario might make it clear that you are excited, happy, and proud?*

    1. **Sitting** quietly in your chair and with a slight smile calmly saying, "I'm so excited and proud."

    2. **Standing up** when they enter the room and giving them a high five and then clasping them on the shoulders as you smile broadly and say, "I'm so excited and proud!"

  - **Imagine being told by a friend that they have just lost their house due to bankruptcy.**

    - ✓ **Ask:** *What type of nonverbal signals are needed in this situation to match your friend's expression?*

(Required) Class Exercise
Reciprocity Matters!

Read aloud the following scenario in a manner that mimics the level of expressed emotional intensity for each person in the story. For the story to work, it is essential for the reader to dramatically act out the lines rather than simply read them. **The lines for the lottery winner** require an excited and happy tone of voice and body movements. **The lines for the friend** should be read using a flat tone of voice, with constricted body movements and little facial expression.

> *Imagine a friend rushes into your office one day with some very good news to tell you. He is very excited. Almost literally jumping up and down, and nearly shouting, he says, "You won't believe what just happened! I just found out that I won the lottery! I am a millionaire! I just won ten million dollars!" You smile slightly and respond, saying, "That's nice…you seem happy about this." Your voice is nondemonstrative; your manner is composed and calm. You have chosen your words carefully so that your friend knows that you understand that this event is a good thing for him.*

Discuss and teach.

  - ✓ **Ask:** *What is missing in the preceding interaction?*

    Recall that nonverbal expressions are usually considered by most people as better indicators of a person's true feelings than what they say. For example, in the preceding scenario, the flat facial affect and voice tone of the listening friend might result in misinterpretation of his true feelings about his friend winning the lottery (for example, envy rather than happiness).

  - ✓ **Ask:** *What would it look like if the friend in the story were to match the lottery winner's emotional signals?*

Instructors may need to demonstrate: "Wow! I just can't believe it!!" or "This is so exciting!" or "Oh my goodness—this is incredible!"

✓ **Ask:** *Can you think of other ways to reciprocally match your friend in the preceding scenario? What would they look like?*

Practice reciprocal matching. Split the class into pairs, and have partners take turns practicing nonreciprocal versus reciprocal matching of emotional signaling with their partner (using the scenario already described or ones created by the class). Remind participants that matching means using differing channels of nonverbal expression, such as voice tone, facial expression (for example, use eyebrow wags), and/or body movements. Make up other scenarios, and have fun!

(Optional) Class Exercise
Validation on Demand

The earlier level 6 exercise of parent and son can also be used to create a game called "Validation on Demand." Tell participants that while the role plays are going on, an instructor will call out a different validation level every few minutes—for example, "Okay, parents, try doing validating using an empathic mind read!" The person playing the parent needs to see if he or she can deliver the new level of validation on demand in a limited amount of time. For example, if "mind read" is called out, the parent might try to say something like "If I were in your shoes, I might be feeling a bit angry that Mom doesn't seem to want to help out." Remind participants that it is perfectly okay to peek at their workbooks as reminders, or the partner can help them out. Mix the exercise up, and create an air of unpredictability—for example, switch things around by having the son have to validate the parent. Smuggle humor and fun whenever possible.

Discuss.

✓ **Ask:** *Which level did you find most difficult to switch to? Were you able to let go of needing to do it perfectly, if only a little? Were some levels easier? Did they feel more natural, or normal? What might this tell you?*

NOTE TO INSTRUCTORS: Remember that the appropriate level is mainly determined by how the son behaves in the situation. For example, it can be hard to validate behavior as normal (see level 5) when the son is behaving petulantly.

(Required) Teaching Point
What About Invalidation?

NOTE TO INSTRUCTORS: Though validation enhances relationships, this does not mean validation must always occur. On the contrary, RO considers it essential to question our personal convictions and perceptions. Sometimes painful feedback is needed in order to grow (see Flexible Mind ADOPTS). As such, invalidation in RO DBT is considered an opportunity for growth and self-enquiry, and sometimes the most effective behavior is to invalidate invalid behavior (for example, a parent would be wise to invalidate their teenager's drinking and driving behavior). Plus, rather than automatically assuming the other person should validate us, RO DBT considers it essential to take responsibility for our personal emotional reactions first (see self-enquiry "how" skills, lesson 13). Instructors can also encourage participants to use Flexible Mind ADOPTS and the twelve questions for accepting or declining feedback to further enhance openness to invalidating feedback.

- **Here's the tricky part—sometimes we need to be invalidated in order to learn, or even survive.** That is, when our behavior is ineffective and we don't know it, or we don't want to know it, we need someone in our tribe to kindly point out our error.

★ **Fun Facts:** *The Story of Oog-Ahh (Sometimes a Cow Is Not a Cow)*

Imagine a mostly nice but sometimes grumpy tribal member known as Oog-Ahh (meaning "Strong One") who lived in Tribe Roc, a Stone Age community living millions of years ago. Over the years, Oog-Ahh had become increasingly nearsighted, a fact that he tried to avoid admitting (sometimes even to himself after smacking into a tree). One day he and his fellow tribe members were out hunting and gathering, as was normal for their way, when suddenly Oog-Ahh froze and pointed excitedly, saying, "Oooga booga buggy tooga!"—that is, "I see a cow!" However, his fellow tribe members said, "Nup, Oog-Ahh, buggy booga teartooga toc!"—that is, "No, Oog-Ahh, it is a tiger—let's run!" Oog-Ahh faced a dilemma—should he believe his own eyes or the eyes of his tribe? Standing firm (as he often had in the past) might mean cow for dinner—for the entire tribe! But then again, listening to his friends might prevent him from being the one who was dinner for someone else. Oog-Ahh chose to eat his pride instead and ran as fast as his legs could carry him. By willingly revealing his observations about nature and listening to the feedback—that is, invalidation of his cow revelation—Oog-Ahh was able to live another day, and the tribe was able to benefit from his excellent mushroom-picking abilities the following morning. (Oog-Ahh was known for his superior sense of smell.) However, in order to save their nearsighted friend, the tribe had to be willing to give him invalidating feedback and tolerate a potential temper tantrum. (Oog-Ahh was sometimes a little scary because he liked to carry around a big stick.) Importantly, to survive, Oog-Ahh had to be able to question his own beliefs after receiving feedback that his cow was not a cow but a tiger. By being open-minded and easygoing (albeit he was known to be grumpy, too), Oog-Ahh survived. And over the years, his telling of his infamous encounter with a man-eating cow, with gleeful self-effacing caricature, became a source of tribal legend and delight for the weans (or "children," as we now know them). The moral of this story is that Oog-Ahh's willingness to openly listen to critical feedback (that is, invalidation) represents a core strength of our species (not an embarrassing artifact). Being able to openly listen and act on critical feedback provided a huge evolutionary advantage because our individual survival no longer depended solely on our personal perceptions. It also helps explain why we are so concerned about the opinions of others.

- *Yet if invalidation is so important for both individual and species survival,* then why do we dislike it so much?

- *We dislike invalidation because (1) we fear social exclusion* (see lesson 8, "Tribe Matters: Understanding Rejection and Self-Conscious Emotions") *and (2) the truth hurts*—invalidation is painful because it often highlights the very place we need to learn from the most (but may be secretly hoping to avoid).

- *From an RO perspective, when we feel invalidated by someone, our goal is to use our discomfort as a reminder to practice self-enquiry first* rather than automatically blaming the world or others and/or expecting the world to change or see things from our perspective. The core question is, *Is there something here for me to learn?*

- *Plus, if invalidation is so useful, then how do we determine when it will be effective to use it?*

- *The good news is, you don't have to worry about when or how to invalidate. Like magic, invalidation happens all by itself!* Recall that from an RO perspective, you cannot make another person feel invalidated (or feel anything); each of us is responsible for how we choose to respond to the world.

- *Thus, healthy interpersonal living involves taking responsibility for our own emotional reactions while recognizing that our behavior also impacts the well-being of other people* (that is, we are responsible not only for how we react emotionally to feedback from others but also for how we behave around others).

- *Phew! That sounds like a lot of responsibility! But you can relax—there is a way forward. It involves being kind;* see worksheet 17. B (Kindness First and Foremost).

- *Kindness differs from validation, yet they both share some features, too.*

  - **Validation** focuses on communicating understanding and acceptance of another's feelings, thoughts, desires, actions, or experience.

  - **Kindness,** as practiced in RO, means lending a hand to help someone or stop unwarranted harm, with humility and without always expecting something in return.

★ **Fun Facts:** *Healthy Interpersonal Living*

- *Just to be different, let's be a little wicked and come up with some rules for healthy interpersonal living.* (Shhhh…don't tell anyone—tee hee ☺; we're supposed to be practicing how not to be so rule-governed!)

  - **Don't** purposefully try to invalidate, niggle, or harm someone because you believe they need to learn a lesson.

  - **Do** purposefully try to understand the other person's perspective and communicate your understanding to them, as best you can.

  - **Don't** assume that it is your responsibility to make the other person feel better.

  - **Do** decide to openly express your emotions and opinions to the other person, with kindness.

  - **Don't** expect others to think or behave like you do.

> - **Do** expect to be invalidated by others, and use the example of Oog-Ahh (Isn't this fun? ☺) to remind yourself to practice self-enquiry before you respond (if possible) and/or make any major decisions.
>
> - **Finally,** if the situation is imminently life-threatening and/or the behavior of the other person is clearly harmful or deceptive, then validation doesn't matter—ethics, fairness, and safety rise to the surface and take precedence. This last rule represents the motivation of the whistleblower. However, before you blow the whistle, seek outside and independent counsel, if at all possible.

(Recommended) Minipractice

Learning How to Learn from Invalidation

> NOTE TO INSTRUCTORS: The purpose of this minipractice is to provide participants a brief opportunity to practice self-enquiry around a recent experience of feeling invalidated. Participants should not pick an event that pertains to one of their RO classmates (that is, the aim is not to try to resolve a current relationship problem with a classmate), albeit it would be okay if they picked a time when they felt invalidated by their therapist (or one of the skills class instructors). As with most other "outing oneself" practices in RO DBT, this exercise DOES NOT involve participants outing themselves in front of the entire class; the exercise is done in pairs and discussed by the entire class afterward. See lesson 13 for more details and principles underlying RO self-enquiry "outing oneself" practices.

Teach. *As we have been learning, a core aim of radically open living is to cultivate an attitude of self-enquiry when confronted with feedback we dislike or personal distress. Research shows that being invalidated by someone triggers automatic emotional distress and reduces prosocial signaling* [Greville-Harris, Hempel, Karl, Dieppe, & Lynch, 2016; Shenk & Fruzzetti, 2011].

Teach. *RO encourages us to practice self-enquiry as our first response when we feel invalidated—rather than automatically blaming the other person, blaming ourselves, defending ourselves, dismissing the feedback, mindlessly giving in, accepting it, or expecting the world to change—in order to learn from the discrepant feedback.*

Instruct. *So think of a recent time you felt invalidated by someone who is not currently present in this room—that is, make sure the event you choose does not involve a fellow member of our class. This helps retain our goal of mutual support as we learn new skills. Plus, it doesn't have to be a big event or traumatic issue. We can learn as much from a minor event (for example, someone not paying attention when we were speaking) as from more dramatic events (for example, someone shouting at us). Here are the steps in brief* (**write each step on a whiteboard or flipchart**).

1. **The person outing themselves attempts to locate their edge** by briefly telling their partner about the emotional event, without justifying, defending, or rationalizing what happened (about one to two minutes).

2. **The listener listens,** without problem solving, assessing, soothing, validating, cheerleading, or encouraging acceptance, and then, after one to two minutes, stops the person outing themselves and asks: *Are you at your edge? If not, then what do you need to do to get there?* The listener writes down their response for their partner on a blank piece of paper.

3. **The listener asks:** *What is it that you might need to learn from this situation?* The listener can also pick a couple of the following questions to help further facilitate the practice.

   - *What might your emotional response to this event be trying to tell you? Is there a chance that what the other person said or did that resulted in the distress may actually represent a core area of growth?*

   - *Is the feedback something you have heard from others before? What might this tell you?*

   - *Is there any possibility that a small part of you is discounting the feedback to purposefully displease or punish the other person? What might this tell you?*

4. The listener writes down the practitioner's responses, without discussing, commenting, validating, soothing, or exploring. Sometimes it can help to ask every so often *Are you still at your edge, or have you regulated?* to help the practitioner learn to notice automatic attempts at regulation (a common occurrence).

After about five minutes, end the practice. The practitioner should attempt to identify the question(s) that most strongly elicited their edge, and the listener records it (them). The sheet of paper containing the self-enquiry questions is then given to the practitioner, and the pair can then share their observations with each other.

Then switch roles—the practitioner becomes the listener, and the listener the practitioner. Conduct the practice in exactly the same manner.

Teach and solicit observations from the entire class.

   ✓ **Ask:** *To what extent did you attempt to justify, explain, or defend yourself during your practice? What might this tell you? To what extent, when you were in the listener role, did you attempt to or desire to soothe, validate, reassure, or problem solve during your partner's practice? What might this mean about how you see the world, yourself, and/or other people?*

For the coming week, assign homework around the self-enquiry questions that arose from the practice. If a class member struggled with finding a question, locating their edge, or willingly practicing self-enquiry, encourage them to use handout 1.3 (Learning from Self-Enquiry), focusing on the questions pertaining to resistance or feeling nothing.

Remind the class that the practices, ideally, should be daily but always brief (no longer than five minutes). Each day, they should gently reask the self-enquiry question they discovered that brought them closest to their edge, and record in their self-enquiry journal what arises each time they ask the question. If a new question emerges, use that one as well.

Remind participants that self-enquiry means finding a good question, not a good answer, and to allow time to discover what might be needed to learn rather than quickly searching for a way to explain things away or regulate. Plus, remind them to practice being suspicious of quick answers or urges to regulate, as these may be masquerading as avoidance.

Lesson 19 Homework

1. **(Required) Worksheet 19.A (Flexible Mind Validates: The Seven Levels).** Ask participants to look for times throughout the week to practice validating others and to record the level(s) used. Encourage participants to see if they can find an opportunity to practice all seven levels. Ask participants to identify specific individuals in their social network who they may be able to practice with. Instructors may need to work on finding situations for practice for some OC individuals, due to isolation or lack of social contact. Participants should be reminded that validation does not have to be done only with people we know well; we can validate anyone.

2. **(Required) Practice being like Oog-Ahh during the week.** Encourage participants to look for opportunities to learn from feedback they find invalidating, using their (secret…shhhh ☺) rules for healthy interpersonal living to help guide them. Instruct them to incorporate Flexible Mind ADOPTS skills to enhance openness.

3. **(Optional) Assign homework around class members' self-enquiry questions that arose from the practice around invalidation** during the coming week. If a class member struggled with finding a question, locating their edge, or willingly practicing self-enquiry, encourage them to use handout 1.3 (Learning from Self-Enquiry), focusing on the questions pertaining to resistance or feeling nothing.

Radical Openness Handout 19.1

Main Points for Lesson 19:
Using Validation to Signal Social Inclusion

1. We are both transmitters and receivers of information.

2. Ruptures in relationships occur when people feel misunderstood. Ruptures are inevitable in close relationships and can be intimacy-enhancing if repaired. Validation is a core means of achieving this.

3. Validation requires us to understand the other person AND to communicate this understanding.

4. The intended receiver must experience the communication as validating, or it is not actually validating.

5. Not everything requires validation—some behaviors are invalid (for example, stealing from others) and require corrective feedback. Plus, from an RO perspective, the discomfort of invalidation serves as a reminder to practice self-enquiry.

Radical Openness Worksheet 19.A

Flexible Mind Validates: The Seven Levels

Look for five opportunities to validate another person. Describe the situations in which you practiced validation, what you said or did, and the aftereffects.

_____

_____

_____

_____

_____

- **Remember,** validation involves (1) understanding the other person, (2) communicating this understanding to them, and (3) the other person confirming that what you communicated was experienced by them as validating.

Level 1. Being Attentive: "You Are a Worthy Tribe Member"

This means using nonverbal signals to ensure that the other person is aware that you are interested and care about them.

Place a checkmark in the boxes next to the skills you practiced.

☐ Used head nods (up-and-down movement) to signal attentiveness.

☐ Matched the other person's emotional expression to signal empathy.

☐ Used eyebrow wags and smiling to signal cooperation.

☐ Used a prolonged shoulder shrug combined with openhanded gestures to signal nondominance and openness.

☐ Turned my body toward them during the conversation to signal interest.

☐ Maintained eye contact to signal interest, caring, or concern.

Other skills.

_____

_____

Level 2. Reflecting Back: "We're in the Same Tribe"

This means simply repeating back to the other person what we heard, with humility.

Place a checkmark in the boxes next to the skills you practiced.

☐ Listened and repeated back what I heard the person saying. I said…

_____

_____

☐ Was open to feedback suggesting that my reflection was not entirely accurate, and then tried again, using an easy manner.

☐ Used Flexible Mind ADOPTS to enhance my openness to the corrective feedback.

Level 3. Empathic Mind Reading: "Welcome Home!"

This means offering helpful guesses about what the other person may be trying to communicate.

Place a checkmark in the boxes next to the skills you practiced.

☐ Began my mind read by saying, "If I were in your shoes, I might be…" and then revealed what I imagined he or she might be experiencing or wanting.

☐ Began by using the Awareness Continuum ("I am aware of imagining that…") and then described what I imagined they might be experiencing or wanting.

☐ Blocked offering solutions or asking questions.

☐ Practiced humility by remembering we don't see things as they are—we see things as we are. Therefore, my mind read may be more about me than it is about them.

☐ Was open to feedback from the other person that my mind read was not entirely accurate or was even completely wrong, and then tried again, with an easy manner, or asked the person to help me understand better.

☐ Used Flexible Mind ADOPTS to be open to corrective feedback.

☐ Apologized if my mind read was experienced as hurtful to the other person, in order to signal that his or her feelings and reactions are important to me.

☐ Remembered that a successful mind read does not mean approval. I can understand someone yet still disagree.

Other skills.

_____

_____

Level 4. "Based on Your History..."

This means signaling to the other person that, given their background or biology, their experience or reaction makes sense.

Place a checkmark in the boxes next to the skills you practiced.

☐ Started by saying "It makes sense that you…," then described my response and continued by saying, "…because of what happened to you in the past," ending with a brief description of the past experience.

☐ Remembered that level 4 validation does not mean approval, and instead communicated, in a warm manner, that the behavior is understandable, given the person's past history or biology.

☐ Was open to being inaccurate, and used Flexible Mind ADOPTS skills to help.

☐ Remembered that it is hard to validate at level 4 if I don't know anything about the person's past history.

Other skills.

_____

_____

Level 5. Normalizing: "You Never Left the Tribe"

This means signaling to the other person that anyone in the same situation would have behaved in a similar fashion.

Place a checkmark in the boxes next to the skills you practiced.

☐ Started by saying "It makes sense that you…," then described the response, ending with "…because anyone would have responded the same."

☐ Was open to feedback from the other person that what I said was not experienced as validating, and asked the person to help me better understand.

Other skills.

_____

_____

Level 6. Signaling Trust: "I Believe in You"

This means genuinely revealing our inner experience, without blaming or trying to control the other person or the situation, and trusting the other person to be able to deal with that.

Place a checkmark in the boxes next to the skills you practiced.

☐ Reminded myself that people trust and prefer to spend time with people who openly reveal their inner feelings, even when the emotions are negative.

☐ Expressed my genuine emotion and inner thoughts, and took responsibility for my reactions rather than blaming my experience on others or the world.

☐ Used the Awareness Continuum to help take ownership and describe my emotions, thoughts, sensations, and images when I was talking with the person (for example, "I am aware of a thought that…," "I am aware of an emotion of…," "I am aware of imagining that…," or "I am aware of a sensation of…").

☐ Trusted the person I was interacting with to be capable of finding his or her own solution rather than telling the person what to do.

☐ Blocked pretending that everything was okay, and revealed what I was genuinely experiencing in the moment, without blaming the other person.

☐ Went opposite to thinking "They won't be able to handle what I truly think or feel" and revealed anyway.

☐ Went opposite to walking on eggshells or trying to control the other person's reaction by revealing my genuine experience in the moment, without blaming the other person for my personal reactions.

Other skills.

_____

_____

Level 7. Reciprocity: "We Are the Same"

This means matching the other person's level of emotional expression or vulnerability.

Place a checkmark in the boxes next to the skills you practiced.

☐ Remembered that people believe nonverbal expressions of emotion to be more truthful than what a person says.

☐ Remembered that matching expressions of emotions (whether positive or negative) communicates that the other person's experience is valid because I am reacting in the same manner.

☐ Practiced matching the level of emotional intensity, vulnerability, or manner of expression of the person I was interacting with.

Other skills.

_____

_____

Enhancing Social Connectedness, Part 1

Main Points for Lesson 20

1. We like people who like us, but to be liked we must take the risk of being disliked.

2. People vary in how much intimacy they desire, and that is okay.

3. We are all dependent on each other, whether we like it or not.

4. Being close to others requires practice. Intimacy requires vulnerability.

5. Old wounds can always be repaired by signaling that we are willing to reengage.

Materials Needed

- Handout 20.1 (Self-Enquiry About Mistrust)

- Handout 20.2 (The Intimacy Thermometer)

- Handout 20.3 (What Characterizes a Genuine Friendship?)

- (Optional) Handout 20.4 (Main Points for Lesson 20, Part 1: Enhancing Social Connectedness)

- Flipchart or whiteboard and markers

(Optional) Teaching Point
Dependency

  ✓ **Ask:** *When you hear the word "dependency," what comes to mind?*

- *Dependency is not a dirty word,* despite what you might have heard.

- *For example, right now we are all depending on the person who made the chairs we are sitting on to have made them strong enough not to break.* We depend on the deliveryperson to bring fresh milk for our coffee or tea. We depend on the farmer to grow healthy food. Doctors depend on their patients to reveal what is ailing them, even when it is embarrassing. We depend on teachers to know what they are doing, and teachers depend on class members to study the material and show up to class. The list goes on and on.

- *Dependency involves trusting another person*—for example, to do what they promised. It is a normal and healthy part of life and relationships. It makes it possible for us to achieve more than one person could ever accomplish alone. Imagine trying to build the pyramids all by yourself.

  ✓ **Ask:** *What are other advantages? What might be some disadvantages?*

(Required) Teaching Point

Friendships Can Be Hard Work

- *We like people who like us, but to be liked we must take the risk of being disliked.* Sitting at home waiting for our knight in shining armor or our beautiful princess to sweep us away works well in the movies, but not in real life.

- *Finding and maintaining a genuinely intimate and mutually caring relationship with another person is hard work!* The effort you put into achieving genuine social connectedness should be equivalent to the effort you would put toward finding and securing a new job.

- *Close friends trust each other.* They are relaxed when together. They feel safe because they trust the other to be nonexploitative.

    ✓ **Ask:** *Who do you feel safe around? What might that tell you about the relationship?*

(Required) Class Exercise

Thinking About Distrust

Refer participants to handout 20.1 (Self-Enquiry About Mistrust).

Ask the participants to think of someone they distrust or are struggling to be open with or self-disclose to. Then ask participants to break into pairs, and have them take turns reading aloud one of the self-enquiry questions found in handout 20.1 (Self-Enquiry About Mistrust) to each other and discussing how relevant the question seems to the distrustful relationship they chose for this exercise.

(Required) Teaching Point

Differences in Desired Intimacy

- *People vary considerably in the strength of their desire for warm, close, and validating experiences with other people* (McAdams, 1985). These differences between people can lead to misunderstanding, confusion, or conflict. The person in a relationship who desires less intimacy is in the power-up position because friendship is something that must be freely given; it cannot be taken. The person desiring more intimacy can be perceived as demanding, needy, or nagging by the person desiring less intimacy (T. R. Lynch, Robins, & Morse, 2003).

- *There is NO right or wrong when it comes to the amount of desired intimacy a person should have.* What is important is the degree of overlap between intimacy needs. When there is little overlap, this can lead to problems. For example, a person needing less intimacy may start to feel smothered, while the person desiring greater intimacy may feel deprived.

- *An important step in improving relationships is to understand, appreciate, and validate the other person's style of intimacy.* This means letting go of harsh judgments about the other person's natural level of desired intimacy or style of relating to others. Remind participants that

419

the person desiring less intimacy can afford to care less or behave in a distant/aloof manner because doing so is *not* incongruent with how they feel. However, this can be experienced by the person desiring more intimacy as hurtful or uncaring. In addition, because the person who desires less intimacy may literally be less concerned about the other person, they may also appear to care less when conflict or disagreement occurs.

(Required) Class Exercise
The Intimacy Thermometer

Refer participants to handout 20.2 (The Intimacy Thermometer).

- **Instructors should draw** three vertical lines, with the names from the handout ("Jill," "Jack," "Julie") above each line, and then label the crosslines—"Jill's (Jack's, Julie's) maximum intimacy," "Jill's (Jack's, Julie's) natural set point," "Jill's (Jack's, Julie's) minimum intimacy"—as in the handout.

- **Ask participants** to take a moment to bring into their awareness a relationship they would like to improve, or a person they would like to get closer to. Ask them to share this with the group, if possible. Depending on time constraints, one or two examples may suffice.

- **Use self-enquiry and discuss.** Ask participants to think of an existing relationship they are in—ideally, a long-term caring relationship, though this is not required. Read aloud the following questions, and then ask participants to quickly write down their first impressions. Use the following questions to facilitate self-enquiry.

  - ✓ **Ask:** *Are there differences in desired intimacy in your relationship? Does one person appear to want more closeness, compared to the other? If so, how does this manifest? Who in the relationship feels most content with the level of closeness? What evidence did you use to answer this?*

  - ✓ **Ask:** *How does this difference in desired intimacy impact your relationship?*

  - ✓ **Ask:** *Does this ever lead to problems or misunderstandings?*

  - ✓ **Ask:** *Would you like to change some of the dynamics of the relationship?*

  - ✓ **Ask:** If unable to answer or unsure how to answer the preceding questions, ask: *What might this mean? What steps would you need to take to find out?*

- **Discuss and teach:** Instructors should use the preceding questions to deepen teaching. Instructors can explain that the good news is that by acknowledging differences in desires for closeness or intimacy in our relationships, we are better able to know how we might help improve the relationship. For example, the person desiring *less* intimacy in a relationship will need to work harder at being more intimate (for example, expressing more, finding time to spend with the other person, looking for shared interests). The person desiring *more* intimacy will need to work at letting go of expectations of achieving their maximum level of intimacy (for example, by practicing acceptance, looking for other means of getting intimacy needs met, and/or appreciating times their partner tries to engage them).

NOTE TO INSTRUCTORS: OC participants will exhibit a range of desires for intimacy. Some may report feeling very little desire, whereas others may report strong desires for intimacy or closeness, and loneliness. Thus, instructors should not presume that the aloof and distant relationships that characterize OC necessarily reflect a lack of desire to be close to others. Often their aloofness is due to a lack of skills in knowing how to get closer to someone. Importantly, not all relationships should (or could) be highly intimate. For example, we might have a family relationship (for example, with a sister or a parent) that is not particularly close, perhaps due to fundamental intimacy differences; however, we can still choose to continue relating to this person and/or honor our prior commitments with them, albeit perhaps with lowered expectations about the degree of closeness possible. Research suggests that we need only one relationship that involves strong feelings of attachment, love, or mutual caring to reap the positive psychological benefits essential for well-being.

(Required) Discussion Point

What Characterizes a Genuine Friendship?

Refer participants to handout 20.3 (What Characterizes a Genuine Friendship?).

NOTE TO INSTRUCTORS: The best way to review handout 20.3 (What Characterizes a Genuine Friendship?) is not to worry about covering every point. This is a good example of a handout that can be used to get everyone in the class speaking and participating when you have quiet classes. Randomly select a class member to read aloud one of the bulleted points on the handout, and then discuss each briefly. If you use the handout for this reason (that is, getting a quiet class to engage) as well as for learning about friendships, then make sure everyone in the class has been given at least one turn to read a statement aloud (OC individuals tend to keep score).

(Required) Teaching Points

Trusting Others

- *Trusting another person can feel scary or unwise BECAUSE...*
  - *Trust requires one to drop one's defenses,* which opens up the possibility of being hurt.
  - *Yet, revealing vulnerability and communicating distress to others is an important part of healthy relationships.* Without it, we would never receive needed help from others or develop close relationships; in fact, communicating painful emotions has been shown to enhance intimacy (Laurenceau, Barrett, & Pietromonaco, 1998).
    - ✓ **Ask:** *What are the pros and cons of being distrustful and the pros and cons of being trustful?*
    - ✓ **(Optional) Ask:** *What behaviors are associated with trusting someone?* (Write them on the board).
    - ✓ **(Optional) Ask:** *What do you typically do to avoid being hurt by someone? Can you identify the hunting dogs and swords you carry with you when you feel distrustful?* (Instructors should be prepared to share examples from their own life).

- **The good news is that you need only one friend (or close relationship).** Research suggests that we need only one relationship that involves strong feelings of attachment, love, or mutual caring to reap the positive psychological benefits essential for well-being.

- **What is important for psychological health is to have one person who you can depend on to be there when you need them.**

- **It is quality that matters, not quantity** (that is, not the number of friends or acquaintances a person has).

- **The skills taught in the next lesson are designed to accomplish this** by providing the steps needed for the development of a close relationship and/or the improvement of an existing one (see Flexible Mind ALLOWs, lesson 21). Yet developing a genuine friend or improving current relationships takes practice—**so you can relax (☺).** The skills we learn today cannot be rushed.

Lesson 20 Homework

1. **(Required) handout 20.1 (Self-Enquiry About Mistrust).** Using handout 20.1, participants should practice self-enquiry and record what they learn in their self-enquiry journal.

2. **(Required) Handout 20.3 (What Characterizes a Genuine Friendship?).** Participants should use handout 20.3 as a guide for how to behave when interacting with friends or people they would like to have as friends. Encourage them to observe their interactions with others. Which principles of friendship are part of their relationships with others? If they find themselves lacking, rather than using this as another opportunity to get down on themselves, give up, or blame others, they should use it as an opportunity to practice self-enquiry. The question is *What is it that I might need to learn?* They should record their observations in their self-enquiry journal.

3. **(Optional) Participants should look for three opportunities in the next week to practice disclosing something at a more personal level than they normally would** (for example, while talking with a grocery clerk, a postal worker, and a neighbor). Instruct them to observe how self-disclosure influences the relationship.

Radical Openness Handout 20.1

Self-Enquiry About Mistrust

Instructions: Use the following sample questions to enhance your practice of self-enquiry about mistrust.

Carry a copy of this list with you, and write down in your self-enquiry journal new questions you discover.

➢ *Is there an alternative explanation for their behavior? How might they describe their behavior?*

➢ *Do I find myself wanting to automatically explain or defend myself? If yes or maybe, is it possible that I am not open to being truly fair-minded?*

➢ *Do I believe the other person must apologize or make amends before I would be willing to consider how I have contributed to the conflict?*

➢ *How open do I want to be in this situation with the person I will be interacting with? What might be holding me back?*

➢ *What is the worst thing that could happen if I express myself more openly?*

➢ *Am I discounting or minimizing positive things about the person or situation in order to punish them? Is it possible that I am not really giving them a chance? What am I afraid might happen if I were to momentarily drop my perspective?*

➢ *Do I believe that further self-examination or work on the relationship is unnecessary because I have already done everything possible?*

➢ *If someone else were watching the person's behavior, would he or she see it differently than me? If yes or maybe, then what might this mean?*

➢ *If the other person appears tense or even hostile when interacting with me, is it possible it has nothing to do with me? Is it possible the person is struggling with other personal issues and not acting out of malice? If so, what might this mean? What is it I need to learn?*

➢ *Is it possible that this other person finds it difficult to regulate emotions or deal with conflict? If so, how might their behavior influence my perceptions of them, and in what way? What might I need to learn?*

➢ *Could the behavior I am seeing be due to past trauma or issues that I don't know about that have influenced their way of responding? Is it possible that they sometimes struggle with empathy toward others or may find it hard sometimes to appreciate how their behavior impacts others?*

Write out the question(s) you found most useful, or other questions that emerged.

_____

_____

_____

_____

_____

- **Remember, keep your self-enquiry practices short in duration**—that is, not much longer than five minutes. The goal of self-enquiry is to *find a good question* that brings you closer to your edge or personal unknown (the place you don't want to go) in order to learn.

- **Remember to record** the images, thoughts, emotions, and sensations that emerge when you practice self-enquiry in your self-enquiry journal.

- **Remember to practice being suspicious of quick answers** to self-enquiry questions. Allow any answers to your self-enquiry practice to emerge over time.

Radical Openness Handout 20.2

The Intimacy Thermometer

Ideally, we find relationships where the intimacy overlap is large.

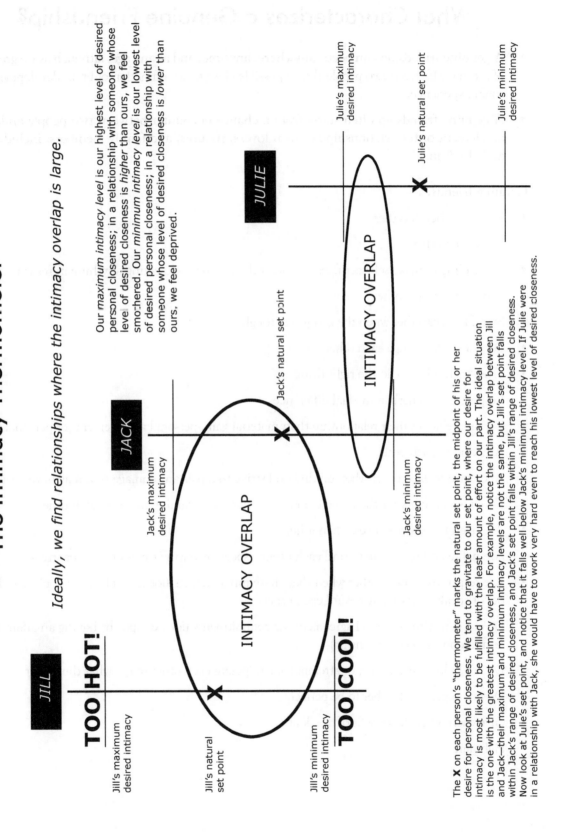

Our *maximum intimacy level* is our highest level of desired personal closeness; in a relationship with someone whose level of desired closeness is *higher* than ours, we feel smothered. Our *minimum intimacy level* is our lowest level of desired personal closeness; in a relationship with someone whose level of desired closeness is *lower* than ours, we feel deprived.

The **X** on each person's "thermometer" marks the natural set point, the midpoint of his or her desire for personal closeness. We tend to gravitate to our set point, where our desire for intimacy is most likely to be fulfilled with the least amount of effort on our part. The ideal situation is the one with the greatest intimacy overlap. For example, notice the intimacy overlap between Jill and Jack—their maximum and minimum intimacy levels are not the same, but Jill's set point falls within Jack's range of desired closeness, and Jack's set point falls within Jill's range of desired closeness. Now look at Julie's set point, and notice that it falls well below Jack's minimum intimacy level. If Julie were in a relationship with Jack, she would have to work very hard even to reach his lowest level of desired closeness.

425

Radical Openness Handout 20.3

What Characterizes a Genuine Friendship?

- **A genuine friendship can occur anywhere, anytime, and at any age,** although as we grow, the type of intimacy between two people that is possible changes as a function of brain development and personal experience.

- **A genuine friendship often starts from a chance encounter between two people and, ideally, is an element of the relationship between lovers, spouses, and family members, including parents and children.**

Genuine friends…

- Feel safe when together

- Trust each other

- Are willing to make self-sacrifices for each other, without expecting anything in return

- Look out for each other

- Stand by each other when the going gets tough

- Do not try to change each other

- Trust each other to do the right thing

- Respect each other's individual differences

- Care more about their relationship than material gain, personal achievement, or personal needs

- Are kind to each other

- Apologize to each other when unkind and strive to repair any damage that may have been done

- Take responsibility for their own emotions rather than blaming them on each other

- Are open to feedback, even when it hurts

- Are polite and respectful toward each other, especially during times of crisis or stress

- Are respectful of each other when they share inner feelings (for example, they don't yell, shout, belittle, or speak sarcastically toward each other)

- Do not betray their mutual agreements or commitments (for example, by having an affair if in a long-term monogamous relationship)

- Do not bully, threaten, lie, or attempt to manipulate each other to get what they want

- Do not expect each other to be perfect

- Give each other the benefit of the doubt

- Fight fair

- Do not automatically assume each other to be in the wrong when they are in conflict
- Admit to each other their own possible contributions to a conflict or disagreement
- Do not hold grudges
- Work out resentments, conflicts, or misunderstandings when they arise rather than walking away, holding on to them, or hoping they will go away
- Work together to solve problems, without keeping track of who has worked harder
- Respect each other's opinions
- Give each other time to express their views and openly listen to each other
- Don't feel self-conscious with each other and can be emotionally uninhibited and loose when together, especially when the context calls for it
- Can drop their guard and relax, and find each other easy to be around
- Look forward to seeing each other
- Protect each other but are also willing to tell each other when they think the other is doing something wrong
- Are open to being wrong about their own opinions
- Revel in and respect their differences rather than expecting to be the same
- Give each other the gift of truth, with kindness, and tell each other what they really think or feel
- See each other as equals
- Are able to tease each other
- Enjoy their time together and miss each other when separated
- Share their successes and failures with each other

Write other ideas.

_____

_____

_____

_____

_____

Radical Openness Handout 20.4

Main Points for Lesson 20, Part 1

Enhancing Social Connectedness

1. We like people who like us, but to be liked we must take the risk of being disliked.

2. People vary in how much intimacy they desire, and that is okay.

3. We are all dependent on each other, whether we like it or not.

4. Being close to others requires practice. Intimacy requires vulnerability.

5. Old wounds can always be repaired by signaling that we are willing to reengage.

Enhancing Social Connectedness, Part 2

Main Points for Lesson 21

1. It is not how many friends you have that matters, it is the quality of your social connectedness.

2. You only need one person in your life who is willing to make self-sacrifices to care for you when you are in distress and make you feel socially safe. Higher levels of intimacy increase social safety.

3. Match + 1 represents a core skill needed to form close social bonds—revealing personal feelings to others fosters reciprocal revelations.

4. Intimate relationships mean knowing not only about the things a person is proud of or does well but also about those areas in life they struggle with and about their inner fears or doubts.

Materials Needed

- Handout 21.1 (Enhancing Social Connectedness, Using Flexible Mind ALLOWs)

- Handout 21.2 (Match + 1 Intimacy Rating Scale)

- Handout 21.3 (Using Match + 1 to Establish New or Improve Existing Relationships)

- (Optional) Handout 21.4 (Main Points for Lesson 21: Enhancing Social Connectedness, Part 2)

- Worksheet 21.A (Practicing Flexible Mind ALLOWs)

- Flipchart or whiteboard and markers

- Video clip showing a range of gestures and facial expressions

- Videoplaying equipment and screen

(Required) Teaching Point

Flexible Mind ALLOWs

Refer participants to handout 21.1 (Enhancing Social Connectedness, Using Flexible Mind ALLOWs).

NOTE TO INSTRUCTORS: As with other RO skills, write out the acronym (ALLOWs) on a flipchart or whiteboard with each letter arranged vertically in a column, but *without* teaching or naming the specific skill that each letter signifies. Next, starting with the first letter in the acronym (A in ALLOWs) teach the skills associated with that letter, using the key points outlined in the following sections, until you have covered all of the skills associated with each individual letter. Importantly, only write out on the whiteboard or flipchart the global description of what each letter actually stands for when you are teaching the skills associated with it.

A **Assess** your commitment to improve the relationship

L **Look** for concrete evidence that mistrust is justified

L **Loosen** your grip on past hurts and fears

O **Out yourself** by revealing inner feelings

W **Welcome** feedback and continue to dialogue

> **NOTE TO INSTRUCTORS:** OC participants will exhibit a range of desires for intimacy. Some may report feeling very little desire, whereas others may report strong desires for intimacy or closeness and loneliness (see also lesson 20). The goal of Flexible Mind ALLOWs is *not* to increase the number of superficial friends or social contacts, but instead to increase the *quality* of intimate relationships, NOT the *quantity* per se.

A Assess *whether you are committed to improving the relationship and are willing to let go of mistrust.*

- Use handout 21.2 (**Match + 1 Intimacy Rating Scale**) to rate both the current level of intimacy in the relationship and the desired level of intimacy.

  - ***Remember that getting closer to someone does not necessarily mean that they must become your best friend*** or that you will get married! Getting closer means improving a relationship. For example, friends are more likely to help each other.

  - ***Practice self-enquiry.*** Ask yourself the following questions:

    ➢ *Am I finding it hard to think about this relationship, question my point of view, or engage in self-enquiry about my feelings when it comes to this relationship? If yes or maybe, then what might this mean?*

    ➢ *What have I found useful or rewarding in the past about this relationship? What do I want from this other person?*

    ➢ *Would an improved relationship help me obtain an important goal or help me to live by my values?*

    ➢ *What are the pros and cons of trusting this person? What are the pros and cons of mistrusting this person?*

    ➢ *What am I afraid might happen if I were to reveal my inner feelings to this person?*

L Look *for concrete evidence that mistrust is justified or the relationship is toxic.*

- Use Flexible Mind SAGE skills to determine if the relationship is toxic.

  - ***Look for Fixed Mind or Fatalistic Mind thinking***—for example, quick dismissal of the importance of the relationship or decisions about possible trustworthiness (Fixed Mind) or feelings of hopelessness or thoughts saying, *Why bother trying? Nothing will ever improve our closeness or the relationship* (Fatalistic Mind).

- *Remember that old hurts and current mood can color how we perceive another person.* We tend to pay attention most to those things that confirm our beliefs, and ignore or dismiss information to the contrary (that is, our perceptions are subject to confirmation bias).

- *Use self-enquiry to open up to the possibility of misperceiving the other person's intentions, beliefs, feelings, or thoughts.*

Refer participants to handout 20.1 (Self-Enquiry About Mistrust).

L Loosen *your grip on past hurts and fears.*

  ✓ **Ask:** *Even if it is true that the person has harmed me in the past, would it be helpful to repair the relationship?*

- *Just because you distrust someone, this does not automatically mean that they distrust you.* He or she may not even know that you feel dislike or distrust; they may feel neutral, and/ or they may even like you.

- *Practice giving them the benefit of the doubt, and assume the person is doing the best they can to cope with life.* (Instructors can model this principle and RO by saying: *I am teaching this point the best I can, right now. But this does not mean that I could not do better. I am sure there might be better ways to make this same point.*) Assuming that someone is doing the best he or she can does not remove the responsibility to work harder, but it does allow us to let go of harsh judgments and expectations.

NOTE TO INSTRUCTORS: Encourage participants to consider the possibility that the distrusted person may have benign or neutral intentions but is perhaps not very good at showing this. Other emotions or past learning may also get in the way.

- *Remember times you thought negatively about someone and later realized you had misjudged the person*—for example, believing that another person's silence meant they disagreed, only to discover later that they agreed but were unsure how to tell you this. People who have the capacity to admit when they are wrong are respected by others. More often than not, admission of a mistake is considered to be a courageous act. Acknowledging when we have been mistaken communicates to others that we value not hurting others (Gold & Weiner, 2000).

- *Remind yourself "Just because I think it, doesn't mean it's TRUE." Go ahead, right now, imagine yourself to be seven feet tall!* Just because you think it, doesn't make it so. (This can be an excellent opportunity to conduct a brief practice of the Oompa-Loompa chant or dance; see lesson 5.)

- *Accept the fact that you can never know what another person is thinking.* Use the required exercise "We Can Never Fully Know," later in this lesson, to augment teaching.

- *Use Flexible Mind Has HEART and forgiveness practices* (see lesson 29) *to let go of past hurts before interacting with the person.* Remember, letting go of distrust does not mean agreement.

(Required) Class Exercise
"We Can Never Fully Know"

The instructor should ask the class to read their mind, using a lighthearted irreverent manner. For example, behave as if you are a famous stage magician challenging the audience. Think of something that is highly improbable for anyone to guess, such as a porpoise swimming through the air in the room, wearing a bowler hat. Be creative! You need to be able to honestly respond that participants' guesses are incorrect. Select participants to guess, and give them another chance…if they want to try again! Make it fun! Ask if anyone else wants the class to try to guess their thoughts. The main point is that we can never truly know what another person is thinking or feeling unless the person reveals it first. And then, of course, you have to trust what they have revealed (remember the first *L* in Flexible Mind ALLOWs: look for concrete evidence that mistrust is justified). Instructors can remind participants that empathic mind reading (taught in lesson 19 validation skills) may appear to contradict the preceding point. However, mind reads are considered helpful guesses about a person's inner experience, not statements of truth or fact.

O **Out yourself** *by revealing inner feelings.*

- **Outing yourself** *means revealing your inner experience to another person* (see lesson 13).

- ***Activate your social safety system before outing yourself.*** For example, use the Big Three + 1 (that is, lean back in chair, closed-mouth smile, take a deep breath, and eyebrow wag) or, if possible, practice loving kindness meditation prior to the interaction.

- ***Self-disclosure communicates to others that you trust them and that you intend them no harm, making it more likely for the other person to reciprocate.*** Recall that we hide our feelings when we feel unsafe or when we distrust someone, and this makes it more likely for others to hide their feelings, too.

  - ✓ **Ask:** *Can you identify a person with whom you can freely express your emotions? What does this feel like? To what extent do they freely express their emotions or inner thoughts to you?*

- ***When you openly express your emotions, the person you are interacting with is likely to mimic your level of self-disclosure and facial expression.*** Research shows that others will match our level of self-disclosure and mimic our facial expressions or body movements during interpersonal exchanges (Savicki, 1972). Thus, if we disclose very little about ourselves, the person we are interacting with is likely to disclose very little, too, whereas if we exhibit high disclosure, the person we interact with will tend to match us.

- ***Use "I" statements when revealing inner experience*** to signal that you are taking responsibility for your emotions, thoughts, and beliefs rather than blaming the other person. Instead of saying *You make me annoyed when you…,* practice saying *I feel annoyed when you…*

- ***Make sure your facial expression matches your words*** (see Flexible Mind Is DEEP, in lesson 10). For example, if talking about a sad event, avoid smiling.

- ***Use the Awareness Continuum to describe your inner experience and perceptions of the other person.*** Begin by saying, *I am aware of imagining…*when talking about someone else's inner experience. This signals you are *not* assuming you know with certainty what the person's inner thoughts, emotions, or motivations are. When revealing your own experience, nonjudgmentally observe, describe, and take responsibility for your perceptions by beginning each observation with *I am aware of an emotion of…, I am aware of imagining that…, I am aware of a thought that…, I am aware of a sensation of…*

- **Be willing to take the lead in outing yourself.** This may be particularly necessary for relationships that have been conflictual in the past.

- **Don't give up. Continue to openly express on multiple occasions, even if at first they don't respond.** Improving damaged relationships takes time. When we feel wronged or hurt by another, it can make it harder to be open-minded to the possibility of change. However, continued practice of open expression and willingness to hear the other person's point of view are the only ways forward if you truly want an improved relationship.

NOTE TO INSTRUCTORS: Remind participants that outing oneself and being open and free in how one expresses emotion do not mean that open expression should be done without awareness or consideration. On the contrary, free expression of emotion is always context-dependent. For example, sometimes the situation calls for inhibited expression (such as a serious business meeting with people you do not know well).

(Optional) Discussion Points
Hiding Versus Revealing

✓ **Ask:** *Can you think of situations that call for emotion inhibition (for example, playing poker) and situations that call for emotional expression (for example, asking someone out on a date)?*

Situations when deliberate control of emotional expression might be effective…

- Being stopped by the police

- Being questioned about our work by a boss who is overcritical

- Being at a funeral

- Being in a meeting where there are competing interests

Situations when free emotional expression might be effective or even expected…

- Watching a football game

- Talking about an emotional film

- Encouraging your child when he or she is playing a sport

- Participating in therapy

W **Welcome** *feedback and continue to dialogue.*

- **Adopt a body stance that signals openness and willingness to hear what the other person has to say.** For example, use the Big Three + 1 (lean back, take a deep breath, closed-mouth smile, and eyebrow wag) while talking. Sometimes simply raising one's eyebrows while listening to the other person is all that is needed to signal open-minded listening and nondefensiveness. In addition, these skills have dual advantages—not only do they signal cooperation to the recipient, they also activate our social safety (see lesson 2).

- *Let go of rehearsing a response when the other person is speaking. Allow them time to complete their sentence before replying.* When we fully listen to another, we are more likely to naturally know how to reply, and we are less likely to misinterpret what they are saying.

- *Give the other person time to adjust to the new information when you disclose something they did not already know about you.* Do not assume that low self-disclosure by the other person means he or she does not desire a close relationship; the other person may need to practice self-disclosure, too! Let go of expectations for the other person to behave the way you would like them to in the situation.

- *Don't give up if the interaction doesn't go as planned. Instead, remain engaged and continue signaling openness.* Remember that intimacy and trust take time to develop. Block automatic action urges to walk away or abandon the relationship. Schedule another time to talk.

- *Remember that conflict can be intimacy-enhancing.* Disagreements are common and natural in close relationships. By staying engaged and working to understand the person from their perspective, we get to know the person better—a process that is essential for deepening a bond with another.

- *Use stall tactics to slow the pace of highly charged emotional exchanges.* A stall tactic allows the other person (and yourself) to save face by allowing for a short break to occur rather than insisting on resolution. When suggesting some time apart, make sure you signal a willingness to take responsibility for your own perceptions and emotions rather than blaming the need to take a short break on the other person. For example, begin by saying: *I am aware of imagining that somehow what I disclosed to you earlier did not make sense to you or was somehow experienced as hurtful. This was not my intention. However, I can see that you might have experienced it that way. If it is okay with you, I would like to take some time apart to think about our discussion and figure out, if possible, how we might be able to go forward in a way that works for both of us, and then get back together. Plus, I would like some time to reflect on what I might have done to contribute to our difficulties and see if I might come up with something to do differently next time we meet. Will that work for you, too?*

- *Use Flexible Mind ADOPTS skills to enhance openness to feedback* and the twelve questions to determine whether to accept or decline the feedback (see lesson 22).

- *Be willing to admit to the other person how your actions may have damaged the relationship, and apologize if an apology is warranted.* Taking responsibility for our actions that may have caused suffering (even if unintended) signals openness, nonarrogance, and a strong desire for an improved relationship. This can be a surefire way to repair a relationship rupture.

NOTE TO INSTRUCTORS: An effective repair or apology is not simple (that is, it doesn't mean simply saying "I'm sorry"). Instructors should be prepared to teach apology skills on an as-needed basis, including (1) accurately identifying the harm done, (2) confirming that your perception of harm is valid with the person you have harmed, (3) blocking rationalization or justification of your harmful behavior, (4) making the repair by ensuring you address the actual damage done (that is, not just saying "I'm sorry" if you have damaged a wall but also finding a way to repair the wall itself), (5) committing to not harm again, and (6) actively working to prevent similar harming behavior in the future.

(Required) Match + 1 Class Demonstration

Self-Disclosure Matters

Instructors should begin the teaching segment for Match + 1 by first demonstrating (that is, acting out) with their coinstructor three interaction styles that impact social closeness: (1) talking with someone who reveals very little personal information (2) talking with someone who asks questions but reveals very little, and (3) talking with someone who does reveal personal information. See the following chart for examples of a role-play script for each of the three interactions.

1	2	3
With your coinstructor, show how nondisclosure shuts down conversation.	With your coinstructor, show how only asking questions limits intimacy.	Show how revealing personal information makes a conversation easy.
Coinstructor: How was your weekend? *Instructor:* Fine. *Coinstructor:* What did you do? *Instructor:* Nothing special. *Coinstructor:* Did you do anything different? *Instructor:* Yes. *Coinstructor:* What was it? *Instructor:* Took a bike ride.	*Coinstructor:* How was your weekend? *Instructor:* Fine. How was yours? *Coinstructor:* Great. I went for a long hike on Sunday with a friend from work. *Instructor:* Where did you hike? *Coinstructor:* Along the Ohio and Erie Canal Towpath Trail, in Cuyahoga Valley National Park. *Instructor:* How long was the hike? *Coinstructor:* Well, we only got as far as the first visitor center, and then we stopped because I had to buy some Band-Aids for a blister. Ha! *Instructor:* Was it fun? *Coinstructor:* All but the blister!	*Coinstructor:* How was your weekend? *Instructor:* It was really nice. I went for a long bike ride to a part of the Cuyahoga Valley area I'd never been to before and came across the Stephen Frazee House along the Ohio and Erie Canal. *Coinstructor:* Wow! I didn't know you loved biking so much. How old is that house? *Instructor:* I looked it up when I got home and found out that it was built sometime between 1825 and 1827. And people say it's haunted! I don't know about that, but I'm a real sucker for the paranormal!

If there is only one instructor in the class, the role play can be conducted with three class participants, each of whom can be asked to simply start by asking the instructor, "How was your weekend?" The instructor then acts out one of the three styles while encouraging the participant to continue the interaction (for example, the instructor replies, "Fine").

It is essential to act out or playact the differing scenarios, not to just intellectually discuss them. Bodily and vocally demonstrating what it looks and feels like to interact with a person in each of the three different styles helps clients viscerally (that is, in their body, not just their mind) understand the core concepts.

Use the following questions to facilitate discussion.

  ✓ **Ask:** *What did you observe? Which demonstration looked or felt more relaxed or intimate?*

  ✓ **Ask:** *How many of you believe that revealing personal information about yourself is a form of bragging?*

  ✓ **Ask:** *What are the consequences of interacting with someone who only asks you questions or never reveals personal information? Who is doing all of the work in this type of interaction? Why doesn't this style of interacting bring people closer? Now that you have seen a demonstration of what it is like to interact with someone who provides very little personal information, does this change your perspective?*

(Required) Teaching Point
Enhancing Intimacy with Match + 1

Refer participants to handout 21.3 (Using Match + 1 to Establish New or Improve Existing Relationships).

- *Match + 1 is the skill for developing or enhancing intimate relationships.*

- *It provides the basic steps for getting to know someone or improving an existing relationship.*

- *It's based on a simple principle—in order to get to know someone, we must reveal personal information about ourselves.* If the person we are interacting with matches our level of self-disclosure, or increases it by revealing more intimate information about themselves than we have revealed, then we can be reasonably sure that they want to get to know us better, too.

- *Recall that revealing personal information says to the other person, "I trust you."*

- *Importantly, the level or degree of personal information revealed varies, depending on how well you already know the person you are interacting with.*

- *When first getting to know someone, less personally revealing interactions are what work best.* For example, when first meeting a new person, it would be inappropriate to start telling them every detail about your personal life, all your doubts and fears, and/or all of your struggles.

  ✓ **Ask:** *How many of you find chitchat difficult, or dislike it? What does chitchat mean to you?*

- *Chitchat is an essential skill that is needed when we first meet another person.* It is a social lubricant that makes interactions go smoother.

- *By using Match + 1 skills, you can transform a relationship that is less intimate or close to something more satisfying* so that chitchat evolves into intimacy.

- *Match + 1 does not mean just asking questions.* Match + 1 means revealing personal information and then nonjudgmentally observing how the other person responds. It is NOT about trying to coerce others to reveal personal information or trying to guess the closeness of the relationship the person wants with you.

- *Remember that when first getting to know someone, the level of personal self-disclosure will naturally be low.* Getting to know someone well takes time, and people vary in how comfortable they are with self-disclosure.

- *Plus, Match + 1, like any other skill, takes practice.* The more you practice, the easier it becomes.

(Required) Class Exercise

Let's Practice Match + 1

Step 1. Revealing Personal Information

Review step 1 of handout 21.3 (Using Match + 1 to Establish New or Improve Existing Relationships).

- *Activate your social safety system before and during the interaction*—for example, use the Big Three + 1.

- *Start by greeting the other person.* For example, say: *Hi. How are you?*

- *Begin Match + 1 by revealing to the other person something about your day, week, or life.* For example, say: *I went on a really nice bike ride today—but PHEW! What a workout!*

- *Listen to how the person responds, and then match his or her level of self-disclosure when you reply.*

- *If you want to get to know the person better, match his or her level of self-disclosure and go one level higher* (Match + 1) by revealing more personal details, genuine opinions, and emotions about yourself.

- *Remember, Match + 1 means revealing personal information about yourself, NOT asking personal questions about another person's life* (though asking questions is okay).

- *Don't forget that when you know a person less well or hardly at all, lower-level personal disclosures are more likely* (for example, talking about sports, politics, school, and low-level emotional opinions).

- *As you practice Match + 1 on multiple occasions with the same person, more intimate self-disclosures become more likely.* So don't rush things unnecessarily, but don't be too inhibited, either.

- *What is important is to keep it up! Don't stop providing details about your life just because the other person does not immediately respond similarly.* Remember that getting to know someone takes time, AND the more you reveal, the more likely it is that a person will reciprocate.

- *All of what we've just been saying applies to real life.* The practice we are about to do will naturally be somewhat artificial. Plus, each practice will also likely be of shorter duration than most of your real-world interactions, so you won't have a great deal of time together. **The point is to use this time to gain some experience with Match + 1** so that you can more effectively use it in your life.

Remind participants to keep it real and to make sure that any information they reveal during the exercise is from their life. They should not try to play a role, pretend they are someone else, or make up stories or information about themselves.

They should feel free to edit what they actually say (this is a normal part of getting to know someone) yet try to be as forthcoming and self-revealing as possible.

Instructors should now split the class into pairs. Explain that each member of the pair will take turns practicing Match + 1 with their partner, and that you will ring a bell or tell them when they should stop and switch. Encourage the class to make it fun and have fun, and to let go of self-judgment.

After two to three minutes, stop the practice, have partners give each other feedback about what happened, and then ask for observations from the entire class to facilitate learning. Use the following questions to enhance discussion.

- ✓ **Ask:** *What did you observe? What was it like to reveal personal information?*

- ✓ **Ask:** *What did you struggle with?*

- ✓ **Ask:** *Were you able to avoid short answers to questions? What validation skills did you use during this exercise?*

- ✓ **Ask:** *Do you feel you know your partner better?*

- ✓ **Ask:** *What does this tell you about interpersonal relationships?*

Step 2. Estimating the Level of Intimacy

Review handout 21.2 (Match + 1 Intimacy Rating Scale) and step 2 of handout 21.3 (Using Match + 1 to Establish New or Improve Existing Relationships).

- *The second step of Match + 1 is helpful but not essential. This step allows us to nonjudgmentally evaluate what we imagine was the level of intimacy of the interaction.* Use handout 21.2 (Match + 1 Intimacy Rating Scale).

- *Remember that closeness takes time.* Practice Match + 1 with someone multiple times in order to obtain a better sense of how close the person may want to be with you.

- *Plus, the ratings are NOT truth, only estimates.* So don't give up on a relationship you really want—keep revealing!

- *Use the following questions after an interaction to deepen your understanding.*

  - *How much personal information did I reveal?*

  - *What level of intimacy do I believe best describes the interaction I had with this person? Use handout 21.2 (Match + 1 Intimacy Rating Scale).*

  - *Did the person I was interacting with match my level of self-disclosure? What did they specifically do or say that helped me make this determination?*

  - *Is there a chance that I am operating from Fixed Mind or Fatalistic Mind when I evaluate the interaction? If so, what might I do to determine this more fully?*

  - *At what levels of intimacy are most of my other relationships?*

  - *What skills do I need to practice to go higher on the Match + 1 Intimacy Rating Scale in my relationships?*

Instructors can now ask participants to repeat the preceding Match + 1 exercise, but with different partners. Practice revealing personal information, as before, and then, after two to three minutes of self-disclosure practice, stop and have participants rate the level of intimacy, using handout 21.2 (Match + 1 Intimacy Rating Scale). After this, have them repractice Match + 1 with a new partner. Instructors should remind participants to keep it real. The goal is NOT to try to force intimacy. Higher intimacy is not necessarily better, particularly if inauthentic. Use the following questions to facilitate discussion. Repeat the exercise, if time permits, with new partners.

✓ **Ask:** *What level of intimacy did you rate the interaction to be at? Did you and your partner have the same rating?*

✓ **Ask:** *Did you find it difficult to determine how close the other person might have wanted to be? What made this difficult?*

✓ **Ask:** *Being able to achieve anything higher than a 5 or a 6 on this scale during this exercise would be unlikely. Why do you think this would be the case? Importantly, there is no right or wrong about the level of intimacy—a higher score does not necessarily mean better. Intimacy is always context-dependent.*

✓ **Ask:** *What did you struggle with?*

✓ **Ask:** *Do you feel you know your partner better?*

✓ **Ask:** *What have you learned?*

End with observations from the entire class, and use this to reteach or discuss how to manage any obstacles or issues arising from the practice.

NOTE TO INSTRUCTORS: The level of self-disclosure may be influenced by a person's mood, how rested or how busy they are, the state of the person's physical health, the topic being discussed, the setting, the degree of privacy, and the person's past relationship history. It may be important to make amends or apologize for past transgressions (see W in Flexible Mind ALLOWs). Thus, instructors should encourage participants to use handout 21.2 (Match + 1 Intimacy Rating Scale) and base evaluations of existing relationships on multiple interactions, particularly if the client is experimenting with using skills to improve the relationship (as the intimacy level is likely to change). The basic principle of Flexible Mind ALLOWs is that the more a person reveals inner feelings, the more likely the other person will be to reciprocate, thereby enhancing the possibility of the relationship becoming more intimate.

Lesson 21 Homework

1. **(Required) Handout 21.1 (Enhancing Social Connectedness, Using Flexible Mind ALLOWs).**

2. **(Required) Worksheet 21.A (Practicing Flexible Mind ALLOWs).** Instruct participants to practice Match + 1 skills on a repeated basis (multiple days) with the same person, using Flexible Mind ALLOWs (O and W skills). Encourage them to observe how using skills influences the relationship.

Radical Openness Handout 21.1

Enhancing Social Connectedness, Using Flexible Mind ALLOWs

A   **A**ssess your commitment to improve the relationship

L   **L**ook for concrete evidence that mistrust is justified

L   **L**oosen your grip on past hurts and fears

O   **O**ut yourself by revealing inner feelings

W   **W**elcome feedback and continue to dialogue

A   Assess *whether you are committed to improving the relationship and are willing to let go of mistrust.*

Practice self-enquiry—ask yourself the following questions.

➢ *Am I finding it hard to think about this relationship, question my point of view, or engage in self-enquiry about my feelings when it comes to this relationship? If yes or maybe, then what might this mean?*

➢ *Is there a part of me that believes it is important for the other person to acknowledge (or apologize) for a past grievance, and that is blocking my willingness to improve the relationship?*

➢ *What have I found useful or rewarding in the past about this relationship? What do I want from this other person?*

➢ *Would an improved relationship help me obtain an important goal or help me live by my values?*

➢ *What are the pros and cons of trusting this person? What are the pros and cons of mistrusting this person?*

L   Look *for concrete evidence that mistrust is justified.*

- **Look for Fixed Mind or Fatalistic Mind biases**—for example, quick dismissal of the importance of the relationship or decisions about possible trustworthiness (Fixed Mind) or feelings of hopelessness or thoughts saying, *Why bother trying? Nothing will ever improve our closeness or the relationship* (Fatalistic Mind).

- **Remember that old hurts and current mood can color how we perceive another person.** We tend to pay attention most to those things that confirm our beliefs, and ignore or dismiss information to the contrary (that is, our perceptions are subject to confirmation bias).

- **Open yourself up to the possibility of misperceiving the other person's intentions, beliefs, feelings, or thoughts.** Use self-enquiry by asking…

    ➢ *Is there an alternative explanation for their behavior? How might they describe their behavior?*

    ➢ *Do I find myself wanting to automatically explain or defend myself? If yes or maybe, then is it possible that I am not open to being truly fair-minded?*

> ➢ *Do I believe the other person must apologize or make amends before I would be willing to consider how I have contributed to the conflict?*

> ➢ *How open do I want to be in this situation with the person I will be interacting with? What might be holding me back?*

> ➢ *What is the worst thing that could happen if I expressed myself more openly?*

> ➢ *Am I discounting or minimizing positive things about the person or situation in order to punish them? Is it possible that I am not really giving them a chance? What am I afraid might happen if I were to momentarily drop my perspective?*

> ➢ *Do I believe that further self-examination or work on the relationship is unnecessary because I have already done everything possible?*

> ➢ *If someone else were watching the person's behavior, would he or she see it differently than me? If yes or maybe, then what might this mean?*

L Loosen *your grip on past hurts and fears.*

> ✓ **Ask:** *Even if it is true that the person has harmed me in the past, would it be helpful to repair the relationship?*

- **Just because you distrust someone, this does not automatically mean that they distrust you.** He or she may not even know that you feel dislike or distrust; they may feel neutral, and/or they may even like you.

- **Practice giving them the benefit of the doubt, and assume the person is doing the best they can to cope with life.** Consider the possibility that the distrusted person *may* have benign or neutral intentions but is perhaps not very good at showing this.

- **Remember times you thought negatively about someone and later realized you had misjudged the person.**

- **Remind yourself "Just because I think it, doesn't mean it's TRUE."** You might think you are seven feet tall, but this doesn't make it so.

- **Accept the fact that you can never truly know what another person is thinking.**

- **Use Flexible Mind Has HEART and forgiveness practices** (see lesson 29) **to let go of past hurts before interacting with the person.** Remember, letting go of distrust does not mean agreement.

O Out yourself *by revealing inner feelings.*

- *Outing yourself* **means taking responsibility for your perceptions** by revealing your inner experience to another person.

- **Outing yourself enhances relationships** because it models humility and willingness to learn from what the world has to offer.

- **Use words to describe what you are feeling to the other person;** allow your facial expression to go with the feelings.

- **Remember, open expression of emotion is contagious and enhances relationships.**

- **Use "I" statements when revealing inner experience,** to signal that you are taking responsibility for your emotions, thoughts, and beliefs rather than blaming the other person. Instead of saying, "You make me annoyed when you…," practice saying, "I feel annoyed when you…"

- **Use the Awareness Continuum to describe your inner experience and perceptions of the other person.** Begin by saying, "I am aware of imagining…" when talking about someone else's inner experience. This signals you are *not* assuming you know with certainty what the person's inner thoughts, emotions, or motivations are.

- **Admit to the other person how your actions may have contributed to a damaged relationship or misunderstanding.**

- **Practice curiosity instead of assuming you already know who another person is.** Listen with an open mind to find out who they see themselves to be, and then reflect back what you hear.

- **You may need to take the lead in revealing personal information, and keep revealing on multiple occasions, if you want to improve the relationship.** This may be particularly important for relationships that have been difficult. Consistency in open-minded and expressive behavior is essential rather than quick decisions to give up because an expected positive response did not occur immediately.

- **Use Match + 1 skills when forming new relationships or wanting to improve a relationship.** Match + 1 enhances mutual self-disclosure and provides a means for estimating the overall level of intimacy in a relationship.

W Welcome *feedback and continue to dialogue.*

- **Adopt a body stance that signals openness and willingness to hear what the other person has to say.** For example, use the Big Three + 1 skills (see lesson 3)—that is, lean back, take a deep breath, closed-mouth smile, and eyebrow wag.

- **Let go of rehearsing a response while mindfully listening to the other person.** When we fully listen to another, we are more likely to naturally know how to reply, and we are less likely to misinterpret what they are saying.

- **Give the other person time to adjust when you disclose something new about yourself.**

- **Do not give up if the interaction does not go as planned—instead, remain engaged and continue signaling openness.** Remember that intimacy and trust take time to develop. Block automatic action urges to walk away or abandon the relationship. Schedule another time to talk.

- **Remember that conflict can be intimacy-enhancing.** By staying engaged and working to understand the person from their perspective, we get to know the person better—a process that is essential for deepening a bond with another.

- **Use stall tactics to slow the pace of highly emotional exchanges.** Stall tactics allow individuals to save face by not insisting on an immediate solution when a disagreement has occurred. But make sure you schedule a time to come back to the discussion.

- **Use Flexible Mind ADOPTS skills to enhance openness to feedback,** and the twelve questions to determine whether to accept or decline the feedback (see lesson 23).

Radical Openness Handout 21.2

Match + 1 Intimacy Rating Scale

Examples of Levels 1-2	Examples of Levels 3-4	Examples of Levels 5-6	Examples of Levels 7-8	Examples of Level 9	Examples of Level 10
Talking about everyday nonemotional events (the weather, traffic conditions, or the taste of a meal) **and/or** stating opinions about nonemotional topics (the service at a restaurant or the color of a room)	Making nonemotional disclosures about personal goals or values (politics, parenting, philosophy) **and/or** making emotional or passionate disclosures about nonpersonal topics (world peace) **and/or** revealing socially acceptable personal preferences ("I love to go mountain biking")	Revealing private feelings or emotional judgments about personal events (one's true feelings about the boss or a coworker) **and/or** revealing possibly socially unacceptable opinions, judgments, or preferences ("I detest disorganized people")	Revealing personal opinions or thoughts about the relationship ("I really like you") **and/or** revealing private feelings or judgments about highly emotional personal events (giving details about one's unhappy marriage) **and/or** engaging in open expression (tears, uninhibited laughter, more eye contact)	Revealing feelings of affection or desire for more intimacy ("I want to spend more time with you") **and/or** sharing stories of shameful or embarrassing experiences that could be damaging if known publicly **and/or** being willing to be highly vulnerable (sharing extreme self-doubt or weaknesses)	Expressing love or intense feelings of caring and desire for a committed long-term relationship **and** being willing to reveal deep-seated vulnerable emotions that one may never have expressed before and to make serious personal sacrifices for the relationship

443

Radical Openness Handout 21.3

Using Match + 1 to Establish New or Improve Existing Relationships

Match + 1 refers to a simple principle: we must reveal personal information in order to get close to another person.

Step 1. Revealing Personal Information

- **Greet the person**—for example, "Hi. How are you?"

- **Begin Match + 1 by revealing to the other person something about your day, week, or life**—for example, "I went on a really nice bike ride today—but PHEW! What a workout!"

- **Mindfully listen to how the person responds.**

- **If you want to get to know the person better, match his or her level of self-disclosure and go one level higher** (Match + 1) by revealing more personal details, genuine opinions, and emotions about yourself.

- **Keep it up! Don't stop providing details about your life just because the other person does not immediately respond similarly.** Remember that getting to know someone takes time, AND the more you reveal, the more likely a person will reciprocate.

- **Match + 1 means revealing personal information about yourself, NOT asking personal questions about another person's life** (though asking questions is okay).

Step 2. Estimating the Level of Intimacy

The second step in Match + 1 is helpful but not essential. This step allows us to nonjudgmentally evaluate what we imagine was the level of intimacy of the interaction.

- **After an interaction with someone you would like to get to know better, use the following questions to encourage self-enquiry.**

  - *How much personal information did I reveal?*

  - *What level of intimacy do I believe best describes the interaction I had with this person?* Use handout 21.2 (Match + 1 Intimacy Rating Scale).

  - *Did the person I was interacting with match my level of self-disclosure? What did they specifically do or say that helped me make this determination?*

  - *Is there a chance that I am operating from Fixed Mind or Fatalistic Mind when I evaluate the interaction? If so, what might I do to determine this more fully?*

  - *At what levels of intimacy are most of my other relationships?*

  - *What skills do I need to practice to go higher on the Match + 1 Intimacy Rating Scale in my relationships?*

- **Next, use the Match + 1 Intimacy Rating Scale** to estimate what level of intimacy you experienced with the other person during the interaction. See handout 21.2 (Match + 1 Intimacy Rating Scale).

- **Remember that closeness takes time.** Practice Match + 1 with someone multiple times in order to obtain a better sense of how close the person may want to be with you.

- **Finally, these ratings are NOT truth, only estimates.** So don't give up on a relationship you really want—keep revealing!

Radical Openness Handout 21.4

Main Points for Lesson 21, Part 2

Enhancing Social Connectedness

1. It is not how many friends you have that matters, it is the quality of your social connectedness.

2. You only need one person in your life who is willing to make self-sacrifices to care for you when you are in distress and make you feel socially safe. Higher levels of intimacy increase social safety.

3. Match + 1 represents a core skill needed to form close social bonds—revealing personal feelings to others fosters reciprocal revelations.

4. Intimate relationships mean knowing not only about the things a person is proud of or does well but also about those areas in life they struggle with and about their inner fears or doubts.

Radical Openness Worksheet 21.A

Practicing Flexible Mind ALLOWs

Think of a relationship that you find difficult and would like to improve, and then practice Flexible Mind ALLOWs. *Describe the problematic relationship.*

_____

_____

_____

A Assess *whether you are committed to improving the relationship and willing to let go of mistrust.*

Answer the self-enquiry questions under A ("assess") in handout 21.1 (Enhancing Social Connectedness, Using Flexible Mind ALLOWs), and complete the pros and cons of trusting the person and/or improving the relationship in the following.

Pros of Trusting or Improving	Cons of Trusting or Improving

L Look *for concrete evidence that mistrust is justified.*

Place a checkbox in the boxes below that best describe the skills you used.

☐ Mindfully observed and described my suspicious and mistrustful thoughts. *Describe* what you observed.

_____

_____

☐ Looked for signs of Fixed Mind or Fatalistic Mind that may have influenced how I evaluated the relationship.

☐ Remembered that old hurts and current mood might influence my perception of the person or the relationship. Used the self-enquiry questions under the first L ("look") in handout 21.1 (Enhancing Social Connectedness, Using Flexible Mind ALLOWs) to understand what might be influencing my perception. *Describe what was learned.*

L Loosen *your grip on past hurts and fears.*

Place a checkbox in the boxes below that best describe the skills you used.

☐ Remembered that letting go of distrust does not mean agreement.

☐ Remembered that the person may not feel the same way that I do about the relationship, and accepted the fact that I can never be certain of what he or she might be thinking or feeling without explicitly being told.

☐ Practiced trusting (to some degree) how the person described the situation, intentions, or personal experience of the relationship rather than automatically assuming that he or she was being deceptive, manipulative, or wrong.

☐ Practiced giving the person the benefit of the doubt.

☐ Remembered times when I thought negatively about someone and later realized that I had misjudged the person.

☐ Tried to see things from the person's point of view. *Describe what you imagined was the point of view.*

☐ Reminded myself that just because I think it, doesn't mean it's TRUE.

☐ Used Flexible Mind Has HEART and forgiveness practices to let go of past hurts or grievances before interacting with the person (see lesson 29).

O Out yourself *by revealing inner feelings.*

Place a checkbox in the boxes below that best describe the skills you used.

- ☐ Used words to describe what I was feeling, and practiced allowing my facial expressions to match my inner feelings.

- ☐ Remembered that open expression of emotion is contagious and enhances relationships.

- ☐ Used "I" statements or the Awareness Continuum when revealing inner experience.

- ☐ Acknowledged to the other person that my actions may have contributed to the misunderstanding or damaged the relationship.

- ☐ Continued practicing open expression and personal self-disclosure with the other person, even during times I thought it might not work.

- ☐ Used Match + 1 skills.

W Welcome *feedback and continue to dialogue.*

Place a checkbox in the boxes below that best describe the skills you used.

- ☐ Adopted a body stance that signals openness and willingness to hear what the other person has to say.

- ☐ Blocked habitual rehearsals of my response when listening to the other person.

- ☐ Gave the other person time to reply by not immediately saying something when silence occurred during the interaction.

- ☐ Did not give up, even though the interaction did not go as I had anticipated. Instead, I remained engaged in the interaction.

- ☐ Reminded myself that conflict can be intimacy-enhancing.

- ☐ Used stall tactics to slow the pace of highly emotional exchanges.

- ☐ Used Flexible Mind ADOPTS skills to enhance openness to feedback, and the twelve questions to determine whether to accept or decline the feedback (see lesson 23).

Other skills.

_____

_____

_____

Learning from Corrective Feedback

Main Points for Lesson 22

1. Highly effective people are open to critical feedback or new information and are able to flexibly alter their behavior (when needed) in order to *learn from* or *adapt to* an ever-changing world.

2. Tension in the body signals that it is time to practice being open.

3. Being radically open to feedback requires a willingness to be wrong, without losing one's perspective or automatically giving in.

4. Use Flexible Mind ADOPTS to facilitate learning from corrective feedback.

5. Use the twelve steps for evaluating feedback to determine whether to accept or decline the feedback.

6. Reward yourself for being open to new information.

Materials Needed

- Handout 22.1 (Being Open to Feedback from Others: Flexible Mind ADOPTS)
- Handout 22.2 (Steps for Evaluating Feedback: Deciding Whether to Accept or Decline Feedback)
- (Optional) Handout 22.3 (Main Points for Lesson 22: Learning from Corrective Feedback)
- Handout 1.3 (Learning from Self-Enquiry)
- Worksheet 22.A (Practicing Flexible Mind ADOPTS)
- Flipchart or whiteboard and markers

(Required) Class Exercise
Recalling a Time We Felt Criticized

The practice we are about to do is designed to help us become better at being open to critical feedback, without losing our point of view. And so, to start, I would like you to sit in a comfortable yet alert position and take a breath with awareness, in order to center yourself into this moment. Notice the rise and fall of your breathing, not trying to change or do anything about it, just being fully present with the full duration of your inbreath and the full duration of your outbreath. [Slight pause.] Now, as best you can, bring into your mind a recent memory of a time you may have felt criticized, misunderstood, or unappreciated. It does not have to be an extremely difficult moment in your life, but the goal of our practice today is to, as best we can, allow ourselves to reexperience a recent time in our life—say, in the past two weeks—when we were given feedback that was upsetting or unwanted. For example, it could be something as simple as a person on a train or bus asking you to give up your seat because they are unwell, or a neighbor telling you that your car is blocking their driveway. Alternatively, it might be more personal, such as a recent argument with your spouse, or a time when you disagreed with your boss. The actual event or memory is not so important. What is more important is for us to see if we can allow ourselves, in this moment, to reexperience what it feels like to be criticized or be given feedback, and to recall the behaviors, thoughts, and emotions that may have occurred. If your mind wanders, without judgment gently guide your attention back to the memory. If you find it difficult to locate a memory, notice that. If you find multiple memories, notice that, too, and then choose a recent memory to focus your attention on, as best you can. Now let us sit silently for a moment and practice observing what arises.

NOTE TO INSTRUCTORS: This practice can be used to strengthen prior teaching that painful experiences or emotions should not be avoided in life, because often they are our greatest teachers.

(Required) Teaching Point
Being Open to Feedback from Others: Flexible Mind ADOPTS

Refer participants to handout 22.1 (Being Open to Feedback from Others: Flexible Mind ADOPTS).

NOTE TO INSTRUCTORS: The best way to review the skills in Flexible Mind ADOPTS is to encourage participants to use their example from the preceding exercise ("Recalling a Time We Felt Criticized") as a reference point, to make the skill being taught more personally relevant. A different example from each class member can be solicited and used to illustrate a differing letter in the acronym ADOPTS. Instructors should be prepared to provide examples of times they have used ADOPTS in their personal lives, in order to further facilitate learning.

- *My grandmother was right—the truth hurts!* Have you ever noticed that you learn the most from the very feedback that you don't want to hear? What makes listening to corrective feedback difficult?

- *Highly effective people are open to critical feedback or new information and are able to flexibly alter their behavior (when needed) in order to learn from or adapt to an ever-changing world.*

- *Flexible Mind ADOPTS represents the core skills for learning how to do this.* Remember these skills by the acronym ADOPTS.

(Optional) Discussion Point
Trying out Feedback

- ✓ **Ask:** *Can you remember a time when you resisted feedback at first but later tried it out and found the new behavior more effective? Skills trainers should be ready to share times from their own lives.*

- ✓ **Ask:** *Think of an example of when you listened to someone else's opinion and it turned out to really be helpful. What does this tell you about being open to feedback?*

- ✓ **Ask:** *When you are giving feedback to someone, what is it about their behavior that tells you they are being receptive or open to hearing your feedback? Does this increase or decrease your positive feelings toward that person? How might openness positively influence relationships?*

Flexible Mind ADOPTS

A   **A**cknowledge that painful feedback is occurring

D   **D**escribe and observe emotions, bodily sensations, and thoughts

O   **O**pen to new information by cheerleading and fully listening

P   **P**inpoint what new behavior is being recommended by the feedback

T   **T**ry out the new behavior

S   **S**elf-soothe and reward yourself for being open and trying something new

A   **A**cknowledge *that painful feedback is occurring.*

- **If you don't notice that you are receiving unwelcome feedback, you can't learn from it.** Unwelcome feedback can be verbal, nonverbal, or situational. It may not involve other people. Sometimes feedback comes from the world (for example, someone honks their horn at you when your car drifts into their lane).

(Optional) Encourage self-enquiry to deepen learning. Remind participants that self-enquiry is not looking for a good answer but a good question that brings a person to their edge (that is, their unknown; see lesson 29). Participants should be encouraged to be suspicious of quick answers to self-enquiry questions. Examples of possible self-enquiry questions related to ADOPTS that could be used in the coming week include…

- ➤ *How skillful do I believe I am at being able to notice or dismiss unwanted feedback? What does my answer to this question tell me about myself?*

- ➤ *How aware am I of my habits for avoiding, blocking, or minimizing unwanted feedback? What might this mean? What is it that I need to learn?*

D   **D**escribe *and observe emotions, bodily sensations, and thoughts.*

Read aloud the following passage.

When someone says something I strongly disagree with, my body is incapable of registering anger or annoyance. At first there is instant denial. I tell myself that I am not bothered and feel a sort of numbness.

*Usually I agree to go along with what they are saying, but inwardly I am silently shouting **NO!** I pretend everything is okay.*

   ✓ **Ask:** *Does this description sound like you? In what ways?*

   ✓ **Ask:** *How do you respond when you feel criticized? What have you noticed in others?*

(Required) Class Exercise
The Many Ways People Respond to Criticism

Instructors should write on a whiteboard or flipchart as many different ways of responding to feedback that the class can come up with. Sometimes it can be helpful to place an A next to those items that are more adaptive and an P next to those items that are more problematic. It is essential for instructors to remind participants that they can only ever imagine or guess that a person's feedback is meant to be critical unless the other person directly identifies it as criticism. Instructors should encourage nonjudgmental self-discovery and self-enquiry, the key point being "You can't change a problem unless you're aware of it first."

Examples include feeling annoyed or frustrated, thinking *I know I'm right* or *They're wrong,* blaming them, feeling ashamed or embarrassed, automatically blaming myself, automatically apologizing, looking away, changing the topic, pretending not to hear, feeling afraid, pretending to listen but inwardly disagreeing, ignoring the feedback, answering a question with a question to put them off guard, immediately rehearsing a rebuttal, researching how they must be wrong, feeling numb, denying that I am disturbed by their feedback, walking away, calling in sick, keeping quiet, smiling and nodding agreement when actually disagreeing, publicly taking the blame in order to block further discussion, attacking the other person, immediately justifying my position, implying they are hurting me or that I will fall apart if they continue, suggesting it is their problem, or bringing up a past hurt to obscure what they are saying.

- **Being open to emotional experience is a goal of flexible and healthy living.** Although we can temporarily block the experience of a particular emotion from our awareness, we still experience it. Even though an emotion may be experienced at a low level of intensity, it still is an emotion. For example, anger can be experienced as low-level frustration.

- **Positive feedback can be as difficult to receive as negative feedback for some people.** For some, being praised is a signal that more will be expected, that they are being manipulated or conned, or that something bad might happen soon.

     ✓ **Ask:** *How do I manage praise or compliments from others? Why might some people find it difficult to accept praise?* For example, some people may believe that being praised is a precursor to conceit. Others may believe praise a form of manipulation—perhaps their family subtly ridiculed people who performed better than they did, or they may have lived with a depressed parent who found happiness in others to be an unwanted reminder of their own personal misery. Sometimes people fear praise because they consider it a way to manipulate someone. Instructors can write on the board the various reasons generated.

- **Positive feedback (for example, praise) and negative feedback (for example, criticism) are both needed to grow, improve, and learn.** When learning anything

---

new (for example, how to play the violin, ride a horse, or even how to be more open to feedback), we need to know not only what we are doing wrong (or incorrectly) but also what we are doing right (or effectively). Imagine a world where no one, not even a child, is praised. What might this world look like? Negative feedback can lead to overcorrection or perfectionism because the person never knows when to stop trying to improve themselves, or it can lead to demoralization because nothing is ever good enough. Instructors can elicit other consequences from participants.

O Open *to the new information by cheerleading and fully listening.*

- *Remember, tension in the body means it's time to practice being open.*
- *Practice self-enquiry when you find yourself resisting being open to the feedback or the new information.*

Refer participants to handout 1.3 (Learning from Self-Enquiry).

NOTE TO INSTRUCTORS: The best way to make use of the handout is to randomly pick a class member to read aloud one of the questions (of their choosing) and then briefly discuss it as a group. Then randomly select a different classmate to do the same. It is not necessary to read aloud each question. The aim is to provide some exposure to the handout in order to encourage participants to use it again later as a source of self-growth. Remind participants that the questions they find most uncomfortable may be the ones they need to learn from the most (see the information about finding one's edge, in lesson 29).

- *Use RO skills to activate your social safety system prior to or during a conversation involving critical feedback.* See handout 3.1 (Changing Social Interactions by Changing Physiology).

- *Nonverbally signal openness—engage the Big Three + 1* by leaning back in your chair (if sitting), taking a deep breath, and closed-mouth smiling with an eyebrow wag when listening to what they have to say. Allow the other person time to speak, and use head nods to signal you are listening.

- *Let go of insisting that you are* **right,** *without automatically assuming that you are* **wrong.** Use the following statements to loosen the grip of Fixed Mind.

  - *There may be something to learn from this feedback.*
  - *There may be some truth in what is being said.*
  - *The feedback isn't saying that I am totally wrong in all situations.*
  - *Perhaps my resistance to this feedback is a sign that I am in Fixed Mind. I can use this feedback to learn more about myself.*
  - *I am working at being more open to the world. I can use this experience as a time to practice openness.*

- *Let go of justifying, explaining, or rebutting.* Remind yourself that being open and listening to feedback does not mean that you must agree with the other's point of view. The goal is to nondefensively attend to what is happening in the moment.

- *Practice enjoying being teased, to be less reactive to critical feedback and learn from social feedback.* Teasing that is healthy is how friends give each other feedback without rubbing the other person's face in it. Practice being open to the feedback that a tease may signal, using Flexible Mind ADOPTS in order to learn.

★ **Fun Facts:** *Teasing and Being Teased*

Teasing is how friends informally point out flaws in each other, without making it a big deal. Essentially, it is Flexible Mind ADOPTS in action, without all the frills. Research shows that it is a useful means for tribes to provide feedback to individual members about minor violations of social norms ("Oops…did you just body-burp?"), to correct mistakes ("Uh-oh, look at this—somebody made popcorn but forgot to clean up. I wonder who that could have been"), or to give feedback about social status or correct inappropriate behavior ("Of course, Your Majesty, we would be delighted to serve you"). Learning how to tease and be teased is an important part of healthy social relationships. A good tease (one that is kind) starts with an apparently hostile comment—delivered with an unsympathetic voice tone (for example, expressionless or arrogant), an intimidating facial expression (such as a blank stare), and a gesture (such as finger wagging) or body posture (for example, hands on hips)—that is quickly followed by appeasement and cooperative playful signals (for example, giggling, gaze aversion, eyebrow wags, and smiling). A good tease momentarily introduces conflict and social distance but quickly reestablishes social connectedness through appeasement and nondominance signals. The nondominance signal is critical for a tease to be taken lightly—that is, as a friendly poke [Keltner et al., 1997]. People who are okay about being teased have an easy manner—they don't take themselves or life too seriously and can laugh (with their friends) at their personal foibles, gaffes, and mishaps. When teasing is playful and reciprocal, it is socially bonding. In fact, teasing is an important component of flirting [Shapiro, Baumeister, & Kessler, 1991].

✓ **Ask:** *To what extent do you enjoy being teased and teasing others? How often do people you know tease each other? To what extent did your family members enjoy teasing each other when you were young? What is it that you might need to learn?*

NOTE TO INSTRUCTORS: It is important for instructors to be sensitive to the fact that teasing can also be done with an intention to harm or control another person or a situation (see Flexible Mind SAGE and Flexible Mind REVEALs). It becomes a problem when it becomes unkind (see lesson 17, "Interpersonal Effectiveness: Kindness First and Foremost"). Unkind teasing can be recognized most frequently by its lack of response to feedback, meaning the tease just keeps on going even though the other person makes it clear (either verbally or nonverbally) that the tease has gone on too long, that they are not enjoying it, and/or that they would like it to stop. Encourage participants to use the questions in Flexible Mind SAGE skills to assess the potential toxicity of the relationship and decide their most likely effective next step.

- *Use the Awareness Continuum when you find it difficult to nonjudgmentally and openly listen to feedback or criticism* (see lesson 12)—for example, *I am aware of imagining that you think I am weak…, I am aware of thinking that I am having difficulty listening to you right now…, I am aware of a feeling of hurt…, I am aware of thinking I am not understood…, I am aware of a feeling of fear as I listen to your point of view.*

(Recommended) Class Exercise

Listening to Criticism

Have the group break into pairs. In each pair, one is the speaker and practices giving feedback about the partner's shoes—one positive and one critical comment. The receiver should practice listening fully and mindfully to the feedback while noticing emotions, thoughts, sensations, and images that arise. Instructors should encourage participants to let go of automatic dismissal or rebuttal of the feedback. The pairs should then switch roles, with the receiver now taking the role of speaker and giving the partner feedback about his or her shoes. Repeat the process, but this time have the receiver purposefully pretend to not listen to the feedback (that is, look away, change the topic, pretend to read a book, and so on). Have fun!

✓ **Ask:** *What was it like giving someone feedback? What emotions did you experience?*

✓ **Ask:** *When being given feedback, what did you find most difficult? Did you find it difficult to not immediately defend your shoes? What might this mean for how you might deal with other, more personally relevant feedback?*

✓ **Ask:** *What was it like to give feedback to someone who appeared to not be listening? What might this tell you about yourself?*

P Pinpoint *what new behavior is being suggested by the feedback.*

- *The goal of pinpointing is to identify what may be the grain of truth in a critical comment,* not to find every possible flaw in the other person's reasoning or to evaluate the utility of the feedback. Knowing whether to accept or decline the feedback is the step *after* pinpointing (and is discussed later in this lesson).

- *Silently ask:* **What, specifically, are they suggesting that I do differently?** What might this new behavior look like?

- *When unclear about what is being suggested, request additional information, with an easy manner* (for example, by raising your eyebrows when making the request).

- *Summarize what you have pinpointed, and verify* with the other person that your summary is accurate. Listen openly and nondefensively to any additional information or clarifications.

- *Incorporate any additional clarifications into your summary,* and verify again by reflecting back what the other person has said. Use an easy manner when summarizing what you have heard.

- *Use stall tactics to give yourself (and the other person) time to regulate when the feedback or discussion becomes heated, but don't completely disengage.* Sometimes it is important to slow down the interaction itself. This allows time for everyone to think a bit before acting or reacting. Plus, you can take this time to practice self-enquiry to further examine personal responses. Regardless, the main point is to feel free to slow down a discussion by asking for a time-out or a cooling-down period. What is most important is that you signal to the other person that you will reengage with the discussion after taking a short break, and then make sure that you do so (that is, don't put off the discussion, despite it being difficult).

NOTE TO INSTRUCTORS: Feedback can feel like a personal attack. This is particularly likely when the feedback includes emotional language that is judgmental or harsh and/or when the other person is vague or unclear about what should be corrected or changed (for example, "You are selfish") or refers to past or future events, not to what is happening in the present (for example, "I don't think you will tell me what you really feel, because you have never done so in the past"), or if the feedback is overly global (for example, "You always repeat yourself"). It is important to mention to participants that obtaining clarity about another person's feedback can be very difficult or sometimes even impossible. Sometimes people are incapable of clearly identifying what they want us to do differently. They may not want us to do anything other than listen better, try to understand them better, and validate them in a manner that feels right to them. As such, participants should be encouraged to listen carefully and openly when attempting to determine what the other person may desire from us. Often, this is a very humbling experience, but the payoff can be great.

(Optional) Class Exercise
Demonstrating Pinpointing

To conduct this exercise, the instructor should (without any forewarning or orientation) simply ask the class for feedback about how he or she might improve teaching Flexible Mind ADOPTS and then use whatever is said to (1) demonstrate how to use the Awareness Continuum to signal openness, (2) demonstrate how to pinpoint and clarify suggested changes by reflecting back what was said, and (3) demonstrate how to verify that the pinpointing was accurate by asking whether or not the summary of suggestions was accurate.

Next, break the class into pairs, and ask each member of the pair to write down on a piece of paper the following statement: *The only one who got everything done by Friday was Robinson Crusoe.* Then ask each member of the pair to take turns practicing giving suggestions (even if silly) about how the listener might change or improve their handwriting while the listener practices pinpointing what was recommended. Then use this as the basis for discussion.

IMPORTANT NOTE TO INSTRUCTORS: Before moving to the next letter in the acronym ADOPTS, (that is, the letter T) instructors should review handout 22.2 (Steps for Evaluating Feedback: Deciding Whether to Accept or Decline) and the teaching points that follow here.

(Required) Teaching Point
Before Trying Out a Suggested Change, Evaluate It

Refer to handout 22.2 (Steps for Evaluating Feedback: Deciding Whether to Accept or Decline).

- *It is important to determine whether to accept or decline the feedback once you have pinpointed it.* Use the twelve questions in handout 22.2 to accomplish this.

NOTE TO INSTRUCTORS: To enhance teaching, ask for a volunteer to share a recent time they felt criticized, and have them briefly describe the circumstances and what the criticism was. Instructors should ensure that the participant has used the "pinpoint" skills before they ask the twelve questions (that is, pinpointing is essential to know not only what is being suggested to change but also to know whether to accept or decline the feedback). Next, using this example, demonstrate how handout 22.2 should be used and how to interpret the scoring guidelines by asking the questions aloud, one by one, and then record the number of YES responses. The rest of the class can be encouraged to follow along while each question is read aloud and then record their answer to each question, using a personal example (for example, they can use the incident they recalled during the required class exercise "Recalling a Time We Felt Criticized"). To facilitate participation from all class members, it can be helpful to have each participant read aloud the question and then have everyone record their answer, using their own personal example. Then ask a different class participant to read aloud the next question. Instructors may need to be prepared to use an example from their own lives. Only after reviewing the steps for evaluating feedback should instructors turn back to handout 22.1 and continue teaching the *T* and *S* in the acronym ADOPTS.

NOTE TO INSTRUCTORS: It is important for instructors to remind participants that answering yes or no to any one of the questions in handout 22.2 is less important than the total score that is derived at the end (that is, after answering all twelve). This can help participants let go of obsessive rumination about getting the correct answer. Instructors must be alert to client answers (usually YES answers) that may represent overlearned self-critical tendencies (that is, Fatalistic Mind) or desires to please the therapist by giving the answer they believe the instructor wants to hear (not what they actually think). The best way to prevent this is for instructors to imagine that they have received the very same feedback in similar circumstances and to then silently ask themselves the same question. If the instructor's answer differs from the client's and/or the therapist believes there may be probable cause that the client's answer may not be warranted, then instructors should gently confront the client's answer and encourage self-enquiry. For example, an overly agreeable client who found it extremely difficult to publicly disagree or state a differing opinion with little hesitation answered YES when asked question 11 during a review of her homework, indicating that she felt tense or frustrated by the feedback. Yet the instructor noted that they had not appeared defensive or angry about the feedback. If anything, they appeared almost happy to automatically accept the feedback as truth. Rather than automatically accepting their answer, the instructor queried the client's response and encouraged self-enquiry by saying: "Hmmm…Jane, do you think it is possible that your quick YES response might actually be another way for you to get down on yourself? That is, is it possible you are being too hard on yourself? I ask this because, frankly, I haven't observed much anger or frustration directed toward the person giving the feedback, or even about the feedback—if anything, you seem happy to accept the blame. What do you think when I say this?" This line of questioning resulted in an animated class discussion about how to discriminate between justified anxiety (linked to reporting in class one's homework) and the type of bodily tension or emotions that might be felt when someone is resisting being open to feedback (that is, Fixed Mind). The client was able to see that she tended to automatically blame herself when conflict or disagreement occurred. Plus, she was able to acknowledge that she had answered YES to question 11 because she thought this was what she was supposed to do in order to be radically open.

The twelve questions in handout 22.2 are listed here, with teaching points embedded after each question. Start by reading each question, and apply it to the sample situation (see the earlier note to instructors). Then ask each participant to answer with their remembered incidents in mind by circling YES or NO on the handout next to the question. Participants should be encouraged to make their best guess when unsure.

1. Does the person have more experience than I do in this area?   **YES/NO**

> NOTE TO INSTRUCTORS: Question 1 refers to whether the person providing the feedback has greater expertise or experience directly in the area the feedback is about. For example, if you are building your own personal computer, does the person giving you feedback know more than you about building computers? Sometimes greater or lesser expertise or experience does not apply to the situation; for example, the statement "You should enjoy the taste of watermelon" represents feedback, but whether or not one likes the taste of watermelon is most likely a matter of personal preference, not experience or expertise per se. Thus, if the person providing the feedback does not have arguably greater experience and/or expertise, the question should be answered NO.

2. Will accepting the feedback help maintain or improve my relationship with the person giving me feedback?   **YES/NO**

> NOTE TO INSTRUCTORS: Question 2 is usually fairly straightforward and easy to answer. In general, accepting feedback from someone we are in an existing relationship with usually helps maintain or improve a relationship (that is, we like it when our suggestions to others are accepted). However, sometimes the person providing the feedback is not in a relationship (of any kind) with the receiver (for example, a taxi driver insinuating that the tip they were given was inadequate), or sometimes whether one accepts or declines feedback is just not pertinent to improving or maintaining the existing relationship (for example, the person providing the feedback genuinely doesn't care whether their feedback is accepted or declined). In addition, sometimes feedback is not coming from a person (or people); it is coming from the environment (for example, a red traffic light sometimes provides unwanted environmental feedback, especially when one is late for a meeting). When there is clearly no relationship or any possibility of a relationship, and/or the feedback is clearly from the environment, then the question should be answered no.

3. Will accepting the advice help me maintain or improve other important relationships?   **YES/NO**

> NOTE TO INSTRUCTORS: Question 3 pertains to the impact accepting or declining the feedback may have on relationships outside of the one with the person providing the feedback. It is designed to help participants distinguish between feedback that may have relatively limited social consequences and feedback that may have broader social consequences. For example, a spouse might tell their partner that they wish they did not always change the topic whenever a topic was discussed involving emotions. Though it is possible that this behavior only occurs within the marriage, it is likely that this behavior (that is, avoiding the discussion of emotional topics) has generalized to other relationships. Acknowledgment of this can be an important step in self-discovery.

4. Am I discounting the feedback to purposefully displease or punish the person?   YES/NO

NOTE TO INSTRUCTORS: Question 4 is purposefully worded in order to capture our tendencies to punish or make life difficult for those who disagree, give us unwanted feedback, and/or do something we perceive as invalidating. It is important for instructors to repeatedly remind participants that feeling invalidated by someone does not automatically mean that the other person should change (that is, "They should validate me"). Instead, RO requires one to first consider (via self-enquiry; see mindfulness "how" skills, lesson 13) the possibility that one's feelings of invalidation may actually represent an important area in life that may need to change. People vary widely in how they may habitually discount or avoid feedback. For example, quick or automatic use of emotion-regulation skills (for example, use of distraction, cognitive restructuring, acceptance) can function as avoidance rather than effective living. Thus, how someone answers this question can be extremely helpful to identify unhelpful envy, bitterness, or resentment toward someone who has provided feedback we dislike. In addition, a YES answer to this question suggests that the receiver of the feedback may not be open to hearing it.

5. If necessary, am I capable of making the changes that are being suggested?   YES/NO

NOTE TO INSTRUCTORS: This question is normally easy to answer. It simply refers to whether or not the recipient of the feedback is actually able to make the suggested change(s). For example, if someone is told that their car is old and ugly, and they have pinpointed and confirmed that the suggestion means "Please buy a new car," a YES answer could only be provided if the recipient of the feedback possessed enough money to actually buy a new car (otherwise, the answer must be NO).

6. Will accepting the feedback help me steer clear of significant problems (for example, financial loss, employment difficulties, problems with the law)?   YES/NO

NOTE TO INSTRUCTORS: Question 6 is important because sometimes the feedback we are given may be linked to potentially significant consequences that are primarily nonrelational in nature.

7. Was the person providing the feedback using a calm and easy manner?   YES/NO

NOTE TO INSTRUCTORS: Question 7 is purposefully designed to give more weight to feedback that is delivered with an easy manner. Instructors should emphasize that the point of this question is not to determine proof of calmness, since it is impossible to truly know another person's inner experience. The goal of this question is to help clients recognize that emotionally charged feedback (for example, sarcastic tone of voice, shouting, or crying) is often, at least to some extent, biased by the emotional experience itself, although strong emotions can also manifest in more subtle ways. Indeed, OC individuals are usually experts at understatement. It is important for instructors to explain that this question is answered NO only when the behavior displayed by the person providing the feedback is clearly emotional in nature (that is, an objective observer would agree that the feedback was emotionally based). This distinction is important for those OC clients who may believe that their personal observations or thoughts are more accurate than others' thoughts and/or that their personal observations or thoughts represent truth (that is, these clients may often operate from Fixed Mind).

8. Does the feedback refer to the actual situation I am in, as opposed to the past or future? YES/NO

> NOTE TO INSTRUCTORS: Question 8 is designed to help participants recognize that feedback that does not pertain to the actual situation the recipient is in may be less relevant and/or biased. For example, feedback about the lectures I gave at my university ten years ago may be less relevant than feedback about a lecture I gave last month. Similarly, feedback about the future (for example, telling someone that they will never change) is also biased and can be demoralizing if believed (since no one can predict the future).

9. Am I in a long-term caring relationship with this person? YES/NO

> NOTE TO INSTRUCTORS: Question 9 is designed to provide extra weight to feedback received from those who have known us for a long time (for example, family members, spouses, long-term friends, children, and partners). Often only those who we live with or come into frequent contact with (over years) truly know our strengths and weaknesses.

10. Is the feedback I am being given something that I have heard from others before? YES/NO

> NOTE TO INSTRUCTORS: Question 10 helps us recognize that feedback delivered from multiple independent sources is more likely to be accurate and/or important to consider.

11. Am I tense or frustrated about this feedback? YES/NO

> NOTE TO INSTRUCTORS: Question 11 helps remind us that feeling tense or frustrated about feedback suggests that we are threatened by the feedback (that is, the fight-or-flight defensive arousal system is activated), making us automatically less open to the feedback. Instructors should encourage participants to consider tension in the body as a signal that it's time to practice openness.

12. Am I saying to myself, *I know I am right*, no matter what the other person says or how things seem? YES/NO

> NOTE TO INSTRUCTORS: Question 12 is usually answered without difficulty. The aim of this question is to help participants recognize that insistence on being correct (at least for most matters) represents closed-mindedness and arrogance.

Next, instructors should ask participants to total up the number of YES responses and use the scoring guide on handout 22.2 to determine whether to accept or decline the feedback. Instructors should encourage participants to use self-enquiry. *Does the score they arrived at match their expectations? If not, what might this mean?*

Declining the Feedback

If you have decided to decline the feedback (score of 4 or lower) then it is important to (1) determine whether or not to tell the person who provided the feedback that their feedback was declined—that is, you have decided to not change your behavior, at least for the time being; (2) remind yourself to be open to new information that might change your decision about the feedback; and (3) commit to practicing self-enquiry about your decision to not accept the feedback, in order to avoid unhelpful Fixed Mind responding.

Accepting the Feedback

A score of 5 or higher on handout 22.2 indicates you should accept the feedback. Importantly, only AFTER determining that the feedback should be accepted should a person actually attempt or try out the suggested change.

Instructors should emphasize this point before returning to handout 22.1 and teaching the last two steps of Flexible Mind ADOPTs.

(Required) Teaching Point

Return to Teaching the Last Two Steps of Flexible Mind ADOPTS, Using Handout 22.1

T **Try out** *the new behavior.*

- *Commit yourself to participate fully in the new behavior or change, without judgment.* The most important step when learning from corrective feedback is to actually try out the suggestion while not giving yourself a hard time. This means practicing the new behavior repeatedly before deciding it doesn't work.

- *If it is not possible to actually do the new behavior in the moment, practice rehearsing it in your mind, or file it away for use later.* Set aside time to practice the new behavior again and again. Use handout 5.1 (Engaging in Novel Behavior: Flexible Mind VARIEs) to strengthen your practice.

S **Self-soothe** *and reward yourself for being open and trying something new.*

- *Reward yourself for being open enough to listen to corrective feedback instead of automatically rejecting, avoiding, or denying it.* See handout 5.1 (Engaging in Novel Behavior: Flexible Mind VARIEs) for examples.

- *Let go of judging yourself* for not having known the new information.

- *Remember, the goal of Flexible Mind ADOPTS is to practice being open, not to practice being perfect.*

- *Use self-enquiry when you find yourself ruminating about your performance or the feedback.*

  ➢ *Am I automatically blaming the other person or the environment for my emotional reactions? If yes or maybe, then is it possible this could represent a way for me to avoid being open to the feedback or learning new behavior?*

  ➢ *What might I need to learn from this?*

461

Lesson 22 Homework

1. **(Required) Handout 22.2 (Steps for Evaluating Feedback: Deciding Whether to Accept or Decline).**

2. **(Required) Worksheet 22.A (Practicing Flexible Mind ADOPTS).**

3. Ask participants to look for times in the coming week when they feel criticized or when things don't go as expected (that is, nonverbal feedback from the environment) and to practice Flexible Mind ADOPTS skills, using worksheet 22.A and handout 22.2.

NOTE TO INSTRUCTORS: Some clients may report that they live such isolated lives that the opportunity for feedback from others is minimal or nonexistent. When this occurs, instructors should be careful not to buy into the client's worldview. Instead, instructors can encourage the client to either actively seek feedback from someone directly (for example, their individual therapist) or to look for nonverbal environmental feedback (for example, when someone cuts in front of them when driving, when their washing machine breaks down, or when they discover that their bank has failed to respond to a request for a new account). Instructors can explain that "feedback," as defined in RO DBT, means anything that elicits an unwanted, disliked, or unexpected experience. Thus, Flexible Mind ADOPTS skills can be applied to both verbal/explicit and nonverbal/implicit feedback.

Radical Openness Handout 22.1

Being Open to Feedback from Others: Flexible Mind ADOPTS

Flexible Mind ADOPTS

A	**Acknowledge** that painful feedback is occurring
D	**Describe** and observe emotions, bodily sensations, and thoughts
O	**Open** to new information by cheerleading and fully listening
P	**Pinpoint** what new behavior is being recommended by the feedback
T	**Try out** the new behavior
S	**Self-soothe** and reward yourself for being open and trying something new

A Acknowledge *that painful feedback is occurring.*

- *Pause* and *notice* that something painful, disconfirming, unexpected, or novel is occurring.

- **Remember, painful feedback can be verbal, nonverbal, or situational.** It may not involve other people. Sometimes feedback comes from the world.

D Describe *and observe emotions, bodily sensations, and thoughts.*

- **Use self-enquiry to compassionately question** automatic responses that might suggest lack of openness.

  - ➢ *Am I talking more quickly—immediately jumping to respond to the other person's feedback or questions?*

  - ➢ *Do I feel a strong desire to explain myself?*

  - ➢ *Do I find myself brooding or ruminating about what happened more than is typical?*

  - ➢ *Am I holding my breath or breathing more quickly? Has my heart rate changed?*

  - ➢ *Am I feeling numb or emotionally shut down?*

  - ➢ *Am I automatically blaming the other person or the environment for my reactions?*

O Open *to new information by cheerleading and fully listening.*

- **Remember, bodily tension means that it is time to practice being open.**

- **Change body posture to facilitate openness**—lean back rather than forward, slow deep breathing, closed-mouth smile, use eyebrow wags.

- **Practice FULLY listening.** Let go of assuming that you know what they are going to say, or stop planning a rebuttal, bringing up past hurts or injuries, or insisting that the other listen to you before you will listen.

- **Stay engaged.** Go opposite to urges to abandon the relationship, walk away, or avoid. Remain in the situation, and thank the person for an opportunity to learn.

- **Encourage openness by silently repeating…**

  - *There may be something to learn from this feedback or what is happening.*

  - *There may be some truth in what is being said.*

  - *Being open does not mean approval or that I must abandon prior beliefs.*

P Pinpoint *what new behavior is being suggested by the feedback.*

- **Clarify exactly what the person would like you to change or do differently.** Use an easy manner; ask for examples.

- **Repeat back what you have heard, to confirm that your perception is accurate.** Be open to the possibility that it is not. Ask the other person to help you understand.

- **Once you have pinpointed the feedback, use handout 22.2 (Steps for Evaluating Feedback: Deciding Whether to Accept or Decline) to determine whether you should accept or decline the feedback.** If your score is 5 or higher, then it is time to try out the new behavior.

T Try out *the new behavior.*

- **Use skills from Flexible Mind VARIEs** (lesson 5) **to enhance your effectiveness.**

- **Practice the new behavior,** again and again.

S Self-soothe *and reward yourself for being open and trying something new.*

- **Let go of judging yourself** for not knowing the new information.

- **Remember, the goal is to *practice* being open, not being perfect.**

Radical Openness Handout 22.2

Steps for Evaluating Feedback: Deciding Whether to Accept or Decline

- Criticism or feedback from another person is not *truth* but a belief held by the other person that may be true, partially true, or not true at all.

- Use Flexible Mind ADOPTS skills to evaluate the feedback you have been given, without automatically rejecting it (Fixed Mind) or automatically accepting it (Fatalistic Mind).

Step 1. Ask the following twelve questions to help determine whether to *accept or decline* the feedback.

1. Does the person have more experience than I do in this area? — **YES/NO**

2. Will accepting the feedback help maintain my relationship with the person giving me feedback? — **YES/NO**

3. Will accepting the advice help me maintain or improve other important relationships? — **YES/NO**

4. Am I discounting the feedback to purposefully displease or punish the person? — **YES/NO**

5. If necessary, am I capable of making the changes that are being suggested? — **YES/NO**

6. Will accepting the feedback help me steer clear of significant problems (for example, financial loss, employment difficulties, problems with the law)? — **YES/NO**

7. Was the person providing the feedback using a calm and easy manner? — **YES/NO**

8. Does the feedback refer to the actual situation I am in, as opposed to the past or future? — **YES/NO**

9. Am I in a long-term caring relationship with this person? — **YES/NO**

10. Is the feedback I am being given something that I have heard from others before? — **YES/NO**

11. Am I tense or frustrated about this feedback? — **YES/NO**

12. Am I saying to myself, *I know I am right*, no matter what the other person says or how things seem? — **YES/NO**

Step 2. Total up the number of YES responses and the number of NO responses.

Then use the following key to guide Flexible Mind in deciding whether to accept or decline the feedback.

11 to 12 YES responses = accept the feedback as accurate and effective, no matter what

9 to 10 YES responses = accept the feedback as likely accurate and effective

7 to 8 YES responses = accept the feedback as possibly accurate and effective; continue to evaluate whether it is useful or true

5 to 6 YES responses = accept the feedback, but very tentatively

3 to 4 YES responses = tentatively decline the feedback, but with an open mind

1 to 2 YES responses = decline the feedback

Radical Openness Handout 22.3

Main Points for Lesson 22: Learning from Corrective Feedback

1. Highly effective people are open to critical feedback or new information and are able to flexibly alter their behavior (when needed) in order to *learn from* or *adapt to* an ever-changing world.

2. Tension in the body signal that it is time to practice being open.

3. Being radically open to feedback requires a willingness to be wrong, without losing one's perspective or automatically giving in.

4. Use Flexible Mind ADOPTS to facilitate learning from corrective feedback.

5. Use the twelve steps for evaluating feedback to determine whether to accept or decline the feedback.

6. Reward yourself for being open to new information.

Radical Openness Worksheet 22.A

Practicing Flexible Mind ADOPTS

- **Use Flexible Mind ADOPTS whenever you receive critical or corrective feedback you do not agree with, are told to change or do something different, or are told something about yourself that you do not like** (for example, by your boss, partner, friend, family member, neighbor, therapist). Flexible Mind ADOPTS can also be used with past memories of critical feedback, so if you cannot find a recent event, use an old one to practice.

- **As you get more practice,** you can start using Flexible Mind ADOPTS with nonverbal feedback (a frown or scowl on someone's face after you voice an opinion) or situations where the world is giving you feedback (for example, you have twice failed a test needed for promotion at work).

- **Use handouts 22.1 and 22.2 to guide your practice** and record your observations.

A **Acknowledge** *that feedback is occurring.*

Pause, notice, and **acknowledge** the painful feedback, without judging yourself or the other person. *Briefly describe the event and the feedback.*

_____

_____

_____

_____

D **Describe** *emotions, bodily sensations, and thoughts.*

Label emotions (for example, *anger, annoyance, sadness, fear*) and action urges (for example, *urge to walk away, urge to retaliate, urge to deny,* or *urge to shut down*). Use the self-enquiry questions from handout 22.1 to help block avoidance or blaming of the other person, the situation, or the world. *Record your observations here.*

_____

_____

_____

_____

_____

O **Open** *to the feedback.*

Place a checkmark in the boxs that best describe the skills you used. Remember, bodily tension means it's time to practice being open.

☐ **Cheer yourself on in practicing openness, using statements like these:**

- *There may be something to learn from this feedback or what is happening.*
- *There may be some truth in what is being said.*
- *Being open does not mean approval or that I must abandon prior beliefs.*
- *Write your own cheerleading statements here.* _____

_____

☐ **Change body posture.** Use eyebrow wags, closed-mouth smile, slow breathing, lean back, open hands, and so on. Describe what you did and how changing your posture influenced you (for example, your emotions, your willingness to listen, your thoughts). *Describe what you did.*

_____

_____

☐ **Practice *fully* listening.** Let go of assuming that you know what the person is going to say. Let go of planning a rebuttal, bringing up past hurts or injuries, or insisting that the person listen to you before you will listen. *Describe what you did.*

_____

_____

☐ **Stay engaged.** Go opposite to urges to abandon the relationship, to walk away, or to avoid. Remain in the situation. Practice thankfulness by remembering that being open to corrective feedback is how we learn. *Describe how you stayed engaged.*

_____

_____

P **Pinpoint** *specifically what the feedback is suggesting, and determine whether you should accept or decline the feedback.*

Check the skills you used.

- ☐ Clarified what specific behaviors the feedback was about and, with an easy manner, asked for examples.

- ☐ Repeated back what I heard, and confirmed that it was accurate. If needed, asked them to help me understand better what they were saying.

- ☐ Used handout 22.2 (Steps for Evaluating Feedback: Deciding Whether to Accept or Decline) after I pinpointed the feedback, to determine whether to accept or decline it. How many YES responses? _____ How many NO responses? _____ Was your score different than you expected? *Record what you decided, and any new learning that emerged.*

_____

_____

_____

T **Try out** *the new behavior if your score on handout 22.2 (Steps for Evaluating Feedback) was 5 or higher.*

Use Flexible Mind VARIEs to enhance your effectiveness. Practice the new behavior, again and again. What happened when you tried it out (either at the time of the feedback or later)? *Record how many times you were able to practice the new behavior. What have you learned?*

_____

_____

_____

S **Self-soothe** *and reward yourself for being open and trying something new.*

Let go of judging yourself for not having known the new information. How did you know that you were less judgmental? *Describe how you plan to use what you have learned in the future. Describe what you did to reward and soothe yourself.*

_____

_____

_____

LESSON 23

Mindfulness Training, Part 1

Overcontrolled States of Mind (Repeated from Lesson 11)

NOTE TO INSTRUCTORS: Lessons 23–26 are a repetition of RO mindfulness training taught earlier in the course. Part 1 (lesson 23) reviews the RO mindfulness states of mind targeting overcontrolled problems (that is, *Fixed*, *Flexible*, and *Fatalistic Mind*; see lesson 11). Part 2 (lesson 24) reviews the "what" mindfulness skills (*observe openly, describe with integrity,* and *participate without planning*; see lesson 12). Parts 3 and 4 review the four mindfulness "how" skills, essential attitudes or mind-sets that RO encourages practitioners to adopt when practicing the "what" skills. Part 3 (lesson 25) reviews the first of the four mindfulness "how" skills (*with self-enquiry*; see chapter 13). Part 4 (lesson 26) reviews the remaining three "how" skills (*with awareness of harsh judgments, with one-mindful awareness,* and *effectively and with humility*; see lesson 14).

Instructors should teach directly from the teaching notes, handouts, and worksheets found for each part of the mindfulness teaching materials in lessons 11–14.

Main Points for Lesson 23

1. Problematic states of mind for overcontrolled individuals are most often closed-minded.

2. These states function to block learning from new information or disconfirming feedback and can negatively impact interpersonal relationships.

3. A closed mind is a threatened mind. Though frequently triggered by nonemotional predispositions for detail-focused processing and inhibitory control, OC problematic states of mind are emotionally driven.

4. Fixed Mind signals that change is unnecessary because I already know the answer. Fixed Mind is like the captain of the *Titanic*, who, despite repeated warnings, insists, "Full speed ahead, and icebergs be damned."

5. Fatalistic Mind says change is unnecessary because there is no answer. Fatalistic Mind is like the captain of the *Titanic*, who, after hitting the fatal iceberg, retreats to his cabin, locks the door, and refuses to help passengers abandon ship.

6. Flexible Mind represents a more open, receptive, and flexible means of responding. It is like a ship captain who is willing to forgo previous plans and change course or reduce speed when icebergs are sighted. There is no abandoning ship or turning completely around at the first sign of trouble.

Materials Needed

- Handout 11.1 (Overcontrolled States of Mind)

- Handout 11.2 (Being Kind to Fixed Mind)

- Handout 11.3 (Learning from Fatalistic Mind)

- (Optional) Handout 11.4 (Main Points for Lesson 11: Mindfulness Training, Part 1: Overcontrolled States of Mind)

- Worksheet 11.A (Being Kind to Fixed Mind)

- Worksheet 11.B (Going Opposite to Fatalistic Mind)

- Whiteboard or flipchart with marker

Mindfulness Training, Part 2

The "What" Skills (Repeated from Lesson 12)

Main Points for Lesson 24

1. In RO DBT, there are three mindfulness "what" skills, each of which represents a differing aspect or way to practice mindfulness. They are *observe openly, describe with integrity,* and *participate without planning.*

2. "Urge-surfing" mindfulness practices facilitate learning how to not respond to every urge, impulse, and desire, such as urges to fix, control, reject, or avoid.

3. The Awareness Continuum is the core RO "describe with integrity" practice and can also be used as an "outing oneself" practice. It helps the practitioner take responsibility for their inner experiences, block habitual desires to explain or justify oneself, and learn how to differentiate between thoughts, emotions, sensations, and images. It is a core means for learning how to step off the path of blame (habitual blaming of self or others).

4. Learning the "participate without planning" skill means learning how to passionately participate in one's life and in one's community and let go of compulsive planning, rehearsal, and/or obsessive needs to get it right.

Materials Needed

- Handout 12.1 ("Describe with Integrity" Skills: The Awareness Continuum)
- Handout 12.2 (Main Points for Lesson 12: Mindfulness Training, Part 2: The "What" Skills)
- Worksheet 12.A ("Observe Openly" Skills)
- Worksheet 12.B (Making Participating Without Planning a Daily Habit)
- Worksheet 12.C (The Three "What" Skills: Daily Practice Log for the "Observe Openly," "Describe with Integrity," and "Participate Without Planning" Skills)
- Whiteboard or flipchart with marker

Mindfulness Training, Part 3

The Core Mindfulness "How" Skill: With Self-Enquiry (Repeated from Lesson 13)

Main Points for Lesson 25

1. In RO DBT, there are four mindfulness "how" skills that represent the kind of attitude or state of mind to bring to a practice of mindfulness. They are *with self-enquiry, with awareness of harsh judgments, with one-mindful awareness,* and *effectively and with humility.* Lesson 13 focuses on the first of these four skills, *with self-enquiry.*

2. *With self-enquiry* is the core RO DBT mindfulness "how" skill. It is the key to radically open living. It means actively seeking the things one wants to avoid or may find uncomfortable in order to learn, and cultivating a willingness to be wrong, with an intention to change, if needed.

3. Self-enquiry involves both willingness for self-examination and willingness to reveal to others what self-examination has uncovered. This process is known as *outing oneself* in RO DBT.

Materials Needed

- Handout 1.3 (Learning from Self-Enquiry)

- Handout 13.1 (The Core Mindfulness "How" Skill: With Self-Enquiry)

- Handout 13.2 (Cultivating Healthy Self-Doubt)

- Handout 13.3 (Practicing Self-Enquiry and Outing Oneself)

- (Optional) Handout 13.4 (Main Points for Lesson 13: Mindfulness Training, Part 3: The Core Mindfulness "How" Skill: With Self-Enquiry)

- Worksheet 13.A (Practicing the Core Mindfulness "How" Skill: With Self-Enquiry)

- Whiteboard or flipchart with marker

Mindfulness Training, Part 4

The "How" Skills (Repeated from Lesson 14)

Main Points for Lesson 26

1. In RO DBT, there are four mindfulness "how" skills that represent the kind of attitude or state of mind to bring to a practice of mindfulness. They are *with self-enquiry, with awareness of harsh judgments, with one-mindful awareness,* and *effectively and with humility.* The core mindfulness "how" skill, *with self-enquiry,* was taught in lesson 13. Lesson 14 focuses on the other three "how" skills.

2. The second "how" skill is *with awareness of harsh judgments.* Judgments become harsh and/or problematic when they are rigidly believed as accurate perceptions of reality; they lead to unhelpful rumination, they make us less open to feedback or new information, and/or they negatively impact how we socially signal or express our intentions and experience to others.

3. *With one-mindful awareness* is the third mindfulness "how" skill. It means doing one thing at a time by purposefully and repeatedly turning one's attention toward the present moment. In RO, one-mindfulness means practicing awareness, with humility. We need humility because what we are aware of in any given moment is an edited version of the present moment, not a true representation of it.

4. *Effectively and with humility* is the fourth RO DBT mindfulness "how" skill and means being able to adapt one's behavior to ever-changing circumstances in order to achieve a goal or live according to one's values, in a manner that accounts for the needs of others. For OC clients, it can mean learning how to *not* always play by the rules, to be less political, to not always base decisions on winning or achievement, to let go of compulsive striving and obsessive self-improvement, and to celebrate ineffective moments as opportunities for growth.

Materials Needed

- Handout 14.1 (The Four RO "How" Skills)
- Handout 14.2 (Using Self-Enquiry to Examine Harsh Judgments)
- (Optional) Handout 14.3 (Main Points for Lesson 14: Mindfulness Training, Part 4: The "How" Skills)
- Worksheet 14.A (Practicing the "How" of RO Mindfulness)
- Whiteboard or flipchart with marker

Envy and Resentment

Main Points for Lesson 27

1. Envy is experienced whenever someone compares themselves unfavorably to others, and unhelpful envy emerges when we believe their advantage over us is unwarranted.

2. Envy is *helpful* when it motivates us to try harder to *achieve our personal goals*, but it can cause problems when it motivates us to *prevent another person from achieving their goals*.

3. Unhelpful envy involves a painful blend of two emotions, *shame* and *anger*, with action urges for *secret revenge*.

4. Changing envy requires going opposite to both shame's urge to hide and anger's urge to attack.

5. To go all the way opposite action to envy, a person must let go of ill will and reveal envious feelings to the envied person.

Materials Needed

- (Optional) Handout 27.1 (Main Points for Lesson 27: Envy and Resentment)

- Worksheet 27.A (Opposite Action to Unhelpful Envy: Flexible Mind DARES [to Let Go])

- Whiteboard or flipchart with marker

(Required) Teaching Point

Envy

The instructor and the coinstructor should read the following dialogue aloud—ideally, using silly voices, such as those of radio announcers.

Instructor:　　I am pleased to announce that the next two lessons will be on your favorite topics, and mine— envy, resentment, bitterness, and revenge. Yeah! Yahoo!

Coinstructor:　We sometimes call this lesson "ERBR." (☺...*tee hee*)

Instructor:　　Importantly, "ERBR" does not mean "little robot from *Star Wars*"—not that I have anything against little robots.

Coinstructor:　Okay, now—that's enough silliness for the day. Let's stop this right now. Stop. Stop. Stop! (*Pause.*) Phew! That's better. So let's begin again...

Without further comment, the instructors should begin teaching again, as they normally would.

- *Envy is experienced whenever we compare ourselves unfavorably to another.* We envy those who are similar to ourselves (for example, same social standing) and who we believe have an advantage we do not have (Smith & Kim, 2007).

- *Envy is a normal human emotion and can involve genuine admiration or appreciation for another person's fortune.* Envy can motivate us to try harder to achieve a desired goal. Benign or helpful envy urges us to emulate or model the person we admire.

- *Benign envy requires humility,* an attitude that most humans value. It involves a willingness to admit to our fallibility, that we don't know everything, and that we have not achieved or succeeded in the way we may have wanted.

- *Envy is unhelpful when it motivates us to prevent others from achieving their personal goals.*

NOTE TO INSTRUCTORS: Unhelpful envy should be differentiated from resentment. Although both require social comparison and a sense of injustice (with accompanying feelings of hostility or ill will), there are important differences. When envious, we know, albeit often without conscious awareness, that others are unlikely to agree with our perception of unfairness (Smith & Kim, 2007). When resentful, we are more likely to believe that others will publicly validate our perception of unfairness. This may help explain the secretive nature of unhelpful envy.

- *Unhelpful envy involves a painful blend of two emotions—shame and anger. Their action urges—to hide and to attack—blend into an urge for secret revenge.*

- *Unhelpful envy also involves a desire for the envied person to fail or experience pain.* There is a word for this, borrowed from German—"schadenfreude"—which means pleasure taken in the pain of others. Whenever we experience secret pleasure in the misfortune of others, we are likely to be envious toward them or the group to which they belong.

- *Revenge can be impulsive, without much forethought* (for example, slashing someone's tires after an argument).

Read the following story aloud, and ask participants about times when they may have acted on revenge impulsively.

I remember a time when my mom got honked at by another driver—she had cut in ahead of him at an intersection. She was furious at him for treating her like a novice driver. So she insisted that all three of us kids look out the back window and stick our tongues out at the driver who had just honked at her.

- *Revenge can also be coldly calculating, performed only after careful preparation*—for example, purposely not inviting the person to an important meeting, sneaking out at night and letting the neighbor's cows loose, purposely throwing out important papers, and stealing the person's mail.

Read the following story aloud, and ask participants about the times when they may have acted on revenge in a calculating way, or with planning.

I fell out with one of my neighbors last year. He thought his garden was so wonderful just because it had won a few silly awards. What does he know? Gardening has been a tradition in my family back to my great-grandmother! Finally I just became fed up with his better-than-thou attitude. So I decided to fix him. I went to the garden store and bought some weed killer and some ice trays. Then I went home and mixed the weed killer with water and made weed killer ice cubes. Every few days I would stroll alongside the fence between our yards and surreptitiously toss a few of my special ice cubes into his garden. Then I just sat back and watched the show from my back porch. He went crazy—it was really funny to watch him scratch his head in confusion. Mr. Green Thumb just couldn't figure out what was creating these small random patches of dead plants. When he mentioned his problem to me one day, I told him that maybe all of his fancy spraying and books about gardening weren't so special after all. And there was no award for him that year.

(Required) Discussion Point
Helpful or Unhelpful Envy?

Ask the class for examples of times they may have experienced envy. Was it helpful envy (admiration) or unhelpful envy? If unhelpful, were the urge for revenge or the actions that followed impulsive or calculating? What did they notice to be different between the two emotional experiences? What was similar about the experiences? What thoughts, action urges, and behaviors did they experience? If someone is struggling with labeling unhelpful envy, ask them whether they have ever experienced secret pleasure when misfortune befell someone. This is a sign that they were experiencing unhelpful envy. Ask participants for examples of times when they may have planned revenge.

NOTE TO INSTRUCTORS: Remind participants that envy is a common emotion, and all humans experience envy. Instructors should be prepared to share personal experiences. Remind participants that envy is a natural consequence of perceiving something to be unfair or failing to achieve a coveted goal that others have achieved. Not achieving goals has real consequences (for example, getting the job or not, being promoted or not, and so on), and thus feeling envy is understandable.

(Required) Teaching Point
Distinguishing Helpful from Unhelpful Envy

- *Feeling envy is part of being human and does not mean you are a bad person.* The question is, does this envy increase or decrease your quality of life? Helpful, benign envy rarely causes difficulties. Helpful envy (admiration) can lead us to try harder in achieving our goals.

- *Unhelpful envy involves desires for revenge and secrecy.*

- *Unhelpful envy, though understandable, is rarely justified and rarely fits the circumstances.* The envied person may rightfully deserve the advantage. He or she may have worked hard to achieve it, and this is why we keep our unhelpful envy secret from others. Unhelpful envy tries hard to keep the other person from achieving his or her goals.

- *Admitting our envy can be difficult, as it is one of the very last emotions that people will admit to feeling; in fact, we are loath to admit envy even privately to ourselves* (Silver & Sabini, 1978). Moreover, people will also go out of their way to avoid being envied by others in order to shield themselves from hostile actions; that is, we fear being envied (Foster, 1972).

- *We hide our envy from ourselves and others because inwardly we know that our desires for revenge are either unjustified or against our own moral values.* We may also recognize our beliefs as irrational (for example, beliefs that the envied person is morally inferior, or that his or her advantage is undeserved), and we may sense that others are unlikely to support our negative thoughts about the envied person.

Read aloud the following story, and use it as a basis for discussion.

One woman considered herself a very caring and a hardworking person. She always strove to do the right thing and play by the rules, especially at work. She often worked longer hours than her colleagues, without complaint or additional pay. One day she was shocked to discover that a younger and flashier colleague had been promoted to a much coveted managerial position over her. Despite strongly believing her rival to have been unfairly promoted, she took pains to keep her beliefs private. She considered her colleagues under the spell of this newcomer, and she wanted to avoid a messy confrontation over what, to her, were obvious shortcomings in her rival. So instead, she downplayed the importance of her rival's promotion and publicly discounted her previously expressed desires to be promoted, but she quietly seethed under a mask of fake smiles. Over time, she found herself feeling more and more like an outsider among her fellow workers and began to harbor increasing bitterness.

- **Changing unhelpful envy requires going opposite to two differing urges—the urge to hide, and the urge to attack.** In order to go all the way opposite action to envy, a person must let go of ill will and reveal the envy to the envied person. The good news is that doing so profoundly changes one's emotional experience while simultaneously improving the relationship with the envied individual.

- *There are five steps for changing unhelpful envy. Remember them with the phrase Flexible Mind DARES.*

(Required) Teaching Point
Flexible Mind DARES (to Let Go)

Refer participants to Worksheet 27.A (Opposite Action to Unhelpful Envy: Flexible Mind DARES [to Let Go]).

> NOTE TO INSTRUCTORS: When teaching Flexible Mind DARES (to Let Go), write out the acronym (DARES) on a flipchart or whiteboard, with each letter arranged vertically in a column, but *without* naming the specific skill that each letter signifies. Next, starting with the first letter in the acronym (*D* in DARES), teach the skills associated with each letter in the acronym, using the key points outlined in the following sections, until you have covered all of the skills associated with that letter. Importantly, only write out on the whiteboard or flipchart the global description of what each letter actually stands for while you are teaching the skills associated with it. This teaching method avoids long explanations about the use of certain words in the acronym and/or premature teaching of concepts.

Flexible Mind DARES

D	**D**etermine if you are experiencing unhelpful envy
A	**A**dmit your envy and decide whether you want to change it
R	**R**ecognize envious thoughts and action urges
E	Go opposite to **E**nvious anger
S	Go opposite to **S**hameful envy

D Determine *if you are experiencing unhelpful envy.*

Use the following questions as a guide.

> NOTE TO INSTRUCTORS: Read aloud each of the following questions, and instruct participants to place a checkmark in each box next to these questions on worksheet 27.A that they think may apply to them. Ask for observations and discuss briefly.

- *Do I feel that I have been wronged, neglected, or passed over by this person or others?*
- *Have I found myself thinking negative thoughts about this person (or group)?*
- *Do I find myself thinking that this person has an unfair advantage over me?*
- *Do I find myself gossiping about this other person frequently?*
- *Do I consider this person a rival or a competitor?*
- *Have I fantasized about getting back at them?*
- *Have I tried to make their life difficult?*
- *Do I desire to punish them, beat them, or prove them wrong?*
- *Do I find myself sometimes secretly enjoying any misfortune that befalls this other person or fantasizing about misfortune occurring?*
- *Do I seek confirmation from others that the person deserves to be punished or has an unfair advantage?*

A Admit *your envy to yourself by labeling it: "I am aware of an emotion of envy."*

- **Labeling the emotion is a good first step toward changing the emotion, because we tend to keep our feelings of envy secret.**
- **Decide whether you want to let go of unhelpful envy.**
- **What are the pros and cons of having envy toward this person (or group)?** Do you really want to change this emotion? Would you like to have a better relationship with the person you feel envy toward? Remember, if you do not want to change envy, then opposite action will not work.
- **Do you truly value the advantage enjoyed by the envied person? Consider whether you actually need it, and ask yourself what is most important in your life. What do you value?** Use self-enquiry to challenge yourself. Is the envied person's coveted advantage something you truly desire? Sometimes we can come to believe that we MUST have something, only to discover later that getting it made us no happier. Remind yourself of times when winning or being right may not have worked. Remember times when coveted advantages, once achieved, may have faded in importance over time. Let go of thinking that you MUST have the advantage.
- **If you decide in your Flexible Mind that you want the same advantage, then look for ways that you can achieve it.** For example, improve your marriage, get that promotion, receive recognition. Determine the first step needed to make this happen, and then take it. Block self-talk that says you will not be able to achieve it. Let go of Fatalistic Mind tendencies to believe that getting what you want is impossible. Remind yourself that achieving advantages often takes time.

R Recognize *the desire for revenge, and label the action tendencies or urges of unhelpful envy.*

- **Notice the action urges for revenge**—for example, urges to get even, make the person's life difficult, or expose the person's moral failings. Desires for revenge are likely when we experience pleasure at the misfortune of an envied person. We may find ourselves speaking in a sarcastic tone or behaving coldly, as if they are not important. We may even feign liking them and insincerely give compliments.

- **Notice the action urges and behaviors associated with shame**—for example, urges to keep your feelings secret, deny your feelings, or relabel them as righteous or correct; becoming numbed out when the person is around you; hiding or avoiding contact with the envied person.

- **Look for action urges to seek validation and confirmation from others** for your beliefs that the envied person does not deserve the advantage. Look for urges to gossip negatively about the envied person.

NOTE TO INSTRUCTORS: Though it is true that we usually avoid seeking social support when envious, the pain of feeling inferior and/or desires for revenge can result in attempts to convince others that our perception of unfairness is correct. Unfortunately, this can be like putting gasoline on an already burning fire. Resentment and righteous indignation can follow, as can mood states that function to confirm our beliefs that harming the other person is justified or even moral.

E *Go opposite to* **Envious** *anger.*

- **Go opposite to the action tendencies of resentment, anger, and desires for revenge directed toward the envied person by taking these steps:**

  1. Take care of yourself
     - Closed-mouth smile, use eyebrow wags, and slow your breathing when thinking about the person you are envious of.
     - Practice being grateful for the things that you have by counting your blessings, and mindfully practice living in the present moment in order to more fully enjoy your life.
     - Use self-enquiry to determine whether what is envied is something you truly value or desire to achieve, and if so, take the first step toward achieving it.

  2. Go opposite to action urges of anger
     - Practice putting yourself in the other person's shoes and seeing the world from the other's perspective.
     - Look for valid reasons why the other person deserves an advantage.

  3. Go all the way opposite action
     - Block looking for negative traits and moral failings in the envied person.
     - Block pleasurable fantasies involving the envied person failing or suffering.
     - Block negative gossip about the envied person.
     - Practice being nonjudgmental and kind and behave decently toward the envied person.

S *Go opposite to* **Shameful** *envy.*

- **Go all the way opposite action to urges to hide your feelings of envy from others** by taking the following steps:

  1. Practice living within your values
     - Behave truthfully by labeling your emotion as envy, and go opposite to urges to justify or pretend the emotion is something else.
     - Repeat the word "envy" aloud to yourself multiple times.
     - Remind yourself that envy is a normal human emotion and that it does not mean you are doing something wrong.

  2. Go opposite to shame
     - Reveal your envy to an objective, caring person, and use the word "envy" when describing your situation.
     - Block attempts by the caring person to label the emotion as something other than envy or to justify your feelings of injustice.

  3. Turn unhelpful envy into admiration *if you desire a closer relationship* with the envied person
     - Remember that revealing vulnerable (even shameful) emotions to others is relationship enhancing.
     - Select a private place to reveal your feelings to the envied person, and use the word "envy" to describe your experience.
     - Apologize for prior negative actions, thoughts, or desires to cause harm or see the person fail.
     - Turn unhelpful envy into admiration by allowing yourself to celebrate the person's success.
     - Reward yourself for living within your values.

NOTE TO INSTRUCTORS: Worksheet 27.A (Opposite Action to Unhelpful Envy: Flexible Mind DARES [to Let Go]) can be given to participants as part of a homework assignment, either in individual therapy or as part of skills training class. Remind participants that the preceding steps may need to be repeated again and again, as envy is an emotion that reappears frequently.

NOTE TO INSTRUCTORS: Revealing our envy to another person is a type of mindfulness "outing oneself" practice (see lesson 13). At first glance, it might appear to be risky. However, rather than getting upset when an envied person is told that they are envied, our clinical experience has repeatedly shown that people usually feel flattered, relieved, and closer to the person outing themselves. Invariably, the envied person has been aware of the envy (albeit he or she may not have consciously labeled it as envy) and may have feared retribution. It is not uncommon for envied people to reveal that they have admired the revealer of envy or may have even felt competitive toward them, too. Outing oneself about our envy enhances relationships because we are signaling vulnerability, and research shows this enhances interpersonal intimacy and reciprocal cooperation. That said, it is important for participants to not *expect* reciprocity from the other person. The goal of opposite action to envy is to change the experience of unhelpful envy and live according to values, not necessarily to enhance relationships (at least directly). In my experience, revealing the unhelpful envy may be the most important step for reducing it because the secretive nature of the emotion prevents the person from gaining any environmental feedback. The secrecy may damage the relationship over time with the envied person via aloofness and distancing. Feeling envy does not mean a person is doing something wrong; indeed, learning to let go of unhelpful envy is a heroic act requiring willingness, humility, and courage.

Lesson 27 Homework

1. (Required) Worksheet 27.A (Opposite Action to Unhelpful Envy: Flexible Mind DARES [to Let Go])

Radical Openness Handout 27.1

Main Points for Lesson 27: Envy and Resentment

1. Envy is experienced whenever someone compares themselves unfavorably to others, and unhelpful envy emerges when we believe their advantage over us is unwarranted.

2. Envy is *helpful* when it motivates us to try harder to *achieve our personal goals,* but it can cause problems when it motivates us to *prevent another person from achieving their goals.*

3. Unhelpful envy involves a painful blend of two emotions, *shame and anger,* with action urges for *secret revenge.*

4. Changing envy requires going opposite to both shame's urge to hide and anger's urge to attack.

5. To go all the way opposite action to envy, a person must let go of ill will and reveal envious feelings to the envied person.

Radical Openness Worksheet 27.A

Opposite Action to Unhelpful Envy: Flexible Mind DARES (to Let Go)

Flexible Mind DARES

D **Determine** if you are experiencing unhelpful envy

A **Admit** your envy and decide whether you want to change it

R **Recognize** envious thoughts and action urges

E Go opposite to **Envious** anger

S Go opposite to **Shameful** envy

D Determine *if you are experiencing unhelpful envy.*

Place a checkmark in the boxes that apply. (*Note:* The more boxes checked, the greater the likelihood you are experiencing unhelpful envy.)

- ☐ *Do I feel that I have been wronged, neglected, or passed over by this person or others?*
- ☐ *Have I found myself thinking negative thoughts about this person (or group)?*
- ☐ *Do I find myself thinking that this person has an unfair advantage over me?*
- ☐ *Do I find myself gossiping about this other person frequently?*
- ☐ *Do I consider this person a rival or a competitor?*
- ☐ *Have I fantasized about getting back at them?*
- ☐ *Have I tried to make their life difficult?*
- ☐ *Do I desire to punish them, beat them, or prove them wrong?*
- ☐ *Do I find myself sometimes secretly enjoying any misfortune that befalls this other person or fantasizing about misfortune occurring?*
- ☐ *Do I seek confirmation from others that the person deserves to be punished or has an unfair advantage?*

A Admit *your envy by labeling it and decide if you want to let it go.*

Place a checkmark in the boxes next to the skills you used.

- ☐ Repeated silently: *I am aware of an emotion of envy* or *The emotion I am feeling is called "envy."*
- ☐ Examined the pros and cons of achieving what the other person or group has achieved.
- ☐ Reminded myself of times when winning or being right may not have worked.
- ☐ Remembered times when I achieved goals, only to discover that their importance faded over time.
- ☐ Used self-enquiry to determine whether what was envied is something I truly value or desire.

R Recognize *and nonjudgmentally label action urges of unhelpful envy.*

Place a checkmark in the boxes next to the urges you observed, and record your observations in the space provided.

- ☐ Action urges to get even with the envied person, to make his or her life difficult, and to expose his or her weaknesses and failings.

- ☐ Urges to avoid using the word "envy," to hide my feelings of inferiority, and to keep my desires for revenge secret.

- ☐ Action urges to avoid contact with the envied person and to shut down or numb out when the person is around.

- ☐ Action urges to harshly gossip about the envied person and seek validation from others that my rival doesn't deserve his or her advantage over me.

Other observations.

_____

_____

_____

_____

E *Go opposite to* **Envious** *anger and desires for revenge.*

Place a checkmark in the boxes next to the skills you used, and record observations in the space provided.

1. **Taking care of myself**

    - ☐ Closed-mouth smiled, used eyebrow wags, and slowed my breathing when thinking about the person I am envious of.

    - ☐ Practiced being grateful for the things that I have by counting my blessings, and mindfully practiced living in the present moment to more fully enjoy my life.

    - ☐ Used self-enquiry to determine whether what was envied was something I truly valued or desired, and, if so, took the first step toward achieving it.

    Describe what steps you took and what other steps will be needed.

    _____

    _____

    _____

2. **Going opposite to action urges of anger**

485

☐ Practiced putting myself in the other person's shoes and seeing the world from the other's perspective.

☐ Looked for valid reasons why the other person deserves his or her advantage.

3. **Going all the way opposite action**

☐ Blocked looking for negative traits or moral failings about the envied person.

☐ Blocked pleasurable fantasies involving the envied person failing or suffering.

☐ Blocked negative gossip about the envied person.

☐ Practiced being nonjudgmental and kind and behaving decently toward the envied person.

Other observations.

_____

_____

_____

_____

S Go opposite to **Shameful** envy and desires to hide your envy from others.

Mark the skills you used, and record observations in the space provided.

1. **Practiced living within my values**

☐ Behaved truthfully by labeling my emotion as envy and went opposite to urges to justify or pretend the emotion was something else.

☐ Repeated the word "envy" aloud to myself multiple times.

☐ Reminded myself that envy is a normal human emotion and that it does not mean I am doing something wrong.

2. **Going opposite to shame**

☐ Revealed my envy to an objective, caring person and used the word "envy" when describing my situation.

☐ Blocked attempts by the caring person to label the emotion as something other than envy; blocked his or her attempts to justify my feelings of injustice.

3. **Turning unhelpful envy into admiration if I desire a closer relationship with the envied person**

☐ Remembered that revealing vulnerable (even shameful) emotions to others is relationship-enhancing.

☐ Selected a private place to reveal my feelings to the envied person and used the word "envy" to describe my experience.

☐ Apologized for prior negative actions, thoughts, or desires to cause them harm or see the person fail.

☐ Turned unhelpful envy into admiration by allowing myself to celebrate the person's success.

☐ Rewarded myself for living within my values.

Other observations.

_____

_____

_____

_____

Cynicism, Bitterness, and Resignation

Main Points for Lesson 28

1. Cynicism is an inclination to believe that people are motivated primarily by self-interest and respond with skepticism to new ideas.

2. Cynics help societies grow by challenging the status quo.

3. Cynics are not easily impressed—they are the skeptics of the world. Yet their natural tendencies to doubt and ask questions help societies grow by challenging the status quo.

4. Pervasive and rigid cynicism often leads to bitterness.

5. Bitterness is characterized by a pessimistic, hateful, discouraged, and resentful outlook on life, a mood that emanates from failures to achieve important goals and/or perceptions that entitlements were wrongfully obtained by others.

6. To change bitterness, one must practice kindness first and foremost, learn how to give and receive help, and practice being thankful for what one has.

Materials Needed

*   (Optional) Handout 28.1 (Main Points for Lesson 28: Cynicism, Bitterness, and Resignation)

*   Worksheet 28.A (Changing Bitterness: Flexible Mind Is LIGHT)

*   Whiteboard or flipchart with marker

(Recommended) Mindfulness Practice

"Who Makes These Changes?"

The Rumi poem "Who Makes These Changes" is a useful mindfulness practice for the start of this lesson because it introduces one of the most common paths to bitterness—that is, trying to control the world. Instructors should use the following script (read it aloud) to guide the practice. (*Note:* The use of a mindfulness bell is optional.)

> *The practice we are about to do will involve listening to a poem I am about to read, and noticing the images, memories, thoughts, sensations, or emotions that might arise, without getting caught up with them. Simply observing what arises and then turning your mind back to listening, again and again. If your mind wanders, notice that, and, without judgment, turn back again to the words being read aloud. I will be reading the poem three times in a row and will ring the mindfulness bell at the end of each repetition. Now sit in a comfortable yet alert position, and take a breath, with awareness, in order to center yourself into*

this moment. Notice the rise and fall of your breathing, not trying to change or do anything about it, just being fully present with the full duration of your inbreath and the full duration of your outbreath. [Slight pause.] I will now ring the bell and begin. As best you can, turn your mind now to the words of the poem, noticing what arises and bringing yourself back to the task of listening.

Who Makes These Changes?

I shoot an arrow right.
It lands left.
I ride after a deer and find myself
chased by a hog.
I plot to get what I want
and end up in prison.
I dig pits to trap others
and fall in.

I should be suspicious
of what I want.

—Mewlana Jalaluddin Rumi, 1230/2004 (Translated by Coleman Barks)

After the mindfulness practice, the instructor can ask participants to share observations and use them as a basis to teach from or for further discussion of the key points described earlier. This poem is also extremely useful in prompting discussion about the pros and cons of controlling the world, other people, or ourselves, and the implications these may have for how a person may choose to live.

NOTE TO INSTRUCTORS: The Rumi poem provides additional opportunities for self-enquiry because it can occasionally trigger defensive arousal or resistance from an OC client. For example, some clients have a strong reaction to the last two lines in the poem, "I should be suspicious / of what I want." Rather than soothing or validating a client when this occurs, instructors should encourage them to use this experience as an opportunity to practice self-enquiry—that is, is there something here to learn? Instructors can help a client begin this process by suggesting a few potentially useful self-enquiry questions (delivered with a warm smile and eyebrows raised): *Is it possible that my bodily tension means that I am not fully open to the concept of healthy self-doubt? If yes or possibly, then what am I afraid of? Or do I find myself wanting to automatically explain or defend myself? What might this mean? Or is it possible that I believe further self-examination would be harmful or unnecessary because I have already completed the necessary self-work? If yes or possibly, then what is it that I fear I may lose?*

(Recommended) Mini–Class Exercise

Fun with Cynicism

✳   *I don't do anger—I just walk away.*   ✳

When conducting this minipractice, instructors should feel free simply to read aloud the following script. Make sure you have extra pens and blank sheets of paper available for participants who may be without.

Instruct (preferably in what you imagine to be a Texas cowpoke accent—tee hee ☺). *Okeydoke, now, ever'body, git a good tight grip on them pens 'n' pencils, an' buckle up yer seat belts real tight, 'cause here comes a big ol' passel o' questions that's gonna ROCK, RUMBLE, 'n' ROLL ya! Ohhh YEAH!* Raise arms high in celebration, then pause in perplexed contemplation.

Continue (now preferably with a posh British accent—tee hee ☺). *Okay, perhaps that was a bit over the top. What I really meant to say is that in a few moments I will be asking you a number of questions. In preparation, please ensure that you have your writing utensils poised and paper available, in order to record any thoughts that may arise. I am confident that you will find it a smashing experience!*

Continue (back to your regular voice—and if that's posh British-speak, that's cool). *Sorry, an overcorrection on my part. Let's start again. What I really, really meant to say is that I am going to read some questions aloud soon, and your job will be to write down the very first thought that pops into your mind on the blank sheet of paper in front of you. We will not be sharing what we write down afterward, so whatever you write is yours and yours alone. You can keep it, throw it away, or use it as part of a self-enquiry practice—the choice is entirely yours. So we can all relax. Are you ready? Here are the questions.*

- ✓ **Ask yourself:** *What does it mean to be a cynic?* (Record the very first thought or word that comes into your mind.)

- ✓ **Ask yourself:** *What is the value of a cynic to society?* (Record the very first thought or word that comes into your mind.)

- ✓ **Ask yourself:** *How cynical am I in this moment? What might this tell me about myself?* (Record the very first thought or word that comes into your mind.)

- ✓ **Ask yourself:** *What are the downsides of being a cynic?* (Record the very first thought or word that comes into your mind.)

- ✓ **Ask yourself:** *What is it that I might need to learn?* (Record the very first thought or word that comes into your mind.)

End. Instructors should end the exercise by leading a brief round of applause (that is, for joining in) while asking for any observations, thoughts, emotions, or experiences that may have occurred during the preceding practice. Instructors should avoid making interpretations about participants' observations and encourage participants to use their experience as an opportunity for self-enquiry in the coming week.

(Required) Teaching Point
Learning from Cynicism

✳ *Life sucks, and then you die.* ✳

- *What is a cynic and why do we need them?*
  - **Cynics help societies grow by challenging the status quo** (for example, defying an unethical order from a superior, exposing wrongdoing in an organization).

  - **Yet, paradoxically, cynicism also protects the status quo,** most often by slowing down premature acceptance of new ideas or potentially risky ventures (for example, declarations of war) until they have had a chance to be refined, debated, or tested by the tribe. Cynics are the guardians of prudence and caution.

- *Cynics don't expect good things to happen—they are not easily impressed, nor are they easily excitable.*

  - ✓ **Ask:** *What types of events or experiences might trigger cynicism? What might reinforce cynicism? Why do most people not aspire to be cynics?*

- *Cynical moods can be a powerful social signal.* Read the following text aloud.

  > *When Mom was in one of her negative cynical moods, everyone in the family knew it, but you weren't allowed to comment on it. She didn't yell. She just would have this look about her that would send people scurrying. If you were smart, you knew to be quiet, do whatever you were supposed to do, and avoid crossing her at all costs until the mood passed, which might take days.*

  - ✓ **Ask:** *To what extent do you use cynical or negative mood states to influence other people?*

- *Finally, habitual cynicism can lead to bitterness—but, fortunately for us, bitterness is our next topic. (☺)*

(Required) Teaching Point

Bitterness

- **Bitterness is a mood state, not an emotion,** meaning that it can last for long periods of time and may subtly taint a person's perceptions (like wearing gray-tinted, not rose-colored, glasses).

- **Bitterness is characterized by a pessimistic, hateful, discouraged, and resentful outlook on life.** It emanates from failures to achieve important goals, or perceptions that entitlements were wrongfully obtained by others.

- **Cynicism is often a precursor of bitterness** (but not always).

- **Bitterness keeps people from joining with community.** Bitter individuals may believe happiness impossible and find it difficult to be grateful for what they have.

- **Changing bitterness involves five steps,** found in Flexible Mind Is LIGHT.

(Required) Teaching Point

Flexible Mind Is LIGHT

Refer participants to worksheet 28.A (Changing Bitterness: Flexible Mind Is LIGHT).

> NOTE TO INSTRUCTORS: When teaching Flexible Mind Is LIGHT, write out the acronym (LIGHT) on a flipchart or whiteboard with each letter arranged vertically in a column, but *without* teaching or naming the specific skill that each letter signifies. Next, starting with the first letter in the acronym (*L* in LIGHT) teach the skills associated with each letter in the acronym, using the key points outlined in the following sections, until you have covered all of the skills associated with each individual letter. Importantly, only write out on the whiteboard or flipchart the global description of what each letter actually stands for while you are teaching the skills associated with it. This teaching method avoids long explanations about the use of certain words in the acronym and/or premature teaching of concepts, since the meaning of each letter is only revealed during the formal teaching of the skills associated with it.

Flexible Mind Is LIGHT

L   **Label** your bitterness, using self-enquiry

I   Notice bitter **Intentions** by examining action urges

G   **Go opposite** to bitter beliefs

H   **Help** others, and allow others to **Help**

T   Practice kindness and being **Thankful**

L **Label** *bitterness by using self-enquiry.*

> **NOTE TO INSTRUCTORS:** Read aloud each of the following questions, and instruct participants to place a checkmark in each box they think may apply to them. Ask for observations, and discuss briefly.

- ☐ *Do I find it difficult to accept help from others (or give help)?*
- ☐ *Do people close to me think that I hold a grudge too long? Is there a past injury that I cannot let go of?*
- ☐ *Do I find it difficult to give compliments to others (or receive them)?*
- ☐ *Do I feel my efforts often go unrecognized?*
- ☐ *Do I find myself ruminating when people don't appreciate what I have done?*
- ☐ *Do I sometimes tell myself that trying to get what I want is just not possible?*
- ☐ *Do I feel resigned to my fate or say to myself, "Why bother?"*
- ☐ *Do I feel that enthusiasm about life or love is misguided or naive?*
- ☐ *Am I a cynic?*
- ☐ *Is it hard to impress me?*
- ☐ *Do I feel that I have not achieved what I should have in life?*
- ☐ *Do I feel life has treated me unfairly and that this happens most of the time?*
- ☐ *Do I frequently find myself questioning the intentions of others?*
- ☐ *Do I find it hard to have empathy for someone who has suffered similar traumatic experiences as I have?*
- ☐ *Do I frequently find myself believing that others judge me or are out to cause me harm?*

I *Notice bitter* **Intentions** *by examining actions, emotions, and thoughts associated with bitterness, such as…*

- *Behaving fatalistically and considering progress impossible or naive.*
- *Being judgmental toward hopeful, optimistic, or enthusiastic people and experiences.*
- *Preventing or minimizing expressions of happiness from self and others.* Bitterness *must* destroy happiness. Happiness signals hope and possibility, whereas bitterness implies futility, cynicism, and blind resistance.

- *Surrounding yourself with cynical, negative stories and entertainment.*
- *Spending time brooding.*
- *Rebuffing help from someone.*
- *Experiencing pleasure when others suffer misfortune,* even if you do not know them.

G Go opposite *to unjustified isolation and cynicism.*

- *Look for uplifting news stories or events that demonstrate altruism, compassion, and mankind's desire to help others.* Research shows that exposure to news stories about moral virtue can spur people to take more positive moral actions, including giving to charity. Purposely avoid books, news, movies, or television shows that focus on strife, conflict, and repeatedly show people hurting others. Remember that what you attend to on a daily basis influences how you feel.

- *Reflect on the commonalities you have with every other human being, and ignore differences.* Repeat silently to yourself while closed-mouth smiling…

  > *Just like me, others are seeking happiness and have known suffering. Just like me, they have harmed others and have been harmed by others. Just like me, they are trying to cope with their lives, as best they can, and yet are still learning.*

- *Interact with individuals who have different ways of dressing, thinking, or acting than you.* Research shows that face-to-face contact with people who are different from us reliably reduces prejudice and judgmental thinking (Pettigrew & Tropp, 2006).

- *Nonjudgmentally listen to opinions from people who hold different values or morals than you.* Research shows that contact with people who have differing views works best when people are on an equal footing, credence is given to the other person's point of view, and both parties treat each other with respect (S. M. Andersen, Saribay, & Thorpe, 2008; Pettigrew & Tropp, 2006). Use handout 22.1 (Being Open to Feedback from Others: Flexible Mind ADOPTS) to practice being open to other perspectives.

NOTE TO INSTRUCTORS: There is some research on intergroup contact suggesting that anxiety must be reduced before increases in empathy, perspective taking, and knowledge of the other group can effectively reduce prejudice or judgmental thinking (Blascovich, Mendes, Hunter, Lickel, & Kowai-Bell, 2001; Pettigrew & Tropp, 2006). Research shows that experiencing a sense of being loved and surrounded by supporting others seems to allow people to open themselves to alternative worldviews and be more accepting of people who do not belong to their own group (Mikulincer & Shaver, 2001). For OC individuals, this suggests the importance of reducing defensive arousal via activation of the social safety system (PNS-VVC) prior to social engagements. To achieve this, instructors should encourage participants to utilize skills designed to change physiology; see handout 3.1 (Changing Social Interactions by Changing Physiology).

H Help *others, and allow others to* Help *you.*

- *Go all the way opposite action to bitterness by helping others and allowing others to help you.*
- *Let go of fears that accepting help will make others see you as weak.*
- *Practice loving kindness meditation to activate your social safety system.*

- *Ask for help and offer help to others, frequently!* One surefire way to become a bitter person is never to allow another person to help you. Go opposite by courageously asking for help when you need it instead of pretending everything is okay. For example, be honest with your doctor about the pain in your side; tell your child that you need them to contribute to the family by being careful of their spending; let someone help you find a dropped contact lens; or allow someone to offer sympathy over the death of a close relative. In addition, look for opportunities to help others, all the while letting go of expectations that your efforts should be appreciated. For instance, help a person struggling with a large load by asking them if you can help carry part of it; look for opportunities to open doors for others or to let others go before you in a long line or queue; help someone look for a lost item; and/or practice nonjudgmentally listening to another person's distress. Remember to thank them (ideally, with a smile) for allowing you the opportunity to help them, or to thank them for helping you.

- *Practice kindness by being frank with others, and encourage them to return the favor.* Kindness is not telling someone yes when you mean no. Practice revealing your inner feelings and thoughts to others (the gift of truth), and encourage them to be frank with you. Frankness does not mean your perspective is correct, yet it does signal genuine caring because you are willing to tell the other person what you really think (that is, frankness is nondeceptive communication).

- *Practice letting go of expectations that self-sacrifices or hard work should be always noticed and appreciated by others, and be kind to yourself while doing so.* Remember, compassion fatigue (loss of empathy) is likely to occur whenever we lack the resources (or energy) to help someone we believe deserving of help. In other words, when we are overwhelmed, depressed, highly anxious, or distressed, our ability to provide support to others is limited; and, consequently, *our desires to help may be less, too.* Low desire to help someone does NOT mean that we are a bad, evil, or uncaring person; instead, these feelings may suggest that we have neglected taking care of ourselves. Compassion arises when we witness another's suffering and desire to help them (Goetz, Keltner, & Simon-Thomas, 2010), but to genuinely care for others, we must also take care of ourselves. Without this, burnout and bitterness are the likely consequences.

NOTE TO INSTRUCTORS: Occasionally participants report that they have never felt gratitude or appreciation toward others. Usually this is because, from their perspective, no one has ever truly helped them, and/or they are "fatally flawed," due to an inability to feel grateful for what others have done to help them. If this happens, instructors should be prepared to validate these experiences as common among individuals who have grown up in difficult or invaliding environments, common among those growing up in cultures valuing independence, or a result of factors that we do not fully understand. Lack of feeling gratitude or thankfulness toward others does not mean that it is not possible. *The real question is whether the participant is willing to try learning how to experience gratefulness or become more grateful.*

- *Practice giving and receiving compliments.* Healthy relationships involve reciprocal positive exchanges. Research shows that the ratio of positive to negative comments in stable marriages is five to one, signifying that an interacting partner needs five positive comments to each negative comment to experience a satisfactory relationship (Gottman, 1994).

- *Increase prosocial behavior.* For example, practice chitchatting with people you hardly know; look for opportunities to join in group activities; say "Thank you" to compliments or praise; practice MATCH + 1, closed-mouth smiles, and eyebrow wags (see Flexible Mind ALLOWs, in lesson 21).

- *"Make meaning" when positive things occur by linking them to your personal attributes or goals.* For instance, when praised by a friend or partner for being available during a time of crisis, instead of dismissing the compliment, use this feedback as evidence for having a kind nature.

When complimented for being on time, link this to the positive attribute of conscientiousness rather than simply assuming that everyone would have behaved similarly.

- **Practice resting after completing a difficult task rather than using this as a means to whip yourself to work harder or simply moving on to the next task.** Build time into each day for some moments that are nonproductive, making sure that you try out new ways to relax; see handout 5.3 (The Art of Nonproductivity and Being Just a Little Bit Silly).

- **Celebrate successes.** Remember to celebrate the positive things in life. Indeed, doing so can be hard work. Look for opportunities to celebrate success or special occasions with others, and go opposite to urges to avoid or isolate.

NOTE TO INSTRUCTORS: Maintaining secure and satisfying relationships can be particularly challenging for OC individuals, as they may doubt whether people sincerely care about them. That said, research suggests that when individuals with low self-esteem were asked to notice a compliment given to them by a partner, and to consider what the praise may have meant for them and the relationship with the partner, they were able to report increased positive feelings about the compliment (Marigold, Holmes, & Ross, 2007).

T *Practice kindness and being* **Thankful** *of self and others.*

✳ *Always be a little kinder than necessary.* ✳

- **Greet each day with thankfulness.** For example, as suggested by the Dalai Lama:

  Today I am fortunate to have woken up, I am alive, I have a precious human life, I am not going to waste it. I am going to use all my energies to develop myself, to expand my heart out to others, to achieve enlightenment for the benefit of all beings, I am going to have kind thoughts toward others, I am not going to get angry or think badly about others, I am going to benefit others as much as I can.

- **Practice kindness first and foremost;** see Flexible Mind ROCKs ON, in lesson 17, and worksheet 17.B (Kindness First and Foremost). "Kindness first and foremost" means treating other people as we would like to be treated. It enhances relationships and appreciates how all things are connected by celebrating our diversity. It signals "We are all the same" to others, and it recognizes our place in the world by acknowledging that we are one of many.

- **Pass it on—pass on the gift of kindness—by looking for small opportunities to practice forgiveness, without expecting acknowledgment or anything in return**—for example, smiling warmly to the harried store clerk, allowing a tailgating car to pass you on the freeway, phoning a sick colleague out of the blue.

- **Engage in anonymous random acts of kindness.** Work in a soup kitchen, make a cake for someone, send money anonymously to a person in need who you do not know, practice forgiving those who fail to appreciate your hard work, be kind in your thoughts by giving others the benefit of the doubt and assuming good intentions on their part. Practice looking for a nonjudgmental interpretation in all situations.

- **Practice genuine humility by letting go of insisting that the world conform to your expectations.** It is arrogant for me to assume that I know the right way or that my perspective is correct. Genuine humility acknowledges that I am flawed, without falling apart.

- ***Use the Big Three + 1 to chill out when around others*** (that is, leaning back in a chair, taking a slow deep breath, closed-mouth smiling, eyebrow wags); see handout 3.1 (Changing Social Interactions by Changing Physiology).

- ***Approach situations that may generate positive emotions.*** Buy a puppy, go to a carnival and ride the Ferris wheel, try out speed dating, or join a running club.

- ***Whistle or sing while doing chores around the house.*** In other words, look for opportunities to practice expressing cheerfulness in everyday life.

- ***Practice forgiveness and let go of grudges*** (use Flexible Mind Has HEART skills, in lesson 29).

Lesson 28 Homework

1. **(Required) Worksheet 28.A (Changing Bitterness: Flexible Mind Is LIGHT)**

2. **(Optional) Practice kindness first and foremost**

Radical Openness Handout 28.1

Main Points for Lesson 28:
Cynicism, Bitterness, and Resignation

1. Cynicism is an inclination to believe that people are motivated primarily by self-interest and respond with skepticism to new ideas.

2. Cynics help societies grow by challenging the status quo.

3. Cynics are not easily impressed—they are the skeptics of the world. Yet their natural tendencies to doubt and ask questions help societies grow by challenging the status quo.

4. Pervasive and rigid cynicism often leads to bitterness.

5. Bitterness is characterized by a pessimistic, hateful, discouraged, and resentful outlook on life, a mood that emanates from failures to achieve important goals and/or perceptions that entitlements were wrongfully obtained by others.

6. To change bitterness, one must practice kindness first and foremost, learn how to give and receive help, and practice being thankful for what one has.

Radical Openness Worksheet 28.A

Changing Bitterness: Flexible Mind Is LIGHT

Flexible Mind Is LIGHT

L   **Label** your bitterness, using self-enquiry

I   Notice bitter **Intentions** by examining action urges

G   **Go opposite** to bitter beliefs

H   **Help** others, and allow others to **Help**

T   **Practice** kindness and being thankful

L   Label *bitterness, using self-enquiry.*

Place a checkmark next to any of the following questions that apply to you, or that you think others might believe apply to you. (*Note:* A greater number of checkmarks = a greater amount of bitterness.)

- ☐ *Do I find it difficult to accept help from others (or give help)?*
- ☐ *Do people close to me think that I hold a grudge too long? Is there a past injury that I cannot let go of?*
- ☐ *Do I find it difficult to give compliments to others (or receive them)?*
- ☐ *Do I feel my efforts often go unrecognized?*
- ☐ *Do I find myself ruminating when people don't appreciate what I have done?*
- ☐ *Do I sometimes tell myself that trying to get what I want is just not possible?*
- ☐ *Do I feel resigned to my fate or say to myself, "Why bother?"*
- ☐ *Do I feel that enthusiasm about life or love is misguided or naive?*
- ☐ *Am I a cynic?*
- ☐ *Is it hard to impress me?*
- ☐ *Do I feel that I have not achieved what I should have in life?*
- ☐ *Do I feel life has treated me unfairly and that this happens most of the time?*
- ☐ *Do I frequently find myself questioning the intentions of others?*
- ☐ *Do I find it hard to have empathy for someone who has suffered similar traumatic experiences as I have?*
- ☐ *Do I frequently find myself believing that others judge me or are out to cause me harm?*

I   Notice bitter **Intentions** *by examining actions, thoughts, and emotions.*

Pick a recent event when you thought bitterness was present. Place a checkmark next to statements that apply to what you experienced, or use the space provided to describe other experience in your own words.

☐ Blocked expressions of happiness or love by others or by myself.

☐ Experienced an urge to tell a person that his or her optimism, love, or desire for happiness was a waste of time, childlike, or naive.

☐ Attempted to avoid people who were expressing hope, optimism, or enthusiasm.

☐ Surrounded myself with cynical, negative, or judgmental stories or entertainment (for example, newspapers, books, TV) or spent time purposefully brooding or writing about melancholic issues.

☐ Rebuffed help from someone.

☐ Secretly desired another person to experience a fate similar to mine.

☐ Found it difficult to feel empathy toward someone who had suffered similarly to the way that I have.

Describe other experiences.

_____

_____

_____

_____

G Go opposite *to unjustified isolation and cynicism.*

Place a checkmark in the boxes next to the skills you practiced.

☐ Looked for uplifting news stories or events demonstrating altruism, kindness, and compassion toward self and others.

☐ Practiced loving kindness meditation in order to activate my social safety system; see handout 3.1 (Changing Social Interactions by Changing Physiology).

☐ Practiced noticing what I have in common with other human beings. Repeated silently: *Just like me, others are seeking happiness and have known suffering. Just like me, others have harmed others and have been harmed by others. Just like me, others are trying to cope with their life as best they can and yet can still learn from what life has to offer.*

☐ Celebrated diversity by nonjudgmentally interacting with people who dress, think, or act differently than I do.

☐ Practiced fully listening without judgment to the opinions expressed by people who I believe to hold different values or morals than I do.

☐ Turned my mind from unhelpful thoughts, such as *If I join with others, then it means my entire life has been a total sham.*

☐ Highlighted positive events or experiences in my life and attributed them to my learning new ways of behaving rather than to coincidence or happenstance.

☐ Remembered times when I experienced warmth or closeness from or toward others (even my therapist).

Describe other skills you practiced or what else you learned.

_____

_____

_____

_____

H   **Help** *others and allow others to* **Help** *me.*

Place a checkmark in the boxes next to the skills you practiced.

- ☐ Engaged in anonymous random acts of kindness.
- ☐ Practiced letting go of fears that if I am kind toward others, they will hurt me or see me as weak.
- ☐ Allowed others to help me (for example, open a door) or asked for help when I needed it.
- ☐ Offered help to others, without expecting that they return the favor.
- ☐ Practiced being frank with others, and encouraged them to return the favor.
- ☐ Practiced letting go of expectations that my self-sacrifices or hard work should be appreciated or noticed by others.
- ☐ Practiced giving and receiving compliments or praise.
- ☐ Increased my prosocial behavior—for example, practiced chitchat with someone, sang with others in church, enthusiastically joined in with others applauding an entertainer, said yes to an offer of tea or coffee or to an invitation to join colleagues after work for a beer.
- ☐ Increased my proactive prosocial behavior—for example, asked others to join me rather than waiting for them to ask me first (for example, to go to a movie, take a walk, visit a museum).
- ☐ Practiced resting and rewarding myself after completing a difficult task rather than telling myself I should get back to work and work harder.

Describe other skills you practiced or what else you learned.

_____

_____

_____

_____

T *Practice* **Thankfulness** *toward self and others.*

Place a checkmark in the boxes next to the skills you practiced.

☐ Greeted each day with thankfulness; for example, repeated to myself: *Today I am fortunate to have woken up, I am alive, I have a precious human life, and I am not going to waste it. I am going to use all my energies to develop myself and be more radically open to what the world has to offer. I will actively seek ways to join with others and accept problems as opportunities rather than obstacles. I am going to have kind thoughts toward others and not think badly about others. I am going to benefit others as much as I can.*

☐ Practiced closed-mouth smiling and eyebrow wags when around others.

☐ Approached situations that generated positive emotions.

☐ Whistled, hummed, or sang while doing chores, and looked for other opportunities to practice expressing cheerfulness in my life.

☐ Practiced humility by not insisting that the world conform to my way of thinking.

☐ Acknowledged that I am one of many while celebrating my uniqueness.

☐ Gave people the benefit of the doubt by assuming good intentions on their part if I had no direct evidence to the contrary.

☐ Practiced forgiveness and letting go of grudges (used Flexible Mind Has HEART skills).

☐ Was grateful for what I have.

Other skills and observations.

_____

_____

_____

_____

Learning to Forgive

Main Points for Lesson 29

1. Forgiveness is not approval or denying the past.

2. Forgiveness does not mean reconciliation.

3. Forgiveness does not mean opening yourself up to being hurt again.

4. Forgiveness means taking care of ourselves and learning to let go of useless anger, resentment, or self-blame.

5. To let go of a past injury or grievance, you must first find your edge that keeps you holding on to the past injury.

6. Forgiveness must be freely chosen. A person cannot be forced to forgive, nor can someone be forced to accept forgiveness when it is offered.

7. Forgiveness requires an ongoing commitment to let go of past hurts in order to grow.

8. We must decide to forgive, and we must decide again repeatedly.

9. To reclaim our life and learn how to forgive, we must grieve the loss of expectations.

10. Practice being thankful for what you have. Remind yourself of all the times in your life when you have needed forgiveness from others.

Materials Needed

- Handout 29.1 (What Forgiveness Is and Is Not)

- Handout 29.2 (Forgiveness Self-Enquiry Questions)

- Handout 29.3 (Strengthening Forgiveness Through Grief Work: Examples of Common Beliefs or Expectations)

- (Optional) Handout 29.4 (Main Points for Lesson 29: Learning to Forgive)

- Worksheet 29.A (Flexible Mind Has HEART)

- Whiteboard or flipchart and markers

(Required) Discussion Point

Understanding Forgiveness

Begin the class by using the following questions to guide a brief discussion (about five minutes at most) about the concept of forgiveness (write on a whiteboard or flipchart what the class comes up with, but don't attempt to generate an exhaustive list).

✓ **Ask:** *What words, images, or emotions arise when you hear the word "forgiveness," "kindness," or "compassion"? How do you define forgiveness?*

✓ **Ask:** *What are the pros and cons of forgiveness?*

> NOTE TO INSTRUCTORS: If concerns or fears about forgiveness are raised by participants during the preceding discussion, instructors should avoid the temptation to engage in long class debates at this point in the teaching and/or to attempt to reassure, appease, or teach what forgiveness is or how to forgive prematurely. Instead, instructors should remind participants that the skills being taught that day will likely address their concerns and encourage them to learn the skill before judging its potential merit.

(Recommended) Mindfulness Practice

Recalling a Time We Needed Forgiveness

Instructors should read the following text aloud to the class and use this as the basis for a mindfulness visualization and self-enquiry practice.

> *To begin this mindfulness practice, I would like you to sit in a comfortable yet alert position. Now take a breath, with awareness, in order to center yourself into this moment. Notice the rise and fall of your breathing, not trying to change it or do anything about it, just simply being fully present with the full duration of your inbreath and the full duration of your outbreath. [Slight pause.] Now, as best you can, try to find a memory of a time when you experienced a strong sense of having been forgiven by another person. The memory does not need to be about a serious offense, and it can be from childhood or any other time in your life. Perhaps there was a time when you accidentally bumped into someone on the street, said something hurtful when angry, hit someone's car while driving, or failed to support someone when the person was most in need. Yet the person forgave you for what happened. What did it feel like to be forgiven? How did your body feel? What emotions did you experience? What thoughts did you have? Were you able to accept the forgiveness? How does your body feel now as you remember this event? What emotions do you feel? If you were going to send a note of gratitude to this other person for the gift of forgiveness, what would you say? [Pause.] Now let's bring our attention back to our breath, noticing how it rises and falls, while letting go of the images, thoughts, memories, emotions, or sensations associated with our practice of finding a time we were forgiven. [Pause.] And now, when you are ready, bring your attention back into this room, and we will discuss any observations you had about this practice.*

Instructors should then end the practice and ask for observations. Use the questions embedded in the preceding script to facilitate discussion and provide opportunities for teaching.

NOTE TO INSTRUCTORS: Sometimes a class participant will report that they have "never been forgiven by anyone—ever!" There is a range of ways to respond to this statement—for example, therapeutically teasing with a smile and eyebrow wag, saying, "Okay, I forgive you for that"; or, "Wow, you mean no one has ever forgiven you, ever? Does this mean you've never done anything bad enough to need forgiveness?" with a slight wink, smile, and eyebrow wag. Alternatively, an instructor might encourage self-enquiry by saying, "Wow. That's really rare, but it can sometimes happen. What do you think this might mean for you? Is there any chance this experience might impact your ability or willingness to forgive others? What is it that you might need to learn from this?" Most often a combination of the two approaches just outlined works best because it smuggles lightheartedness to a subject many people find difficult while simultaneously encouraging self-discovery via self-enquiry.

(Required) Teaching Point
What Is Forgiveness?

Refer participants to handout 29.1 (What Forgiveness Is and Is Not).

- *Forgiveness is not approval or denying the past.* Forgiveness does not mean forgetting what happened and moving on. Wishing a past hurt away never works—the hurt keeps resurfacing, and the more you try to deny its existence, the more it seems to impact your life.

- *Forgiveness does not mean opening yourself to being hurt again.* Deciding to reengage with someone who has hurt you is separate from deciding to forgive or not.

- *Practice self-enquiry…*

  ➢ *What will move you closer to how you would like to live, and what is more in line with your personal values—forgiveness or revenge?*

  ➢ *What do you fear you might lose if you were to practice forgiveness?*

  ➢ *Are you holding on to the past injury for other reasons?*

- *Forgiveness means taking care of ourselves.* Letting go of unhelpful or ineffective anger, resentment, guilt, shame, or self-blame is freeing and helps us live more fully in the present. Forgiveness can also open up opportunities for new or improved social connections and experiences because we are focusing on present events, relationships, and opportunities rather than engaging in unhelpful brooding or rumination about a past grievance.

- *We admire those who are able to forgive and often desire to be close to them.* For example, most people would like to meet the Dalai Lama (he attracts large crowds of people), not so much because he can eloquently talk about the importance of forgiveness but because people viscerally experience the depth of his kindness and forgiveness when in his presence.

- *Find your forgiveness heroes*—for example, Mahatma Gandhi, Martin Luther King Jr., Nelson Mandela, the Dalai Lama, Saint Teresa of Calcutta (Mother Teresa), Thich Nhat Hanh, Saint Francis of Assisi, Rumi. *What characteristics do these people share? Why do people admire people who are able to forgive? Would you like to behave similarly? What might this say about your values?*

- *We forgive more than we know.* For example, have you ever told someone who bumped into you on the subway or on a street that it was okay (even if they failed to apologize) and really meant it?

  ✓ **Ask:** *What might this tell us? Is it possible that all people are capable of forgiveness? Is it possible that you forgive more than you realize? How might this knowledge help you?*

NOTE TO INSTRUCTORS: Experiencing fear, trepidation, or anger when thinking about a past injury does not mean one is incapable of forgiveness. Instructors can point out that being able to name a forgiveness hero tells us that the person values forgiveness, because they admire those who are able to practice it. Plus, any experience in the past in which a person forgave someone, even for a minor mistake (for example, being bumped on the subway), also suggests that the person likely values forgiveness. A surefire way to feel bad about oneself is to not live according to one's values. Instructors can use these observations to encourage clients who are struggling with the idea of forgiveness. Forgiveness means living according to your values. You might only need more practice.

NOTE TO INSTRUCTORS: It is important to validate fears that forgiveness could somehow make a person less vigilant for future harm (see "Offer Forgiveness Training," in chapter 9 of the RO DBT textbook). Having memories of past harms or painful experiences helps protect us. However, at the same time, research shows that we never *unlearn* anything (Bouton, 2002); we only lay down new learning or new associations over old learning. Thus, a past injury will never be fully forgotten, but it can fade from memory, to the extent that it seems nearly nonexistent. However, if the right reminders appear, then the memory will reappear, too (albeit with less emotional intensity), thereby allowing us to respond appropriately in the moment (for example, protect ourselves, if needed). Instructors should remind participants that forgiveness does not mean forgetting.

(Required) Class Mindfulness Exercise
Finding a Past Injury

Guided mindfulness instructions (read aloud):

Begin by simply taking a breath—with awareness—not trying to change the breath or fix it in some way, just being fully present with the full duration of the inbreath and the full duration of the outbreath. Now, as best you can, bring into your awareness a time when you felt hurt, injured, or transgressed upon. It could be a recent event or something happening long ago. The goal of this exercise is to locate a past grievance to use as a practice ground for learning forgiveness. Notice the emotions, sensations, images, or thoughts associated with your recollection. Allow yourself to rest here and now—with the images associated with this past hurt—as best you can. Not trying to change it or make it go away, simply opening and softening to the experience, right here and now. [Pause for about ten seconds.] Now gently bring your awareness back into this room, allowing this past memory to fade, as best you can. Reminding yourself that no matter how painful this past experience was or how difficult this practice may have seemed, reencountering a painful event is the only way to let it go, and this is the first step toward forgiveness.

- ✓ **Ask:** *What did you observe?*

- ✓ **Ask:** *If you were to use one word to describe this, what would it be? For example, did you feel disappointed, misunderstood, betrayed, wrongfully criticized, or dealt with unfairly?*

NOTE TO INSTRUCTORS: Participants should be encouraged to share the past hurt they identified in the preceding mindfulness practice, and instructors should be prepared to help those finding it difficult to identify one. Instructors should first encourage participants to focus on events that are of low-level or moderate-level emotional intensity. It is best to start small and build toward mastery prior to attempting high-intensity practices (that is, when first learning to swim, don't start by jumping in the deep end). Sometimes it can be helpful for instructors to share examples of grievances, either their own or those they may have heard about from others. These can trigger memories for those who struggled locating a specific incident. Once each person in the class has identified a past hurt, instructors should ask participants to keep this event in their awareness throughout the lesson and to use this experience as a basis for practice during class. Instructors should alert individual therapists when particular participants have strong reactions (for example, arguing, shutting down, or being unusually quiet) following this mindfulness practice. My clinical experience suggests that this type of response is rare. However, it is important for therapists to be sensitive that discussions involving forgiveness can be difficult, especially for individuals who may have had multiple or extreme traumatic past experiences. The format of the skills training group does not allow the time or emotional space for the type of support that may be needed when dealing with high-intensity traumas, long-held grievances involving deliberate transgressions, or highly charged and complicated emotional events. Participants should be encouraged to discuss these more serious or severe grievances with their individual therapist and work out the best course of action and/or skills needed.

(Required) Teaching Point

Flexible Mind Has HEART

Refer participants to worksheet 29.A (Flexible Mind Has HEART).

NOTE TO INSTRUCTORS: Introduce Flexible Mind Has HEART to participants by writing the acronym (HEART) on a whiteboard or flipchart. Explain that the acronym HEART is designed to remind them of the skills for forgiveness. Each letter of the word HEART is a step toward healthy forgiveness. Instructors should then start teaching the letter *H* in the acronym. Instructors can note aloud to participants that they already demonstrated willingness and took the first step when they participated in the mindfulness exercise that was just completed.

Flexible Mind Has HEART

H   Identify the past **Hurt**

E   Locate your **Edge** that's keeping you stuck in the past

A   **Acknowledge** that forgiveness is a choice

R   **Reclaim** your life by grieving your loss and practicing forgiveness

T   Practice **Thankfulness** and then pass it on

H *Identify the past* **Hurt***, grievance, or injury you are holding on to.*

- *Forgiveness is most needed whenever we find ourselves unable to let go of a painful past experience.*

- *Identify the areas in your life that may require forgiveness, using the following questions.*

Instructors can read each of the following questions aloud and, without necessarily encouraging further discussion, ask participants simply to record silently in their self-enquiry journal what arose.

✓ **Ask:** *Is there a past experience, event, or interaction that I find myself repeatedly thinking about or cannot stop thinking about?*

✓ **Ask:** *Is there a particular event or experience that I want to avoid, pretend never happened, or try to forget?*

✓ **Ask:** *What past experiences do I blame the world or others for?*

✓ **Ask:** *What events or experiences in my life do I harshly blame myself for?*

✓ **Optional:** *What events or experiences in my life do I feel shame or embarrassment about and/or attempt to hide from others?*

✓ **Optional:** *Are there events in my life that I have purposefully lied about or that I avoid talking about?*

✓ **Optional:** *Is there a particular person or set of people that I hold a grudge about or have felt betrayed by?*

✓ **Optional:** *Who in my life do I feel or believe has wronged me and I have been unable to forgive? What in my life have I done that I find impossible or difficult to forgive myself for?*

✓ **Optional:** *Is there a particular person or set of people that I have desires to hurt or get back at and/or would feel happy if they experienced failure?*

NOTE TO INSTRUCTORS: The preceding questions correspond to the descriptors found under *H* in worksheet 29.A (Flexible Mind Has HEART). They are designed to trigger memories of painful past experiences. It is common for clients to identify a range of past injuries (for example, five or more). Instructors should be alert to avoid smuggling anti–RO DBT notions implying that painful emotions, past traumas, or negative past experiences are inherently dangerous or scary. Instead, instructors should remind participants that obstacles, traumas, and painful experiences are experienced by everyone—no one is immune— albeit some may have had more severe or intense experiences than others. A core RO DBT principle is that obstacles in life are part of life, and each time they are encountered, they can become opportunities for self-growth. Thus, if a participant reports disliking the first step of Flexible Mind Has HEART, or that they experienced distress and/or are fearful of experiencing distress if they allow themselves to recall a past injury, instructors should encourage the client to practice self-enquiry about their reaction—for example, by asking "What is it that I might need to learn from my reaction?" rather than immediately assuming that distress should be avoided, soothed, validated, regulated, or automatically accepted.

NOTE TO INSTRUCTORS: Encourage participants to get into the habit of noticing small grievances (for example, rumination/anger about a rude gesture that appeared to be directed to them by the driver of a car passing them on the freeway) to practice forgiveness with, not just waiting for the big ones to come along.

- *Record in your self-enquiry journal all the past injuries you identified, and rank-order them according to severity and/or avoidance* (with 1 representing the most severe or most avoided).

- *Pick the past hurt or injury you want to practice forgiveness with.* Remember, when you are learning forgiveness to start with the lower levels first, with an intention to work toward higher-severity issues over time.

NOTE TO INSTRUCTORS: Instructors should encourage participants to resist the temptation to rush forgiveness out of a sense of duty or desire to fix things quickly. For example, some clients may report that they want to begin with their most painful past injury. Though this may seem sensible or courageous, it can often lead to unforeseen problems that make learning forgiveness more difficult. Instructors can ask participants to imagine a first-time skier insisting on starting out on the most dangerous slope. How likely is it that they will have a positive first-time experience?

E   Locate your **Edge** *that's keeping you stuck in the past.*

- *To let go of a past injury or grievance, you must first find your edge that keeps you holding on to the past injury.* Our edge is where self-growth occurs. It is most often described as a feeling of tension or resistance, embarrassment, a desire to avoid, or a sense of numbness. It usually involves things in our life that we don't want to think about or admit to.

- *Start this process by noticing...*

  - *Desires to explain, justify, or defend...*

    - What happened
    - Your responses
    - Another person or people

  - *Desires to blame yourself, blame others, or blame the world...*

    - For the event itself
    - For not getting what you want
    - For your suffering
    - For having to cope
    - For not living according to your values
    - For making it happen or not preventing it

NOTE TO INSTRUCTORS: In general, the fact that a client finds it difficult to let go of a painful past experience suggests that an edge may be present. Importantly, self-enquiry means being open to the possibility that one does not have an edge about a particular past injury while retaining an understanding of one's fallibility and a willingness to further question oneself if circumstances change (see more on self-enquiry in lesson 13).

Refer participants to handout 29.2 (Forgiveness Self-Enquiry Questions), and direct their attention to the subheading "Finding Your Forgiveness Edge." Instructors should randomly pick a participant to read aloud one of the questions from this list and then encourage class members to place a checkmark in the box next to the question if it appears to bring them closer to their edge. The instructor can then randomly pick another participant to read aloud one of the other questions and ask the class to do the same. Importantly, it is not necessary to read aloud all of the questions on the handout; the point is to introduce participants to several of them and then to encourage them to use the handout and the questions to enhance self-enquiry when practicing forgiveness.

- *Practice self-enquiry to deepen awareness of your edge, using the questions in handout 29.2 as a guide.*

- *Remember that self-enquiry means finding a good question that brings you closer to your edge (that is, your unknown), not a good answer.* Allow yourself time to discover what you might need to learn rather than quickly searching for a way to explain things away or regulate.

- *Each day, gently re-ask the self-enquiry question you discovered that brought you closest to your edge, and record what arises each time you ask.*

- *Practice being suspicious of quick answers or urges to regulate, as they may be masquerading as avoidance.* Keep your self-enquiry practices short (for example, five minutes in duration). Short and frequent (for example, daily) practices, using the same question or a new question that emerged from the previous day, are usually more effective. Longer practices can sometimes be secretly motivated by desires to find an answer or a solution.

- *Observe and record in your self-enquiry journal how your practice of self-enquiry about the past injury changes over time.*

A Acknowledge *that forgiveness is a choice.*

- *Forgiveness requires a conscious decision to let go of painful experiences* or past grievances because holding on to them is no longer effective.

- *Forgiveness must be freely chosen.* A person cannot be forced to forgive, nor can someone be forced to accept forgiveness when it is offered.

- *Acknowledge that forgiveness is a choice that only you can make—it is ultimately your decision.*

- **Not deciding** *is still making a choice.*

NOTE TO INSTRUCTORS: We often believe that punishment will make things better, yet the punisher is the one who may be most likely to suffer in the end (for example, by triggering rumination about the punishment or the past event and/or refiring painful emotions). Plus, most OC clients are characterized by high moral certitude (that is, there is a right and wrong way of doing things), and this is often linked to beliefs that good deeds should be rewarded and evil deeds punished. Punishing the transgressor restores a person's faith in a just world. A just world is one where actions and occurrences have predictable and appropriate consequences and people get what they deserve, depending on how they behave. This helps explain why many people find it so difficult to forgive—it can feel morally wrong not to punish the transgressor. This also explains why OC clients can find it difficult to forgive themselves for past wrongs—in order to restore their faith in a just world, they must first punish themselves (see also "Dealing with Suicidal Behavior and Self-Harm," in chapter 5 of the RO DBT textbook). To assess "just world" beliefs linked to punishment, instructors can ask, "To what extent do you believe that noble actions should be rewarded and evil actions punished?" Common sayings or phrases linked to "just world" thinking include "You got what was coming to you," "You reap what you sow," and "What goes around comes around" (see Furnham, 2003, for a review of the research surrounding the "just world" phenomenon).

- *Holding a grudge against someone is like drinking poison every day with hopes of punishing your enemy.* It just doesn't work; it only creates more suffering for ourselves by refiring useless anger, and it wastes precious time dwelling on a past event that cannot be redone or remade.

- *Let go of thinking that somehow the transgressor will get away with what they did wrong if you stop feeling anger.*

- *Remember that punishing a transgressor punishes ourselves because it keeps us stuck in the past* and wastes precious time dwelling on a past event that cannot be redone or remade.

- *Every time you find yourself wanting to think about how to punish the other person (or yourself), practice self-enquiry instead* (refer participants to handout 29.2, and direct their attention to the questions under the subheading "Self-Enquiry About Punishment").

NOTE TO INSTRUCTORS: When teaching self-enquiry questions, randomly pick participants to read aloud some of the questions, and briefly discuss and/or ask participants to record what they observed following each question in their self-enquiry journal.

- *Surrender your arrogance by acknowledging the fallibility inherent in all humans.*

- *Let go of insisting that all past injuries must be vindicated by acknowledging the impossibility of this task.*

- *Stop insisting that the world conform to your moral code or values by celebrating diversity among people* (for example, different cultural, linguistic, religious, genetic, and family backgrounds).

- *Practice seeing the world from the perspective of the person who hurt you,* using self-enquiry by asking…

  ➤ *Is it possible that when the transgression occurred, those involved never intended harm and/or that they regret their behavior now?*

> ➤ *Even if the other person appears to not regret their behavior, is it possible that they were not fully aware or capable of understanding how harmful their behavior was?*

> ➤ *Is it possible that major problems or past traumas in their life may have made them (or myself) more vulnerable to the painful event?*

- **Practice accepting that something hurtful happened that was outside of your control** while remembering that acceptance does not mean approval or resignation.

R Reclaim *your life by grieving your loss and practicing forgiveness.*

> NOTE TO INSTRUCTORS: Remind participants that it is impossible to NOT think about something—for example, try not to think about a pink giraffe. It is impossible to block any form of thought or image about it, because to not think about something, you have to first think about it. The same applies to past injuries or grievances—trying not to think about them almost always backfires.

- **When we have been injured, our belief in a just world is shaken.** Our confidence in being able to predict what will happen and engage in effective, goal-driven behavior may feel threatened.

- **To forgive and reclaim our life, we must first grieve our loss of our expectations and beliefs about the world, ourselves, or other people.** Sadness helps us recognize that we cannot control the world.

- **Grieving means allowing yourself to feel the sadness or disappointment associated with a loss and then letting the sadness go.** Grieving does not mean wallowing in sadness, ruminating about the past event, or building your house in the cemetery. Grieving means allowing yourself to fully experience the sadness, over days and weeks—for brief periods of time—and then going about your business as usual.

- **Grief work clears out old ways of thinking and allows us to be more open to what's happening now.**

  - ✓ **Ask:** *What part of myself or what belief about the world did this past injury damage?*

  - ✓ **Ask:** *What is it that I need to grieve?*

> NOTE TO INSTRUCTORS: Grief work helps a person's brain recognize that the world has changed; it is like updating your computer with the latest software in order to improve its functioning. When we attempt to avoid the sadness associated with a loss, we never allow our computer (our brain) the time to improve how we see the world by downloading the latest information about important events that happened in our life. This makes it more likely for us to become upset, angry, or hurt again whenever we encounter a memory of the past event, because our brain is still running on the old software that still expects the world to be the same as prior to the injurious event.

- *Prior to each practice, remind yourself what forgiveness is and is not.*

  - **Forgiveness does not mean reconciliation.** You can forgive and restore the relationship or forgive and not restore the relationship. You can forgive without ever seeing the person again.

  - **Forgiveness does not mean approval.**

- **Forgiveness does not mean opening yourself to being hurt again.** Our brains will retain the ability to react to what is harmful and take steps to avoid it or deal with it. Thus, you can afford to let go of your past hurts without fear of losing your ability to cope with future threats.

- **Forgiveness means taking care of ourselves.** Holding on to a past injury keeps us stuck in the past—our lives become trapped in what was, not grounded in what is.

Refer participants to handout 29.3 (Strengthening Forgiveness Through Grief Work: Examples of Common Beliefs or Expectations).

NOTE TO INSTRUCTORS: Read several examples aloud from handout 29.3 and then ask participants to take a moment to place a checkmark in the box(es) next to the expectation(s) or belief(s) they may need to grieve for the past injury they identified in the earlier mindfulness practice. Encourage them to refer to this handout each time they practice forgiveness on a different past injury, because often what needs to be mourned varies, depending on the event. The examples provided in handout 29.3 represent only a subset of possible beliefs or expectations about the world, other people, or oneself. Instructors should encourage participants to look for others when none seem to apply to their unique circumstances. **Examples include** an expectation for a parent to be loving and caring; a belief that a spouse or partner should be faithful; a belief that others will work as hard as yourself; a belief that people should be straightforward or honest; a belief that you will always do the right thing; a belief that you are always kind or considerate; a belief that others will play fair; a belief that others will value or appreciate your hard work or efforts to help; a belief that others will be kind; a belief that other people will treat you with respect; a belief that the world should be stable or orderly; a conviction that you are able to accurately predict what will happen in the future; a conviction that you can know the intentions of others; a belief that others will be polite; a belief that a parent, spouse, or family member will not purposefully attempt to harm you; a belief in your ability to overcome any obstacle or solve any problem, no matter where or how it may appear.

(Required) Class Exercise

Practicing Forgiveness

Instructors should ask participants to write down or highlight on handout 29.3 the loss just identified. Instructors should point out that each participant will likely have a different loss to use in the practice that is about to commence, because each person's past injury is uniquely their own. For example, if the past injury involved a person unjustly accusing someone in an unkind or disrespectful manner, then the loss inserted into the following script for this person might read: "I need to grieve the loss of my expectations that others will treat me fairly and with kindness." Instructors should then begin the practice by reading aloud the forgiveness script that follows.

To start, sit in a comfortable yet alert position, and take a breath, with awareness, in order to center yourself into this moment. Bring into your awareness the memory of the past grievance or injury you have chosen and the loss you need to grieve. Now silently repeat after me...

I recognize that to forgive and reclaim my life, I must first grieve my loss of my expectations or beliefs about the world, myself, or other people. For today's practice, I need to grieve the loss of my expectations that...[Name the expectation requiring grief work; see handout 29.3.] By grieving this loss, I am learning to recognize that I cannot avoid the pain of this past injury—it is not something that I can ignore, deny, or pretend never happened—as this only creates more suffering. My sadness helps me recognize that the world is not always as I expect it to be. By allowing myself to experience the sadness of my loss—without getting down on myself, falling apart, or blaming others—I take the first step toward forgiveness and genuine healing. I recognize that forgiveness is freely chosen. And so, with full awareness, I freely choose to forgive.

Turn your mind to the area in your life needing forgiveness. Take a slow deep breath, raise your eyebrows, closed-mouth smile. Say…

I forgive you. [Deep breath.] *I forgive you.* [Deep breath.] *I forgive you.* [Deep breath.] *I recognize that this brief practice of forgiveness means taking care of myself, and that by repeating this practice frequently, I am freeing myself from useless anger, resentment, or rumination and reclaiming my life by taking a step toward living more fully in the present.*

NOTE TO INSTRUCTORS: Activation of the social safety system (for example, via an eyebrow wag, closed-mouth smile, slow deep breath) when saying the words "I forgive you" in the preceding script is essential because it helps pair social safety with forgiveness.

Instructors should repeat the forgiveness script three times in a row before ending the practice, and then solicit observations.

- ✓ **Ask:** *What did you observe during this practice?*
- ✓ **Ask:** *Were you able to feel the sadness of your loss? How did that influence your willingness to forgive?*
- ✓ **Ask:** *Were you able to forgive? What was that like? How do you feel now?*
- ✓ **Ask:** *If you found it difficult to grieve or forgive, what might this mean? What is it that you need to learn?*

Instructors should remind participants that the preceding script can be used to forgive a person, oneself, or the world. Encourage participants to make a commitment to use the forgiveness script in handout 29.3 or to create their own each time they practice. Encourage participants to practice on a daily basis until the memory of the past injury no longer triggers a strong reaction, desires for revenge, or urges to avoid.

(Required) Teaching Points

Forgive Again and Again

- **Remember that forgiveness is a process, not an end point—it requires ongoing commitment and practice with the same event.** The good news is that each time we forgive, we loosen the grip of unhelpful resentment or anger.

- *Decide to forgive again each time you encounter a reminder of the past injury, and then practice, practice, practice.*

- *Repeat your grief statement each time you find yourself thinking about the past injury.*

- *Repeat your forgiveness practice about a past injury again and again until you are able to think about the past hurt without falling apart or attempting to avoid it.*

- *Let go of expecting quick results.*

- *Forgive yourself for struggling with forgiveness.*

NOTE TO INSTRUCTORS: Remind participants that they cannot escape the pain of a past injury. They will have pain if they try to avoid grieving the loss, and they will have pain if they allow themselves to experience the sadness that is associated with the loss. Encourage self-enquiry—for example, by asking, "Which pain gets me closer to how I want to live?" Ideally, we should enter the practice of forgiveness with the understanding that we may never fully resolve the pain. Acknowledgment of this facilitates self-compassion.

T *Practice* **Thankfulness** *and then pass it on.*

- *Be thankful when an opportunity for forgiveness arises.* Remind yourself of all the times in your life when you have needed forgiveness from others.

- *Practice being thankful for what you have now.* For example, you are alive, you have a roof over your head, you have a place to sleep, you have food to eat and clean water to drink, you have clothes to wear, and you are learning new skills.

- *Pass it on. Pass on the gift of forgiveness by looking for small opportunities to practice forgiveness, without expecting acknowledgment or anything in return.* For example, you can practice forgiveness for the person tailgating you on the freeway, the rude salesperson on the telephone, the family member who forgot your birthday.

- *Practice kindness first and foremost* (refer participants to worksheet 17.B) *by...*

  - *Engaging in random acts of kindness, without expecting anything in return.* For example, smile warmly at the harried store clerk, allow the tailgating car to pass you on the freeway, phone a sick colleague out of the blue.

  - *Giving people the benefit of the doubt. Look for benign explanations for another person's behavior before assuming the worst.* For example, consider that they may be late because their car broke down, that they may be speeding because their child has been in a serious accident, that they are not smiling because they may be in physical pain or may have had a very bad day, that they may be praising you because they really mean it.

  - *Acknowledging that all people (even you) are doing the best they can at any given moment,* even when what they are doing appears ineffective—for example, the street person begging for money, the person yelling across the street, the priest who curses, the math teacher who miscalculates.

- *Practice radical forgiveness by remembering that humans share a common bond of suffering (we have all harmed, and we have all been harmed),* and therefore we all deserve forgiveness. No small child ever aspires to be evil when they grow up.

> NOTE TO INSTRUCTORS: Some clients may insist that saying "We all deserve forgiveness" is Pollyannaish or unrealistic, supporting their argument with examples of individuals for whom forgiveness would appear wrong (for example, pedophiles or Hitler). Others will want to change the wording of the phrase "all people deserve forgiveness" to something less arousing or confrontational—for example, "I can (should) be capable of forgiving all people." Changing the wording retains a "just world" view implying that control is possible while exacerbating common OC problem behaviors associated with excessive striving. When these types of objections emerge, instructors should not attempt to convince or persuade the client otherwise. Instead, instructors should smile and, with an eyebrow wag, remind the client that forgiveness is a choice. Plus, forgiveness does not mean reconciliation, approval, or forgetting the past. One can forgive a person (for example, for a horrendous act), but that doesn't mean you have to hang out or spend time with the person. Instructors can remind participants that in many ways forgiveness is a selfish act. By forgiving someone, I take care of myself by letting go of useless anger, shame, or self-criticism.

- *Use self-enquiry to help loosen hypervigilant scanning for potential wrongdoing.* **Refer participants to handout 29.2** and the subheading "Self-Enquiry About Your 'Probation Officer'"; read aloud a few examples, and discuss.

- *Acknowledge that forgiveness is hard work.* For example, it requires a person to take responsibility for their personal reactions to the world when things don't go their way, without falling apart or blaming others.

- *Observe how your practice of forgiveness influences your relationships.*

  ✓ **Ask:** *When I engage in forgiveness, do I feel more or less like being around other people? What might this mean?*

  ✓ **Ask:** *Have my relationships changed in any way since I have been practicing forgiveness? What have I noticed?*

- *(Optional) Notice secret desires to be recognized, acknowledged, or appreciated when practicing forgiveness, and practice self-enquiry in order to learn.* **Refer participants to handout 29.2** and the subheading "Self-Enquiry About Pride" to facilitate this. Recognize that it is normal for pride to emerge when practicing forgiveness. Feeling good about working hard and living according to your values is an important part of healthy living.

  - *Reveal any secret pride about your forgiveness practice by admitting it,* first to yourself and then to a friend or fellow practitioner (that is, out yourself).

Lesson 29 Homework

1. **(Required) Worksheet 29.A (Flexible Mind Has HEART).** Encourage participants to work with their individual therapists around particular difficulties that might arise in completing this worksheet.

2. **(Optional) Handout 29.3 (Strengthening Forgiveness Through Grief Work: Examples of Common Beliefs or Expectations).** Instruct participants to practice grieving a loss each day. They should look for small instances where things did not go as expected, planned, or predicted. Using handout 29.3 as a guide, they should identify the loss needing to be grieved and record their observations in their self-enquiry journal.

3. **(Optional) Instruct participants to practice forgiveness when negative, unexpected, or problem events occur** (for example, if someone shows up late for an appointment, tailgates them on the freeway, or doesn't say "Thank you"). Participants should practice giving people the benefit of the doubt and block automatic blaming of others' character or personality.

4. **(Optional) Random acts of kindness.** Encourage participants to do something kind for people they don't know, or to direct kind thoughts toward someone they are having a conflict with, someone they dislike, or someone they find difficult (for example, they can bring the person a cup of coffee or tea, smile at the person as they pass, let the person go ahead of them at a lunch counter, say "Good morning," give them a compliment, and so on). Participants should record their observations in their self-enquiry journal.

Radical Openness Handout 29.1

What Forgiveness Is and Is Not

Forgiveness is Not...

- Approval or denying the past
- Holding on to prior grievances, grudges, or desires for revenge
- Opening yourself to being hurt again

Practice Self-Enquiry

- ➤ *What will move me closer to how I would like to live, or what is more in line with my personal values?*
- ➤ *Which path leads to more suffering?*
- ➤ *What do I fear I might lose if I were to practice forgiveness? Is this fear justified?*
- ➤ *Would my life be more fulfilling if I were able to relax vigilance about the past hurt or grievance?*
- ➤ *Am I holding on to my fear or anger for other reasons (for example, secret desire for revenge)?*

Forgiveness is...

- Taking care of ourselves
- A way to help us save face because it signals we are taking responsibility for our emotional reactions
- Living in line with our values
- Staying focused on the present
- A voluntary choice
- Dependent on an ongoing commitment (we must decide to forgive, and we must redecide repeatedly)
- Remembering that as humans we have all harmed, and we have all been harmed
- Letting go of the past in order to not be controlled by it
- Gaining freedom from the burden of the past
- A process that takes time

Radical Openness Handout 29.2

Forgiveness Self-Enquiry Questions

Practice self-enquiry to deepen awareness of your edge, using the following questions.

Finding Your Forgiveness Edge

➢ *How does your body feel when thinking about the past injury? Do you find your muscles tightening, teeth clamping together, mouth tightening, face flushing, or do you feel rigid or numb?*

➢ *Do you find yourself ruminating about the event or not sleeping because you can't stop thinking about the event?*

➢ *How willing are you to look at the past injury? Do you find yourself avoiding things in order to not think about the past grievance? Do you ever try not to think about the past injury or hope it will go away by itself? Is there any information, memory, or emotion about the past injury that you secretly don't want to remember? What might this tell you about the event or experience?*

➢ *What is it that you are afraid would happen if you were to forgive? To what extent are you telling yourself that it is unfair, wrong, or damaging to recall a past injury or to even be asked to consider recalling it?*

➢ *Do you believe it would be inappropriate or wrong to let go of this past grievance? What is it you fear might happen if you let go?*

➢ *Who are you hurting or helping by holding on to this grievance?*

➢ *What do you think keeps you from letting go of this grievance?*

➢ *What was your perspective when the injury occurred in the past? Has it changed over time? What might this tell you about your willingness to forgive?*

➢ *What was the perspective of other people involved at the time of the injury? What might their reactions tell you about your pain and desires to hold on to the memory of the injury?*

➢ *Is forgiveness, gratitude, or compassion toward others a behavior that you admire? What might this tell you about yourself or your personal values?*

If you find yourself resisting self-enquiry to find your edge, use self-enquiry to explore your resistance.

➢ *What might my resistance be trying to tell me? What is it I need to learn?*

➢ *What does my resistance tell me about myself or my willingness to engage in learning this new skill?*

➢ *What am I resisting? Is there something important for me to acknowledge or recognize about myself or the current moment? What is it I need to learn?*

Self-Enquiry About Punishment

➤ *Is this really worth my time? Who am I really hurting when I think like this?*

➤ *Who's really winning in the long run when I spend my life thinking about my enemy or the person that hurt me? What is it that I need to learn?*

➤ *What am I afraid might happen if the individual went unpunished? What is it I need to learn?*

➤ *Is it possible that my insistence on not forgetting the past injury, or my desire to find a way to punish the transgressor, means that I am giving them the power to control my life, even if they don't know it?*

➤ *Is it possible that by letting go of my desires for revenge I will be the one winning because I will no longer be holding on to the past? What do I need to learn from this?*

Self-Enquiry About Your "Probation Officer"

➤ *Am I refusing to consider alternative explanations for the other person's behavior? Is it possible I am neglecting potential factors or causes outside of the other person's control that may have led to the painful event?*

➤ *Is it possible that I am misreading a flat face or blank expression as hostile or disapproving when it may stem from factors unrelated to me, intense concentration on their part, or a habit of not showing emotions? If so or possibly, then what is it I need to learn?*

➤ *Am I assuming that the other person's reaction or behavior is solely a reflection of his or her personality or moral failure?*

➤ *Have I given the other person the same consideration or benefit of the doubt that I might extend myself when I am in similar circumstances, or if I had a history similar to the wrongdoer's? If not, what might this mean?*

Self-Enquiry About Pride

➤ *What might my pride tell me about my practice of forgiveness? Is it possible that I am wearing my forgiveness as a badge of honor? What might this mean?*

➤ *Is it possible that I secretly believe that my forgiveness practice is better, more genuine, more real, or more difficult than that of others? Do I secretly look down on others who I imagine are less able to forgive? What might this mean?*

➤ *Do I secretly desire my forgiveness to be acknowledged or appreciated by the person I am extending it toward? When I practice forgiveness, do I feel that the other person owes me? Do I only practice forgiveness when I believe I will get something in return? What might this mean? What do I need to learn?*

➤ *What am I afraid would happen if I allowed myself to experience pride about my forgiveness work? Is it possible that I am being too hard on myself? What do I need to learn?*

➤ *Am I using self-enquiry practice to punish myself or to prove that I am always working hard? If yes or maybe, what is it I need to learn? For what do I deserve punishment? For whom am I working hard? What is preventing me from feeling good about my forgiveness practice? What is it I need to learn?*

Radical Openness Handout 29.3

Strengthening Forgiveness Through Grief Work: Examples of Common Beliefs or Expectations

Place a checkmark in the boxes next to the expectations or beliefs you may need to grieve for a past injury.

☐ An expectation for a parent to be loving and caring

☐ A belief that a spouse or partner should be faithful

☐ A belief that others will work as hard as yourself

☐ A belief that people should be straightforward or honest

☐ A belief that you will always do the right thing

☐ A belief that you are always kind or considerate

☐ A belief that others will be kind and considerate

☐ A belief that others will play fair

☐ A belief that others will value or appreciate your hard work or efforts to help

☐ A belief that others will be kind

☐ A belief that other people will treat you with respect

☐ A belief that the world should be stable or orderly

☐ A conviction that you are able to accurately predict what will happen in the future

☐ A conviction that you can know the intentions of others

☐ A belief that others will be polite

☐ A belief that a parent, spouse, or family member will not purposefully attempt to harm you

☐ A belief in your ability to overcome any obstacle or solve any problem no matter where or how it may appear

Forgiveness Script

To start, sit in a comfortable yet alert position, and take a breath, with awareness, in order to center yourself into this moment. Bring into your awareness the memory of the past grievance or injury you have chosen and the loss you need to grieve.

Read the following script aloud three times in a row.

I recognize that to forgive and reclaim my life, I must first grieve my loss of my expectations or beliefs about the world, myself, or other people. For today's practice, I need to grieve the loss of my expectations that... [Name the expectation requiring grief work.] *By grieving this loss, I am learning to recognize that I cannot avoid the pain of this past injury—it is not something that I can ignore, deny, or pretend never happened—as this only creates more suffering. My sadness helps me recognize that the world is not always as I expect it to be. By allowing myself to experience the sadness of my loss—without getting down on myself, falling apart, or blaming others—I take the first step toward forgiveness and genuine healing. I recognize that forgiveness is freely chosen. And so, with full awareness, I freely choose to forgive.* [Turn your mind to the area in your life needing forgiveness. Take a slow deep breath, raise your eyebrows, closed-mouth smile.] *I forgive you.* [Deep breath.] *I forgive you.* [Deep breath.] *I forgive you.* [Deep breath.] *I recognize that this brief practice of forgiveness means taking care of myself, and that by repeating this practice frequently, I am freeing myself from useless anger, resentment, or rumination and reclaiming my life by taking a step toward living more fully in the present.*

Radical Openness Handout 29.4

Main Points for Lesson 29: Learning to Forgive

1. Forgiveness is not approval or denying the past.

2. Forgiveness does not mean reconciliation.

3. Forgiveness does not mean opening yourself up to being hurt again.

4. Forgiveness means taking care of ourselves and learning to let go of useless anger, resentment, or self-blame.

5. To let go of a past injury or grievance, you must first find your edge that keeps you holding on to the past injury.

6. Forgiveness must be freely chosen. A person cannot be forced to forgive, nor can someone be forced to accept forgiveness when it is offered.

7. Forgiveness requires an ongoing commitment to let go of past hurts in order to grow.

8. We must decide to forgive, and we must decide again repeatedly.

9. To reclaim our life and learn how to forgive, we must grieve the loss of expectations.

10. Practice being thankful for what you have. Remind yourself of all the times in your life when you have needed forgiveness from others.

Radical Openness Worksheet 29.A

Flexible Mind Has HEART

Flexible Mind Has HEART

H   Identify the past **Hurt**

E   Locate your **Edge** that's keeping you stuck in the past

A   **Acknowledge** that forgiveness is a choice

R   **Reclaim** your life by grieving your loss and practicing forgiveness

T   Practice **Thankfulness** and then pass it on

Instructions: Pick the past hurt or injury you want to practice forgiveness with, using the following skills. Remember, it doesn't have to be something big. Each letter of the word HEART is a step toward healthy forgiveness.

H *Identify the past* **Hurt**, *grievance, or injury you are holding on to.*

Place a checkmark in the box next to each statement that helps you locate a past hurt, grievance, or injury.

- ☐ An event or interaction occurred, either recently or in the distant past, that I find myself repeatedly thinking about.

- ☐ Thoughts, images, or feelings about the event keep popping up in my mind, despite my attempts to prevent this from happening.

- ☐ I often wish that the event had never happened, or that things had gone differently.

- ☐ I have tried to hide what happened from others by changing the topic or attempting to avoid discussing it.

- ☐ I have lied to others about the event or pretended it never happened.

- ☐ The event pertains to a time when I was harmed or betrayed by someone.

- ☐ The event pertains to a time when I harmed or betrayed another person.

- ☐ I believe that a particular person or group of people should be punished for what happened and cannot stop thinking about it.

- ☐ I blame myself for what happened and/or believe I should be punished because of what happened.

- ☐ I believe I should be punished for what happened.

- ☐ When I think about the event, I sometimes want to give up.

- ☐ I believe that the event is further proof that I am a failure or flawed.

Other hurts, grievances, or injuries.

_____

_____

_____

_____

Describe the event you want to practice forgiveness with in the space provided. _If you have more than one event, rank-order them from most avoided/disliked (1) to least avoided/disliked, and place a checkmark next to the event you want to work on this week._

_____

_____

_____

_____

E _Locate your_ **Edge** _that's keeping you stuck in the past._

To let go of a past injury or grievance, you must first find your edge that keeps you holding on to the past injury. Our edge is where self-growth occurs. It is most often described as a feeling of tension or resistance, embarrassment, a desire to avoid, or a sense of numbness. It usually involves things in our life that we don't want to think about or admit to.

Place a checkmark in the boxes next to the statements that best describes the skills you used.

- ☐ Observed urges to explain, justify, or defend…

    - ☐ What happened in the first place

    - ☐ How I responded during or after the event

    - ☐ How others responded during or after the event

Record in the space provided what you actually did.

_____

_____

_____

☐ Observed urges to blame myself, blame others, or blame the world...

    ☐ For the event itself

    ☐ For making it happen or not preventing it

    ☐ For not doing the right thing

☐ Used handout 29.2 (Forgiveness Self-Enquiry Questions) to help locate my edge.

Record in the space provided what you discovered about your edge.

_____

_____

_____

☐ **Practiced self-enquiry about my edge.** _Place a checkmark in the boxes next to the statements that best describes the skills you used._

    ☐ Remembered that self-enquiry means finding a good question that may lead to new learning, rather than an explanation or way to feel better.

    ☐ Practiced daily or over several days and remembered to keep practices brief (five minutes) in order to block automatic tendencies to fix or find solutions.

    ☐ Practiced being suspicious of quick answers to self-enquiry questions.

    ☐ Recorded the thoughts, emotions, memories, and sensations that arose following or during each self-enquiry practice in my self-enquiry journal.

    ☐ Following multiple practices over multiple days, used my self-enquiry journal to help "make meaning," find a solution, or gain new insight about my edge.

Record in the space provided what you learned.

_____

_____

_____

A Acknowledge *that forgiveness is a choice.*

Place a checkmark in the boxes next to the statements that best describes the skills you used.

☐ **Acknowledged that forgiveness is a choice that only I can make—it is ultimately my decision.** No one can be forced to forgive, nor can someone be forced to accept forgiveness when it is offered. *Not deciding is still making a choice.*

☐ **Reminded myself that holding on to a past grievance or grudge against someone is like drinking poison every day with hopes of punishing my enemy.** It creates more suffering for myself.

☐ **Practiced letting go of imagining that somehow the transgressor will get away with what they did wrong if I stop feeling anger toward them.**

☐ **Remembered that punishing a transgressor punishes myself in the long term because it keeps me stuck in the past,** and it wastes precious time dwelling on a past event that cannot be redone or remade.

☐ **Practiced self-enquiry whenever I noticed desires to punish the other person (or myself);** for example, I used the "Self-Enquiry About Punishment" questions in handout 29.2.

☐ **Practiced surrendering arrogance by acknowledging the fallibility inherent in all humans, including myself.**

☐ **Practiced letting go of insisting that all past injuries must be vindicated by acknowledging the impossibility of this task.**

☐ **Celebrated diversity rather than assuming everyone should behave or think like I do.**

☐ **Practiced seeing the world from the perspective of the person who hurt me,** and used self-enquiry to facilitate this by asking…

➤ *Is it possible that when the transgression occurred, those involved never intended harm and/or that they regret their behavior now?*

➤ *Even if the other person appears to not regret their behavior, is it possible that they were not fully aware or capable of understanding how harmful their behavior was?*

➤ *Is it possible that major problems or past traumas in their life may have made them (or myself) more vulnerable to the painful event?*

☐ **Practiced accepting that something hurtful happened that was outside of my control** while remembering that acceptance does not mean approval or resignation.

R Reclaim *your life by grieving your loss and practicing forgiveness.*

To reclaim our life, we must first grieve the loss of our expectations and beliefs about the world, ourselves, or other people.

• **Grieving means allowing oneself to feel the sadness or disappointment associated with a loss for a brief time, and then letting the sadness go.** Grieving does not mean wallowing in sadness or ruminating about the past event.

• **Sadness helps us recognize that we cannot control the world.** It helps us stop expecting life to be the same by blocking useless denial. It helps us grow because it updates our "computer," or brain, by allowing the loss to be fully acknowledged.

- Grief work clears out old ways of thinking and allows us to be more open to what's happening now.
  - ✓ **Ask:** *What part of myself or belief about the world did this past injury damage?*
  - ✓ **Ask:** *What is it that I need to grieve?*

Use handout 29.3 (Strengthening Forgiveness Through Grief Work: Examples of Common Beliefs or Expectations) and note in the space provided what you need to grieve.

_____

_____

_____

_____

Place a checkmark in the boxes next to the statements that best describes the skills you used.

- ☐ Reminded myself what forgiveness is and is not (see handout 29.1).
- ☐ Checked my resolve to forgive, and recommitted, if needed. *Describe how you noticed that your resolve had wavered.*

_____

_____

_____

- ☐ Practiced forgiveness by grieving my loss, using the script provided in handout 29.3.
- ☐ Activated my social safety system while allowing the past memory to emerge into my awareness.
- ☐ Held the image of the past grievance in my mind and repeated silently "I forgive you" three times while mindfully breathing.
- ☐ Remembered that forgiveness requires a conscious decision to forgive again each time we encounter a reminder of the past injury.
- ☐ Repeated my grief statement each time I found myself thinking about the past injury.
- ☐ Forgave myself for struggling with forgiveness.

T *Practice* **Thankfulness** *and then pass it on.*

Place a checkmark in the boxes next to the statements that best describes the skills you used.

- ☐ Practiced *radical forgiveness* by remembering that humans share a common bond of suffering (*we have all harmed, and we have all been harmed*), and therefore we all deserve forgiveness.

☐ **Practiced loosening hypervigilant scanning for wrongdoing,** using the questions from handout 29.2 under the subheading "Self-Enquiry About Your 'Probation Officer.'"

☐ **Practiced being thankful when an opportunity for forgiveness arose.**

☐ **Practiced being thankful for what I have now.**

☐ **Passed on the gift of forgiveness** by looking for small opportunities to practice forgiveness, without expecting acknowledgment or anything in return.

☐ **Practiced kindness first and foremost, using worksheet 17.B.**

☐ **Acknowledged that forgiveness is hard work.**

☐ **Observed how practicing forgiveness influenced my relationships.** *Record any observations in the space provided.*

_____

_____

_____

RO Integration Week

Main Points for Lesson 30

1. None! (tee hee ☺) The idea is to have fun!

2. Okay, maybe one main point: "Don't forget to wash behind your ears."

3. Okay, okay—a real main point, I promise… hmmm. "Yes, the main purpose of RO Integration Week is to **integrate all of our skills and be creative in how we do this**." Some of it might involve reteaching key concepts or covering optional material.

4. RO Integration Week is designed partly as a catch-up lesson, making it possible for instructors to teach or reteach material they were unable to cover in prior lessons and/or reteach certain key principles. Thus, there is no real curriculum or set of goals to achieve. So feel free to be creative! This lesson offers some ideas for games, role plays, exercises, and new teaching not covered in other lessons (the materials listed as "needed" are only necessary for those exercises that you choose to use from the list of suggestions). Instructors should feel free to pick and choose between the ideas in this lesson and feel free to be creative.

Materials Needed

- Handout 30.1 (The Asch Experiment)

- Photocopies of the Mimicry Game cards on page 510 (prepare in advance by cutting along the dotted lines to create enough cards for all participants; for game instructions, see "The Mimicry Game," later in this lesson)

- Photocopies of the Facial Affect Guessing Game cards on page 511, or make your own cards showing emotions like envy, glee, happiness, contentment, rage, embarrassment, humiliation, love, or curiosity (prepare in advance by cutting along the dotted lines to create enough cards for all participants; for game instructions, see "The Facial Affect Guessing Game," later in this lesson)

- Photocopies of the six "Read My Mind" Game cards on page 512 (prepare in advance by cutting along the dotted lines to create the six cards; for game instructions, see "The 'Read My Mind' Game," later in this lesson)

The Mimicry Game

To make cards, use scissors to cut along the dotted line.

Scenario 1

You have just discovered that you lost your entire savings because your bank failed. You are about to meet a friend, and you decide to tell your friend about what happened and to express how horrible it is. You are feeling angry, outraged, and betrayed by your bank for mishandling your money. Underneath, you also feel fear and some despair.

During the role play, try to exaggerate your facial expressions, body movements, and voice tone to reflect your feelings of outrage, great despair, and confusion. Have fun with it—and remember, the more you can exaggerate your responses, the greater an opportunity you give your partner to practice.

Scenario 2

You are an independent film director and screenwriter with a passion for telling stories involving social issues. You have just heard that a proposal you sent to an agent five months ago has been picked up by Steven Spielberg, and he is flying you first class to Hollywood to discuss your idea for a possible movie. You are extremely excited about this news and can't wait to tell a good friend about it.

During the role play, try to exaggerate your facial expressions, body movements, and voice tone to reflect your feelings of excitement and joy. Have fun with it—and remember, the more you can exaggerate your responses, the greater an opportunity you give your partner to practice.

The Facial Affect Guessing Game

Instructions: *Cut along dotted lines and use these "cards" to play the game.* Mimic the expression on your partner's face and see if you can guess what emotion they are trying to express.

FEAR	GUILT
JOY	*SAD*
SHAME	DISGUST
ANGER	*SURPRISE*

The "Read My Mind" Game

Instructions: Ask for a volunteer, then have them sit in a place where other members of the class will not be able to read the card that you show them. Show the volunteer one card at a time making sure to hide the "Truth" or "Lie" instructions from the rest of the class and then read out loud the question. The class should then try and guess whether the volunteer was telling the truth or lying. Make up new questions yourself and have some fun!

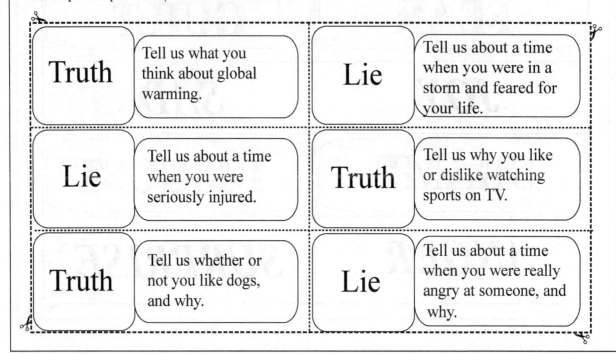

Truth — Tell us what you think about global warming.

Lie — Tell us about a time when you were in a storm and feared for your life.

Lie — Tell us about a time when you were seriously injured.

Truth — Tell us why you like or dislike watching sports on TV.

Truth — Tell us whether or not you like dogs, and why.

Lie — Tell us about a time when you were really angry at someone, and why.

NOTE TO INSTRUCTORS: The idea of RO Integration Week originated from research applying RO DBT to severely underweight adult anorexia nervosa patients on the Haldon Unit Eating Disorders Service in southwest England (see T. R. Lynch et al., 2013).

Integration Week Practice Examples Designed to Loosen Inhibitory Control

The "Inhibit Versus Express" Game

Show a short clip of an emotional scene from a movie or music video (for example, a scene from the movies *Aliens* or *Meet the Fockers*), or instructors may wish to read an emotional story or poem. Ask participants to pair off and to practice expressing their feelings, thoughts, and reactions as they normally would for about one minute. Then stop the interaction and instruct participants: *Now do the very same thing, only this time show no facial expression, eyebrow wags, head nods, or gestures when you talk to your partner.* Instructors can then...

- ✓ **Ask:** *Which style of expression did you prefer engaging with?*

- ✓ **Ask:** *How did it feel to interact with someone who completely masked his or her expression of emotion?*

- ✓ **Ask:** *How free did you feel expressing your emotions when your partner was inhibiting theirs?*

The "Let's Be a Mirror" Game

This exercise augments skills taught during lesson 3 (that is, to strengthen client practices involving big gestures). The game involves splitting the class up into dyads (pairs) and then assigning one member of each dyad to be the lead in the upcoming exercise. The lead begins the game by simply moving their hands, arms, and legs in unexpected ways—for example, waving arms, wiggling fingers, pointing up at the ceiling, flapping one's arms like a chicken, fidgeting and picking at invisible spots on one's clothes, scratching one's nose, pulling one's ears, smiling then frowning, standing up and then sitting down quickly, and so on. The goal of the game is for their partner to try and match the lead's body and facial movements, like a mirror. After about one minute of mimicking, ask partners to switch roles and repeat the game. Instructors can playfully introduce this game by purposefully employing large and dramatic gestures and facial expressions during their initial explanation of the game while coinstructors, standing to one side and slightly behind, silently mimic their body gestures and movements. This type of introduction almost always results in raucous bouts of glee and laughter, especially when the instructor suddenly notices the coinstructor's behavior and then engages in fervent demands (with wild gestures, which are continually mimicked by the coinstructor) of "Stop mimicking me!" and/or mock-scolds the coinstructor by saying, "You are behaving in a silly manner!" or implores, "Take life more seriously!" Instructors should ask participants to switch roles several times (with each minipractice lasting one minute). The quick pace allows for multiple exposures while making it harder to think too much about what one might do. After two to three switches, instructors should end the practice and solicit observations and discussion.

- ✓ **Ask:** *What was the point of this practice?* Instructors should be prepared to explain to participants that the primary goal of this exercise is to break down overlearned OC inhibitory barriers to free expression of emotion.

- ✓ **Ask:** *Why is it important for OC individuals to practice breaking down inhibitory barriers?* Instructors can remind participants that practicing big gestures, even when they may feel awkward or phony, helps override their brain's natural tendency to desire control. Learning to be more expressive and candid is essential for OC clients to rejoin the tribe.

The Mimicry Game

This game resembles the "Let's Be a Mirror" Game but has additional components (such as verbal behavior) related to the impact that social signaling has on empathic understanding of another.

Needed: Cut-up photocopies of the Mimicry Game cards on page 530.

Game instructions: Split the group into pairs. Provide one member of each dyad with a copy of scenario 1, and explain to their partners that their goal is to mimic their partners' expressions, body movements, and voice tones. The instructor and the coinstructor can demonstrate what mimicry might look like. After about one to two minutes, the partners switch roles and play again, with the mimicker from scenario 1 now acting out the description from scenario 2. After playing both scenarios, switch dyads and repeat the practice once more. Instructors should end the practice by soliciting observations and discussion.

✓ **Ask:** *What was your experience like? Did you experience any emotions or judgmental thoughts?*

✓ **Ask:** *Are there times that someone would not want to match another (for example, when showing disapproval, or when disagreeing with their approach)?*

✓ **Ask:** *How might this help in real life?* Instructors should point out that this practice helps further break down overlearned inhibitory barriers.

Mimicking While Watching TV

For this exercise, instructors should find a short video clip that shows someone making a range of different gestures and facial expressions. Play it on a TV monitor or computer screen that can be seen by all class members. Everyone in the class, including instructors, is to mimic the movements, gestures, and facial expressions shown in the video as it plays. Doing this as a group helps minimize self-consciousness. A favorite clip we have used, available free on YouTube, is "You Can Call Me Al," featuring Paul Simon and Chevy Chase and based on Simon's 1986 album *Graceland*. If this video is used, participants should practice mimicking Chase's movements, including his dance moves. Instructors should encourage participants to use their mindfulness participation skills and to practice letting go of judgmental thoughts. Have fun exaggerating the movements or creating new ones. Participants can be encouraged to practice at home, mimicking gestures of people while watching TV as a way to further help expand their repertoire.

The Facial Affect Guessing Game

Needed: Cut-up photocopies of the Facial Affect Guessing Game cards on page 531 (or cut-up copies of your own cards showing emotions like envy, glee, happiness, contentment, rage, embarrassment, humiliation, love, and curiosity).

Game instructions: Split the group into pairs and give each member of each dyad a different card. Instruct them not to share what is written on their cards. Partner A begins by nonverbally expressing the emotion given on his or card, using facial muscles. Partner B's job is to see if he or she can mimic the expression and then guess the emotion. Instructors should allow about ten to fifteen seconds and then ask the class what the emotion was. Partner B then nonverbally expresses the emotion on the card while partner A mimics the expression and guesses the emotion. Distribute the next cards with different emotion words and play the game again. Make this a fun and fast-moving game with no winners or losers. Give everyone a chance to play with expressing emotions. Repeat again and as often as time permits. Have fun! Use the following questions for discussion after the last round of the game.

✓ **Ask:** *Which emotions are more difficult to express or guess?*

✓ **Ask:** *Why do you think some emotions are harder than others to express (or guess)?*

✓ **Ask:** *What might this mean when we interact with others?*

✓ **Ask:** *Was it easier to guess the emotion when you mimicked the expression?* Instructors should remind participants that research shows that we micromimic (in milliseconds, most often without awareness) the facial expressions of others, and this process helps facilitate empathic understanding of how others feel (see lesson 2).

✓ **Ask:** *How easy or difficult was it to exaggerate the expression?*

Integration Week Practices and Teaching Designed to Enhance Relationship IQ

Being Liked Versus Being Correct: Class Discussion

Refer participants to handout 30.1 (The Asch Experiment).

Social psychologists have long studied two motivating factors among humans: a motivation to be correct in their judgments, and a motivation to be accepted and liked by others (Insko, Drenan, Solomon, Smith, & Wade, 1983). When these two motivations are in conflict, tension can occur. Research has shown that individuals who rigidly prioritize one of these motivations regardless of circumstance can damage relationships and/or experience or cause psychological distress (T. R. Lynch et al., 2003). Instructors can describe the classic study examining social pressure and perception originally conducted by Solomon Asch (1951) by reading aloud the following text:

> *Imagine yourself in the following situation. You sign up for a psychology experiment. On a specific date, you and seven others arrive and are seated at a table in a small room. You assume the other seven are also volunteer subjects like you, but they are actually associates of the experimenter, and their behavior has been carefully scripted. You're the only real subject. The experimenter arrives and tells you that the study in which you are about to participate concerns people's visual judgments. She places two cards before you. The card on the left contains one vertical line. The card on the right displays three lines of varying lengths. The experimenter asks each person, one at a time, to choose which of the three lines on the right card matches the length of the line on the left card. The task is repeated several times with different cards, and each time it happens you are almost always the last person to be asked your opinion. On some occasions the other "subjects" unanimously choose the wrong line. It is clear to you that they are wrong, but they have all given the same answer.*

> ✓ **Ask: What do you think you might do in this situation?** *Would you go along with the majority opinion, or would you stay firm and trust your own eyes?* To the experimenter's surprise, thirty-seven of the fifty subjects conformed to the majority at least once, and fourteen of them conformed on more than six of the twelve trials, and this has been replicated multiple times over the years. The tendency to conform can be strong. People tend to conform for two main reasons in this experiment: because they want to be liked by the group, and because they believe the group is better informed than they are.

• *Evaluate the pros and cons of being relationship-focused and the pros and cons of being correctness-focused.* Solicit ideas from the class, and write them on the flipchart or whiteboard. Either focus can be problematic when rigidly held.

- *Encourage self-enquiry by asking:* *What do I value more, being correct or being liked? To what extent is my behavior influenced by one or the other of these motivations? Is there one of these motivations (that is, being liked versus being correct) that I strongly dislike? If so, what might this mean? What is it that I need to learn?*

Being Correct or Being Liked: Class Exercise

Instructors should request participants to rate, on a 10-point scale, the importance of being correct versus being liked (1 = low importance, and 10 = high importance). Instructors should remind participants that there is no right way to complete this self-assessment. Indeed, the more a person struggles with rating themselves, the more they may value being correct (since they are fixating on how to rate themselves, presumably in the correct way), and the less concerned they may be about complying with instructions given by the skills instructor (that is, the less concerned they may be with relationships). Some participants will rate both dimensions the same—equally high, equally low, or equally moderate. Most people want to be *right* and *liked* at the same time, but it is hard to have both *all* of the time. Encourage self-enquiry while validating comments that the context or situation can strongly influence how one behaves in the moment; for example, when on a romantic date, the relationship might take priority over being correct, whereas the reverse may be true when taking an algebra test.

- ✓ **Ask:** *Is it possible that my struggle with completing this task stems from a secret wish to be perfect or balanced? If yes or maybe, then what might this mean? Which of these dimensions (being liked versus correct) do I most not want to consider as important? What might this mean?*

- ✓ **Ask:** *What do my ratings tell me about how I might respond to criticism? If someone prioritized correctness over relationships, what type of feedback might they tend to avoid or find difficult to hear? If someone valued relationships over being correct, what type of feedback might they tend to dislike?*

- ✓ **Ask:** *How might hypervigilance for criticism, or fear of making mistakes, impact relationships? If people worry about being competent or correct, could this influence how they listen to others? How comfortable might they feel revealing vulnerable emotions to someone?*

- ✓ **Ask:** *If people worry whether they are liked or approved of by others, could this influence how comfortable they are disagreeing with someone, or their ability to stand up for themselves? Is there a chance that they may feel that their needs are never met? Could this lead to burnout because they try to please others all of the time?*

> NOTE TO INSTRUCTORS: Participants who are focused on relationships might struggle sometimes to stand up for themselves or maintain their self-respect in interactions. They might need to practice asking for what they want, saying no to what they don't want, and sticking to their values. Refer them to worksheet 18.A (Being Assertive with an Open Mind: Flexible Mind PROVEs) to learn how to assert with humility and still get what they want.

The Empathic Mind Reading Game

Split the group into pairs. Person A should tell partner B about a time when they had to take care of someone, or a time when someone had to take care of them (for example, a broken ankle). Ask B to read the partner's thoughts, emotions, or experience during the conversation—for example, "If I were in your shoes…" or "I'm aware of imagining…" Then swap roles. The idea is for participants to practice making helpful guesses or accurately mind reading their partner's experience in a manner that is perceived as supportive (not phony), and without trying to fix or solve anything. Participant B should practice saying "Oops" or "Sorry" and try again when participant A reports that the mind reading is not quite accurate. Have fun!

- ✓ **Ask:** *How successful were you in generating empathic mind reading?*

- ✓ **Ask:** *Was any of your mind reading experienced as judgmental or less supportive?*

- ✓ **Ask:** *How hard was it to not offer solutions?*

- ✓ **Ask:** *How often did you find yourself asking questions rather than performing empathic mind reading?*

The "Read My Mind" Game

Needed: Cut-up photocopies of the six "Read My Mind" Game cards on page 532

Game instructions: Each of the six cards is made up of a "Tell us…" instruction and either the word "truth" or the word "lie." Ask for a volunteer, and then tell the volunteer that you are going to pose a question to which he or she will have to respond with either a lie or the truth, depending on what the card indicates. You then give the volunteer a card, without letting the class see what is on it. Ask the volunteer the question, and have him or her answer. The rest of the class, including the coinstructor, guesses whether the volunteer is lying or not. This can be great fun!

★ **Fun Facts:** *We May Be Good Social Safety Detectors,*
But We're Not So Good at Lie Detection

Humans are expert social safety detectors—our brains are hardwired to detect the extent to which another person is feeling genuinely relaxed versus tense, uncomfortable, or self-conscious during interactions. Our brains have developed ways to reliably detect the extent to which another person is prosocial and likely to engage in reciprocal cooperative behavior. Research shows that we can recognize another's prosocial intent through emotion-based touching, smiling, and overall level of emotional expressivity [Boone & Buck, 2003; Brown & Moore, 2002; Hertenstein et al., 2006; Schug et al., 2010]. We are adept at knowing whether a smile is genuine or phony, and we can accurately detect tension in the voice of a person, even over the telephone [Ekman, 1992a; Pittam & Scherer, 1993].

However, research shows we are not very good at detecting whether someone is lying [O'Sullivan & Ekman, 2004]. In general, most people are about 50 percent accurate (like flipping a coin) in guessing correctly about whether someone is lying or telling the truth.

- ✓ **Ask:** *What's the difference between detecting social safety (that is, knowing whether a person is uptight or not) and detecting lies? Why might we be good at social safety detection but not at detecting lies? [Answer: Lies involve words, whereas detecting social safety depends on nonverbal signals.]*

NOTE TO INSTRUCTORS: The idea of this exercise is to have fun. If someone does exceptionally well at guessing when someone is lying, the instructors should take a relaxed stance toward this. Ekman and his colleagues (Ekman & O'Sullivan, 1991; Ekman, O'Sullivan, & Frank, 1999; O'Sullivan & Ekman, 2004) have identified some individuals who are highly accurate at detecting deception. A number of factors differentiate the accurate lie detectors from the inaccurate ones. First, the accurate lie detectors reported using different and more varied verbal and nonverbal cues, in particular the latter. Second, the accurate lie detectors were able to identify microexpressions of emotion. Third, the accurate lie detectors had a high level of interest in lie detection. They practiced their skill and sought feedback about their performance to improve their abilities. This suggests they would not be misled by the widely held stereo-types of a liar. Further, the majority of O'Sullivan and Ekman's "wizards" reported that from a very early age they were aware of changes in the emotional levels of others. Many had experienced some sort of childhood trauma, such as alcoholism in the family, a highly emotional mother, or not speaking English until grade school (O'Sullivan, 2005; O'Sullivan & Ekman, 2004).

The Milgram Experiment

Read the following text aloud.

Imagine two people arriving at a psychology laboratory to take part in a study of memory and learning. One of them is designated a teacher, and the other a learner. The experimenter explains that the study is concerned with the effects of punishment on learning.

The learner is escorted into a room and seated in a chair; his arms are strapped to prevent excessive movement, and an electrode is attached to his wrist. He is informed that his task is to learn the word pairs on a sheet in front of him, and he is told that whenever he makes an error, he will receive electric shocks of increasing intensity. However, the real focus of the study is to examine the behavior of the teacher. The shocks themselves are faked, and the learner in the experiment is in fact a paid actor who simulates the effects of the shocks, depending on the voltage. For example, at 120 volts, the actor complains verbally; at 150 volts, he demands to be released; and as the shocks escalate, he becomes increasingly vehement and emotional, uttering agonized screams and eventually becoming nonresponsive.

This was an actual experiment, and it was designed to determine whether the teacher would be willing to harm another person simply because they are told to do so by someone. Experts surveyed prior to the experiment believed that only a very small percentage of people (1 to 3 percent of the subjects) would actually choose to deliver the maximum level of shock, and those people were thought to be pathological or psychopathic. Actual results were contrary to these predictions: 65 percent of teachers (the true experimental subjects) administered the final 450-volt "DANGER—SEVERE SHOCK," despite clearly being uncomfortable doing so. This experiment has been repeated multiple times, and overall the results suggest that most humans are capable of committing harmful and even horrible acts toward other people when requested by an authority figure.

Instructors should use this story to help deepen class participants' understanding that people under stress can some-times engage in behavior that goes against their core values. Use the following questions to enhance discussion.

✓ **Ask:** *How do you think you would respond in this situation?*

✓ **Ask:** *What might this tell us about how people behave when under stress?*

✓ **Ask:** *How might we use these findings to enhance our practice of forgiveness?*

✓ **Ask:** *Do you think compliance in the experiment just described represents a form of Fatalistic Mind? What might this tell us about Fatalistic Mind?*

✓ **Ask:** *What type of evolutionary advantage would compliance with authority provide for a species?*

Lesson 30 Homework

Since there is no required material for RO Integration Week, homework assignments will vary, depending on what was taught or practiced. Homework can include anything from no homework (☺) up to practicing as many RO skills as you can the entire next week (☺). Usually it pertains specifically to practicing the principles or material that the instructors chose to teach that day. In some ways, especially for any class members who started with lesson 1 and worked all the way through to lesson 30 (that is, Integration Week), the class this day is like graduation day. Thus, if possible, the lesson should be celebratory as well as educational.

Handout 30.1

The Asch Experiment

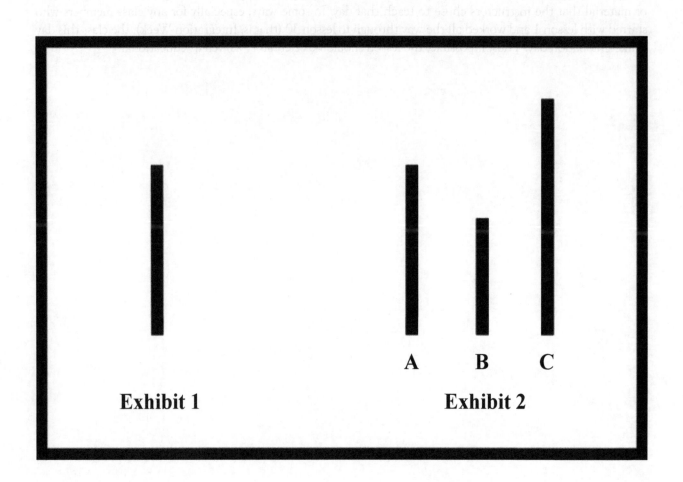

References

Adolphs, R. (2008). Fear, faces, and the human amygdala. *Current Opinion in Neurobiology, 18*(2), 166–172. doi:10.1016/j .conb.2008.06.006

Aloi, M., Rania, M., Caroleo, M., Bruni, A., Palmieri, A., Cauteruccio, M. A., … Segura-García, C. (2015). Decision making, central coherence, and set-shifting: A comparison between binge eating disorder, anorexia nervosa and healthy controls. *BMC Psychiatry, 15*(6). doi:10.1186/s12888–015–0395-z

Ambady, N., & Rosenthal, R. (1992). Thin slices of expressive behavior as predictors of interpersonal consequences: A meta-analysis. *Psychological Bulletin, 111*(2), 256–274. doi:10.1037/0033–2909.111.2.256

Ambady, N., & Rosenthal, R. (1993). Half a minute: Predicting teacher evaluations from thin slices of nonverbal behavior and physical attractiveness. *Journal of Personality and Social Psychology, 64*(3), 431–441. doi:10.1037/0022–3514.64 .3.431

Andersen, H. C. (1837/2004). *The emperor's new clothes.* Boston, MA: Houghton Mifflin Harcourt.

Andersen, S. M., Saribay, A., & Thorpe, J. S. (2008). Simple kindness can go a long way: Relationships, social identity, and engagement. *Social Psychology, 39*(1), 59–69. doi:10.1027/1864–9335.39.1.59

App, B., McIntosh, D. N., Reed, C. L., & Hertenstein, M. J. (2011). Nonverbal channel use in communication of emotion: How may depend on why. *Emotion, 11*(3), 603–617. doi:10.1037/a0023164

Asch, S. E. (1951). Effects of group pressure on the modification and distortion of judgments. In H. Guetzkow (Ed.), *Groups, leadership and men: Research in human relations* (pp. 177–190). Pittsburgh, PA: Carnegie Press.

Beermann, U., & Ruch, W. (2011). Can people really "laugh at themselves"? Experimental and correlational evidence. *Emotion, 11*(3), 492–501. doi:10.1037/a0023444

Berntson, G. G., Cacioppo, J. T., & Quigley, K. S. (1991). Autonomic determinism: The modes of autonomic control, the doctrine of autonomic space, and the laws of autonomic constraint. *Psychological Review, 98*(4), 459–487.

Bieling, P. J., & Kuyken, W. (2003). Is cognitive case formulation science or science fiction? *Clinical Psychology: Science and Practice, 10*(1), 52–69. doi:10.1093/clipsy/10.1.52

Blascovich, J., Mendes, W. B., Hunter, S. B., Lickel, B., & Kowai-Bell, N. (2001). Perceiver threat in social interactions with stigmatized others. *Journal of Personality and Social Psychology, 80*(2), 253–267. doi:10.1037/0022–3514.80.2.253

Boone, R. T., & Buck, R. (2003). Emotional expressivity and trustworthiness: The role of nonverbal behavior in the evolution of cooperation. *Journal of Nonverbal Behavior, 27*(3), 163–182. doi:10.1023/a:1025341931128

Bouton, M. E. (2002). Context, ambiguity, and unlearning: Sources of relapse after behavioral extinction. *Biological Psychiatry, 52*(10), 976–986. doi:10.1016/S0006–3223(02)01546–9

Bracha, H. S. (2004). Freeze, flight, fight, fright, faint: Adaptationist perspectives on the acute stress response spectrum. *CNS Spectrums, 9*(9), 679–685.

Brown, W. M., & Moore, C. (2002). Smile asymmetries and reputation as reliable indicators of likelihood to cooperate: An evolutionary analysis. In S. P. Shohov (Ed.), *Advances in psychology research* (Vol. 11, pp. 19–36). Hauppauge, NY: Nova Science Publishers.

Butler, E. A., Egloff, B., Wilhelm, F. H., Smith, N. C., Erickson, E. A., & Gross, J. J. (2003). The social consequences of expressive suppression. *Emotion, 3*(1), 48–67.

Carson, J. W., Keefe, F. J., Lynch, T. R., Carson, K. M., Goli, V., Fras, A. M., & Thorp, S. R. (2005). Loving-kindness meditation for chronic low back pain: Results from a pilot trial. *Journal of Holistic Nursing, 23*(3), 287–304. doi:10.1177/0898010105277651

Chen, E. Y., Segal, K., Weissman, J., Zeffiro, T. A., Gallop, R., Linehan, M. M., ... Lynch, T. R. (2015). Adapting dialectical behavior therapy for outpatient adult anorexia nervosa: A pilot study. *International Journal of Eating Disorders*, *48*(1), 123–132. doi:10.1002/eat.22360

Davidson, R. J., & Irwin, W. (1999). The functional neuroanatomy of emotion and affective style. *Trends in Cognitive Sciences*, *3*(1), 11–21. doi:10.1016/S1364–6613(98)01265–0

DePaulo, B. M., & Kashy, D. A. (1998). Everyday lies in close and casual relationships. *Journal of Personality and Social Psychology*, *74*(1), 63–79. doi:10.1037/0022–3514.74.1.63

DeScioli, P., & Kurzban, R. (2009). Mysteries of morality. *Cognition*, *112*(2), 281–299. doi:10.1016/j.cognition.2009.05.008

De Waal, F. B. M. (1996). Macaque social culture: Development and perpetuation of affiliative networks. *Journal of Comparative Psychology*, *110*(2), 147–154. doi:10.1037/0735–7036.110.2.147

Eisenberger, N. I., & Lieberman, M. D. (2004). Why rejection hurts: A common neural alarm system for physical and social pain. *Trends in Cognitive Sciences*, *8*(7), 294–300. doi:10.1016/j.tics.2004.05.010

Ekman, P. (1972). Universal and cultural differences in facial expressions of emotion. In J. Cole (Ed.), *Nebraska symposium on motivation, 1971* (pp. 207–283). Lincoln: University of Nebraska Press.

Ekman, P. (1992a). An argument for basic emotions. *Cognition and Emotion*, *6*(3–4), 169–200. doi:10.1080/02699939208411068

Ekman, P. (1992b). Are there basic emotions? *Psychological Review*, *99*(3), 550–553. doi:10.1037/0033–295X.99.3.550

Ekman, P. (1993). Facial expression and emotion. *American Psychologist*, *48*(4), 384–392. doi:10.1037/0003–066X.48.4.384

Ekman, P., & O'Sullivan, M. (1991). Who can catch a liar? *American Psychologist*, *46*(9), 913–920. doi:10.1037/0003–066X.46.9.913

Ekman, P., O'Sullivan, M., & Frank, M. G. (1999). A few can catch a liar. *Psychological Science*, *10*(3), 263–266. doi:10.1111/1467–9280.00147

English, T., & John, O. P. (2013). Understanding the social effects of emotion regulation: The mediating role of authenticity for individual differences in suppression. *Emotion*, *13*(2), 314–329. doi:10.1037/a0029847

Feinberg, M., Willer, R., & Keltner, D. (2012). Flustered and faithful: Embarrassment as a signal of prosociality. *Journal of Personality and Social Psychology*, *102*(1), 81–97. doi:10.1037/a0025403

Feldman, C., & Kuyken, W. (2011). Compassion in the landscape of suffering. *Contemporary Buddhism*, *12*(1), 143–155. doi:10.1080/14639947.2011.564831

Ferguson, T. J., Brugman, D., White, J., & Eyre, H. L. (2007). Shame and guilt as morally warranted experiences. In J. L. Tracy, R. W. Robins, & J. P. Tangney (Eds.), *The self-conscious emotions: Theory and research* (pp. 330–348). New York, NY: Guilford Press.

Foster, G. M. (1972). The anatomy of envy: A study in symbolic behavior. *Current Anthropology*, *13*, 165–202.

Fox, E., Lester, V., Russo, R., Bowles, R. J., Pichler, A., & Dutton, K. (2000). Facial expressions of emotion: Are angry faces detected more efficiently? *Cognition and Emotion*, *14*(1), 61–92. doi:10.1080/026999300378996

Fox, S. J. (1977). A paleoanthropological approach to recreation and sporting behaviors. In B. A. Tindall & P. Stevens (Eds.), *Studies in the anthropology of play*. West Point, NY: Leisure Press.

Fruzzetti, A., & Worrall, J. M. (2010). Accurate expression and validating responses: A transactional model for understanding individual and relationship distress. In K. T. Sullivan & J. Davila (Eds.), *Support processes in intimate relationships* (pp. 121–150). New York, NY: Oxford University Press.

Furnham, A. (2003). Belief in a just world: Research progress over the past decade. *Personality and Individual Differences*, *34*(5), 795–817. doi:10.1016/S0191–8869(02)00072–7

Goetz, J. L., Keltner, D., & Simon-Thomas, E. (2010). Compassion: An evolutionary analysis and empirical review. *Psychological Bulletin*, *136*(3), 351–374. doi:10.1037/A0018807

Gold, G. J., & Weiner, B. (2000). Remorse, confession, group identity, and expectancies about repeating a transgression. *Basic and Applied Social Psychology*, *22*(4), 291–300. doi:10.1207/15324830051035992

Gottman, J. M. (1994). *What predicts divorce? The relationship between marital processes and marital outcomes.* Hillsdale, NJ: Erlbaum.

Greville-Harris, M., Hempel, R., Karl, A., Dieppe, P., & Lynch, T. R. (2016). The power of invalidating communication: Receiving invalidating feedback predicts threat-related emotional, physiological, and social responses. *Journal of Social and Clinical Psychology, 35*(6), 471–493. doi:10.1521/jscp.2016.35.6.471

Gross, J. J. (2007). *Handbook of emotion regulation.* New York, NY: Guilford Press.

Gross, J. J., & John, O. P. (2003). Individual differences in two emotion regulation processes: Implications for affect, relationships, and well-being. *Journal of Personality and Social Psychology, 85*(2), 348–362. doi:10.1037/0022-3514.85.2.348

Gruenewald, T. L., Dickerson, S. S., & Kemeny, M. E. (2007). A social function for self-conscious emotions: The social self preservation theory. In J. L. Tracy, R. W. Robins, & J. P. Tangney (Eds.), *The self-conscious emotions: Theory and research* (pp. 68–87). New York, NY: Guilford Press.

Happé, F., & Frith, U. (2006). The weak coherence account: Detail-focused cognitive style in autism spectrum disorders. *Journal of Autism and Developmental Disorders, 36*(1), 5–25. doi:10.1007/s10803-005-0039-0

Havas, D. A., Glenberg, A. M., Gutowski, K. A., Lucarelli, M. J., & Davidson, R. J. (2010). Cosmetic use of botulinum toxin-A affects processing of emotional language. *Psychological Science, 21*(7), 895–900. doi:10.1177/0956797610374742

Hertenstein, M. J., Verkamp, J. M., Kerestes, A. M., & Holmes, R. M. (2006). The communicative functions of touch in humans, nonhuman primates, and rats: A review and synthesis of the empirical research. *Genetic, Social, and General Psychology Monographs, 132*(1), 5–94. doi:10.3200/MONO.132.1.5-94

Hofmann, S. G., Grossman, P., & Hinton, D. E. (2011). Loving-kindness and compassion meditation: Potential for psychological interventions. *Clinical Psychology Review, 31*(7), 1126–1132. doi:10.1016/j.cpr.2011.07.003

Houk, P. G., Smith, V., & Wolf, S. G. (1999). Brain mechanisms in fatal cardiac arrhythmia. *Integrative Physiological and Behavioral Science, 34*(1), 3–9.

Hughes, J. W., & Stoney, C. M. (2000). Depressed mood is related to high-frequency heart rate variability during stressors. *Psychosomatic Medicine, 62*(6), 796–803.

Hutcherson, C. A., Seppala, E. M., & Gross, J. J. (2008). Loving-kindness meditation increases social connectedness. *Emotion, 8*(5), 720–724. doi:10.1037/a0013237

Insko, C. A., Drenan, S., Solomon, M. R., Smith, R. H., & Wade, T. J. (1983). Conformity as a function of the consistency of positive self-evaluation with being liked and being right. *Journal of Experimental Social Psychology, 19*(4), 341–358. doi:10.1016/0022-1031(83)90027-6

Kashy, D. A., & DePaulo, B. M. (1996). Who lies? *Journal of Personality and Social Psychology, 70*(5), 1037–1051. doi:10.1037/0022-3514.70.5.1037

Kaul, T. J., & Schmidt, L. D. (1971). Dimensions of interviewer trustworthiness. *Journal of Counseling Psychology, 18*(6), 542–548. doi:10.1037/h0031748

Keltner, D., & Harker, L. (1998). The forms and functions of the nonverbal signal of shame. In P. Gilbert & B. Andrews (Eds.), *Shame: Interpersonal behavior, psychopathology, and culture* (pp. 78–98). New York, NY: Oxford University Press.

Keltner, D., Young, R. C., & Buswell, B. N. (1997). Appeasement in human emotion, social practice, and personality. *Aggressive Behavior, 23*(5), 359–374. doi:10.1002/(SICI)1098-2337(1997)23:53.0.CO;2-D

Keogh, K., Booth, R., Baird, K., & Davenport, J. (2016). A Radically Open DBT informed group intervention for over-control: A controlled trial with 3-month follow-up. *Practice Innovations, 1*(2), 129–143.

Kernis, M. H., & Goldman, B. M. (2006). A multicomponent conceptualization of authenticity: Theory and research. In M. P. Zanna (Ed.), *Advances in experimental social psychology* (Vol. 38, pp. 283–357). San Diego, CA: Academic Press.

Khurana, R. K., Watabiki, S., Hebel, J. R., Toro, R., & Nelson, E. (1980). Cold face test in the assessment of trigeminal-brainstem vagal function in humans. *Annals of Neurology, 7*, 144–149.

Kraus, M. W., & Keltner, D. (2009). Signs of socioeconomic status: A thin-slicing approach. *Psychological Science, 20*(1), 99–106. doi:10.1111/j.1467-9280.2008.02251.x

Kuyken, W., Fothergill, C. D., Musa, M., & Chadwick, P. (2005). The reliability and quality of cognitive case formulation. *Behaviour Research and Therapy, 43*(9), 1187–1201. doi:10.1016/j.brat.2004.08.007

Lang, K., Lopez, C., Stahl, D., Tchanturia, K., & Treasure, J. (2014). Central coherence in eating disorders: An updated systematic review and meta-analysis. *World Journal of Biological Psychiatry, 15*(8), 586–598. doi:10.3109/15622975.2014.909606

Laurenceau, J., Barrett, L. F., & Pietromonaco, P. R. (1998). Intimacy as an interpersonal process: The importance of self-disclosure, partner disclosure, and perceived partner responsiveness in interpersonal exchanges. *Journal of Personality and Social Psychology, 74*(5), 1238–1251. doi:10.1037/0022-3514.74.5.1238

Leary, M. R., Haupt, A. L., Strausser, K. S., & Chokel, J. T. (1998). Calibrating the sociometer: The relationship between interpersonal appraisals and state self-esteem. *Journal of Personality and Social Psychology, 74,* 1290–1299.

Lee, J. J., & Pinker, S. (2010). Rationales for indirect speech: The theory of the strategic speaker. *Psychological Review, 117*(3), 785–807.

Lerner, M. J. (1997). What does the belief in a just world protect us from: The dread of death or the fear of undeserved suffering? *Psychological Inquiry, 8*(1), 29–32. doi:10.1207/s15327965pli0801_5

Linehan, M. M. (1993a). *Cognitive-behavioral treatment of borderline personality disorder.* New York, NY: Guilford Press.

Linehan, M. M. (1993b). *Skills training manual for treating borderline personality disorder.* New York, NY: Guilford Press.

Linehan, M. M. (2015a). *DBT skills training manual* (2nd ed.). New York, NY: Guilford Press.

Linehan, M. M. (2015b). *DBT skills training: Handouts and worksheets* (2nd ed.). New York, NY: Guilford Press.

Linehan, M. M., Bohus, M., & Lynch, T. R. (2007). Dialectical behavior therapy for pervasive emotion dysregulation: Theoretical and practical underpinnings. In J. Gross (Ed.), *Handbook of emotion regulation* (pp. 581–605). New York, NY: Guilford Press.

Livingstone, M. S. (2000). Is it warm? Is it real? Or just low spatial frequency? *Science, 290*(5495), 1229. doi:10.1126/science.290.5495.1299b

Lopez, C., Tchanturia, K., Stahl, D., & Treasure, J. (2008). Central coherence in eating disorders: A systematic review. *Psychological Medicine, 38*(10), 1393–1404. doi:10.1017/S0033291708003486

Lopez, C., Tchanturia, K., Stahl, D., & Treasure, J. (2009). Weak central coherence in eating disorders: A step towards looking for an endophenotype of eating disorders. *Journal of Clinical and Experimental Neuropsychology, 31*(1), 117–125. doi:10.1080/13803390802036092

Losh, M., Adolphs, R., Poe, M. D., Couture, S., Penn, D., Baranek, G. T., & Piven, J. (2009). Neuropsychological profile of autism and the broad autism phenotype. *Archives of General Psychiatry, 66*(5), 518–526. doi:10.1001/archgenpsychiatry.2009.34

Lynch, M. P. (2004). *True to life: Why truth matters.* Cambridge, MA: MIT Press.

Lynch, T. R. (2018). *Radically open dialectical behavior therapy: Theory and practice for treating disorders of overcontrol.* Oakland, CA: New Harbinger.

Lynch, T. R., Gray, K. L., Hempel, R. J., Titley, M., Chen, E. Y., & O'Mahen, H. A. (2013). Radically open–dialectical behavior therapy for adult anorexia nervosa: Feasibility and outcomes from an inpatient program. *BMC Psychiatry, 13*(293). doi:10.1186/1471-244x-13-293

Lynch, T. R., Hempel, R. J., & Clark, L. A. (2015). Promoting radical openness and flexible control. In J. Livesley, G. Dimaggio, & J. Clarkin (Eds.), *Integrated treatment for personality disorder: A modular approach* (pp. 325–344). New York, NY: Guilford Press.

Lynch, T. R., Hempel, R. J., & Dunkley, C. (2015). Radically open–dialectical behavior therapy for disorders of overcontrol: Signaling matters. *American Journal of Psychotherapy, 69*(2), 141–162.

Lynch, T. R., Lazarus, S. A., & Cheavens, J. S. (2015). Mindfulness interventions for undercontrolled and overcontrolled disorders: From self-control to self-regulation. In K. W. Brown, J. D. Creswell, & R. M. Ryan (Eds.), *Handbook of mindfulness: Theory, research, and practice* (pp. 329–347). New York, NY: Guilford Press.

Lynch, T. R., Robins, C. J., & Morse, J. Q. (2003). Couple functioning in depression: The roles of sociotropy and autonomy. *Journal of Clinical Psychology, 59*(12), 1349–1359. doi:10.1002/jclp.10226

Marigold, D. C., Holmes, J. G., & Ross, M. (2007). More than words: Reframing compliments from romantic partners fosters security in low self-esteem individuals. *Journal of Personality and Social Psychology, 92*(2), 232–248. doi:10.1037/0022–3514.92.2.232

Mauss, I. B., Shallcross, A. J., Troy, A. S., John, O. P., Ferrer, E., Wilhelm, F. H., & Gross, J. J. (2011). Don't hide your happiness! Positive emotion dissociation, social connectedness, and psychological functioning. *Journal of Personality and Social Psychology, 100*(4), 738–748. doi:10.1037/a0022410

McAdams, D. P. (1985). Motivation and friendship. In S. Duck & D. Perlman (Eds.), *Understanding personal relationships: An interdisciplinary approach* (pp. 85–105). Thousand Oaks, CA: Sage.

Mikulincer, M., & Shaver, P. R. (2001). Attachment theory and intergroup bias: Evidence that priming the secure base schema attenuates negative reactions to out-groups. *Journal of Personality and Social Psychology, 81*(1), 97–115. doi:10.1037/0022–3514.81.1.97

Montgomery, K. J., & Haxby, J. V. (2008). Mirror neuron system differentially activated by facial expressions and social hand gestures: A functional magnetic resonance imaging study. *Journal of Cognitive Neuroscience, 20*(10), 1866–1877. doi:10.1162/jocn.2008.20127

Morris, D. (2002). *Peoplewatching*. London, England: Vintage.

Murray, S. L., Griffin, D. W., Rose, P., & Bellavia, G. M. (2003). Calibrating the sociometer: The relational contingencies of self-esteem. *Journal of Personality and Social Psychology, 85*(1), 63–84.

Öhman, A., Lundqvist, D., & Esteves, F. (2001). The face in the crowd revisited: A threat advantage with schematic stimuli. *Journal of Personality and Social Psychology, 80*(3), 381–396.

O'Sullivan, M. (2005). Emotional intelligence and deception detection: Why most people can't "read" others, but a few can. In R. E. Riggio & R. S. Feldman (Eds.), *Applications of nonverbal communication* (pp. 215–253). Mahwah, NJ: Erlbaum.

O'Sullivan, M., & Ekman, P. (2004). The wizards of deception detection. In P.-A. Granhag & L. Strömwall (Eds.), *The detection of deception in forensic contexts* (pp. 269–286). New York, NY: Cambridge University Press.

Pellegrini, A. D. (2009). *The role of play in human development*. Oxford, England: Oxford University Press.

Perls, F. S. (1969). *Ego, hunger and aggression: The beginning of Gestalt therapy*. New York, NY: Random House.

Pettersson, E., Boker, S. M., Watson, D., Clark, L. A., & Tellegen, A. (2013). Modeling daily variation in the affective circumplex: A dynamical systems approach. *Journal of Research in Personality, 47*(1), 57–69. doi:10.1016/j.jrp.2012.10.003

Pettigrew, T. F., & Tropp, L. R. (2006). A meta-analytic test of intergroup contact theory. *Journal of Personality and Social Psychology, 90*(5), 751–783. doi:10.1037/0022–3514.90.5.751

Pittam, J., & Scherer, K. R. (1993). Vocal expression and communication of emotion. In M. Lewis & J. M. Haviland (Eds.), *Handbook of emotions* (pp. 185–197). New York, NY: Guilford Press.

Porges, S. W. (1995). Orienting in a defensive world: Mammalian modifications of our evolutionary heritage: A polyvagal theory. *Psychophysiology, 32*(4), 301–318.

Porges, S. W. (2001). The polyvagal theory: Phylogenetic substrates of a social nervous system. *International Journal of Psychophysiology, 42*(2), 123–146.

Porges, S. W. (2003). Social engagement and attachment: A phylogenetic perspective. In J. A. King, C. F. Ferris, & I. I. Lederhendler (Eds.), *Roots of mental illness in children* (pp. 31–47). New York, NY: New York Academy of Sciences.

Porges, S. W. (2007). The polyvagal perspective. *Biological Psychology, 74*(2), 116–143.

Porges, S. W. (2011). *The polyvagal theory: Neurophysiological foundations of emotions, attachment, communication, and self-regulation*. New York, NY: Norton.

Ross, L. (1977). The intuitive psychologist and his shortcomings: Distortions in the attribution process. In L. Berkowitz (Ed.), *Advances in experimental social psychology* (Vol. 10, pp. 174–221). New York, NY: Academic Press.

Rumi, Mewlana Jalaluddin. (1230/2004). "Who makes these changes?" In C. Barks (Ed. and Trans.), *The essential Rumi, new expanded edition*. San Francisco, CA: HarperSanFrancisco.

Salzberg, S. (1995). *Lovingkindness: The revolutionary art of happiness* (1st ed.). Boston, MA: Shambhala.

Sarra, S., & Otta, E. (2001). Different types of smiles and laughter in preschool children. *Psychological Reports, 89*(3), 547–558. doi:10.2466/PR0.89.7.547–558

Savicki, V. (1972). Outcomes of nonreciprocal self-disclosure strategies. *Journal of Personality and Social Psychology, 23*(2), 271–276. doi:10.1037/H0033038

Schaefer, C. E., & Reid, S. E. (2001). *Game play: Therapeutic use of childhood games* (2nd ed.). New York, NY: Wiley.

Schauer, M., & Elbert, T. (2010). Dissociation following traumatic stress: Etiology and treatment. *Zeitschrift für Psychologie/ Journal of Psychology, 218*(2), 109–127. doi:10.1027/0044–3409/a000018

Scherer, K. R., & Wallbott, H. G. (1994). Evidence for universality and cultural variation of differential emotion response patterning. *Journal of Personality and Social Psychology, 66*(2), 310–328. doi:10.1037/0022–3514.66.2.310

Schneider, K. G., Hempel, R. J., & Lynch, T. R. (2013). That "poker face" just might lose you the game! The impact of expressive suppression and mimicry on sensitivity to facial expressions of emotion. *Emotion, 13*(5), 852–866. doi: 10.1037/a0032847

Schug, J., Matsumoto, D., Horita, Y., Yamagishi, T., & Bonnet, K. (2010). Emotional expressivity as a signal of cooperation. *Evolution and Human Behavior, 31*(2), 87–94. doi:10.1016/j.evolhumbehav.2009.09.006

Schupp, H. T., Öhman, A., Junghöfer, M., Weike, A. I., Stockburger, J., & Hamm, A. O. (2004). The facilitated processing of threatening faces: An ERP analysis. *Emotion, 4*(2), 189–200. doi:10.1037/1528–3542.4.2.189

Shapiro, J. P., Baumeister, R. F., & Kessler, J. W. (1991). A three-component model of children's teasing: Aggression, humor, and ambiguity. *Journal of Social and Clinical Psychology, 10*(4), 459–472.

Shaw, A., & Olson, K. R. (2012). Children discard a resource to avoid inequity. *Journal of Experimental Psychology: General, 141*(2), 382–395. doi:10.1037/a0025907

Shenk, C. E., & Fruzzetti, A. E. (2011). The impact of validating and invalidating responses on emotional reactivity. *Journal of Social and Clinical Psychology, 30*(2), 163–183. doi:10.1521/jscp.2011.30.2.163

Silver, M., & Sabini, J. (1978). The social construction of envy. *Journal for the Theory of Social Behaviour, 8*(3), 313–332. doi:10.1111/j.1468–5914.1978.tb00406.x

Simic, M., Stewart, C., Hunt, K., Konstantellou, A., & Underdown, S. (2016, May). *Experiential workshop: Radically open dialectical behavior therapy for adolescents following partial response to family therapy for anorexia nervosa.* Paper presented at International Conference on Eating Disorders, San Francisco, CA.

Smith, R. H., & Kim, S. H. (2007). Comprehending envy. *Psychological Bulletin, 133*(1), 46–64. doi:10.1037/0033–2909 .133.1.46

Steklis, H., & Kling, A. (1985). Neurobiology of affiliative behavior in nonhuman primates. In M. Reite & T. Field (Eds.), *The psychobiology of attachment and separation* (pp. 93–134). Orlando, FL: Academic Press.

Tangney, J. P., Miller, R. S., Flicker, L., & Barlow, D. H. (1996). Are shame, guilt, and embarrassment distinct emotions? *Journal of Personality and Social Psychology, 70*(6), 1256–1269.

Tsoudis, O., & Smith-Lovin, L. (1998). How bad was it? The effects of victim and perpetrator emotion on responses to criminal court vignettes. *Social Forces, 77*(2), 695–722. doi:10.2307/3005544

Van der Gaag, C., Minderaa, R. B., & Keysers, C. (2007). Facial expressions: What the mirror neuron system can and cannot tell us. *Social Neuroscience, 2*(3–4), 179–222. doi:10.1080/17470910701376878

Weijenberg, R. A. F., & Lobbezoo, F. (2015). Chew the pain away: Oral habits to cope with pain and stress and to stimulate cognition. *BioMed Research International*, article ID 49431. doi:10.1155/2015/149431

Williams, L. M., Liddell, B. J., Kemp, A. H., Bryant, R. A., Meares, R. A., Peduto, A. S., & Gordon, E. (2006). Amygdala-prefrontal dissociation of subliminal and supraliminal fear. *Human Brain Mapping, 27*(8), 652–661. doi:10.1002 /hbm.20208

Williams, L. M., Liddell, B. J., Rathjen, J., Brown, K. J., Gray, J., Phillips, M., … Gordon, E. (2004). Mapping the time course of nonconscious and conscious perception of fear: An integration of central and peripheral measures. *Human Brain Mapping, 21*(2), 64–74. doi:10.1002/hbm.10154

Wirth, J. H., Sacco, D. F., Hugenberg, K., & Williams, K. D. (2010). Eye gaze as relational evaluation: Averted eye gaze leads to feelings of ostracism and relational devaluation. *Personality and Social Psychology Bulletin, 36*(7), 869–882. doi:10.1177/0146167210370032

Thomas R. Lynch, PhD, FBPsS, is professor emeritus of clinical psychology at the University of Southampton school of psychology. Previously, he was director of the Duke Cognitive-Behavioral Research and Treatment Program at Duke University from 1998–2007. He relocated to Exeter University in the UK in 2007. Lynch's primary research interests are understanding and developing novel treatments for mood and personality disorders using a translational line of inquiry that combines basic neurobiobehavioral science with the most recent technological advances in intervention research. He is founder of radically open dialectical behavior therapy (RO DBT). Lynch has received numerous awards and special recognitions from organizations such as the National Institutes of Health-US (NIMH, NIDA), Medical Research Council-UK (MRC-EME), and the National Alliance for Research on Schizophrenia and Depression (NARSAD). His research has been recognized in the Science and Advances Section of the National Institutes of Health Congressional Justification Report; and he is a recipient of the John M. Rhoades Psychotherapy Research Endowment, and a Beck Institute Scholar.

Index

MORE BOOKS *from*
NEW HARBINGER PUBLICATIONS

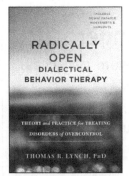
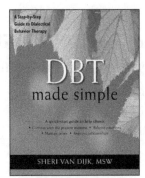
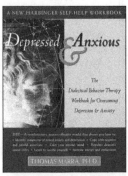
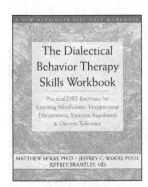
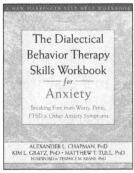
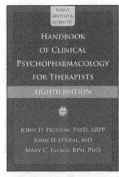

Register your **new harbinger** titles for additional benefits!

When you register your **new harbinger** title—purchased in any format, from any source—you get access to benefits like the following:

- Downloadable accessories like printable worksheets and extra content

- Instructional videos and audio files

- Information about updates, corrections, and new editions

Not every title has accessories, but we're adding new material all the time.

Access free accessories in 3 easy steps:

1. Sign in at NewHarbinger.com (or **register** to create an account).

2. Click on **register a book**. Search for your title and click the **register** button when it appears.

3. Click on the **book cover or title** to go to its details page. Click on **accessories** to view and access files.

That's all there is to it!

If you need help, visit:

NewHarbinger.com/accessories

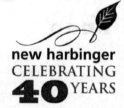
new harbinger
CELEBRATING
40 YEARS